High Risk Maternity Nursing Manual

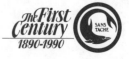

High Risk Maternity Nursing Manual

edited by

Kathleen Buckley
Nurse Consultant (Midwife)
New York State Department of Health
New York, New York

Nancy W. Kulb
Certified Nurse Midwife
Maternity Infant Care/Family Planning Project
New York, New York

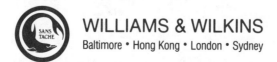

WILLIAMS & WILKINS
Baltimore • Hong Kong • London • Sydney

Editor: Susan M. Glover
Associate Editor: Marjorie Kidd Keating
Copy Editor: Sandra Tamburrino
Designer: BETS Ltd.
Illustration Planner: Ray Lowman
Production Coordinator: Charles E. Zeller

Accurate indications, adverse reactions, and dosage schedules for drugs are provided in this book, but it is possible that they may change. The reader is urged to review the package information data of the manufacturers of the medications mentioned.

Printed in the United States of America

Library of Congress Cataloging in Publication Data

High risk maternity nursing manual / edited by Kathleen Buckley, Nancy
   W. Kulb.
      p.   cm.
   Includes index.
   ISBN 0-683-09558-7
   1. Obstetrical nursing—Handbooks, manuals, etc. 2. Pregnancy,
Complications of—Handbooks, manuals, etc. I. Buckley, Kathleen
II. Kulb, Nancy W.
   [DNLM: 1. Obstetrical Nursing—methods.   2. Pregnancy
Complications—nursing.   WY 157 H6375]
RG951.H539   1989
610.73′678—dc19
DNLM/DLC
for Library of Congress   89-5389
                                                                            CIP

90 91 92 93
1 2 3 4 5 6 7 8 9 10

This book is dedicated to
Florence Schomen,
to David, Alan, and Carolyn Kulb,
and of course,
to Tia and Ralph,
who ate the manuscript as fast as we could produce it.

 # Preface

Health care professionals in obstetric practice today have a changing and ever-expanding body of knowledge on which to base their practice. This is especially true in the care of high risk maternity clients. Dramatic advances in theoretical knowledge and in diagnostic and treatment modalities have contributed greatly to decreasing maternal and neonatal mortality rates. As this knowledge base has grown, the clinical judgments and intensive care skills required of the practitioner have become more complex. *High Risk Maternity Nursing Manual* evolved out of the need for a practical, in-depth reference of clinical information concerning high risk maternity nursing care. It is intended for obstetric nurses, nurse practitioners, and other health professionals who are actively involved in the care of the high risk maternity client. It will serve as a reference for nurse clinicians in primary health care settings who are challenged to assess maternal and fetal risk, and sometimes, unexpectedly, to provide maternal intensive care. Primarily, this text is for practitioners in tertiary care settings and for graduate maternity/perinatal nursing students.

The substantive content assumes a basic knowledge of anatomy and physiology, as well as obstetric nursing practice—principles and skills. The focus is on theoretical content and technical skills that practicing obstetric nurses (especially in tertiary care settings) are called on to use, but will not learn in school or even in practice in a primary or secondary obstetric care setting.

The book is unique in its focus on *maternal* rather than fetal or neonatal complications, since it provides in-depth, comprehensive information about maternal deviations from the norm and suggests specific nursing actions for each one. Philo-

sophically, this focus has grown out of the conviction that the best possible outcome for mother and baby is achieved by high quality prenatal care, intensive antenatal screening for and management of complications when they occur, and intensive monitoring of maternal and fetal status during labor, delivery, and the postpartum period. Although this text deals with maternal deviations, the intent is to focus on the client—the mother and her family—in need of expressive nursing care as well as technical competence. The vast majority of pregnancies are normal, and all women and families with high risk pregnancies require the same supportive nursing care for their normal needs as that given to women and families with normal pregnancies. The focus on deviations in this book is intended to enhance care concerning a deviation from normal without detracting from the expert care required to manage normal aspects of each pregnancy.

We believe that the nurse is in a unique position to identify complications early, and to coordinate the efforts of the health care team in achieving the best possible outcomes for both mother and baby. We envision the obstetric nurse's role as being that of an essential partner in provision of health care for the high risk client—a partner with other health care professionals who are committed to promoting the health and well-being of the mother, infant, and family, and who work with the client in meeting her health care goals. The fact that the nurse works with mothers from different cultures in a variety of settings is also recognized.

We hope that this book will contribute to the health and well-being of mothers, babies, and families by enhancing the knowledge base of the health care professionals who serve them.

# Contributors

Kathleen Buckley, C.N.M., M.S.N.
Nurse Consultant (Midwife)
New York State Department of Health
New York, New York

Nancy Campau, C.N.M., M.S.
Nurse-Midwife
State University Hospital
Health Science Center at Brooklyn
Brooklyn, New York

Nina Mimoni Daratsos, R.N.C., M.S.N.
Maternal Child Health Consultant Nurse
New York State Department of Health
Albany, New York

Barbara Decker, C.N.M., Ed.D.
Faculty
Maternal-Newborn Nursing/Nurse Midwifery
   Program
Yale University School of Nursing
New Haven, Connecticut

Nancy De Vore, C.N.M., M.S.N., M.S.
Director, Women's Health Center
Bronx Municipal Hospital Center
Director, Midwifery Practice
Albert Einstein College of Medicine
Bronx, New York

Tina Duperret, C.N.M., M.S.N.
Nurse-Midwife
Medical Care Associates-Health Key Medical
   Group
St. Louis, Missouri

Mary C. Fallon, R.N., M.S.N.
Assistant Director of Nursing
Maternal-Child Division
San Francisco General Hospital
San Francisco, California

Peggy Gallagher, C.N.M., M.S.
Certified Nurse-Midwife
Hudson Valley Associates
Rhinebeck, New York

Barbara J. Greitzer, R.N.C., P.N.P., M.S.
Neonatal Care Coordinator
Department of Nursing
Beth Israel Medical Center
New York, New York

Aliza Holtz, Ph.D.
President
Holtz Communications, Inc.
New York, New York

Nancy W. Kulb, C.N.M., M.S.
Certified Nurse Midwife
Maternity Infant Care/Family Planning Project
New York, New York

Joanne Middleton, Ph.D., C.N.M.
Director, Nurse-Midwifery Service
State University Hospital
Health Science Center at Brooklyn
Brooklyn, New York

Margherita Modica-Hawkins, R.N., M.S.
Director of Education
Columbia-Presbyterian Medical Center Regional
   Perinatal Network
New York, New York

Patricia Aikins Murphy, C.N.M., M.S.
Certified Nurse-Midwife
Prevention of Prematurity Program
Harlem Hospital Center
New York, New York

Debra Brook Paparo, C.N.M., M.S.
Aspen, Colorado

Hilda Pedersen, M.B., Ch.B., F.F.A.R.C.S.
Associate Professor of Clinical Anesthesiology
College of Physicians and Surgeons of Columbia
   University
New York, New York

Angela Portale, R.N., M.S.
Department of Obstetrics and Gynecology
Harlem Hosital Center
New York, New York

Tina Quirk, R.N., M.S.N.
Certified Clinical Specialist-Psychiatric Nursing
New York, New York

Dale Bierschenk Scorza, C.N.M., M.P.H.
Faculty and Private Practice
University of Colorado/St. Luke's Hospital
Denver, Colorado

Suzanne M. Smith, C.N.M., M.S., M.P.H.
Midwife, Private Practice
C.B.S. Midwifery, Inc.
New York, New York

Nola Geraghty Snyder, R.N., M.S.N.
Lecturer-Clinical Instructor
University of Massachusetts School of Nursing
Amherst, Massachusetts

Joyce E. Thompson, C.N.M., D.P.H.
Associate Professor and Director of Nurse-
   Midwifery
University of Pennsylvania School of Nursing
Philadelphia, Pennsylvania

Henry O. Thompson, M. Div., Ph.D.
Adjunct Associate Professor of Ethics
University of Pennsylvania School of Nursing
Philadelphia, Pennsylvania

Linda V. Walsh, C.N.M., M.P.H.
Lecturer in Nursing
University of Pennsylvania School of Nursing
Philadelphia, Pennsylvania

Contents

Section 1: General Considerations

Chapter 1
Perinatal Care
Nancy W. Kulb, C.N.M., M.S. and Aliza Holtz, Ph.D.

INTRODUCTION

The ultimate goal of perinatal care is a healthy mother and a healthy baby. In order to provide effective care for maternity clients, the nurse must not only understand the physical and psychological aspects of care but also the context in which the care is provided. This chapter discusses perinatal statistics, recommendations for improving maternal and newborn health care services, and the nurse's role in planning and providing care.

Analysis of outcome data is a crucial first step in developing comprehensive nursing services as well as public health policy for cities, states, and the nation. Definition of the following terms will help clarify perinatal statistics (1).

Birth: The complete expulsion or extraction of the fetus from the mother, regardless of whether or not the umbilical cord has been cut or the placenta is attached. (Often, a fetus of less than 20 weeks' gestation or 500 g is considered an abortus rather than a birth.)

Birth rate: The number of births per 1000 people.

Fertility rate: The number of live births per 1000 females ages 15–44.

Live birth: Birth of an infant who shows any signs of life (e.g., heart beat, spontaneous breathing, spontaneous movement of voluntary muscles).

Stillbirth: Birth of an infant that shows no signs of life at or after birth.

Neonatal death: Early neonatal death is death of a live-born infant during the first 7 days of life. Late neonatal death is death of a live-born infant after 7 days but before 29 days of life.

Stillbirth rate: The number of stillborn infants per 1000 infants born.

Fetal death rate: Synonymous with stillbirth rate.

Neonatal mortality rate: The number of neonatal deaths per 1000 live births.

Perinatal mortality rate: The number of fetal deaths plus neonatal deaths per 1000 total births.

Infant mortality rate: The number of deaths of infants prior to 1 year of age per 1000 live births.

Low birth weight: Birth weight less than 2501 g.

Term infant: An infant born from 37 completed weeks of gestation through 41 completed weeks of gestation. (Alternatively, it is suggested that 38–42 weeks' gestation might reflect more accurately the optimum time of delivery.)

Preterm: An infant born before 37 completed weeks of gestation.

Postterm infant: An infant born at 42 or more weeks of gestation.

Abortus: A fetus or embryo expelled from the uterus at 20 weeks' gestation or before, or a fetus weighing less than 500 g or measuring less than 25 cm in length.

Direct maternal death: Death of a mother resulting from obstetric complications of the pregnancy, delivery, or puerperium.

Indirect maternal death: Death of the mother from a disease that developed before or during the pregnancy or puerperium and that was aggravated by the maternal physiologic adaptation to the pregnancy.

Maternal death rate: Number of maternal deaths that occur as the result of the reproductive process per 100,000 live births.

3

MATERNAL AND CHILD HEALTH OBJECTIVES

In 1979 the United States Surgeon General established national infant health objectives as goals to be met by the year 1990. These goals seemed modest at the time and certainly achievable based on the trends of the 1970s. However, several of them no longer appear reachable by 1990 or for several decades to come unless the rate of progress improves. The objectives pertinent to maternity care include the following (2):

1. The national infant mortality rate should be reduced to no more than 9 deaths per 1000 live births, with no county or racial or ethnic subgroup having a rate in excess of 12 deaths per 1000 live births.
2. The neonatal mortality rate (deaths of infants less than 28 days old) should be reduced to 6 per 1000 live births.
3. The postneonatal mortality rate should be reduced to 2.5 per 1000 live births.
4. Low birthweight births should constitute no more than 5% of all births, with no county or racial or ethnic subgroup having a proportion in excess of 9%.
5. At least 90% of all pregnant women should begin prenatal care within the first 3 months of pregnancy.
6. Virtually all women and infants should be served at levels appropriate to their needs through a regionalized system of primary, secondary, and tertiary care for prenatal, maternal, and perinatal health services.

Examination of current vital statistics reveals that some of these goals are far from being met and that certain segments of the population fare far worse than others.

VITAL STATISTICS

The most recent available statistics in the United States are those from 1986, a year that marked a new low in the continuing long-term trend of decreasing infant mortality (see Fig. 1.1). Although the trend toward lower infant mortality—now at 10.4 deaths per 1000 live births—is encouraging, the rate of progress has slowed during the 1980s, and the United States' rank compared to other countries has deteriorated over time. In 1986 the United States ranked 18th, behind such countries as Hong Kong and Singapore (see Table 1.1).

For the second year in a row, the black infant mortality rate did not improve at all (Fig. 1.1). The difference between white and black infant mortality rates is the greatest it has ever been since 1940, when rates began to be reported by race. In 1986 black infants were 2.02 times more likely to die before 1 year of age than their white counterparts (3). The discrepancies in infant deaths between blacks and whites and among various socioeconomic strata also point out that much work is left to be done with respect to improving perinatal health care, with special attention given to the prevention of low birth weight.

Infant death rates resulting from congenital anomalies, which usually are not preventable, are essentially the same for black and white infants. Causes of death that are considered preventable through adequate maternity and infant health care are largely responsible for the discrepancy in mortality rates. For example, black infants were nearly four times as likely as white infants to die from prematurity or low birth weight and twice as likely to die from maternal and newborn complications and newborn infections (Table 1.2).

Three-quarters of neonatal deaths result from low birth weight, either prematurity or intrauterine growth retardation. The rate of low birth weight births in 1986 was 6.8%—the same as in 1980. The percentage of very low birth weight babies (less than 1500 g) increased to 1.2% in 1986. The percentage of preterm births increased in 1986 to 17.7% among black babies and 8.4% among white infants. There was a slight improvement in neonatal mortality rates in 1986, presumably because of improvements in neonatal care rather than because of the birth of healthier babies. Since low birth weight, either directly or indirectly, is responsible for so many neonatal deaths, it is clear that its prevention is of highest priority.

In 1986 postneonatal infant mortality rates decreased slightly overall. However, for the second year in a row, the rates for black infants increased, possibly in part because of prolonging the life of unhealthy infants beyond 28 days of life and partly because of an increase in accidents (3, p 9).

Statistical data by geographic region indicate trouble spots. Certain southern states continue to have high black infant mortality rates, and South Dakota had a significant and disturbing increase in infant mortality in 1986, with a nonwhite (primarily Native American) infant mortality rate of 27.5 (3, p 15).

Rural areas have a slightly higher mortality rate than the national averge, but "babies born in the urban core of America's largest cities are at the

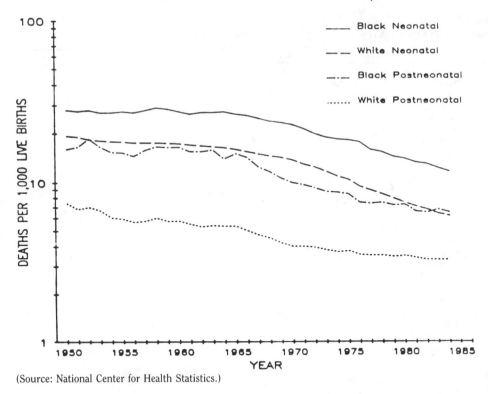

(Source: National Center for Health Statistics.)

Figure 1.1. Infant mortality rates, by race, United States, 1978–1986.

highest risk of death during infancy among all American children" (3, p 22). In general, black urban infant mortality rates are much higher than white. While there has been some improvement in urban infant mortality rates in the 1980s, progress has been sporadic, with some areas actually showing an increase.

The proportion of births to teens continued to drop in 1986, down to 12.6% of all births. This is a reflection of both the smaller number of teens in the population and a lower teenage birth rate (number of live births per 1000 teenage women). However, the teenage birth rates among blacks increased in 1986, and 22.8% of black births were to teenagers—more than twice the proportion for whites. The proportion of births to older women (over 30 years old) has increased in recent years as women have continued to postpone childbearing.

Births to unmarried women continued to rise in 1986 to the highest level ever seen in the United States (23.4%). The rate of births to unmarried black women (61.2%) remains higher than to unmarried white women (15.7%), but the gap is narrowing. Many births to unmarried women are planned and wanted, a factor that certainly affects the disposition of the infant. However, unmarried

women are more likely to be poor and receive inadequate prenatal care.

The maternal mortality rate has decreased remarkably over the last 50 years—down from 582.1 per 100,000 live births in 1935. The decline in maternal mortality can be attributed to many factors, including safe blood transfusions, antibiotics, and the maintenance of fluid-electrolyte and acid-base balance with the serious complications of pregnancy and during labor. Also very important is the increased training and competence of obstetric personnel and the increased availability of the facilities required for good obstetric care. There remains a greater than threefold difference in maternal mortality rates between black and white women. In 1986 the maternal mortality rate for blacks was 18.8, for nonwhites was 16.0, and for whites was 4.9 (3, p 10). It is postulated that the difference is due to unfavorable social, economic, and health care factors, such as relative lack of skilled personnel and adequate health care facilities, lack of prenatal care, lack of family planning services, and perhaps poor dietary intake and poor hygiene.

The four leading causes of maternal death (Table 1.3) are considered preventable. Especially notable is ectopic pregnancy, which has increased more than fourfold from 1970 to 1985, from 4.8 to

Table I.I.
INFANT MORTALITY RATES, SELECTED COUNTRIES, 1986[a]

RANK	COUNTRY	RATE[b]
1	Japan	6
1	Finland	6
1	Sweden	6
4	Denmark	7
4	Switzerland	7
4	Norway	7
7	Netherlands	8
7	France	8
7	Canada	8
10	Hong Kong	9
10	Singapore	9
10	German Democratic Republic	9
10	Belgium	9
10	Germany, Federal Republic	9
10	United Kingdom	9
10	Spain	9
10	Ireland	9
	U.S. (White)	*9*
18	Austria	10
18	Australia	10
18	United States	10
21	Italy	11
21	New Zealand	11
23	Greece	12
24	Israel	14
24	Czechoslovakia	14
26	Cuba	15
26	Bulgaria	15
28	Poland	18
28	Hungary	18
28	Portugal	18
28	Costa Rica	18
	U.S. (Black)	*18*

[a]Source: UNICEF. Data from Hughes D, et. al., *The Health of America's Children*. Children's Defense Fund, Washington DC, 1989, p 14; from Grant JP: *The State of the World's Children 1988*, UNICEF, Oxford University Press, 1988.
[b]Deaths per 1000 live births.

20.9 per 1000 live births. This dramatic increase parallels an increase in sexually transmitted diseases, especially gonorrhea and *Chlamydia*, that cause pelvic inflammatory disease—a frequent cause of ectopic pregnancy. Ectopic pregnancies are increasing among both black and white women, but while the ectopic rate is 50% higher in black women, the maternal mortality rate because of ectopic pregnancy is 600% greater than that of white women (3, p 12).

UTILIZATION OF PRENATAL CARE

In 1986 75.9% of infants were born to women who received early prenatal care (i.e., in the first trimester of pregnancy). This represents a decline from 76.2% in 1985 and 76.3% in 1980 (3, p 50). Overall, 6% of all births were to women with late

(third trimester) or no prenatal care, up from 5% in 1985. The proportion of births to white women receiving early prenatal care decreased slightly, while the proportion receiving late or no prenatal care increased. In 1986 the proportion of births to black women receiving late or no prenatal care increased for the fifth time since 1980; 1 in 10 received late or no prenatal care (3, p 51).

These trends in mortality rates and utilization of prenatal care are disturbing. There is widespread agreement that prenatal care is effective in improving pregnancy outcomes and that it is especially important for women at high risk, either medically or socially. Many other countries with better infant mortality rates than the United States (e.g., Japan and most Western European countries) have a health care system that ensures and encourages adequate, early maternity care, with few barriers to that care; thus, very high proportions of women in those countries seek prenatal care early. Prenatal

Table 1.2.

INFANT MORTALITY RATES[a] FOR 15 OF THE LEADING CAUSES OF INFANT DEATH, BY RACE, UNITED STATES[b]

ALL CAUSES	ALL RACES	WHITE	NONWHITE BLACK	NONWHITE TOTAL	RATIO OF BLACK TO WHITE
	1035.3	894.3	1803.5	1568.1	2.0
1. Congenital anomalies	219.5	219.5	232.1	219.4	1.1
2. Sudden infant death syndrome	140.5	123.0	233.6	206.6	1.9
3. Respiratory distress syndrome	90.6	81.5	144.2	124.8	1.8
4. Disorders related to short gestation and low birthweight	86.4	60.3	225.4	185.1	3.7
5. Maternal complications of pregnancy	36.1	31.9	61.0	51.8	1.9
6. Intrauterine hypoxia and birth asphyxia	26.2	22.2	47.6	41.3	2.1
7. Infections specific to the perinatal period	24.4	20.7	44.1	38.7	2.1
8. Complications of placenta, cord, or membranes	22.3	19.6	37.8	32.4	1.9
9. Accidents and adverse effects	24.2	20.3	43.1	39.1	2.1
10. Pneumonia and influenza	17.6	14.2	35.9	30.8	2.5
11. Neonatal hemorrhage	9.2	7.4	18.8	16.2	2.5
12. Septicemia	8.0	6.4	16.7	14.4	2.6
13. Homicide	7.4	5.4	18.2	15.0	3.4
14. Birth trauma	7.1	6.3	12.1	9.9	1.9
15. Meningitis	5.9	4.5	11.9	10.8	2.6

[a]Deaths per 100,000 live births.
[b]Source: National Center for Health Statistics.

Table 1.3.

THE FOUR LEADING CAUSES OF MATERNAL MORTALITY[a], BY RACE, 1986[b]

CAUSE OF DEATH	TOTAL	WHITE	BLACK	OTHER NONWHITE	RATIO OF BLACK TO WHITE
Complications of the puerperium	2.0	1.4	5.0	4.2	3.6
Toxemia of pregnancy	1.1	0.6	3.4	2.7	5.7
Ectopic pregnancy	1.0	0.5	3.1	2.5	6.2
Hemorrhage of pregnancy and childbirth	0.7	0.5	1.4	1.4	2.8

[a]Deaths per 100,000 live births.
[b]Source: National Center for Health Statistics.

care has been demonstrated to be cost effective. The Institute of Medicine in a 1985 report estimated that each dollar spent on prenatal care for low income, poorly educated women could reduce medical care costs for care of their low birth weight infants by $3.38 during the first year of life (4). Therefore, it seems reasonable to direct resources into encouraging adequate and timely prenatal care.

There are several demographic risk factors associated with insufficient prenatal care: minority status, age (especially less than 15 years old and more than 40 years old), low education level, multiparity (with more dramatic decrease in prenatal care for fourth and fifth children), unmarried status, poverty, and geographic location (either inner cities or isolated rural areas). Many women have several of these risk factors, and they have a disproportionate share of insufficient prenatal care and poor obstetrical outcome (4, pp 3–4).

The Institute of Medicine in a 1988 report identified four categories of obstacles or barriers to full participation in prenatal care (4, pp 4–7):

1. Financial problems with private insurance or Medicaid, or complete lack of health insurance.
2. Inadequate capacity in prenatal care systems.
3. Problems in the organization, practices, and atmosphere of prenatal services.
4. Personal and cultural factors that limit use of services.

The financial barrier to prenatal care is somewhat unique to this country, for we do not have a national health system ensuring access to prenatal care. Financial concerns also underlie many of the system, provider, and patient barriers to care. Although private health insurance may cover normal maternity care, often the coverage is optional and costly or may require substantial out-of-pocket copayment. It may not even be available in employer-based group insurance. Medicaid has allowed low income individuals to increase their use of medical services since it was enacted in 1965, but it has certainly not solved all the problems. The enrollment process is so time consuming that a woman may be well into the pregnancy before her application is approved. The types of clinics used by Medicaid clients often are overutilized or understaffed, resulting in long waiting times for appointments. Some physicians do not accept Medicaid patients because of the low reimbursement, which further restricts access to care. Also, some of the poor are not eligible for Medicaid. Congress has expanded Medicaid eligibility in the mid 1980s, but still an estimated 26% of women of childbearing age have no maternity coverage at all, and the number is likely to increase (4, pp 5–6). Other financial aspects of prenatal care, often overlooked, are additional expenses such as transportation to the clinic and child care.

The American Nurses' Association (ANA) Consensus Conferences on Access to Prenatal Care identified the following nonfinancial barriers to prenatal care (5):

1. Policy or system barriers (e.g., uncoordinated care, inconvenient time and place, long waiting times, limited availability of appointments, inflexible rules, confusing eligibility requirements, professional liability insurance crises [resulting in fewer maternity care providers], inadequate outreach and follow-up, lack of transportation or child care).
2. Provider barriers (e.g., negative personal characteristics; inadequate teaching, communication, and counseling skills; poor communication between providers; turf battles; lack of confidentiality; inadequate knowledge and use of community resources).
3. Patient barriers (e.g., fear, denial, or ambivalence about pregnancy; informational deficits; pride of the "new poor;" unhealthy life-style habits; cognitive and emotional impairments; lack of support).

The Institute of Medicine and the ANA each established recommendations for reducing the barriers to prenatal care. The Institute of Medicine report has 14 major recommendations, some of which are summarized briefly here: The nation should adopt the principle that all pregnant women should be provided access to prenatal, labor and delivery, and postpartum services according to their needs. National leaders, from both the public and private sector, should commit themselves to a new maternity care system—not merely changes in the existing system—designed to draw all women into prenatal care and should provide them with appropriate health and social services throughout the childbearing cycle. Elimination of identified barriers to prenatal care, with top priority given to financial barriers, should be an immediate goal. Services should be plentiful enough to allow prenatal appointments within 2 weeks to providers close to the patient's home. Prenatal services should have minimal bureaucratic requirements and a welcoming atmosphere. Follow-up of missed appointments should be routine. Long-term, high quality public information campaigns should be implemented, emphasizing the importance of early prenatal care for healthy mothers and infants; specific information on where to go or call for prenatal services always should be provided. Outreach activities should exist in a well-designed, well-functioning, accessible maternity health care system. Programs providing prenatal care to high risk and often low income groups should provide social support services, with home visits available (4, pp 13–16).

The ANA Consensus Conferences issued one overall recommendation: All pregnant women should be assured access to timely, comprehensive, high quality maternity care (5, p 57). Policy recommendations to implement that goal include the following (5, pp 57–60):

1. A national system of public maternity financing should be developed, and it should be supported through a combination of federal and state revenues administered by the states and implemented at the community level.
2. Funding for Community and Migrant Health Centers programs and Title V maternal and child health block grant programs should be increased and targeted for perinatal services.
3. Programs should be developed or expanded to give pregnant women all of the nutrition assistance and other forms of public support they need.
4. All health professional schools should be required to incorporate into their curricula theory and practice related to health education, counseling, and the social and cultural aspects of patient care.
5. All federal public assistance programs should have identical eligibility criteria for pregnant women; the criteria should measure only financial need; application forms should be

6. Reimbursement under Medicaid, Title V, and other public and private programs should be based on uniform standards to ensure that pregnant women receive all the necessary components of care and that care is accessible and of high quality.
7. An equitable system of malpractice compensation should be maintained.
8. Federal and state governments and the private sector should launch a nationwide effort to educate the public, policy makers, and pregnant women about the importance, effectiveness, and cost effectiveness of timely, high quality maternity care.
9. Federal and state governments and the private sector should support research related to low birth weight.
10. State nursing practice laws should be unified to permit practice to the maximum extent possible by certified nurse-midwives and nurse-practitioners.
11. Federal tax laws should be amended to require all employers to furnish parental leave to employees.

The ANA conference participants called for improvements in accessibility to prenatal care as an important step in decreasing the incidence of low birth weight and mortality in the United States, but they recognized that basic life needs such as food, clothing, and shelter also must be met to improve the health of our next generation.

PERINATAL CARE

In recent years perinatal care has undergone dramatic changes; technology has expanded, giving the health care team new modalities for diagnosis and treatment (e.g., electronic fetal monitoring, ultrasonography, amniocentesis, chorionic villi sampling, and even fetal surgery). At the same time, however, consumers have begun to reject these interventions and have demanded a return to natural childbirth in a simple, caring environment. The two trends seem paradoxical. Progress has been made and needs to continue toward the development of a standard of care that views pregnancy, labor, and delivery as natural phenomena, requiring little intervention, as long as the process is normal. However, observation of the process must be astute so that when deviations from normal occur, precise diagnosis and appropriate immediate inter-

(top of right column) ...brief, uniform, and easily accessible; and applications should be processed within 2 weeks.

vention can be instituted so that maternal and fetal/neonatal health can be regained.

Often, in the past, more emphasis has been placed on treating disease than on preventing it. For example, care of very small and/or very sick neonates has advanced more rapidly than prevention of the delivery of low birth weight and sick babies. In recent years, however, increased emphasis has been placed on identification of patients at risk for pregnancy complications and on early intervention to prevent those complications from causing serious sequelae for mother and baby. Much research needs to be done in this area.

In the past, perinatal care has focused primarily on improvements in fetal testing and advances in newborn care. Recently, more attention has been given to the fact that the mother is a part of a much wider social system that involves her family, community, cultural group, and society as a whole. Significant events that occur in her environment affect her health, and that of her baby. It is clear that financial, psychological, educational, and social support services are an integral part of adequate perinatal care.

Because of the rapidity of change in perinatal care, it is clear that not every practitioner in every setting can (or should) maintain the expertise and equipment needed to provide "state-of-the-art" care for their patients. In order to provide the best utilization of personnel and equipment, regionalization of care has emerged. The concept of regionalization involves the idea that different institutions within a given geographical area are needed to provide different levels of care. Thus, some hospitals provide care for essentially normal obstetric patients (level I), some to patients with intermediate complications (level II), and some have complete technology to provide state-of-the-art care for high risk women and neonates (level III). It is the responsibility of providers of prenatal care to ensure that patients are referred to the institution providing the level of care necessary. There must be an easy flow of patients back and forth, for the level of care needed may change during the pregnancy or neonatal period.

NURSING MANAGEMENT

The maternity nurse has a unique and pivotal role in providing obstetric care. Maternity nurses function at all levels in the provision of perinatal care: preconception counseling, in the prenatal office or clinic, in the antepartum unit of the hospital, in labor and delivery, in the normal and intensive care nurseries, and on the postpartum unit. Care may be provided in level I, II, or III hospitals; in birth centers; or at home. Thus, it is clear that maternity nurses have many opportunities to influence the care of the mother and/or baby and can assist in planning and providing services that will help meet the national goals for improved pregnancy outcome.

Nursing generally focuses on health promotion rather than disease. Prevention is a key concept, and it occurs on three levels:

1. Primary—intervention *before* disease occurs.
2. Secondary—early treatment of disease to retard or stop it, thus preventing complications.
3. Tertiary—intervention to inhibit the progression of sequelae of the disease.

Screening for high risk pregnancy is an important step in primary and secondary prevention. Ongoing, continuous assessment and evaluation of all of the factors that predispose a patient to potential complications are required. Table 1.4 details initial and ongoing screening criteria. Factors that influence outcome are multietiologic in nature, including past reproductive performance, genetic makeup, exposure to environmental hazards, age, presence of acute or chronic disease, nutritional status, and emotional health.

Because so many factors may influence maternal and infant outcome, standardized risk assessment tools have been devised to formalize the risk assessment process. The patient's risk factors are evaluated at the first prenatal visit and, depending on the number or the severity of conditions found, a score of low, moderate, or high risk is assigned. A plan of care based on the risk status is developed. The risk status is reevaluated at the 28th week of gestation. A patient's risk score may escalate from low to moderate or high risk. However, the score is never reduced from high to moderate or low, because even if a condition such as nutritional status has improved, its presence during the first two trimesters will continue to impact on pregnancy outcome. The plan of care is revised according to the updated score. Table 1.5 an example of such a risk tool.

Table 1.4.
CRITERIA FOR IDENTIFICATION OF HIGH RISK PREGNANCY[a]

Characteristics of the patient
Age
   Teenage: under 18 years at conception
   Elderly: 35 years or older at conception

Weight
   Underweight: 100 pounds or less
   Overweight: more than 20% over standard weight
   Gain: over 30 and under 15 pounds

Height
   Short stature: 60 inches or less

Race (specific problems affecting specific races, i.e., Tay-Sachs, sickle cell anemia, cystic fibrosis)

Marital status
   Single
   Separated/divorced
   Widowed

Culture (specific cultural practice affecting pregnancy, i.e., pica)

Education/occupation
   Less than high school diploma
   Other than skilled or professional workers

Economics (lack of money for pregnancy care, housing, and environment)

Available emotional supports (if none, may have emotional and other additional stressors)

Drug addiction or ingestion

Alcoholism

Smoking (two packs plus per day)

Emotionally stressed
   Fear
   Anger
   Hostility
   Anxiety and tension
   Lack of support
   Ambivalence
   Family problems
   Patient perceptions ("I know something is wrong")

Characteristics of the father
Age
   Teenage: under 18 (lack of support and/or responsibility)
   Elderly: 40 years or older (increased incidence stillborn)

Table I.4. (continued)
CRITERIA FOR IDENTIFICATION OF HIGH RISK PREGNANCY[a]

Blood group
   Rh-positive baby with Rh-negative mother
   ABO incompatibilities

Family history
   Genetically transferred conditions
   Genetically predisposed conditions

Chronic disease
   Drug addiction
   Alcoholism
   Diabetes mellitus

Previous pregnancy history
Parity
   Grand multipara (seven or more pregnancies over 20
     weeks or 500 g)
   Primigravida

Previous surgical delivery
   Cesarean section
   Version
   Vacuum extraction
   Mid to high forceps
   Breech extraction

Previous outcomes
   "Early" fetal loss (two pregnancies terminated before
     28 weeks)
   "Late" fetal loss (one or more at 28 weeks plus)
   Live prematures (two or more under 2500 g)
   "Early" neonatal death (one or more before 7 days)
   "Early" fetal loss and live premature (one fetal loss
     before 28 weeks in last two pregnancies plus one
     live premature [any pregnancy])
   "Large" infant (one or more larger than 4000 g)
   "Damaged" or traumatized infant (one or more living
     or not)
   Infants small for gestational age

Pregnancy occurrence
   Less than 3 months after last delivery
   More than 5 years after last delivery

Labor length
   Prolonged or dystocia
   Precipitate

Medical/surgical history during nonpregnancy period,
   previous pregnancy, or present pregnancy)
Hypertensive disease
Renal disease
Diabetes
Cancer in past 5 years
Thyroid disease

Hereditary disorders
Cardiovascular disease
Respiratory disease
Blood factor sensitization
Severe malnutrition
Psychiatric disorder
Neurologic disease
Drug addiction or ingestion
Alcohol addiction or ingestion
Mental retardation
Lupus erythematosus
Infectious disease
Infertility
Gynecologic complication

Additional medical complications (during previous or
   present pregnancy)
Toxemia
Bleeding
Rubella
Anemia
   Hemoglobin 8 g or less
   Hematocrit 30% or less
   Sickle cell anemia
   Cooley's anemia
Multiple pregnancy
Abnormal positional problems
   Abnormal presentation
   Abnormal lie
   Abnormal position

Indifference to health needs
   Missed appointments (three or more)
   Failure to follow recommendations consistently

Nutrition
   Weight loss and/or crash dieting, fasting
   Weight gain (less than 15 pounds or more than 30
     pounds)

Progression
   Incompatible fundal height with gestation
   Small for gestational age fetus
   Large for gestational age fetus
   Multiple pregnancy
   Incorrect calculation of dates
   Hydramnios or oligohydramnios

Other
   General anesthesia or surgery
   Abdominal x-rays
   High altitude
   Stressors
   Decreased fetal movement

[a]Reprinted with permission from Kinney M, et al., *AACN's Clinical Reference for Critical Care Nurses*. New York, McGraw-Hill, 1981.

Table 1.5.
SAMPLE RISK TOOL[a]

Patient Name _____

PRENATAL RISK ASSESSMENT
Prevention of Low Birth Weight Program

I. INITIAL EVALUATION   Weeks Gestation_____

Moderate Risk Factors		High Risk Factors		Very High Risk Factors	
Age (≤17 or ≥35)	☐	A. Diabetics (insulin req.)	☐	Drug Addiction	☐
Race (nonwhite)	☐	Cardiac (class III or IV or arrhy)	☐	≥2 Prior Low Birthwt. Infants	☐
Marital Status (cur. unwed)	☐			≥2 Section B High Risk Factors	☐
Height (<5'1")	☐	Rh Sensitization (titer ≥1/8)	☐		
Weight (<100 or >255 pounds)	☐	Prior Neurologically Damaged Infant	☐		
Anemia (<11 g)	☐				
Smoking (>½ pack per day)	☐	Prior Infant with Major Anomaly	☐		
Poor Socioeconomic Cond.	☐				
Suspected Poor Nutrition	☐	B.-Uterine Abnorm. or Incomp. Cervix	☐		
Substance Abuse	☐	*1 Prior Low Birthwt. Infant (<5½ pounds, 2500 g)	☐		
Prior Cesarean Section	☐				
Cardiac (class I or class II or MVP)	☐	*Hypertension (>160/95 or req'g meds)	☐		
Epilepsy	☐	*Renal Disease (chronic, serious)	☐		
Endo. Infertility or Other Chronic Med. Illness	☐	*Hx of ≥2 Spont. Early Fetal Death or ≥2 ITOPs	☐		
Hx of Rx with DES	☐				
Sought Prenatal Care > 20 Weeks		*Prior Spont. Late Fetal Death (20 weeks gestation to delivery)	☐		
		*Prior Neonatal Death (from delivery to 28 days)	☐		
		*Prior Infant Req'g ICU	☐		
		C. ≥4 Moderate Risk Factors	☐		

Outcome of Risk Assessment: Low _____ Moderate _____ High _____ Very High _____

Additional Notes:

By: _____ Date _____

Table 1.5. (continued)
SAMPLE RISK TOOL[a]

II. REEVALUATION   Weeks Gestation _____

Moderate Risk Factors	High Risk Factors	Very High Risk Factors
Weight Gain (avg. <½ or >2 pounds/week) ☐	A*Rh Sensitization (titer >1/8 ☐	Multiple Pregnancy ☐
Anemia (<10 g) ☐	*Suspected Hydramnios ☐ *Suspected Viral Inf. ☐	Mid and/or 3rd Trimester ☐ Bleeding
Smoking—reg. (≥½ packs per day) ☐	*Uterine Irritability ☐	Toxemia (including chronic ☐ hypertension—BP >160/95
Clinical U. Infection ☐	B*Other (specify) ☐	or req'g meds)
Other Infection(s) (specify) ☐	*>2 moderate Risk Factors ☐	Ruptured Membranes ☐
+ Glucose Tol. Test ☐		Cervix Effacing > 40% ☐
Poor or Noncompliance ☐ Following Advice, Appts., Meds.		Cervix Dilated >2 cm ☐
		Tocolytics Req. ☐
Excess Use of Drugs (including ☐ alcohol)		Suspected Poor Fetal Growth ☐
		≥2 Section A High Risk Factors ☐
Working Mother ☐		
Maternal Stress ☐		

Outcome of Risk Assessment: Low _____ Moderate _____ High _____ Very High _____

Additional Notes:

By: _____ Date _____

[a]From: New York State Department of Health. Prevention of Low Birth Weight Program Risk Scoring Tool.

Women identified as high risk should receive intensive services in a setting that is able to support complex obstetric and neonatal problems. In the United States the tertiary or level III facilities (also called perinatal centers) are the proper site of care for all high risk patients and should provide the following services (6):

1. Early identification and treatment of high risk pregnancy;
2. Intensive labor and delivery care;
3. Ability to accept high risk patients in transfer;
4. Comprehensive support services, including medical consultation, nursing care, social services, extensive laboratory testing, health education, nutrition counseling, and home follow-up; and
5. A system to evaluate services, including a system to process and evaluate outcome data.

The nurse is most often the one not only to identify risk factors that impact on outcome but also to complete the standardized scoring system. Thus, she is in an ideal position to coordinate the efforts of the entire health care team in order to provide restorative care with the goal of maximizing not only physical but also psychological outcome (7). The ANA has defined the scope of practice for nurses providing high risk perinatal care. Practice is provided within the framework of the nursing process and includes but is not limited to the following:

1. Assessment—Assessing the psychosocial and physiological status of the high risk childbearing family by differentiating the level of perinatal risk; by initiating and utilizing multiple sources and assessment tools for data collection, such as histories, physical examination, and appropriate laboratory data; and by interpreting data that lead to nursing diagnoses.
2. Plan of care—Establishing an appropriate plan of intervention with the high risk perinatal family based on nursing diagnoses by collaborating with the family and other health care providers; by differentiating immediate and long-term health care goals with the family; and by determining and coordinating the plan of action to meet these identified goals.

3. Intervention—Implementing the interventions with the high risk perinatal family that are based on the plan of care, including initiating technical procedures and therapeutic regimes; maintaining a therapeutic environment; intervening in life-threatening situations; teaching, counseling, and facilitating family development; preventing further complications; and promoting optimum health development of the high risk perinatal family.

4. Evaluation—Evaluating the plan of care of the high risk perinatal family by evaluating the interventions; evaluating the effects of the interventions on the family; evaluating the family's progress toward the identified goals; and initiating changes in the plan of care based on new data and resources and on the environment.

PSYCHOLOGICAL EFFECTS OF HIGH RISK PREGNANCY

Normal pregnancy is a time of stress as the family members prepare to accept new roles and responsibilities and to evaluate their supportive relationships surrounding the pregnancy. This stress is exaggerated further when the diagnosis of high risk pregnancy is confirmed. Fear of death and anxiety about the outcome for both mother and baby may lead to long-term emotional problems for the mother and/or her significant others. Chapter 2 discusses these problems in depth.

Exposure to intensive perinatal care services may leave a woman overwhelmed and dehumanized. It is the high risk perinatal nurse who must not only provide expert care but also uphold the patient's right to dignity—even in an emergency situation. The nurse must be ever mindful of the humanity of the patient, assist in maintaining family integration, and provide emotional and psychological support for the entire family.

REFERENCES

1. Pritchard JA, MacDonald PC, Gant NF: *Williams Obstetrics,* ed 17. Norwalk, CT, Appleton-Century-Crofts, 1985, p 2.
2. Healthy People: The Surgeon General's Report on Health Promotion and Disease Prevention, 1979. Washington, DC, U.S. Department of Health, Education and Welfare, pp 21–31.
3. Children's Defense Fund: *The Health of America's Children: Maternal and Child Data Book.* CDF, May 1989, p 3.
4. Committee to Study Outreach for Prenatal Care: *Prenatal Care: Reaching Mothers, Reaching Infants.* Institute of Medicine, Washington, DC, National Academy Press, 1988, p 2.
5. Report of Consensus Conferences, American Nurses' Association: *Access to Prenatal Care: Key to Preventing Low Birthweight.* Kansas City, MO, American Nurses' Association, 1987, pp 24–32.
6. Vestal K, McKenzie C; *High Risk Perinatal Nursing.* Philadelphia, WB Saunders, 1983, p 15.
7. *A Statement on the Scope of High Risk Perinatal Nursing Practice.* American Nurses' Association, No. MCH-12, 1980, p 2.

Chapter 2
Maternal Psychosocial Adaptations to High Risk Pregnancy

Nancy DeVore, C.N.M., M.S.

Helene Deutsch has stated that "the processes of pregnancy are the concern of biology, psychology, and social science" (1). Certainly, the many stresses of the perinatal period can be classified in this manner. A few of these normal concerns are as follows:

1. Physical stresses
   a. Hormonal changes
   b. Fatigue, exhaustion, sleep deprivation
   c. Pain
2. Psychological stresses
   a. Fear of pain, disability, disfigurement, death
   b. Fear of labor and delivery
   c. Ambivalence about pregnancy and life changes
3. Socioeconomic stresses
   a. Financial concerns
   b. Social isolation
   c. Alterations in family responsibilities and relationships

In an uncomplicated pregnancy the list is endless, and the effect is a cumulative one of multiple stresses. When a pregnancy is designated "high risk," the stresses certainly can multiply and intensify.

In the high risk maternity patient, physical concerns may also include obstetrical or medical problems and medicinal effects. Hemorrhage from a placenta previa, placental abruption, or postpartum uterine atony; infection from premature or prolonged rupture of membranes; lacerations from a midpelvis forceps delivery; electrolyte imbalance from hyperemesis gravidarum; changes in the metabolism of nutrients from hiatal hernia; and tachycardia associated with ritodrine therapy for premature labor are some of the physical stresses that may deplete maternal reserves and jeopardize adjustment to the maternity experience. The frequent prohibition on exercise for the high risk patient precludes an effective normal outlet for excess tension.

A high risk pregnancy has its own list of psychological stresses. When the woman has had a poor reproductive history, such as spontaneous abortion, premature labor, congential anomaly, stillbirth, or neonatal death, her anxiety may be quite high for fear of repeat poor outcomes. Discussions of dreams and fantasies often will make concrete the otherwise nebulous fear of doom. A review of the woman's total obstetrical history is imperative. The mention of a prior elective abortion should alert all to a possible source of anxiety (2, 3)—the fantasy of having harmed her body or having incurred God's punishment so that a future pregnancy is destined to fail.

In a high risk population, fear of labor and delivery, fear of a damaged baby, or fear of death is much intensified beyond such anxieties in a normal group. The course of labor, which is monitored by the most advanced technology and scrutinized by a high risk specialist, has little chance of being anxiety free. Although machinery used and tests performed may be reassuring to some women, to others they are sources of physical and psychological discomfort—constant reminders of the danger inherent in this process that both mother and baby must be protected against (4, 5). In addition, the constant threat of cesarean section exists: major surgery with the potential for pain, disfigurement, and complications, including death.

Although all pregnant women fear delivering a less than perfect infant, high risk women may be fearful more realistically of this outcome. Those who have sustained a perinatal infection (e.g., rubella in the first trimester, active herpetic lesions near term), those in their late 30s and early 40s (when the risk of chromosomal abnormalities escalates), those who have abused alcohol, and those with chronic hypertension that has led to decreased uterine blood flow are examples of women who may have an increased fear of delivering a damaged baby. An intensified fear of death for the infant may be anticipated in those women fighting premature labor or in those whose babies show signs of fetal distress. Fear of death for oneself is most often found in women with severe medical or obstetrical problems—uterine rupture, severe preeclampsia, ruptured appendix.

Finally, a major psychological stress during this period is the impaired self-image that is frequently found in women with high risk pregnancies. The inability to conceive, carry, and deliver successfully a normal infant may result in a feeling of inadequacy as a woman. The body is seen as defective and, hence, undesirable. This is often reflected by a deterioration of the marital relationship. When the pregnancy is complicated by a chronic illness, the self-image may be impaired yet again. Enforced dependency—e.g., when severe preeclampsia or premature labor requires bedrest—may conflict with a woman's need to be self-sufficient. Anxiety and resentment may then emerge.

The socioeconomic stresses of a high risk pregnancy include financial concerns, social isolation, and alterations in family responsibilities and relationships. Financial concerns may include both loss of income (the high risk problem may preclude the woman's continuing her usual work) and additional costs for the mother (special tests, increased hospitalization, medication), for the baby (prolonged hospitalization, often with the high cost of a special care nursery), and for the family (transportation to the hospital, assistance with housework, or care of the other children).

Social isolation becomes a stress when the high risk problem dictates retreating from usual activity and cloistering in the home or hospital. Boredom as well as loss of the ongoing support of family, friends, and community may lead to increased anxiety. Unless the care provider keeps such concerns in mind, efforts at treatment may be thwarted. For example, bedrest in the hospital may seem like the ideal treatment for the preeclamptic patient; however, it is doomed to failure if the mother is anxious about who is watching her toddler at home.

Finally, a high risk pregnancy may cause severe strain on the family unit. As the mother is confined to bed or moved to the hospital, roles must change to meet the family's needs of daily life. Often, the partner assumes some of the more domestic functions, such as caring for the home and children. When added to his usual activities, such work may engender anxiety and anger—a feeling that he is doing everything and the woman is doing nothing. Further, within the marital relationship, certain high risk problems (e.g., placenta previa, premature labor, premature rupture of membranes) may necessitate the avoidance of usual sexual activity. More anxiety and anger may occur.

The strain of high risk problems on the family most clearly is seen in the form of impaired communication. The woman's anxiety may be translated into anger that is often expressed toward the partner or the pregnancy. The parnter's fears often go unrecognized and unvoiced. Unfortunately, a cyclic form of miscommunication often results: the original anxiety produces impaired communication, which produces more anxiety, and so on. Awareness of this potential problem is essential for all those providing care in high risk settings.

ADAPTATIONS TO STRESS

One can hypothesize that the outcome of negotiating the stresses of a high risk pregnancy will be determined by the individual's constitutional and acquired traits. Where the underlying personality structure is fragile, the potential for more severe reactions exists.

In most women the stresses of the perinatal period can be anticipated to activate unconscious intrapsychic conflict, to stimulate emotional reorganization, and to cause a reordering of priorities—changes necessary for becoming a mother. For example, ambivalence about pregnancy may cause the woman to deal with unresolved conflicts about her own dependence and independence. The uncovering of her feelings about these basic states is important if she is to undertake the care of a totally dependent infant and to assist the child in the struggle to achieve a measure of independence.

At times, however, the normal response to stress does not occur. Instead, a neurotic, psychotic, or psychophysiologic response ensues, impairing the course of pregnancy and adaptation to the mothering role.

A neurotic response to stress may be manifested in a variety of forms. The woman who has experienced premature labor may appear extremely tense, angry, depressed, or withdrawn. If she is tense, her anxiety is unchanneled, diffuse, and free floating. She may feel that she is living with a time bomb—a sense of impending danger and doom—and she may display difficulties in sleeping, eating, and concentrating.

A high risk pregnancy also may engender an angry response to stress. A diethylstilbestrol (DES) daughter who has a history of incompetent cervix may blame outright her own mother for her poor reproductive outcomes. A woman who has a baby with sepsis in neonatal intensive care unit may be furious with her practitioner for not having diagnosed and treated the premature rupture of her membranes more aggressively.

Depression may occur if the woman feels angry and turns her anger inward rather than expressing it. An uncontrolled diabetic patient whose infant has been noted to have a major cardiac anomaly may cry and evidence disturbances in sleeping and eating. Externally, she displays depression. Internally, she may be furious about her physical illness, her doctor's inability to control the problem, the loss of her fantasy of a perfect infant, and the socioeconomic disturbance this affliction may cause her family.

Another major mechanism of the high risk patient for dealing with anxiety is denial. Displaying a definite lack of anxiety, the woman may intellectualize her fears. She may describe in great detail the pros and cons of amniocentesis for a woman 39 years old, and she may add without a trace of anxiety that she has decided not to have the test because she would not abort if the results showed a defective child. By displaying an attitude that "I will cope with whatever adversity befalls me," she is able to intellectually control her anxiety.

Noncompliance is a manifestation of denial to which many professionals respond with frustration and anger. Failure to take medications as prescribed, to abstain from coitus after premature rupture of membranes, or to keep regular prenatal appointments despite discussion of the importance of such activity may appear initially to be an angry gesture toward the care provider and the baby. In actuality it may represent a defense against severe anxiety associated with her high risk pregnancy.

Suppression and isolation are two other defenses similar to denial that may be employed as a neurotic response to stress. By suppressing normal fantasies about the source of her anxiety, such as the pain of the labor and delivery experience or the possible abnormality of her infant, the woman may avoid facing the associated anxiety. By isolating her feelings of fear, repugnance, and sadness as she touches her newborn with a cleft palate, the woman is able to function for the moment. Unfortunately, although both defenses have a momentary protective value, when persistent they become pathologic and seriously interfere with the bonding process that is so vital to the role of mothering.

PSYCHOTIC RESPONSE

A few women respond to the stress of a high risk pregnancy with a psychotic or psychophysiologic response (see chapter 15).

FAMILY SYSTEM RESPONSE

In addition to these individual responses to stress, a high risk pregnancy may precipitate a family system response. In a positive vein, relationships within the family may be strengthened by the crisis. The marital pair may support each other physically and emotionally—voicing their fears and disappointments both verbally and nonverbally. In addition, concerns may be shared with and support sought from older children and other members of the extended family.

When the family system is weak, the crisis of a perinatal problem may be manifested in the disintegration of tenuous bonds and the failure to establish new sources of support. Alliances may be challenged as the parents misdirect their frustations toward each other, make scapegoats of their other children, or alienate other family members or friends.

NURSING ASSESSMENT

A systematic history is essential to understand the maternal psychosocial adaptations to a high risk pregnancy. Items of interest might include the following.

Family of Procreation

What is the nature of the relationship with the spouse or partner—close? cordial? distant? combative? How long has this relationship persisted? Has the couple previously faced any crisis? What was the nature of that concern? How was the problem eventually solved? How is the partner responding or expected to respond to the present crisis? How might he best be helped?

Are there any other children of this union? Does either partner have children by someone else? Which children live with the family? Where do the others reside and how frequently are they seen? How old are all of the children? Do any have any physical or emotional problems? How are the children responding or expected to respond to the present crisis? How might they best be helped with the current problem?

What is the nature of the relationship with the family of origin of each parent? With which members is the patient close? cordial? distant? combative? Where do they reside? How frequently are they in contact physically? by phone? by letter? What type of problems has the family of origin faced previously as a group? How were such concerns resolved?

Has either partner experienced death of a family member, either of origin or of procreation? Who? When? From what cause? How did the patient respond? How did the family react as a group?

Friends and Other Supports

Which friends or neighbors does the patient feel comfortable asking for help from in times of crisis? Has she ever previously asked them for support? Which type of request can she address to which people? Who will help physically? emotionally? financially?

Does the patient belong to a church or any community organizations? What is the degree of closeness with the members of these groups? Has she previously asked them for support?

Social Responsibilities

Does the patient have regular employment? What is the nature of her work? How long has she been in the job? What is the importance of her work to her and her family? Is there much pressure for her to return to work? Does the pressure come from herself? her family? her boss? her coworkers?

What is the financial situation of this family? What are their sources of income? Do they have medical insurance, and what are the limits of their coverage? Do they anticipate financial problems because of this pregnancy crisis? What solutions are available?

What is the nature of the patient's family responsibilities—housework? child care? care of other individuals or pets? What priorities can she establish with these functions? What alternatives exist for meeting the family's needs?

Interests

What are the patient's usual daily activities? What does she do for exercise? What recreational activities does she enjoy? Does her high risk problem preclude any of these outlets? What alternative interests might she develop in light of her maternity problem?

Response to Stress

What types of crises has the patient experienced previously? How has she responded to such stress? What types of crises has her family experienced previously? How has the family responded to such stress? Has the patient or any other family member been treated for an emotional problem? What was the nature of the problem? Was hospitalization needed? If the same problem were to occur today, would the individual respond in a less severe manner? What new strengths or supports would allow this different response?

KEYS TO DEVELOPING INDIVIDUALIZED NURSING ACTIONS

With the preceding understanding of maternal adaptations of high risk pregnancy, the nurse should be able to plan care that meets the individual psychosocial needs of each of her patients. In a systematic manner she should

1. Recall normal stresses of the perinatal period;
2. Identify those concerns that have been intensified by the high risk problem of her patient;
3. Recall the usual individual and family system responses to stress;
4. Identify the responses manifested by the patient and her family at the present time;
5. Take a comprehensive psychosocial history of her patient;
6. Integrate the data gathered to help the patient and family define the present stress, their response, past methods of coping, and past and current supports; and

7. Assist the patient and family to determine alternatives of care in the present setting, thus supporting some need for self-determination.

REFERENCES

1. Deutsch H: *The Psychology of Women.* New York, Grune & Stratton, 1945, vol. II, p 134.
2. Kumar R, Robson K: Previous induced abortion and antenatal depression in primiparae; a preliminary report of a survey of mental health in pregnancy. *Psychol Med* 8:711–715, 1978.
3. DeVore N: The relationship between previous elective abortions and postpartum depressive reactions. *JOGN* 8:237–240, 1979.
4. Beck CT: Patient acceptance of fetal monitoring as a helpful tool. *JOGN Nurs* 9:350–353, 1980.
5. Shields D: Maternal reactions to fetal monitoring. *Am J Nurs* 78:2110–2112, 1978.

Chapter 3
Grief and Loss

Joanne Middleton, C.N.M., Ph.D. and Tina Quirk, R.N., C.N.M., M.S.

Pregnancy loss often is treated as a nonevent (1). Miscarriages occur in 10–20% of all pregnancies, and stillbirths occur in 1 in 100 deliveries (2). Still, many health professionals, family, and friends of the bereaved couple find dealing with the tragedy overwhelming and thus withdraw emotionally and physically from the couple. This tragic loss in place of joyful life leaves bereaved parents without the usual supports of bereaved persons: comforting family and friends; established rituals such as wakes and funerals; and, most important, society's acknowledgment that someone special has died and its permission to grieve openly.

Yet, perinatal death is a significant loss to the parents, siblings, grandparents, and other close family members and friends. It is a crisis for all, especially the bereaved mother and father; and it is a loss that, to be resolved in a healthy way, must be grieved. Whether the loss is a miscarriage, stillbirth, or neonatal death, certain factors should be understood in order for health professionals to help bereaved parents and family. These factors are as follows:

1. A true crisis prevails and should be managed to a healthy resolution.
2. Grieving is a healthy function and should be facilitated and supported by health professionals, families, and friends.
3. A parent experiencing perinatal bereavement has certain special needs and considerations particular to this situation.
4. Health professionals who are close to the death experience also need permission and an opportunity to grieve.

CRISIS THEORY

A crisis is defined as a perceived physical, psychological, or social threat, that may come from an external or internal source (3). Common psychological or social stressors may be role changes brought on by marriage, by the birth of a child, from new job demands, from a promotion at work, or from the death of a loved one. Crisis can be defined further as maturational or situational. A maturational crisis represents internal psychobiological changes such as pregnancy or menopause (4); a situational crisis constitutes a significant external event such as death of a loved one, loss of a limb, or loss of employment (5).

If an individual is responding to a maturational or situational crisis, anxiety levels rise to an uncomfortable level, which stimulates problem-solving abilities, thus moving the individual toward a healthy resolution or unhealthy disorganization. According to Caplan (3), healthy resolution of a crisis involves

1. A reality orientation that accommodates the changing circumstances of the crisis;
2. Awareness and verbalization of feelings to allow release of tension and expression of anger; and
3. Skill in using available resources or support systems.

In working with the client in crisis, the crisis therapist has the interpersonal growth of the client as a goal (6). This goal is facilitated by listening actively, and empathically, assuming a moderately directive role, and helping the client set realistic goals. Healthy resolution of a crisis is realized when the client assumes new roles, develops new realistic life goals, and resumes appropriate socialization patterns.

Pregnancy as a crisis has been studied from both sociopsychological and psychoanalytic perspectives. Pregnancy, as a maturational crisis, stimulates an intense examination of the woman's self-esteem, her feelings about her own childhood, her relationship with her mother, her relationship with the baby's father, and her accomplishments and goals in life. These and many more individual issues must be resolved emotionally in order to accommodate her new role as a mother.

The psychoanalyst Deutsch described pregnancy as fulfilling the deepest yearnings of a woman by confirming her ability to nurture and protect, and therefore confirming her essential womanliness (7). Thus, pregnancy carries both the reward of success and, conversely, the burden of failure if the baby dies. Deutsch theorized that women fear death at childbirth as deeply and as unconsciously as men fear castration (8). This fear usually remains unconscious, except when revealed in dreams; however, its presence affects the process of resolving the maturational crisis of pregnancy, especially if the outcome is death.

GRIEF THEORY

The classic paper "Symptomatology and Management of Acute Grief," by Lindemann, established a conceptual framework for grief theory (9). He defined grief as a syndrome with five categories of symptoms:

1. Somatic distress—i.e., tightness of chest and throat, shortness of breath, digestive problems, lack of muscular power, tendency to sighing and crying.
2. Preoccupation with the image of the deceased, a feeling of unreality that the person is dead, and increased emotional distance from others.
3. Guilt—a strong preoccupation with failure to have done right by the deceased.
4. Hostile reactions, irritability, and anger, which make the person feel uncomfortable about him/herself.
5. Loss of patterns of conduct, aimlessness, and inability to initiate organized activity.

Resolution of grief (Table 3.1) occurs following a period of grief work or mourning lasting from 4 to 6 weeks and during which the bereaved emancipate themselves from bondage to the deceased, re-

Table 3.1.
STAGES OF GRIEF: ELISABETH KUBLER-ROSS[a]

1. Denial—Characterized by shock, disbelief, "no, not me." May be manifested by refusing to talk about or tell others about the diagnosis; refraining from asking questions about the diagnosis, prognosis, or treatment; attributing the baby's symptoms to a minor condition; seeking opinions from multiple physicians; acting very happy or optimistic.
2. Anger—Characterized by hostility, envy, or resentment directed at oneself or others. May recur throughout the grief process.
3. Bargaining—The attempt to postpone the inevitable death. May attempt to bargain with oneself, a significant other, or God.
4. Depression—The realization of the inevitability of the death and the necessity to say goodbye.
5. Acceptance—Characterized by the resolution of denial, anger, and depression, leaving inner peace and perhaps the desire for solitude.

[a]Adapted from Kubler-Ross E: *On Death and Dying*. New York, Macmillan, 1969.

adjust to the environment from which the deceased is missing, and form new relationships. Distortions of grief include delayed or postponed grief reaction; precipitation of a former unresolved grief reaction; emergence of inappropriate behavior (e.g., euphoria, tearlessness, or a psychosomatic illness); expression of extreme hostility against specific persons; extreme social isolation; agitated or deep depression with feelings of worthlessness; and self-punishment behavior (Table 3.2).

Anticipatory grief is the grief work that begins when the threat of death is apparent and ends when the death actually occurs or is confirmed (10). This time of anticipatory grieving is filled with ambivalent feelings as the person wishes for the loved one to be alive but also wants an end to the uncertainty causing such emotional turmoil. Anticipatory grief can help prepare a person for the inevitable loss and provide a transition time before the death, but it does not replace the acute grief process that begins when the death occurs.

PERINATAL BEREAVEMENT

Theory and Research

Parents who have lost an infant in the perinatal period exhibit the symptoms of acute grief described by Lindemann (9). They describe a feeling of emptiness in the body, pain in the chest, a "broken heart," and arms aching to hold their baby. They recall the delivery and the death of their baby in vivid detail.

Table 3.2.
MORBID GRIEF REACTIONS[a]

MORBID REACTION	CHARACTERISTICS
Delay or postponement of grief	None of the expected psychosomatic reactions of grief immediately after the death
	Grief for an unresolved earlier loss rather than for the current one
	Initiation of grief reaction on a significant "anniversary" date
	Postponement of grief while sustaining the morale of others
Distorted reactions	Overactivity without a sense of loss
	Acquisition of symptoms related to the last illness of the deceased
	Acquisition of a recognized psychosomatic illness (e.g., ulcers, asthma)
	Conspicuous alteration in relationship to friends and relatives—usually social isolation
	Furious hostility toward specific persons
	Repression of hostility, resulting in altered affect and conduct
	Lasting loss of patterns of social interaction, especially lack of decision and initiative
	Altered behavior that is detrimental to social and economic existence (e.g., unjustified generosity)
	Agitated depression, with danger signs of suicide.

[a]Adapted from Whaley L, Wong D: *Nursing Care of Infants and Children*, ed 3. St. Louis, Mosby, 1987, p 965, and based on Lindemann E. Symptomatology and management of acute grief. *Am J Psychiatry* 101:141–148, 1944.

Parents often visit or telephone the hospital, inquiring about the baby after it has died. Women describe dreams about the baby and experiences of hearing the baby cry or feeling the baby kicking still within the uterus.

Grieving parents also express a great deal of responsibility about the child's death, blaming themselves for having done something wrong during the pregnancy. Some interpret the baby's death as a punishment for a previous elective abortion, for having ambivalent feelings about the expected baby, or for wanting the baby too much.

Respondents in one survey of mothers experiencing perinatal loss recalled the following reactions during the first 6 weeks following the loss: sadness, emptiness, depression in 80% of respondents; grief-related dreams of pregnancy, delivery, and the wished for child in 33% of respondents; headaches, fatigue, nausea, and vomiting in 25% of respondents; and lack of energy for activities of daily living in 10% of respondents (Middleton, unpublished observations).

Thullen reports that mothers and fathers grieve differently (11). Mothers respond verbally and usually immediately, reviewing the experience of pregnancy, labor, and delivery with clarity. When they see another baby or put away the baby clothes and crib, acute grief symptoms appear. Periods of depression and apathy occur. Resolution is indicated by a decision to return to work or when previous activities and contacts with friends resume.

Fathers, Thullen believes, are not as verbal in releasing their deep feelings because of society's expectations of a stoic male image. Their behavior often is task oriented: collecting information, arranging for the mother's return home, and informing relatives of the death. Fathers attempt to assist the mother to feel better without fully expressing their own grief; communication between the couple lacks depth and fullness in the sharing of grief. Fathers find escape from sadness and grief when they must necessarily return to work. Thus, their span of grieving, although less intense, is prolonged and sometimes never resolved fully.

The time frame and intensity of normal grieving for parents experiencing perinatal loss varies according to each individual's life situation and previous experiences with death and crisis. Kennell et al. (12) observed that the mourning response in parents is present whether or not an infant was viable, the pregnancy was planned, or the infant was touched by the parents. Lindemann (9) and Marris (13) found that deaths of infants and young children often triggered long and intense mourning reactions.

A prevailing attitude among health professionals and the public is that those who have had miscarriages experience a less intense grief process than those with other perinatal losses. Peppers and Knapp (14) investigated the intensity of grief in 65 self-selected women who had experienced miscarriage, stillbirth, or neonatal death. Among the three groups, there was no difference in the women's perception of the intensity of grief. In addition, if at a later date a healthy child was born, the intensity of grief decreased, whereas difficult subsequent pregnancies increased the intensity of grief. One explanation for this finding is that bearing a healthy child can help parents resolve their grief feelings for the original loss; continuing "failures" in childbearing result in further losses and exacerbate the grief process.

Stack (15) found that there was often a psychological neglect of families who experienced spontaneous abortion if any of the following factors were present:

1. Friends did not know the woman was pregnant.
2. The bereaved woman felt embarrassed about the loss.
3. Unresolved material or ambivalence existed from the narcissistic stage of pregnancy.
4. The bereaved woman did not see the fetus.
5. There was no ritualistic ceremony.
6. Care providers failed to recognize the event as significant.
7. Support persons encouraged parental denial instead of expression of grief.
8. Maternal or paternal guilt or helplessness resulted in depression.

Two retrospective psychiatric studies evaluated grief resolution after perinatal loss. One-third of 56 women were reported by Cullberg (16) to have experienced serious mental health symptoms, including death anxiety, psychosis, cancer phobia, deep depression, and obsessive thoughts. Eleven women who had initially denied their feelings experienced acute grief symptoms over a longer period of time than those who grieved immediately. Marital conflict or other social complications were noted by one-third of the women studied. Cullberg viewed the family support systems, the significance of object loss, and the degree of sexual identification as pertinent factors in analyzing women's reactions to perinatal loss.

Wolff and Nielson (17) studied 40 women from the immediate postpartum period to 3 years after the loss and found no significant psychiatric difficulties present. The researchers suggested that their interviews over the years had given the women the opportunity to ventilate their grief feelings and had, in fact, encouraged expression of feelings when other defensive symptoms, such as denial, might have occurred instead. Fifty percent of the mothers resolved the loss of the pregnancy within 3 years. Return to employment, academic studies, or intensive household activities were cited as resolution hallmarks by some women.

In J. Middleton's retrospective survey of women who had experienced perinatal loss 1 to 2 years prior to interview (unpublished observations), 34% claimed to have had acute grief symptoms lasting 6 weeks or less, 40% lasting between 6 weeks and 6 months, and 26% lasting longer than 6 months. In those women (10%) reporting no early grief symptoms, one-third had grief symptoms 1 to 2 years after the loss. Fifty percent of the women

Table 3.3.
COMMON FACTORS AFFECTING THE EXPERIENCE OF PERINATAL GRIEF

FACTORS	EXAMPLES
1. Emotional significance of pregnancy	Creativity
	Femininity
	Lack of other options
	First or last childbearing
2. Mental health	Level of maturity
	Degree of ambivalence
	Preexisting mental health status
	Coping ability
	Presence of personal and professional support systems
	Preexisting stress levels
3. Physical health	Age
	Preexisting health status
	Presence of chronic, debilitating disease
	Presence of severe medical complications
	Malnutrition
	Physical handicap
4. Point of loss	Miscarriage
	Fetal demise
	Neonatal death
	Relationship to other pregnancy losses

reported that the fathers initially had been withdrawn emotionally, while the mothers had shown upset feelings. Thirty-three percent of the mothers said that their mates had expressed anger and sadness 1 to 2 years after the loss.

Factors Affecting the Perinatal Grief Experience

There are many factors that affect the experience of the perinatal bereavement crisis. Although each bereaved family has its own constellation of individual meanings and needs, there are some common factors that may heavily influence the outcome of the grief experience (Table 3.3). Significant factors are discussed here.

Psychologic Factors in Perinatal Grief

Motivation for pregnancy is a complex issue that Rabin (18) divides into the following four categories:

1. Altruistic: parents have an unselfish desire for parenthood with positive feelings for children.
2. Fatalistic: man exists to procreate and perpetuate the species.
3. Narcissistic: parents anticipate that children reflect glory upon the parent, thus boosting their masculine or feminine identity.

4. Instrumental: the child has the power to achieve unmet parental goals, such as preservation of the marriage.

Although the motivation for pregnancy usually involves a combination of all of these motivating factors, perinatal death can provoke extreme feelings of anger, anxiety, and fear in parents who are unaware or unable to cope with their deeply hidden, unrealistic, or immature inducements toward parenthood.

Ambivalence is a normal part of pregnancy, even if the child has been planned by caring, concerned parents. Increased responsibility, self-denial, and revision of a comfortable family system are sources of an ambivalence that may not be acknowledged. However, this unexpressed ambivalence may add feelings of guilt to the couple who experiences the loss of a baby.

In addition to other factors, very young parents have their own immaturity and inexperience in problem-solving and in positive crisis resolution. They may never have experienced a death before; their baby's death may be the first. Parents who, because of age or medical condition, have no future prospects for pregnancy have to work through this closure of their childbearing period, which in itself is a loss of an integral body function. When a pregnancy is lost or a child is damaged because of maternal illness or substance abuse, the parents must acknowledge deep feelings of guilt, loss of self-esteem, and anger in order to proceed with grieving.

Self-esteem and maturity are challenged severely by perinatal loss. Conflicting feelings about one's good and bad self as well as doubts about one's femininity and masculinity may emerge. Those parents with well-developed egos and a confident sense of self will weather the crisis best and experience emotional growth because of it.

Social Supports

Religious beliefs may have a great influence on the number of children a couple chooses to have. If their religion and community support having children, the parents' loss also will be the community's loss, and the couple will be comforted by the community's supportive actions. Less supportive social situations may make the perinatal death an isolating experience.

Point of Pregnancy Loss

Miscarriage

When a miscarriage occurs, it is important for persons supporting the bereaved parents to understand that miscarriage often is viewed as a phenomenon that happens to others—not to oneself. When miscarriage is accompanied by heavy vaginal bleeding, a frightening trip to a hospital emergency room will add to the emotional and physical distress. Often, the woman will be discharged quickly after a uterine dilatation and curretage, and she will experience little supportive professional interaction. The pregnancy is suddenly over, the physical problem resolved, and everything is expected to return to normal. The bereaved father often goes back to work immediately, and the bereaved mother either sits at home alone wondering why she feels so upset or goes back to her work place where colleagues may not even have known she was pregnant. She often feels isolated and confused by her feelings of loss. A miscarriage may be a very traumatic event to the mother who has bonded to her fetus. The father, family, and friends, who have not bonded, may urge her to "get over" her emotional distress quickly.

Bereaved parents need to be reminded that the public, including their friends and family, often view miscarriage as a common, rather insignificant event that deserves no more than a quick "I'm sorry." A source of comfort for bereaved parents is other couples who have experienced a similar loss.

In an ectopic pregnancy the loss of a fallopian tube potentially means the loss of the ability to conceive. The couple therefore experiences a double loss: the fetus and the potential to have other babies. This double loss certainly can intensify the grief reaction.

Fetal Demise

When a fetus dies, medical management may range from terminating the pregnancy immediately after diagnosis to waiting for labor to begin spontaneously. Having a dead baby within the womb is extremely difficult for many pregnant women, while others wish to hold on to the pregnancy and fear giving up the fetus at delivery. If there is no medical emergency, the timing of the pregnancy termination should be individualized according to the parents' emotional as well as physical needs. Bereaved parents need different periods of time to work through the shock and denial of fetal demise and to begin anticipatory grieving before the death actually is confirmed at delivery.

When a pregnant woman arrives at a hospital in labor and is informed by the hospital staff that there is no fetal heartbeat, usually she is stunned, even if she has detected no fetal movement for several days. The emotional shock, denial, and confusion that the parents experience is a protective defense and indeed the first stage of grief. Professional staff, wishing to avoid the anger and misery of the parents, often have great difficulty telling them the bad news. However, gentle telling of the truth and warm emotional support will set the tone of open communication so that both parents and the health professionals may begin the grief work. Overmedication of a mother about to deliver her stillborn child only strengthens her defense of denial and increases her confusion while protecting the hospital staff from the necessary obligation of sharing her pain. It is important that the father accompany the mother through the labor and delivery in order to support her and allow him to share the experience with her.

Neonatal Death

When a questionably viable fetus is born, it is very important for the parents to see and touch their infant to begin the bonding process before the infant is transferred to the neonatal unit. The bonding process is very important even if the baby dies eventually, because the parents then have a focus for their grief. It is very difficult to grieve normally for someone never seen.

When parents observe the care of their infant, including resuscitation efforts, they usually feel reassured that everything possible has been done for the child.

Many parents are forever grateful for a photograph of their live child, especially one of them holding the child. When survival is no longer possible, holding the child as it dies can provide great comfort.

If the child dies, detailed follow-up explanations about the child's medical condition and treatment should be provided by the nursing and medical staffs. In addition, the health professional should discuss practical details, such as burial choices, viewing by the family, obtaining a footprint sheet, and application for a death certificate, and the health professional also should counsel the parents about the normal grieving process.

Multiple Pregnancy

When a woman loses one child of a multiple pregnancy, she experiences grief and joy simultaneously, even if she did not know she was carrying more than one fetus. In this situation of divergent feelings, the mother must be supported as she grieves a death, while taking comfort and joy from the live birth. Health professionals should tell the parents that these mixed feelings, while painful, are normal and sometimes include strong feelings of guilt. It is important to explain that the children are individuals and that the death or survival of one had no influence upon the other sibling's death or survival, since parents may unconsciously blame the live child for the death of its sibling. As with other grieving parents, the health professional should encourage expression of feelings and open communication about the tragedy.

Relationship to Other Pregnancy Losses

Whether the loss occurs during the first pregnancy or the tenth seems to have no effect on the intensity or the length of grief. Bourne (19) reports that mothers claimed that the first loss was greater if they experienced multiple losses. Anxiety and fear for the baby are the most common phenomena of a pregnancy that occurs subsequent to a perinatal loss. It is critical for the caregiver during a subsequent pregnancy to take a history of perinatal losses. The nurse then can evaluate where the parents are in resolving their grief over their previous loss(es), explore their current needs, and help them anticipate the feelings of ambivalence, anxiety, and fear that are certain to accompany this current pregnancy.

Reactions of Family Members

Fathers

Little research has been reported on fathers' reactions to pregnancy loss. In our society the strong male image seems to demand little or no show of emotion. The father's expected role is that of providing support for the grieving mother. At the Downstate Medical Center Bereavement Clinic, a survey of fathers 4 weeks after their loss showed the following (J. Middleton, unpublished observations):

1. Difficulty finding an outlet for generalized emotional distress;
2. Difficulty dealing with the anger related to the loss; and
3. Problems interacting with their wives or the baby's mother.

In counseling sessions these fathers were encouraged to talk to the physicians and nurses involved, to increase physical exercise or other tension-relieving activities, and to communicate with the grieving mother by sharing their own sad and angry emotions as well as their supportive understanding. It is apparent that many fathers require permission to grieve.

Siblings

Hiding a miscarriage or stillbirth from young siblings remains a common practice because it is viewed as a means of protecting them from emotional trauma. However, most young children are very aware of their parents' emotional states and can sense trouble. Simple explanations about the loss by loving parents can help the child express emotions instead of repressing them. Occasionally, young siblings experience nightmares for a period of time after the loss. These expressions of emotional distress may be a component of the child's grief work; however, if they are prolonged and intense, they may require professional intervention.

Grandparents

Bereaved mothers and fathers naturally often look to their own parents to provide support for them. However, the grieving parents need to remember that their parents have lost a grandchild and will be experiencing a personal grief reaction of their own. Therefore, they may be unable to provide the support the parents want and expect.

The Health Professional's Grief

The literature, in general, avoids the topic of the professional's feelings of grief. Most staff members, both professional and nonprofessional, work with maternity patients because of the joy of birth. When death intervenes, each staff person must confront his or her own mortality, concept of success and failure based upon personal beliefs and society's expectations, and ability to deal with the bereaved's emotional trauma as well as personal feelings of grief. This is a heavy assignment, and the tendency is to avoid the patient, deny the problem, and put aside one's own feelings. The staff members' awareness and acceptance of their own feelings of grief is the first step toward providing an emotionally healthy and supportive environment for both staff and parents. A sharing of feelings and mutual support among staff members are essential if the staff is to be able to provide assistance and counseling to parents who are in the throes of grief.

BIRTH OF THE ABNORMAL OR SICK BABY

When a mother gives birth to a baby that lives but is abnormal in some way (e.g., premature, birth defects), she and her family experience grief over the loss of the "perfect" baby they had fantasized about throughout the pregnancy. They may work through many or all aspects of the grief process, and they may experience anticipatory grief if they do not yet know whether the infant will survive. The mother may wonder if she did something wrong to cause the baby's problem, or she may feel she is a failure because she did not deliver the expected healthy baby. If the baby requires intensive care, this feeling of failure may be heightened by her inability to care for all of the baby's needs. She

may have difficulty investing energy in bonding with the baby if she feels she contributed to the baby's condition or if she feels the baby may die (20).

While the mother and family are grieving, they also may have many questions and concerns about the baby's diagnosis, treatment, and ultimate prognosis. The health professional must be prepared to answer questions honestly, simply, and perhaps repeatedly as the parents work through their grief and learn to care for the child with special needs. Providing repeated contact with the parents, reinforcing information with written material or visual aids, encouraging parents to practice care-giving activities as much as possible, and referring parents to groups of parents with babies who have the same or similar problems may help parents resolve their feelings of helplessness, anger, and grief. Continued contact after hospital discharge and the provision of a telephone number to call if questions arise also will assist the family in adjusting to the new baby with special needs (21).

REFERENCES

1. Lewis, E: Management of stillbirth: coping with an unreality. *Lancet* ii:619–620, 1976.
2. Pritchard J, MacDonald P, Gant NF (eds): *Williams Obstetrics*, ed 17. New York, Appleton-Century-Crofts, 1985, p 467.
3. Caplan G: *Principles of Preventive Psychiatry*. New York, Basic Books, 1964.
4. Caplan G: Patterns and parental response to the crisis of premature birth. *Psychiatry* 23:265–274, 1960.
5. Erikson E: Identity and the life cycle. *Psychol Issues*. Monograph 1, 1959.
6. Aguilera D, Messick J: *Crisis Intervention–Theory and Methodology*. St. Louis: Mosby, 1974.
7. Deutsch H: *The Psychology of Women I*. New York, Grune & Stratton, 1944.
8. Deutsch H: *The Psychology of Women II*. New York, Grune & Stratton, 1945.
9. Lindemann E: Symptomatology and management of acute grief. *Am J Psychiatry* 101:141–148, 1944.
10. Aldrick C: The dying patient's grief. *JAMA* 184:329, 1963.
11. Thullen J: When you can't cure, care. *Perinatol/Neonatol* Nov/Dec: 1–16, 1977.
12. Kennell J, Slyter H, Klaus M: The mourning response of parents to the death of a newborn infant. *N Engl J Med* 283:344–349, 1970.
13. Marris P: *Widows and Their Families*. London, Routledge and Kegan Paul, 1958.
14. Peppers L, Knapp R: Maternal reactions to involuntary fetal/infant loss. *Psychiatry* 43:155–159, 1980.
15. Stack J: Spontaneous abortion and grieving. *Am Fam Physician* 21:99–102, 1980.

16. Cullberg J: Mental reactions of women to perinatal death. In Morris N (ed): *Proceedings of International Congress of Psychosomatic Medicine in Obstetrics and Gynecology*. New York, Karger, 1972.

17. Wolff J: The emotional reactions to a stillbirth. In Morris N (ed): *Proceedings of International Congress of Psychosomatic Medicine in Obstetrics and Gynecology*. New York, Karger, 1972.

18. Rabin A: Motivation for parenthood. *Projective Techniques in Personality Assessment* 29:405–411, 1965.

19. Bourne S: The psychological effect of stillbirths on women and their doctors. *J R Coll Gen Pract* 16:103, 1968.

20. Klaus M, Kennell J: *Parent-Infant Bonding*, ed 2. St. Louis, Mosby, 1982.

21. Frost N: Counseling families who have a child with a severe congenital anomaly. *Pediatrics* 67:321–324, 1981.

Chapter 4
Ethical Considerations in High Risk Pregnancies

Joyce E. Thompson, C.N.M., D.P.H., and Henry O. Thompson, M.Div., Ph.D.

INTRODUCTION TO BIOETHICS

Definitions

Ethics, Bioethics, and Morals

There are several ways to define the terms used in ethics. Common usage interchanges the words ethics and morals. Their original meanings in Greek and Latin were approximately the same, so this is appropriate. An alternative is to view morals as the rules by which people live; those rules come from the experience of society, religion, philosophy, and individuals. *Ethics* is then a reflection upon the rules. Theologians and philosophers ask for reasons and try to understand why a rule exists. Sometimes a rule is seen as no longer valid, and sometimes the rule is viewed as expressing a higher principle that remains valid but needs a new form of expression.

People may, of course, ask why a principle exists and then ask again and again in an unending series of "Why?" Eventually, some people reach an end or ultimate. This carries one into the realm of *metaethics*. The Greek *meta* means "beyond." Theists may find this ultimate in God; others find it in Nature. Some define metaethics as the concern with what ethics is or as the question "Why be ethical in the first place?" If ethics is reasoning about morals, metaethics is reasoning about ethics.

Some theorists have suggested there is only one ethics—human ethics. Others suggest that the one ethics is the will of God. Yet others see many ethics—e.g., legal ethics and business ethics, professional ethics, theoretical ethics, and applied ethics. Nursing ethics has been called an applied ethics, yet some theorists do not think there is a nursing ethics but only a medical ethics involving nursing situations. Others see nursing ethics as health care ethics applied to nursing, just as medical ethics usually is thought of as health care ethics applied to physicians and the care they provide. Ethics may be seen as applicable to all of life, as in *bioethics*, from the Greek *bio* meaning "life." Originally, this term was coined for the environment; more recently, it has been restricted to health care ethics.

Ethical Theories and Principles

Philosophically, there are two major systems of ethics in bioethics. The *utilitarian* says the end justifies the means. Maintaining a high risk pregnancy may cause inconvenience, pain, or suffering for all involved, but the bottom line is the intent or purpose of improving the outcomes for mother and infant. Utilitarians also are concerned with the greatest good for the greatest number. This has been used to justify hospitalization for all births, including those with no high risk factors.

The second major approach is called *deontology*, from the Greek word *deon*, which means "rules" or "principles." Principles include autonomy, informed consent, confidentiality, truth telling, quality of life, sanctity of life, allocation of resources, and euthanasia. There is no limit to the number of principles, but some arise in high risk pregnancy more often than others.

Values and Value Clarification

Many of the ethical issues surrounding care of high risk pregnancies are of recent origin and are a direct result of new technological advances, such as amniocentesis, ultrasonography, chorionic villi biopsy, surrogate motherhood, in vitro fertilization, improved management of diabetes in pregnancy, and neonatal intensive care units. When one discusses the issues raised in modern health care and specifically during high risk pregnancies, there are a variety of views about what should be done (the morals of the situation). These views often represent the individual value preferences of clients and providers and may result in conflict in deciding what is the best thing to do in a particular situation.

Values are a person's beliefs about the truth, beauty, or worth of a thought or behavior put into practice during one's life. Values come from a variety of people and sources, including parents, teachers, and other authority figures, as well as through personal reflection and life experience. Values are learned, and they can be changed, providing the individual chooses to do so. Thus, health care professionals can alter their value perspectives on ethical issues, if deemed appropriate, through discussion with others, moral reasoning, or introspection and personal growth to the next stage of moral development.

Nurses who care for women experiencing high risk pregnancies are highly educated and skilled in the newest technologies, yet they may also disagree on when to use that technology. They come face to face with this and other ethical issues in high risk pregnancy care on a daily basis. We live in a pluralistic society in which freedom to decide who shall live and who shall die engenders a variety of responses. These responses represent the variety of value positions held by the persons involved. High risk pregnancies often require such decisions on life and death. Facing ethical issues, such as abortion of genetically defective fetuses, rights of women to health and life versus rights of fetus to life, or equity in the allocation of expensive, scarce health resources to relatively few pregnant women or neonates, often leads to exploration of what the nurse as an individual and professional believes or values in the situation. Ethical nursing practice requires self-knowledge and an understanding of others' values. Clarification of one's personal values on the ethical issues in high risk pregnancy care contributes to understanding one's responses to the issues as well as understanding others' value perspectives. Better health care is then the result.

Bioethical Decision Making and Nurses

The Moral Reasoning Process

Ethical nursing is not just a matter of mechanically plugging in principles when one is called upon to make a decision in care. It is rather a reasoning process. The process includes reviewing the situation at hand with as much accurate clinical data as possible, and it includes the feelings and personal considerations of the individual patient and family, as well as those of the health care providers. The reasoning process considers the whole of society and the ethical standards of society and the health care professions. Some people suggest we need to consider both principles and consequences in light of the total situation to the extent any of this can be known. Where it cannot be known, the principle of respect for persons requires caution before and in proceeding to action.

Moral Development

The Swiss child psychologist Jean Piaget believed that children develop intellectually through stages that involve quite different kinds of reasoning. A similar finding appeared when he studied moral development. Lawrence Kohlberg confirmed and extended this theory into adulthood. There are six stages of development divided into three levels: preconventional, conventional, and postconventional. The conventional level is where most people are; the ethics at this level are those of consensus or of conventional morality.

The levels move from self-centered to societal to a universal concern with humanity. Each level has two stages. Stage 1 says might makes right. The concern is reward or punishment from others. In stage 2 the person realizes that others must be considered in order to get what one wants. This is the common political consideration of "You scratch my back and I'll scratch yours." Stage 3 recognizes authority—parents, teachers, physicians, head nurses, peer groups. Whatever the authority says is right, regardless of consequences, is considered right. Stage 4 abstracts this authority in terms of law or moral rules. Stage 5 is the level of the United States Constitution. It is a utilitarian concern for the greatest number. Stage 6 is concerned with justice and fairness for all. It has been suggested that the American Nurses' Association (ANA) *Code for Nurses* (Fig. 4.1) basically is at stage 5. Its concern with equal treatment for all clients is stage 6.

Cultural Aspects of Ethical Decisions

In one situation a couple wanted a home birth. There were complications, and the baby died. The

CODE FOR NURSES

(1) The nurse provides services with respect for human dignity and the uniqueness of the client unrestricted by considerations of social or economic status, personal attributes, or the nature of health problems.
(2) The nurse safeguards the client's right to privacy by judiciously protecting information of a confidential nature.
(3) The nurse acts to safeguard the client and the public when health care and safety are affected by the incompetent, unethical, or illegal practice of any person.
(4) The nurse assumes responsibility and accountability for individual nursing judgments and actions.
(5) The nurse maintains competence in nursing.
(6) The nurse exercises informed judgment and uses individual competence and qualification as criteria in seeking consultation, accepting responsibilities, and delegating nursing activities to others.
(7) The nurse participates in activities that contribute to the ongoing development of the profession's body of knowledge.
(8) The nurse participates in the profession's efforts to implement and improve standards of nursing.
(9) The nurse participates in the professional's efforts to establish and maintain conditions of employment conducive to high quality nursing care.
(10) The nurse participates in the profession's effort to protect the public from misinformation and misrepresentation and to maintain the integrity of nursing.
(11) The nurse collaborates with members of the health professions and other citizens in promoting community and national efforts to meet the health needs of the public.
(From *Code for Nurses with Interpretive Statements.* Kansas City, MO, American Nurses' Association, 1976.)

Figure 4.1.

parents accepted this by saying it was the will of God. Others, however, responded that they killed their infant by choosing to deliver out of the hospital setting. In another situation a premature infant was born at the lowest edge of viability. The parents wanted no heroic measures to save the child. Hospital personnel, however, convinced the parents to sign a paper allowing movement of the infant to a tertiary care unit. Here the baby was put on a respirator and numerous procedures were undertaken. In the 6 months of his life, many iatrogenic problems developed, and the baby eventually died from heart failure. Yet the hospital personnel considered the parents bad people for wanting to be merciful and let the baby die shortly after birth.

These examples involved people within the same culture, but their subcultures carried different values or ethical perspectives. There are both common ethical perspectives and different ones across cultural lines. Some cultures or religions would view a seriously ill or deformed neonate as a bad omen and respond to it accordingly. Some see high risk pregnancies as the will of the gods or as fate. Some third world health countries have accused the West of racism and elitism. The West spends more money on high risk pregnancies and defective neonates than these countries have for all health care, including all pregnancies. Consideration of cultural perspectives is another component

of ethical decision making and ethical nursing practice.

American Nurses' Association *Code for Nurses* and the Role of the Nurse

As nurses work with women and families experiencing a high risk pregnancy, knowledge of both the ethical issues and the components of bioethical decision making is a helpful tool. A review of the ethics embodied in the ANA *Code for Nurses* is useful for the nurse interested in practicing in an ethical manner. A code of ethics is a professional group's attempt to define the moral conduct of the members of that profession. This behavior is required of all members of the profession and may be interpreted as the ethical framework for professional practice and decision making. The ANA *Code for Nurses*, therefore, can provide direction for the nurse in working with clients and colleagues.

The ANA code of ethics addresses the following concerns: respect for persons; autonomy and self-determination of the client; provision of care without discrimination; maintenance of confidentiality; and protection of clients from the unethical, illegal, or incompetent practice of others. The code also expects competent nursing practice and responsibility and accountability for nursing judgment and actions. All of these ethical principles are important to the care of women and families experiencing a high risk pregnancy.

A primary goal of nursing practice is to provide the best care for clients. The role of the nurse caring for families experiencing a high risk pregnancy embodies this nursing goal. Because of the variety of ethical issues raised by high risk pregnancies, however, definition of what is "best" and "for whom" may be difficult at times. The nurse caring for any pregnant woman also essentially is caring for at least two individuals, the woman who is pregnant and the fetus. Others might also include the father of the fetus and other significant family members in their definition of "client." Focusing one's nursing efforts on more than one individual simultaneously may raise ethical conflicts in care—e.g., who receives priority in care and decision making at any given time? While the ANA *Code for Nurses* cannot offer specific direction for ethical decision making, it does provide general guidelines for the nurse to consider in the care of clients.

Overview of Major Ethical Issues in High Risk Pregnancy

There are many major ethical issues involved in the management of care of women with high risk pregnancies. They include the ethical and legal concept of informed consent and informed decision making based on client self-determination (autonomy). Other ethical concerns include risk/benefit considerations, such as value of the life and health of the woman and the fetus (quality of life versus sanctity of life) and how much emotional and familial disturbance can be tolerated, abortion as an option, and truth telling. All of these ethical issues or concerns may be framed within the concept of the ethics of caring for persons in a high technology environment.

GENETIC SCREENING, COUNSELING, AND DIAGNOSIS

Informed Choice and Consent for Procedures

Tests during pregnancy, such as amniocentesis, chorionic villi biopsy, or blood tests, normally require, both ethically and legally, the informed consent of the pregnant woman. Some think every pregnant woman should have amniocentesis, suggesting that this compulsory screening would promote the greatest good for the greatest number. This perspective, however, denies client autonomy and violates informed consent for the pregnant woman. Compulsory amniocentesis also raises the issue of the allocation of

scarce resources, e.g., money spent on amniocentesis may further limit money for health. This limitation may then affect the availability of prenatal care for all pregnancies, especially those of poor women, and thus contribute to more premature and high risk pregnancies.

There are several concerns here. The word "informed" is an accordion word that expands and contracts. At what point is a person really informed? Some say only professionals with many years of education are informed. Health care has developed so rapidly in recent decades that a degree dated yesterday may not be a guarantee that even professionals are "informed." In spite of the difficulties, however, professionals both ethically and legally are required to inform their patients.

At one point the law accepted the concept of an effort appropriate for "the reasonable professional." The law is now moving toward a standard of "the reasonable patient." Both concepts may be a fiction, but the law marches on. One ethical concept here is that of equity. By definition, the professional is more knowledgeable than the lay person. Knowledge is power, so the professional has power and the lay person is powerless or less powerful. The ethical obligation is to help the lay person rise to greater equity, i.e., to more power with more knowledge.

The concept of choice is an ethical concern for the autonomy and the dignity of the individual. We are not autonomous and self-determining without choice. Without choice, of course, there is no freedom to choose. Consent for procedures, in turn, cannot be genuine without informed choice.

This ethic is complicated by the common knowledge that some people do not want to be informed and some do not want a choice. They are sick, and they want to be well. They have a problem, and they want it solved or cured. Their autonomy may cause a dilemma for the health care provider, who is ethically and legally obligated to inform them and who may not be able to proceed legally unless the patient is informed. On the one hand, health care providers have an obligation to respect the patient, while, on the other hand, they also have an obligation to society and to themselves. On rare occasions, patients have turned around later and sued the health care provider for lack of informed consent.

Confidentiality in Screening and Counseling

Screening programs have computerized their data. In the past this information occasionally has become available to others, such as insurance companies and employers. The effect sometimes has been that people who may be carriers of genetic abnormalities that do not affect their health or their ability to work have, through either ignorance or supercaution, been burdened with higher insurance costs or no insurance at all, with restrictions on jobs or no job ap all. Several studies have shown how genetic carriers may be stigmatized and suffer social ostracism or discrimination. These are practical reasons for maintaining confidentiality, but this is an ethical end in itself that must be upheld if screening programs are to be ethical.

Other studies have shown that screening is largely ineffective if people do not receive counseling. It may even be counterproductive. Premarital screening may limit marital choices. Prepregnancy screening may indicate potential problems. Pregnancy screening has great value, but it is limited in the information it can give. On the one hand, people may not realize this without adequate counseling. On the other hand, they may magnify the problem unnecessarily, causing anxiety, pain, and suffering without adequate counseling. The counselor must present factual data, with both the condition and the options, as honestly as present clinical knowledge allows.

Truth Telling

Truth telling is a major ethical concern in genetics. At times, genetic procedures result in information not asked for or anticipated. What to do with that information is of ethical concern. For example, newer techniques in ultrasound allow for determination of the sex of the infant at times. Many prospective parents do not want this information before birth, yet the professionals may insist on giving it. It is also important to realize that the truth can be told in several ways. It may be brutal without adequate compassion or consideration for the feelings of the person. This may cause unnecessary pain and suffering.

Counseling involves adequate information that is honestly and sensitively presented. Professionals may be tempted to present their own views, e.g., prolife or prochoice. This may not be strictly forbidden, but it might violate the concepts of adequate information and honesty. It might also be a matter of paternalism that imposes the professional's view in a way that violates the client's autonomy. Some procedures used in genetic screening, such as ultrasound, appear to have no risks. In the past, however, procedures that appeared safe have later proved deleterious. This suggests caution in the use of tests without longevity to indicate safety as well as discussion of such risks with the pregnant woman during the informed consent process.

Role of the Nurse in Screening and Counseling

Nurses working with high risk pregnant women and families may participate to varying degrees in genetic screening and counseling. One of the primary nursing roles is as a support person during early pregnancy when women/families are deciding whether to proceed with genetic screening. Once this decision is made, the nurse continues in a listening, supportive, informative role as the family awaits test results and then decides how to proceed with their pregnancy. Some nurses with special training also assume the role of genetic counselor with all it entails. As with any aspect of counseling and support in nursing, the nurse develops skills in listening, in guiding others in decision making, and in avoiding the imposition of his or her own values. Even when asked what he or she would do in a particular situation, the nurse often chooses not to answer with personal experience but rather with examples of the variety of decisions made in similar situations. These may afford the pregnant women/couples with new information or with questions to consider in their deliberations.

SPECIAL PREGNANCIES

Artificial Insemination

Artificial insemination is impregnation of a woman by sperm from the husband (AIH) or from a donor (AID). The sperm for these procedures is collected by masturbation, which some groups consider immoral. AID has been called adultery, also considered wrong by some groups. The legal history of AID turns on this issue of adultery. A few states require adoption by the woman's husband, while others require signed statements of agreement to AID in advance.

Some people look upon these procedures as different, strange, and unnatural. By the ethical standard of natural law, they consider the unnatural unethical. It has been pointed out, however, that nature is not simply an open book, rather, it is interpreted, and what is called unnatural merely may be different. Thus, if it is unnatural, it will not work and obviously, AIH and AID work; thousands of babies have been conceived by these procedures. Therefore, other groups do not see these procedures as immoral.

Test Tube Babies

Test tube babies are conceived in glass Petri dishes (in vitro), not test tubes. The sperm is obtained by masturbation and is under the same legal and moral strictures as AIH and AID. The egg is obtained by medical procedures, which obviously are not natural in the sense that they do not occur spontaneously in nature. The different, the strange, and the technical may be perceived as unnatural and thus in violation of natural law. In addition, some groups consider conception the beginning of life. In the course of the effort to create a test tube pregnancy, a number of fertilized eggs are wasted. This procedure therefore carries the same objection as abortion, and right-to-life groups that espouse conception as the beginning of life oppose this process. Others do not consider the conceptus a life.

The procedure is expensive, however, and raises the ethical issue of allocation of resources. Millions of babies conceived through sexual intercourse are unwanted, uncared for, starving to death, malnourished, ill fed, ill clothed, ill housed, and existing or dying with a quality of life ranging from low to zero. Some would suggest it is immoral to waste thousands of dollars on modern technology to add to the population explosion when such money could help take care of the children the world has already but does not want.

Surrogate Motherhood

When a woman is unable or does not want to carry a pregnancy, surrogate motherhood may be an option. It is an ancient custom. For instance, in Bible history Sarah was unable to bear children, so she had her maid, Hagar, act as a surrogate. Abraham's grandson Jacob followed a similar process with his two wives' maids. The difference today is that, instead of natural intercourse, the surrogate mother is impregnated by sperm supplied through masturbation. A woman bearing another man's child may also be considered an adultress. This issue again raises the legal problems of AID. The husband of the surrogate could even get a divorce on this ground. Here, too, the new and different is considered unnatural and a violation of natural law. Additional problems appear. After a woman has a baby, she may decide it is hers and want to keep it. Do the contracting parents have a legal right to take the baby away from the "natural" mother? Defective surrogate babies already have appeared. Neither of the parents wants such a child. Who is legally responsible? The ethics of producing an unwanted child thus become part of the issue. Some states are considering legally regulating surrogate motherhood.

Role of the Nurse

Nurses caring for women or couples choosing AID or AIH, in vitro fertilization, or surrogate motherhood should examine their own values and responses to these choices. This examination hope-fully will lead to a reasoned choice to work or not work with such clients, depending on one's views. Those professionals who do care for women choosing these options face the major ethical issue of confidentiality in all aspects of care.

DECISION TO ABORT A HIGH RISK PREGNANCY

If tests indicate a fetus with abnormalities or genetic problems, one option is abortion. Some even insist that unless the person is prepared to have an abortion, there is no point in having the expensive genetic tests. Others suggest that knowing is easier to live with than the uncertainty of not knowing. Adequate preparations can be arranged in advance if parents decide to carry a defective fetus to term. Abortion raises a number of issues such as quality of life and sanctity of life for the pregnant woman and the fetus.

Quality of Life versus Sanctity of Life

In the legal field, lawsuits for wrongful life in the past have not been recognized for fear such actions would clog the courts. Legal experts have been pointing out for years that this fear is not sufficient legal grounds for dismissing such suits. In more recent years several actions have been accepted for review by the courts, which often have adjudicated in favor of the wronged person. Parents or legal guardians have taken action against health care providers, laboratories, and so on. Other suits have been by children against parents, such as the case in which a 33-year-old person with spina bifida sued the parents for $33 million.

Ethics also has had its debates. While many insist that life—any kind of life—is sacred, others insist on considering the quality of life. A recent survey of nurses included the statement that they have "Do not resuscitate!" tattooed on their chests lest they receive unwanted prolongation of dying. A recent book described the prolonged dying of a neonate. The prognosis for life was almost nil, but the neonatal intensive care unit strung out the infant's life for months in a research/experimental triumph that gave residents needed training.

In Jewish tradition there are several cases of rabbis who would allow contraception or abortions for the sake of the woman. Some high risk pregnancies seriously threatened the life of the woman, and abortion was considered an acceptable action to take. Abortion was not allowed for fear of a defective child, however. The argument for abortion was that who knows whether a handicapped life is better than no life at all, which was one basis for the legal argument noted above. But with the advent of machinery, antibiotics, and other procedures that can keep a body minimally functioning for indefinite periods of time, some have become more and more concerned with the quality of life. One basic argument is that life without any meaning is not worth living. Many handicapped infants, however, can survive to a meaningful life; meaningful is another accordion term, of course. What is meaningful to one may not be meaningful to another.

The allocation of scarce resources is a major concern here also. Maintaining the life of a sick or handicapped neonate may cost hundreds of thousands of dollars. Likewise, high risk pregnancy care is very costly, often including days and months of hospitalization. If the parents cannot pay, society pays through insurance or taxes. It is one thing to decide to do something that will cost oneself time, suffering, money, and so on. It is another thing entirely when the decision costs someone else. Some think there are limits to what we can require or demand that others pay without their consent. Early abortion obviates these costs.

Conflict of Rights: Woman, Fetus, Family, Man, Society

In times past, women were considered chattel. If a woman died, a man could always get another, depending on his ability to pay. The Protestant Reformation leader, Martin Luther, said that if having too many children killed a woman, so be it. That is what she is for. Children were a form of immortality and, more importantly for this earth, a form of insurance. They could take care of you in your old age when you were no longer able to care for yourself. Thus, in any choice between the woman and the child, the child had precedent. A religious perspective that supported this was that the woman was baptized and, time permitting, could receive the last rites. An infant needed baptism to get into heaven. In the event of death or a threatened death in the womb, special instruments were available to baptize the fetus. In the event of a difficult birth, the child would be favored over the woman. Note that this is not sanctity of life. The woman's life did not matter. The child's life was valued for its labor or insurance.

These values are still present in our society: the innocent child has not had a chance to live its life, etc. However, there has been a growing insistence in modern times that women are human beings, in contrast to earlier attitudes. Some insist, as in some abortion decisions, that the woman should have priority, a

complete turn from older traditions. Others believe that both the pregnant woman and the fetus have equal rights. In the event of a conflict, there must be some effort to balance these rights. Some would allow abortions under some conditions, such as rape, incest, or the ill health of the woman.

In the past the father and husband was *pater potestes*, the all-powerful father with the authority of life and death over his children and, frequently, his wife as well. Current thought favors considering the father as one part of the family; siblings and the extended family also may be considered. Moving beyond the family, some think society has some rights too. Others think that society only has the responsibility to pay the bills.

Client Autonomy/Self-Determination

Who Is/Are the Client(s)?

Western society has tended toward individualism in contrast to other traditions that focus on the tribe or the people. Health care as it has developed in the West has tended to focus on the individual. In recent years there has been a shift in some quarters that has extended health concerns to the family. The father more and more has been included in childbirth. The whole family is affected by a handicapped child. Some health care providers are beginning to consider the family as the patient rather than only the individual who happens to be the locus of the immediate health concern. This raises questions about autonomy. There have always been limits on autonomy, as there are limits on rights. In the case of the family as patient, the individual's autonomy is interwoven with that of the family. The family's autonomy is independent of the health care system and needs to be considered accordingly. Others would move to yet a larger picture and point out that society also is affected by what a family does or does not do. Thus, society should be considered the client or as part of the client picture when decisions about such issues as abortion are made.

Should the Fetus Have an Advocate?

Many think so. The pregnant woman normally is the advocate for the fetus. However, some women are abusers—drug addicts, alcoholics, etc.—of substances known to harm a fetus. Some women are malnourished and are not able to get proper prenatal care because of poverty, powerlessness, ignorance, isolation, and so on. In these latter cases it may be the women who need the advocate, but the fetus is a part of the advocacy. In abortion decisions those who oppose abortion may take the position of advocate for the fetus. The ethical concerns supporting abortion may be for the quality of life of the future child or the pregnant woman. There may be concern for the society that will pay for the future care or that will lack the future contributions of people whose potential was diminished by harmful substances in utero. In abortion decisions the concern may be for life itself for those who consider the fetus a person with a right to life.

Who Should Decide?

This is an ethical decision itself, and it may also be a political one. (Some, such as Helen Holmes, have noted that politics is ethics.) George Annas, M.D., J.D., claims that the government's recent attempts to make clinical decisions about defective neonates is political ethics rather than bioethics. In the tradition of autonomy and informed consent, the primary decision maker should be the patient—not the health care providers. During pregnancy and for neonates, this means that the parents to be or parents should make the decisions. The Supreme Court has ruled that a pregnant woman does not need her husband's consent to get an abortion; this then points to the pregnant woman as the primary decision maker.

Others, however, claim that the fetus has a right to life and/or that abortion is wrong. Thus, the parent or parents are not the decision makers or at least are not the sole decision makers. Indeed, in the paternalistic or maternalistic tradition of health care, health care providers claim the right to make the decisions. "Just do what the doctor ordered" or "Do what the nurse says" are old standards that some claim still hold. These positions may violate the patient's autonomy, but others hold that that autonomy is limited. When it is in conflict with other goods (other goods might include the rights of health care providers or of society), the right of autonomy is restricted.

If morals are the rules and ethics are the reasons behind the rules, one perspective is that the question of who decides is determined by the ethical reasoning process. When all of the principles are considered, the decision maker may become apparent. Others note that if the ethical process is followed adequately, who makes decisions may be irrelevant, for the final decision will be ethical.

Role of the Nurse in Abortion Decisions and Care

Nurses caring for pregnant women who decide to terminate their pregnancy face the many ethical issues surrounding abortion. They also confront the varying views on what is right and wrong about this decision. Nurses who, for personal reasons, cannot in good conscience support abortion for any reason may find it better to work in other areas of health care so

that they do not have to compromise their deeply held belief. Others, who may not personally choose abortion, may effectively support and counsel those pregnant women who have made the choice to terminate a pregnancy. The nurse should be aware of her own value position on abortion. Nurses who care for women choosing abortion need to provide counseling and support before, during, and after the procedure. One needs also to remain sensitive to the woman's (couple's) need for further professional counseling and make the necessary referral.

DECISION TO MAINTAIN A HIGH RISK PREGNANCY

Client Choice and Informed Decision Making

A choice to maintain a high risk pregnancy should be self-determined and informed. One basis for these two principles is autonomy—i.e., the person's own choice. Autonomy is not absolute; consideration for others is a major ethical issue. One of the limits on autonomy is suicide. Some think that people have a right to risk or sacrifice their own lives and even to take their own lives. Others claim there are limits to this.

The high risk pregnancy classification may be based on many different medical, obstetrical, or fetal complications. Thus, the impact of continuing a high risk pregnancy on mother and fetus will vary. The major point is that pregnant women need full, truthful information and support as they weigh the risks and benefits of continuing the pregnancy. They must also be willing to accept responsibility for their choice, as noted earlier. To carry a pregnancy that endangers the life of the woman or to choose to carry and deliver an infant with severe genetic disease raises ethical issues such as the value of a woman's life and the quality of life of the infant. The emphasis in informed decision making, however, is sufficient information for the decision to be truly informed and sufficient freedom for the choice to be genuinely autonomous.

Quality versus Sanctity of Life in Maintaining Pregnancy

There is considerable debate about quality of life. Since people insist that it should never be considered. Others insist that it must be. In some cases this issue is clearer than in others; the suffering, the number of operations, the cost of maintaining life, and the meaningfulness and the productivity of life of either mother or infant are part of the concern. The most debatable element, however, is rationality, which, along with intellectual ability, is a major value in some cultures.

Sanctity of life is a relatively recent consideration in health care. While some theists continue to hold God as the ultimate, others consider life the ultimate. In this view life is the highest good, regardless of any cost in suffering, money, or personal relationships, especially when the cost is someone else's. Some insist that money should be no consideration in health care.

Responsibilities of Client

A major responsibility for a woman with a high risk pregnancy is following recommended procedures. Health care providers cannot enhance a good outcome without the client's cooperation. Women facing long hospitalizations during pregnancy, separated from friends and family, may become less willing to follow the medical regimen as time goes on. Grief over the loss of the perfect pregnancy or child contributes to depression and may interfere with the woman's willingness to take care of herself or her fetus.

Competence of Professional Staff and the Ethic of Caring

Staff competence in caring for high risk pregnancies and neonates is essential. Anything less is unethical. Competence includes keeping up with technology as well as providing caring, sensitive, family-centered health care. Physicians and nurses working with high risk pregnant women and families also must be skilled communicators, counselors, and motivators.

The ethic of caring is central to any health care. It is doubly so in care of high risk pregnancies—for the women themselves and their families. Professionals have been said to focus on the machinery or the technology used to diagnose and monitor rather than on the persons for whom this machinery is supposedly being used. Sometimes science and technology become ends in themselves and the patients get lost in the system. The ethic of caring requires great sensitivity and respect for persons along with competence in high technology.

Allocation of Technology and Personnel Resources

One of the ethical principles listed earlier was the just allocation of scarce resources. The allocation of resources, according to one theory, must be based on human need with considerations of equity. The wealthy or powerful have the resources to get health care. The poor do not. Women who are poor more often have poor outcomes of pregnancy than women who are able to pay for pregnancy care. Networking tertiary referral centers and neonatal intensive care nurseries has improved access to high risk care in recent years. Questions remain as to whether these costly services are beneficial to society as a whole. Again, society usually is expected to pay for these expensive services.

Others would suggest that while society can pay for high technology, the poor do not have the resources to care for traumatized women or infants. Even if the outcomes are good, the poor may not have the resources for normal care, let alone high technology care when the pregnancy leaves mother or fetus in need of it. It is suggested that society should pay for everything, including, if necessary, the institutionalization of the infant for life. Others point out that if society paid for normal prenatal care, premature births would be reduced by as much as two-thirds. Technology may be a status symbol or carry a value of its own in human culture, quite apart from concern for the health or well being of people.

Role of Nurse in Resource Allocation

Recently, some nurses have been involved in regional planning efforts where the allocation of hospital beds for high risk care, the choice of populations to be served, and the type of services are determined. Nurses have their greatest input on allocation decisions when they participate in the care of an individual family or sick neonate. These are micro decisions on allocation and often are made without regard for their impact on the larger community or society as a whole. Some ethicists claim these latter concerns should never enter into decisions for care of an individual. Others suggest that our health care resources are finite and must be distributed with justice and equity. The latter includes honoring the rights of society as well as the individual. Should access to tertiary care be based on need? Who determines the need? If access is limited, how should we decide who will receive high risk care? These are but a few of the justice concerns in high risk pregnancy care.

Chapter 5
Nursing Theoretical Framework for Care of the High Risk Maternity Patient

Barbara Decker, C.N.M., M.Ed.

WHAT IS THEORY?

A theory is a description—an explanation of an event or a series of events. It is characteristic of human beings to construct theories to explain everyday events. Scientists construct theories in formal ways so they can be tested and built upon to advance knowledge.

Scientific theory building is a systematic process of observation, analysis, hypothesis making, and testing. For example, the germ theory of disease was constructed on a base of hundreds of years of observation of the nature of illness and was dependent on the invention of the microscope and the subsequent discovery of microorganisms. Pasteur made the theoretical correlation between the presence of organisms and changes in organic processes and then tested that hypothesis. Lister strengthened the theory when he demonstrated that the use of antiseptic techniques reduced the incidence of infection. The germ theory laid the basis for the construction of later theories that enabled the control we now have on the incidence of infectious diseases.

The importance of having a theoretical basis for practice is illustrated by the case of Semmelweiss. He had, before Lister did his work, advocated the use of handwashing to reduce the incidence of puerperal fever. Even though Semmelweiss could demonstrate good results with handwashing, he did not propose a theoretical base for the practice as Lister later did. Semmelweiss's work was not accepted until after his death and the

general acceptance of germ theory. Good ideas and effective clinical practices therefore need theoretical bases to gain acceptance from the scientific and health care communities.

Scientific theory describes a limited number of events or phenomena. Everything in the universe cannot be explained by one meaningful theory. The theorist must make the crucial decision about which phenomena are important to observe. For example, our pre-Bronze age ancestors did not include sexual intercourse in their theories about how babies are conceived. They did include, logically, events that were more closely connected in time and emotion to childbirth. Their theories were wrong to the extent that they ignored a vital phenomenon. The problem of selecting events to be observed is very important in our time as well: do we know all the phenomena to be observed to build a theory about the causes of preeclampsia? Not yet.

Theory also is logical. Two opposite logical processes can be used to construct theory. Induction is used to draw a conclusion from observations. For example, Semmelweiss observed that the incidence of puerperal fever was great when birth attendants recently had been performing autopsies. He theorized that there was a principle or agent that was being transferred from the autopsy room to the birthing room. Inductive theories are created when the theorist does not know why or how something is happening but makes an educated guess based on a cluster of observations.

The opposing logical process used to construct theory is deduction, which is used when a general principle is known and a specific theoretical conclusion is drawn from it. An example is Lister's work. He knew that certain organisms are present in certain types of diseases. He theorized that the use of antiseptics would kill the organisms and prevent the occurrence of those diseases. Both inductive and deductive reasoning are necessary to theory construction. The choice is determined by how much is known in the area to be studied.

WHAT IS NURSING THEORY?

Every scientific discipline has a theory base. That base is global theory delineating the areas of study for the particular discipline. Nursing theory attempts to describe the phenomenon of nursing. Nurses are constructing a theory of nursing to focus work and research on topics that are of primary concern for nurses rather than for other professionals. Nurses still have not reached an agreement on what is or is not nursing.

Nursing is following a pattern of development that has occurred in all other scientific disciplines. As the discipline matures, scientists accumulate observations and are able to theorize about phenomena of particular interest to their discipline. As theories are proven and disproven, specialized knowledge accumulates and new questions for study arise. Practice disciplines like nursing and medicine face special problems that pure scientific disciplines do not, because practitioners are called upon to apply theories in human rather than laboratory situations.

Every nurse has a theoretical base for practice whether or not she has been educated in nursing theory. The reason why this must be so is because nursing theory is a description of what nursing is. It is not possible to practice nursing without making some assumptions about the work to be done. Or, said more positively, a nurse knows what to do because he or she knows what nursing practice is. That knowledge is a theory of nursing.

IS THERE AN ACCEPTED THEORY OF NURSING?

There is no agreement on a single theoretical basis for nursing practice. Instead, many theories have been developed as nurses struggle to describe systematically the myriad of nursing activities and concerns that exist. Some of the published theories have received a great deal of professional attention because they are imaginative, insightful, relevant to a wide audience, or sometimes because their authors make them widely known. The works of Rogers (1), Roy (2), and Orem (3), among others, are known by many nurses.

Nursing theories vary both in structure and in operation. There is some agreement in the literature about basic structural elements that should be part of every nursing theory. These are called common elements or commonplaces and can be thought of as the skeleton of a theory. Stevens identifies these commonplaces as nurse, patient, health, and the relationships between them (4). These structures are found in most developed theories, but there is surprising variation among theorists in the forms their skeletons take. The nurse may be the primary figure in one theory and the patient in another. For some theorists health is a practical goal, while for others it is an unattainable ideal. See Chinn and Jacobs (5) for comparison of the structures of some well-known theories.

The operation of a theory is governed by the method of thinking the theorist uses and that gives direction to the relationships between the structural elements. Operation can be thought of as the muscle and flesh that gives power and shape to the skeleton. There are four types of thinking evident in published nursing theories.

Dialectical Thinking

Understanding comes through relating something to its apparent opposite to see that it is part of a larger whole. Birth and death are both parts of life. Sickness can be understood as a different way of being, and maybe a constructive way of being, rather than as just the opposite of health. Much of Eastern philosophy is based on dialectical thinking, and general systems theory is based on dialectical thinking.

Logistical Thinking

Understanding comes through study of the smaller and smaller parts of the whole. Understanding of human labor comes from knowledge of gross anatomy, the structure and function of the uterus, the biochemistry of uterine muscle contractility, the behavior of molecules in living systems, and the myriad other components of a woman in labor. Logistic reasoning is the primary method of Western science.

Problematic Thinking

Understanding comes through identification of a problem, collection of information about it, and work toward resolution of the problem. Two things are different about this kind of thinking: the person who defines the problem is part of the process, and the process comes to a conclusion when resolution is achieved. Governments use problematic thinking as they act to identify and resolve societal problems. Problem-oriented charting is based on this kind of thinking.

Operational Thinking

Understanding comes through making finer and finer distinctions between events or things. Differential diagnosis is an example of operational thinking. A symptom can be subjected to a data collection process that yields a possible set of diagnoses. Each possibility is then ruled in or out by finer discriminations (more precise data) until a final selection of diagnosis and treatment is made. Orem is an operational thinker.

To understand the operation of a theory or how it should work in practice, the written theory must be read carefully and analytically.

HOW IS NURSING THEORY USED?

Some nursing services, educational programs, and individual nurses have found great appeal and practical relevance in one or another of these theories. They have then used that developed theory in its entirety as the theoretical basis for their work. Other institutions and individual practitioners have used a more eclectic approach in building their own theories. Ideas from published theory may be useful in part but in some respect are unsatisfactory. For example, the reader who examines Orem's theory closely may find that it seems excellent in providing maternity nurses with a theoretical basis for health teaching and preventive care but that the theory is weak in recognizing the importance of sexuality in human life and in providing a clear theoretical basis for nursing practice in that area. So, one may keep Orem's theory and expand upon it to define the place of sexuality in the self-care needs of people and the role of the nurse in relation to sexuality needs. Adapting existing theory must be done with care to avoid stretching borrowed and new concepts beyond coherence. When that happens, the theory statement is confusing to read and lacks relevance to nursing practice.

HOW CAN ONE CHOOSE A NURSING THEORY?

Many theoretical bases for nursing are possible. The theory chosen should be consistent with the nurse's own philosophy of life and nursing. Descriptions of patient, nurse, health, and so on should fit with the nurse's ideas and experience. Often, very careful analysis of a theory is necessary to determine that consistency. For example, examination of Nightingale's *Notes on Nursing* shows that her idea of "patient" is a passive person who is managed by the nurse and others (6). Nurses who believe that "patients" are people active in their own health care could not accept that part of Nightingale's theory, although they might be able to accept Nightingale's notion that it is the nurses' responsibility to provide the patient with a comfortable and healthy environment.

A second criterion for an acceptable nursing theory is that it must be consistent with the theory of the practice setting or institution. An institution devoted solely to the treatment of disease may not provide staffing or space for health education efforts. A nurse whose theory includes health education will find it difficult or impossible to practice in such a setting. That nurse may choose to change employment or, better, to work with other nurses to change institutional practices to permit nursing practice based on an agreed upon nursing theory.

A final criterion for an acceptable theory is that it should enable the nurse to give excellent care measured by any standard: client preferences, health outcomes, local standards of practice, etc. A good theory is broad in scope to allow for the different kinds of service that nurses provide. It also is socially relevant—able to be put into practice according to current societal expectations for health care.

AN EXAMINATION OF TWO DIFFERENT THEORETICAL BASES FOR PRACTICE

Two bases for high risk maternity nursing practice are examined here. They represent two ends of a spectrum of possible theories that can be useful, and they are presented to help the reader fit the content of this book into a framework that will be individually and professionally relevant for practice.

Dorothea Orem is a nurse who has developed a theory for nursing practice used by many schools and institutions (3). Ludwig von Bertalanffy was a biologist who developed a theory about the nature of life—General Systems Theory—intended for use by all those who study and work with the processes of life (7). Nurses, psychologists, and others have borrowed from his theory.

Orem is an operational thinker. She uses logic to make choices between different courses of action and bases those choices on finer and finer discriminations. Bertalanffy was a dialectical thinker who looked at larger pictures to explain apparent differences.

In terms of scientific philosophy, Orem is a reductionist. Reductionists attempt to explain phenomena by reducing them to their simplest forms; ideally, that form is a mathematical equation. Bertalanffy was a holist in that he believed that a key to understanding phenomena is in looking at how things are organized. For example, one cannot understand man by looking only at his cells, plasma, and organs. One must look at the relationship between those things and at man in his relationship with the world around him. Understanding comes with knowledge of relationship and patterns of organization.

Orem and Bertalanffy also differ in the ways in which their theories are used. Orem is goal oriented, and the goal is self-care. Bertalanffy's theory is process oriented, and systems processes are the subjects. Orem's theory is a well-developed nursing theory. Bertalanffy's theory is rudimentary in its applicability to nursing practice.

Dorothea Orem

Dorothea Orem's work is special in that patient education and self-care and patient responsibility for health are stressed. Orem's theory of nursing has been selected for application to high risk maternity nursing practice because it is widely known and is being used by many educational programs and nursing services.

According to Orem, nursing is a social institution set up to meet the personal needs for care that people cannot meet themselves. Orem calls these needs self-care requisites. There are three categories of self-care needs. Universal self-care requisites are common to all human beings and include needs that support physical life processes (e.g., air, food) and social and psychological functions. Developmental self-care requisites are those associated with various life cycle stages and events such as infancy and pregnancy. Health deviation self-care needs arise from any kind of deviation from health and

normal functioning and from medical diagnostic procedures and treatment (3, p 41).

Following are complete lists of the three categories of self-care requistes according to Orem.

Universal Self-Care Requisites

1. The maintenance of a sufficient intake of air.
2. The maintenance of a sufficient intake of water.
3. The maintenance of a sufficient intake of food (nutrients).
4. The provision of care associated with elimination processes and excrements.
5. The maintenance of a balance between activity and rest.
6. The maintenance of a balance between solitude and social interaction.
7. The prevention of hazards to human life, human functioning, and human well-being.
8. The promotion of human functioning and development within social groups in accord with human potential, known human limitations, and the human desire to be normal. *Normalcy* is used in the sense of that which is essentially human and that which is in accord with the genetic and constitutional characteristics and the talents of individuals (10, p 42).

Developmental Self-Care Requisites

1. The bringing about and maintenance of living conditions that support life processes and promote the processes of development—i.e., human progress toward the higher levels of the organization of human structures and toward maturation during:
   a. The intrauterine stages of life and the process of birth;
   b. The neonatal stage of life when (1) born at term or prematurely and (2) born with normal birth weight or low birth weight;
   c. Infancy;
   d. The developmental stages of childhood, including adolescence and entry into adulthood;
   e. The developmental stages of adulthood; and
   f. Pregnancy either in childhood or adulthood.
2. Provision of care either to prevent the occurrence of deleterious effects of conditions that can affect human development (type 2.1) or to mitigate or overcome these effects (type 2.2) from such conditions as:
   a. Educational deprivation;

b. Problems of social adaptation;
c. Failures of healthy individuation;
d. Loss of relatives, friends, or associates;
e. Loss of possessions or loss of occupational security;
f. Abrupt change of residence to an unfamiliar environment;
g. Status-associated problems;
h. Poor health or disability;
i. Oppressive living conditions; and
j. Terminal illness and impending death (3, p 47).

Health Deviation Self-Care Requisites

1. Seeking and securing appropriate medical assistance in the event of exposure to specific physical or biological agents or environmental conditions associated with human pathological events and states, or when there is evidence of genetic, physiological, or psychological conditions known to produce or to be associated with human pathology.
2. Being aware of and attending to the effects and results of pathological conditions and states.
3. Effectively carrying out medically prescribed diagnostic, therapeutic, and rehabilitative measures directed to the prevention of specific types of pathology, to the pathology itself, to the regulation of human integrated functioning, to the correction of deformities or abnormalities, or to compensation for disabilities.
4. Being aware of and attending to or regulating the discomforting or deleterious effects of medical care measures performed or prescribed by the physician.
5. Modifying the self-concept (and self-image) in accepting oneself as being in a particular state of health and in need of specific forms of health care.
6. Learning to live with the effects of pathological conditions and states and the effects of medical diagnostic and treatment measures in a life-style that permits continued personal development (3, pp 50–51).

The Nursing Care Plan: Orem

Orem's version of the nursing care plan is called a nursing system and is derived from her theory. Here, Orem's theory is put into operation, and the practical significance of the abstract theoretical statements becomes obvious. The nursing system that results from following these operations will be very different from the traditional nursing care plan. Client preferences, habits, and values will necessitate a much more individualized plan than is usual.

The process in this theory originates with the patient. The patient has primary responsibility for identifying self-care needs with which he or she needs assistance. If the person is unable because of illness, immaturity, or ignorance to identify need, then family, friends, physicians, or nurses can assist in that process. Once the nurse and patient are in professional contact, the two work out a complete list of self-care needs particular to the patient in order to arrive at a statement of the therapeutic self-care demand. This is analogous to the nursing care plan. The therapeutic self-care demand will fall into one of three nursing systems that categorize the degree to which the nurse helps the patient to meet his or her needs. These are (1) wholly compensatory systems in which the patient is totally unable to engage in self-care activities, (2) partly compensatory nursing systems in which the client can perform some activities, and (3) supportive-educative (developmental) nursing systems in which the patient can and should perform all self-care activities. The therapeutic self-care demand is an identification of client needs, and the nursing system gives direction for the roles and activities of nurse and patient in meeting the needs. The demand and the system will change as needs are met and as patient status changes.

The nurse, in Orem's theory, is a person specifically educated to help people meet their self-care needs. The nurse is not defined by specific nursing acts performed but by social designation as the person responsible for ongoing self-care when the patient is unable. An act becomes a nursing act when the nurse does it.

Orem's theory is very logical and consistent in that all its parts fit together. It is a deficit theory. That means that health care needs are seen as deficiencies from some standard of health. If all the needs can be met, the nursing system will come to rest. The system that Orem describes is a cybernetics or computer-type system in which the data entered are needs, the process is action by patient and nurse to meet the needs, and the output is improved health status.

The strength of Orem's theory is in providing a clear rationale for education and for patients taking an active role in their own health care. The fact that diagnosis of deficits and formation of the plan are performed with the client ensures that the individual needs and preferences of each client will be taken into account. The contractual nature of the process works to increase the patient's sense of responsibility for it and, hopefully, his or her ability to follow it.

Ludwig von Bertalanffy

Bertalanffy is the originator of the General Systems Theory (7). When he began his work as a biologist, the discipline was split into two camps. The mechanist camp derived its concept of living things and its methods of research from the field of physics; the mechanists believed that eventually the laws of chemistry and physics would be able to answer all questions about living things. The vitalist group, on the other hand, believed that a separate vital principle existed in all living things that carried the goal of development and existence within itself. The soul is one idea about the vital principle in man. Neither mechanists nor vitalists were able to account for all that is observable in man or other living things without recourse to concepts that are separate from man or animals: metaphysics or the soul.

Bertalanffy developed general systems theory as a tool to be used to explain aspects of life that could not be explained by the mechanistic theory or relegated to the unknowable by the vitalists.

The general systems concept is one of wholeness. Living things are open to and continuously exchanging energy with the environment. They can be understood only in terms of their organization, which gives direction to the forces of change.

To approach this concept more concretely, consider the red blood cell. The erythrocyte contains hemoglobin, which binds to iron, which binds to oxygen, and this process must occur if the cells of the body are to receive enough oxygen for life. The next level of organization for the erythrocyte is the blood; if the flow is blocked or if the blood pressure is too low, oxygen still will not be delivered to the cells. One can go to ever higher levels of organization to look for answers to problems in delivering oxygen to cells, and these levels are not often included in the nursing data base: if society does not make iron-rich foods available to a person, sufficient oxygen may still not be delivered to cells. If acid rain destroys the crops that feed the farm animals that provide dietary iron, etc., the process still will fail.

In his insistence that we look at wholeness, Bertalanffy does not negate the value of studying parts but maintains that an understanding of living systems can only be achieved by doing both. We must look at parts but also at how parts and higher levels of parts are organized. And we must remember that a single part, say a person, exists in many simultaneous relationships or kinds of organiza-

tion. A person may be a patient in the health care system, a parent in a family system, and a criminal in the legal system, for example.

The study of systems is arranged in a hierarchical order, with the study of basic units representing only one level. Bertalanffy presents the hierarchical model as a series of concentric circles, the smaller embedded in the larger to represent dynamic energy interchange between them. Nonliving closed systems may also import or export energy, but the process is not dynamic. In a closed system that is not capable of dynamic interchange with the environment, the second law of thermodynamics pertains: there will be progressive entropy (tendency toward stasis), a final state of maximum chaos will result, and the process will come to a halt. For example, if two gases are mixed in a container, the molecules will reach a state of statistically random dispersion at statistically predicted distances from each other.

It is Bertalanffy's contention that science has viewed organisms and especially man as closed systems. If pain is experienced, the reflex is to withdraw. Satisfied, the system comes to rest. This stimulus-response pattern is what Bertalanffy calls the robot view of man (8). It does not account for why people willingly tolerate pain or how pain can be used as the stimulus for artistic expression. In what parts of the human machine can we find the apparatus of love, creativity, or self-denial?

General systems theory opens the door to a new discussion of the intrinsic characteristics of man: individuality and creativity. The data base mandated by this theoretical foundation for nursing practice is expanded tremendously. If we look at the organization of a person not only internally but at the level of familial, societal, and physical world interaction, then almost no question that could be asked would be irrelevant.

Applying General Systems Theory to Nursing Practice

The idea of a nursing care plan is not holistic in Bertalanffy's sense of the word. Instead, it is a reductionist idea and process: the patient is analyzed for needs or deficits, or whatever theory dictates is the basis for giving nursing care. The whole person loses wholeness (on paper at least), and attention is focused on his or her component parts. Nursing care plans are used successfully in practice because our health care system uses reductionist, analytical science as the basis for practice. It is very difficult to apply holistic theory in the dialectical meaning of the word in standard health care settings if, and this is an important qualification, the holistic view is the sole basis for practice. Our society insists that safe practice is based on the use of scientific/analytic data.

General systems theory allows for the study of living organisms at all levels of organization. The functioning of the erythrocyte is not less important because we are also concerned with how a person's creativity may be related to his or her illness. The nurse can use both analytical and holistic thinking in practice.

Bertalanffy is quoted here from a talk on general systems theory that he gave to a class of student nurses. He said that an "important problem is that modern medicine is using a mechanistic approach, treating the patient like an injured machine rather than applying the humanistic-systems-organismic approach" (9).

The addition of general systems theory to the more traditional theoretical basis for nursing practice can enhance nursing practice greatly. That is because it increases the number of relevant questions we can ask about a person and so increases our understanding of that person and, eventually, all people. The questions asked can be the basis for new and different kinds of research to improve health care.

A Clinical Example

A young woman is admitted for dilatation and curettage following a spontaneous abortion. Good, safe care is incomplete unless we understand how this fetal loss is a part of this woman's life. To help both the woman and the care givers reach that understanding, some nontraditional questions need to be asked about this situation:

1. Will the loss of this fetus affect the mother's biological functioning in any positive way?
2. If there are negative physical effects for the mother, what purpose could they serve?
3. What are the possible positive or negative effects of this event in any of the woman's social and family systems?

These kinds of questions ignore much of what analytical scientific theory provides as a base for collecting data about this woman's needs. Accepted psychological theory can lead us to assume that this loss is an entirely negative event in the woman's life because it is not normal. Dialectical reasoning enables the care giver to go beyond questions about normal and abnormal and to look for

perhaps more valid explanations for this event. Suppose, for example, that this woman became pregnant to fill some unconscious need of her mother's and that pregnancy would not be constructive now in her own life. We know that emotions exert powerful effects on physical functioning and can assume that in some way not yet understood that could be the case here. Further exploration of this and other possibilities could provide the basis for much more effective health care in preventing physically debilitating repeat miscarriages, enabling further psychological maturation and individuation, and reducing the need for costly medical treatment.

SUMMARY

The challenge for the practicing nurse is to articulate a theoretical basis for practice that will serve clients well and be consistent with current knowledge and personal professional experience. Nursing theorists have provided excellent resources by articulating their own ideas about what nursing is. Even rudimentary theories provide the nurse with the opportunity to think about and evaluate the ideas and beliefs of fellow professionals. Outside the nursing sphere, Bertalanffy and others concerned with the nature of man have valuable ideas to contribute to nursing's search for better ways to work with people.

REFERENCES

1. Rogers M: *An Introduction to the Theoretical Basis of Nursing*. Philadelphia, F.A. Davis, 1970.
2. Roy C: The Roy adaptation model. In Riehl J, Roy C (eds): *Conceptual Models for Nursing Practice*, ed 2. New York, Appleton-Century-Crofts, 1980.
3. Orem D: *Nursing: Concepts of Practice*, ed 2. New York, McGraw-Hill, 1980.
4. Stevens B: *Nursing Theory Analysis, Application, Evaluation*, ed 2. Boston, Little, Brown, and Company, 1984, pp 11–14.
5. Chinn PT, Jacobs MK: *Theory and Nursing: A Systematic Approach*. St. Louis, Mosby, 1983, pp 34–39.
6. Nightingale F: *Notes on Nursing*. New York, Dover Publications, 1969.
7. Bertalanffy L von: *General System Theory*. New York, George Braziller, 1968.
8. Bertalanffy L von: *Robots, Men and Minds–Psychology in the Modern World*. New York, George Braziller, 1967.
9. Davidson M. *Uncommon Sense*. Los Angeles, Tarcher, 1983, p 121.

Chapter 6
Assessment of Fetal Status

Patricia Aikins Murphy, C.N.M., M.S.

INTRODUCTION AND OVERVIEW

Recent decades have seen a change from viewing the fetus as a passive passenger in the mother's body to accepting the fetus as a patient in its own right. Obstetrical advances have made it possible to diagnose, manage, and even treat potentially threatening conditions in the unborn baby. As it has become more common for women with medical and obstetrical problems to successfully conceive, carry, and give birth to children, clinical and technological assessment of the fetus plays a more prominent role in the care of these women. Nurses involved in the care of the high risk maternity patient need to be aware of these assessment procedures in order to enhance their nursing diagnoses and to involve the pregnant woman and her family more fully in her care.

Assessment of the fetus should be carried out continuously during pregnancy. Together, clinical assessment and technological tools can provide a composite picture of the fetus in terms of its health, well-being, or maturity. Clinical management decisions are made more easily when based on a variety of assessment data.

CLINICAL ASSESSMENT

Clinical assessment begins at the first prenatal visit and continues throughout the pregnancy. A comprehensive history and physical examination are the foundation for nursing management of pregnancy. Thorough evaluation of history of medical or family illness, surgery/trauma, obstetrical or gynecological problems, contraceptive history, social habits, environmental factors, and life-style will identify areas of potential concern. An intensive history of the present pregnancy from the probable date of conception may highlight additional factors. Any deviation from expected findings on physical or laboratory examination will complete the initial risk assessment. The woman and her family should be aware of risk factors and their probable management in order to participate actively in the patient's care.

Subjective Parameters of Fetal Assessment

Subjective parameters of fetal assessment should include the following:

1. The estimated date of confinement (EDC) is calculated from the first day of the last normal menstrual period (LNMP) by adding 280 days—or 9 months plus 7 days—to that date (Naegele's rule). The key factor is determining the last normal menses, a task that often requires some probing. The resulting EDC is a rough estimate, since the calculations are based on a 28-day menstrual cycle with ovulation on day 14. Many women do not regularly follow this pattern or have altered it with hormonal contraception. If, however, the LNMP is certain and the client's average cycle is 28–30 days in length, the calculated EDC will be fairly reliable. With the EDC established, use of a "gestation wheel" will enable the clinician to determine the approximate weeks of gestation on any given date during the pregnancy.

2. Quickening denotes the first perception of fetal movement by the mother. Generally, it occurs between 16 and 22 weeks of pregnancy.

3. Fetal movement counts are established as a useful adjunct in monitoring the well-being of the fetus. Several researchers have studied fetal move-

ment patterns and have noted a gradual increase from the time of quickening, reaching a maximum in the third trimester (28–36 weeks) with a slight decrease in the last weeks before delivery (1). A client may be taught to monitor fetal movement in the late third trimester in one of several ways. In general, she should be instructed to report any lessening or cessation of movement.

Sadovsky recommends recording fetal movement for 30–60 minutes three times a day (morning, afternoon, and evening). These totals are extrapolated to reflect a 12-hour count. If there are three or fewer fetal movements in any 1 hour, the patient should continue to count for 6–12 hours. Marked reduction in fetal movement is a "movement alarm signal." Four or fewer movements in a 12-hour period is indicative of a severely distressed fetus (2). Other reports have used a similar method with slight alterations in the time spent counting fetal movements.

Another method is the "Cardiff Count To Ten," in which the client records on a chart the time at which the tenth fetal movement of the day is felt (3) (Fig. 6.1). The client is instructed to report any 12-hour period with fewer than 10 movements. If this occurs, the client is referred for further evaluation.

A sudden increase in fetal movements followed by a marked reduction in fetal activity is thought by some to indicate cord accidents or placental abruption (2) and should be evaluated vigorously.

One controlled clinical study of fetal movement counts in a large number of patients suggests that monitoring fetal movement counts is beneficial as a screening test, in spite of the poor predictive value of positive tests (4). However, the trial was not randomized, so further clinical studies are necessary to determine the actual value of the test. The test does have the advantages of simplicity, safety, low cost, convenience, and no need for specialized equipment or personnel (5).

Objective Parameters of Fetal Assessment

Objective parameters of fetal assessment will include the following:

1. Evaluation of uterine size is done at each prenatal visit to provide a rough estimate of fetal growth. The size of the uterus is estimated in early gestation via a bimanual examination. After the uterus has risen out of the pelvis, the height of the uterine fundus is measured in relation to body landmarks, such as the symphysis pubis xyphoid, or umbilicus, using finger breadths, tape measure, or calipers (Fig. 6.2). The most precise of these is a measurement taken from the symphysis pubis to the top of the fundus, in centimeters, by the same examiner at each visit. The client should be supine, with bladder empty, and the measurements should be taken with the legs straight to prevent upward rotation of the symphysis.

Rough clinical guidelines call for the measurement in centimeters to approximate the weeks of gestation after about 22 weeks. Fundal height is not an absolute measure of gestational age but relative, according to the population served. Measurements falling below the 10th percentile established for a given population will indicate slow growth (which may be normal or abnormal); those falling above the 90th percentile indicate rapid growth. This method has been found to be very effective in pinpointing abnormal uterine growth patterns (6–8).

2. The fetal heart can be heard via unamplified fetoscope by a careful and experienced examiner between 17 and 22 weeks' gestation if the woman is not obese. The fetal heart should be auscultated at each subsequent visit. If at least 20 weeks have passed since the FH was first heard via stethoscope, the pregnancy probably will be at term.

3. Abdominal palpation carried out at each prenatal visit (after 24–28 weeks) should provide information on the growth of the uterus, position of the baby, fetal movement, amount of amniotic fluid, and estimated fetal weight.

4. Amnioscopy may be employed in certain circumstances to evaluate the amniotic fluid in a term pregnancy. A cone-shaped endoscope is inserted into the vagina, the tip resting in the cervical canal. The membranes then can be visualized for the presence of meconium or blood in the fluid. The cervix must be accessible and partially dilated to accomplish this, and the procedure is contraindicated in the presence of an unstable lie, third trimester bleeding, vaginal or cervical infection, or gestation of less than 34 weeks. There is a 2–3% risk of rupturing the membranes (9, 10). Positive amnioscopy always warrants further assessment. The incidence of false-negatives (fetal or neonatal compromise following negative amnioscopy) is difficult to assess, because the frequency of performing the test varies in different studies from daily to weekly. Proponents say it must be done at least every 48 hours to be valuable (11). In addition, some reports of neonatal compromise following negative amnioscopy may be due to intrapartal asphyxia or other factors that cannot be predicted by antepartal amnioscopy (12).

The limitations of clinical assessment tools lie mainly in their subjectivity and lack of precision.

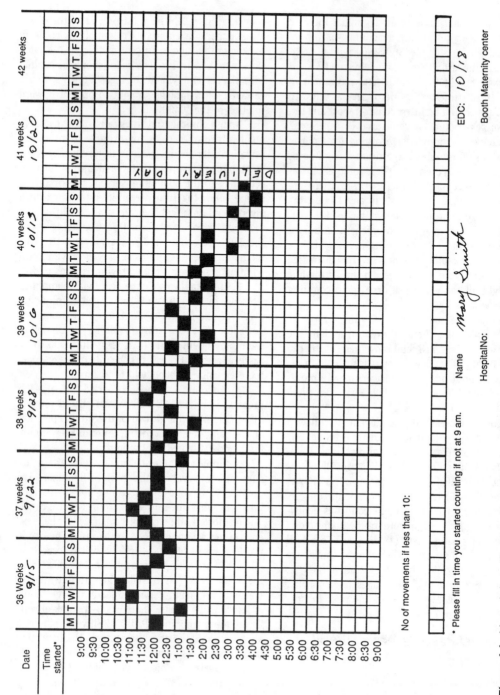

No of movements if less than 10:

* Please fill in time you started counting if not at 9 am.   Name   Mary Smith

HospitalNo:

EDC: 10/18

Booth Maternity center

Figure 6.1. Normal chart. (Reprinted by permission of Elsevier Science Publishing Co., Inc., from Fetal movement and fetal outcome in a low risk population by Fischer S, Fullerton J, Trezise L, *Journal of Nurse-Midwifery* 26(1): 29. Copyright 1981 by The American College of Nurse-Midwives.)

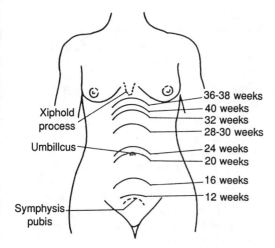

Figure 6.2. Normal location of the height of the fundus during pregnancy. (From Buckley K, Kulb N: *Handbook of Maternal-Newborn Nursing.* New York: John Wiley & Sons, 1983, p 5.)

These can be minimized by accurate assessment and examination by the same care provider at each visit.

Studies of clinical assessment of gestational age have attempted to ascertain their reliability in controlled situations. Table 6.1 shows one analysis of clinical factors in descending order from the most to least reliable, followed by the mean intervals from each clinical event to delivery. If the LNMP is unknown, the EDC can be projected by averaging the remaining three clinical parameters (13, 14).

In high risk pregnancies, clinical assessment tools often are not the sole criteria for determining fetal age or well-being. Technological assessments are used to complement and further refine clinical assessments.

Table 6.1.
CLINICAL FACTORS DETERMINING
GESTATIONAL AGE[a]

EVENT	MEAN INTERVAL TO DELIVERY
Known LMP	284 days ±14 days
Uterus at level of umbilicus	141 days ±15 days
1st fetal heart with fetoscope (unamplified)	136 days ±17 days
Quickening	156 days ±18 days

[a]Adapted from Anderson F: Gestational age assessment II. *Am J Obstet Gynecol* 140(7):770, 1981.

TECHNOLOGICAL ASSESSMENT

Ultrasound Assessment

Ultrasound is a technique that employs intermittent high frequency sound waves, inaudible to the human ear, to generate an image of the contents of the pregnant uterus. A transducer made of piezoelectric crystals is applied to the abdominal wall with liberal use of a coupling agent such as mineral oil, and a pulse of sound waves is transmitted through the soft internal tissues. When these waves reach structures of differing densities, some of the energy is reflected back to the transducer, which "listens" to the echoes and converts them into an image on a screen. Clinical obstetrics uses several types of ultrasound:

1. Continuous wave Doppler, which will detect the fetal heart by 10–12 weeks' gestation and which is used to monitor the fetal heart in labor or during certain test procedures.
2. Static scanners, which provide large images of good quality and definition. They produce A-mode or B-mode images that measure along a single line of sight and assess tissue consistency along that line. Pulses from the returning echo are marked in spikes (A-mode) or dots (B-mode) along a vertical axis. A B-scan combines B-mode display on a time baseline to produce a tomographic effect that can outline organs and masses or measure consistency and density variables (15).
3. Real-time ultrasound, which requires multiple, sequential pulse-echo systems, adds time and motion to B-scan techniques, allowing observation of fetal movement and certain physiological events, such as umbilical vessel pulsation, cardiac valve function, or fetal breathing movements, in addition to routine sonographic findings. Real-time equipment is smaller and more mobile and will provide information for most obstetrical needs. A static B-scan may be preferred for a panoramic view of the pelvis or a large field of vision (16).

The risks of ultrasound are still unclear. At present, the "majority of animal studies and human observations do not indicate that ultrasound exposures at diagnostic levels produce harmful or permanent effects" (17). In 1984 a consensus development conference convened by the National Institutes of Health (NIH) studied the use of ultrasound in pregnancy and concluded that ultrasound

Table 6.2.

AVERAGE ULTRASOUND MEASUREMENTS OF CROWN-RUMP LENGTH (CRL), BIPARIETAL DIAMETER (BPD), AND FEMUR LENGTH (FL) ACCORDING TO WEEKS' GESTATION[a]

WEEKS' GESTATION[b]	CRL (mm)	BPD (mm)	FL (mm)
6	5	—	—
7	9	—	—
8	15	—	—
9	22	10	—
10	31	13	—
11	41	17	—
12	53	21	—
13	—	25	12
14	—	28	15
15	—	32	18
16	—	36	21
17	—	39	24
18	—	43	26
19	—	46	29
20	—	50	32
21	—	53	35
22	—	56	37
23	—	59	40
24	—	62	43
25	—	65	45
26	—	67	48
27	—	70	50
28	—	73	53
29	—	75	55
30	—	77	58
31	—	80	60
32	—	82	62
33	—	85	65
34	—	87	67
35	—	89	69
36	—	91	72
37	—	93	74
38	—	95	76
39	—	—	78
40	—	—	80

[a]Adapted from Chervenak F, Jeanty P, Hobbins J: Fetal age and growth assessment. *Clin Obstet Gynecol* 10:424–426, 1983.
[b]Weeks' gestation rounded to nearest completed week of gestation.

can improve patient management and outcome when there is an accepted medical indication. The NIH conference reviewed many of the studies reporting on the safety of ultrasound in humans and found many of them inadequate because of technical problems with the research. There are some studies suggesting adverse effects in animals, leading to a decision to withhold recommendation for routine ultrasound screening (18, 19). More research, more sensitive indicators of fetal damage, and extensive long-term follow-up will be necessary before a final evaluation can be made.

The benefit of ultrasound clearly is its usefulness in assessing the previously inaccessible fetus. It provides a wealth of information that may be crucial in evaluating the high risk pregnancy. Anecdotal evidence suggests that visualization of the fetus may enhance the formation of the prenatal bond with the infant; nurses may find this useful when assisting the client to adjust to her "high risk" status (20).

Stage I Sonography

Stage I or level I ultrasound provides basic information on fetal presentation, fetal growth, placental grade and location, amount of amniotic fluid, and gestational age; it may also detect gross anomalies. It is best performed when the client has a full bladder because it improves resolution, provides an anatomical landmark, and elevates the fetus out of the pelvis.

Gestational Age

Gestational age is determined by a variety of sonographic measurements and with varying degrees of accuracy (Table 6.2). The crown-rump length of the fetus, when measured between 8 and 13 weeks, is thought to be accurate within ±5 days. A single biparietal diameter (BPD) measurement, if taken prior to 26 weeks' gestation, may be accurate ±11 days. After 26 weeks there is increasing variation; at term, a single BPD may have a standard error of 3 weeks. Some authorities will accept a single BPD of 9.3 cm or greater as evidence of a gestational age of 36 weeks and fetal weight over 2500 g, but more supportive evidence is desirable (21). Growth-adjusted sonographic age is a technique that tries to account for differences in the rate of BPD growth among fetuses. It requires a first BPD before 26 weeks and a second prior to 32 weeks; the fetus is categorized as small, average, or large based on these, and the EDC is adjusted to account for the rate of growth. The standard error is then reduced to ±3–5 days, according to proponents (22, 23).

Femur length may be predictive within ±7 days if measured prior to 23 weeks (24). The ratio of femur length to BPD in normal pregnancies is approximately 78% ± 8%; findings outside this range might indicate the presence of skeletal or cranial abnormalities. Other researchers have studied humerus length or biocular distance as measures of fetal age (25).

Suspected abnormalities in fetal growth are evaluated further by serial BPDs, which may show consistent growth rates below the 10th percentile, or a "late-flattening" growth rate, where head growth slows at the end of pregnancy (26). Since the fetal head is the last parameter affected in growth retardation, the abdominal circumference also may be evaluated. This is measured at the upper fetal abdomen to include the liver and subcutaneous tissues and will detect asymmetric, head-sparing growth retardation. The head-abdomen ratio should decline as gestation progresses due to the increase in fetal fat and subcutaneous tissue. The head-abdomen ratio generally is greater than 1.0 until 36 weeks and less than 1.0 approaching term (27); findings outside this range may be useful in predicting intrauterine growth retardation (IUGR), macrosomia, or some anomalies such as hydrocephaly or microcephaly.

Fetal Growth

Excessive or rapid fetal growth also may be evaluated. Fetal macrosomia may be symmetric, where head, trunk, and femur length all are above the 90th percentile; this usually is genetic or in gestations over 41 weeks. Asymmetric macrosomia, where head and femur are below the 90th percentile and the excess weight is from soft tissue, may be seen in class A or B diabetes (28).

Total intrauterine volume (TIUV) measures the volume occupied by the fetus, placenta, and amniotic fluid. Decrease in any one parameter is reflected by a lower TIUV and may indicate growth retardation. Due to the difficulty of evaluating the entire intrauterine contents on one ultrasound picture, this measure often is replaced by other parameters. Some sonographers will use estimated fetal weight, calculated from fetal measurements, to evaluate fetal growth compared with gestational age.

Amniotic Fluid Volume

Amniotic fluid volume (AFV) can be estimated by ultrasound, and oligo- or polyhydramnios may be detected in the second half of pregnancy. If the largest pocket of amniotic fluid measures less than 1.0 cm in its broadest diameter, oligohydramnios is present (29) and may be an indicator of IUGR. AFV also is used in evaluating the postterm pregnancy; if oligohydramnios is present, it is considered an indicator of increased perinatal risk (30, 31). Polyhydramnios is readily detected on sonogram when large fluid-filled spaces are seen within the uterus. Its discovery should be followed by a search for fetal anomalies (see Chapter 30).

Placental Assessment

Placental localization is imperative prior to intrauterine procedures and in evaluating any vaginal bleeding during pregnancy. Placental grading is an adjunct measure in dating pregnancy and assessing fetal maturity based on the theory that the placenta should mature in a similar fashion to fetal organs. These maturational changes occur in specific areas—not always sequentially. They may be delayed in class A or B diabetes or RH isoimmunization and

Table 6.3.
PLACENTAL GRADE[a]

Grade 0	Homogeneous immature placenta with no calcifications; may be seen after 32 weeks in diabetes or Rh isoimmunization. There is minimal correlation with fetal lung maturity.
Grade I	One major change, echogenic densities, appears in the placenta; appears at about 31 weeks; 40% will remain grade I until term; rarely seen after 42 weeks.
Grade II	Two major changes: calcifications and indentations of the chorionic plate; appears at about 36 weeks; 45% will remain grade II until term; 70–90% chance of fetal lung maturity.
Grade III	Multiple indentations on placenta, causing "Swiss cheese" pattern; appears at about 38 weeks; may appear before 35 weeks in IUGR, hypertension, preeclampsia. Due to a spurt of maturation at 40–41 weeks' gestation, 45% will be grade III at 42 weeks. If present, there is a >90% chance for fetal lung maturity.

[a]Adapted from Grannum P: Ultrasound examination of the placenta. *Clin Obstet Gynecol* 10(3):464, 1983; and Gottesfield K: Clinical role of placental imaging. *Clin Obstet Gynecol* 27(2):327, 1984.

may be accelerated in hypertensive disease or class C diabetes (32–34) (Table 6.3). A grade III placenta may indicate fetal lung maturity, but the false-positive rate ranges from 7–25%, and further assessment is needed (35).

Stage II Sonography

Stage II or level II ultrasound examination is an in depth search for evidence of congenital anomalies. An experienced sonographer usually is able to detect the following:

1. Craniospinal anomalies, such as spina bifida, hydro-, micro-, or anencephaly; and encephalocele.
2. Cardiothoracic anomalies, such as cardiac or pulmonary lesions and diaphragmatic hernia.
3. Gastrointestinal lesions, such as duodenal or esophageal atresia.
4. Urinary tract anomalies, such as renal dysplasia.
5. Skeletal anomalies.

Fetal Heart Rate Assessment

Nonstress and contraction stress tests use continuous wave Doppler ultrasound to monitor the fetal heart, allowing the clinician to make judgments about fetal condition. See Table 6.4 for selected indications for fetal heart rate testing and Tables 6.5

Table 6.4.

INDICATIONS FOR ANTEPARTUM FETAL
HEART RATE TESTING[a]

Hypertensive disorders
Diabetes mellitus
Cyanotic heart disease
History of previous stillbirth
Suspected intrauterine growth retardation
Postdate pregnancy
Decreased fetal activity
Meconium in amniotic fluid on amniocentesis or
   amnioscopy

[a]Adapted from Scalone R: Determination of fetal status. In Buckley K, Kulb NW (eds): *Handbook of Maternal-Newborn Nursing.*
New York, John Wiley & Sons, 1983, p 195.

and 6.6 for sample protocols. A nonstress test
(NST) is based on the theory that, in a healthy fetus, fetal movement will be accompanied by transient accelerations of the fetal heart rate. An external fetal monitor is used, and fetal movement is
recorded on the graph paper by noting "spikes" of
movement sensed by the tocodynamometer or by
having the mother or an observer mark the paper
when movement is felt. In general, a normal fetal
response consists of good fetal heart rate variability
(6–10 bpm) with three or more fetal movements accompanied by accelerations of the fetal heart of at
least 15 bpm, lasting 15–30 seconds or more in a
20-minute period. (Institutions may have slightly
different interpretations of normal fetal response.)
A reactive NST generally is predictive of continued
fetal health for 2–7 days depending on the type or
severity of obstetric risk identified in the client.

A nonreactive NST may be *abnormal,* when fetal accelerations either are absent or do not meet
the above criteria, or *unsatisfactory,* when no fetal
movement is appreciated or the tracing is of poor

quality. Lack of fetal movement may be due to a
transient fetal sleep state lasting approximately 20
minutes, the effect of certain drugs (phenobarbital
or central nervous system depressants), or fetal
compromise. An attempt may be made to elicit fetal
movement by stimulation or manipulation, by giving the mother food or drink, or by waiting for the
end of the sleep cycle or drug effect. Continued inability to elicit fetal movement is an abnormal NST
that requires further evaluation.

A contraction stress test (CST) measures fetal
response to uterine contractions and thus evaluates
uteroplacental sufficiency. It may be used to further evaluate the fetus after a nonreactive NST and
is preferred by some clinicians as the primary fetal
evaluation test. An external fetal monitor is applied,
and a baseline monitor strip is obtained. Contractions may occur spontaneously or be induced by
nipple stimulation (36, 37) or oxytocin infusion.
(Individual institutions will have approved protocols for the oxytocin challenge test or OCT.) For
proper interpretation there must be three contractions lasting 40–60 seconds in a 10-minute period.
A negative CST will show good fetal heart rate variability and no decelerations with contractions and
is thought to predict fetal health for 1–7 days, depending on the obstetric risk factors.

A positive CST will show persistent late decelerations with contractions. A suspicious CST shows
a few late decelerations that do not persist. Other
categories include the hyperstimulated CST, where
contractions are too frequent or last too long to allow valid interpretation (this can occur with nipple
stimulation as well as with oxytocin) (38, 39) and
an unsatisfactory CST, where the tracing is of poor
quality or the clinician is unable to establish a pattern of three contractions in 10 minutes. These
must be repeated in order to obtain correct data on

Table 6.5.

PROTOCOLS FOR NONSTRESS TEST[a]

 1. Explain the procedure to the patient, including the amount of time involved (usually 30 minutes to 1 hour).
 2. Instruct the patient to eat a meal before the test.
 3. Have the patient change into a gown and empty her bladder before the test.
 4. Place the patient in a semi-Fowler's position at a 30- to 45-degree angle with a slight left tilt (which can be
    facilitated by a folded blanket or sheet placed under the right hip).
 5. Place the patient on an external monitor and use an ultrasound transducer or a phonotransducer to record the
    fetal heart rate. A tocodynamometer should be used to document fetal movement.
 6. Record the patient's blood pressure initially and at 5- to 10-minute intervals.
 7. Instruct the patient to indicate each time fetal movement occurs by pressing the record button on the monitor.
 8. Readjust the ultrasound transducer and tocodynamometer as necessary to obtain the best possible tracing.
 9. Obtain a 20-minute graph of the fetal heart rate and fetal movement.
10. If the tracing is nonreactive, stimulate the fetus by abdominal palpation, and continue monitoring for another 20
    minutes. If it is still nonreactive, inform the physician at once.
11. Record all results and consultations on the patient's prenatal chart.

[a]Adapted from Scalone R: Determination of fetal status. In Buckley K, Kulb NW (eds): *Handbook of Maternal-Newborn Nursing.* New York,
John Wiley & Sons, 1983, p 196.

Table 6.6.

PROTOCOLS FOR CONTRACTION STRESS TEST[a]

1. Rule out contraindications to the contraction stress test: high risk for preterm labor or conditions in which uterine contractions may be dangerous (e.g., placenta previa).
2. Explain the testing procedure to the patient, including the amount of time involved (usually about 90 minutes, but may take 3 hours or more).
3. Have the patient change into a gown and empty her bladder.
4. Place the patient in a semi-Fowler's position at a 30- to 45-degree angle with a slight left tilt (which can be facilitated by a folded blanket or sheet placed under the right hip).
5. Place an external monitor on the patient. A phonotransducer or an ultrasound transducer is used to record the fetal heart rate, and a tocodynamometer is used to measure uterine contractions.
6. Record the patient's blood pressure initially and at 5- to 10-minute intervals.
7. Obtain a baseline recording of fetal heart rate for at least 10 minutes, and observe for spontaneous uterine contractions.
8. If there are no spontaneous contractions, in some institutions the patient may be asked to use nipple stimulation to try to induce contractions. Protocols vary, but one suggested protocol is given here. The patient is given a towel and asked to rub one nipple for 30 seconds. If no contractions are observed after 5 minutes, she is instructed to repeat the procedure. If there are no contractions after 5 minutes, she is instructed to try on the other side for 30 seconds. If there are no contractions after 5 minutes, she is instructed to rub the nipple with the towel for one minute. If contractions adequate for the CST are not induced, proceed with oxytocin infusion.
9. Start an intravenous infusion of 500 cc of 5% dextrose in water as a primary line to keep the vein open.
10. Prepare the oxytocin infusion:
    a. Five units of oxytocin are added to 250 cc of normal saline (0.9% solution). This yields a solution with a concentration of 20 mU of oxytocin per milliliter (to be used with a Harvard pump), *or* 2.5 units of oxytocin are added to 500 cc of normal saline (0.9% solution). This yields a solution with a concentration of 5 mU of oxytocin per milliliter (to be used with an IMED or a 2620 Harvard pump).
    b. Prepare the infusion pump.
    c. Set the infusion pump according to the dosage of oxytocin ordered by the obstetrician.
    d. Start the infusion (secondary line) by inserting the needle into the connector of the primary line. Be sure to keep the primary line running at a slow rate.
    e. Start with 0.2 mU/minute oxytocin. The oxytocin infusion may be increased every 15–20 minutes according to the following dosage schedule, until three moderate contractions occur within a 10-minute period:
       Start infusion at 0.2 mU/min
       0.4 mU/min
       1 mU/min
       2 mU/min
       4 mU/min
       8 mU/min
       10 mU/min
    f. The patient must be evaluated by the obstetrician when the dosage of oxytocin reaches 10 mU/min. If the oxytocin infusion is to be continued according to the obstetrician's orders, it is increased as follows:
       12 mU/min
       16 mU/min
       20 mU/min
11. Discontinue the oxytocin infusion if:
    a. Adequate stress is achieved (three moderately firm uterine contractions in 10 minutes);
    b. Hyperstimulation occurs (i.e., uterine contractions lasting longer than 60 seconds or less than 2 minutes apart); or
    c. Definite repetitive late decelerations are seen with uterine contractions.
12. After the oxytocin infusion has been discontinued, continue monitoring until:
    a. The fetal heart rate returns to a stable baseline; and
    b. Uterine contractions are decreased to the baseline level.
13. Review all results with the obstetrician and record them on the patient's prenatal chart.

[a]Adapted from Scalone R: Determination of fetal status. In Buckley K, Kulb NW (eds): *Handbook of Maternal-Newborn Nursing*. New York, John Wiley & Sons, 1983, pp 197–199.

fetal condition. A summary of the steps of fetal heart rate testing is given in Figure 6.3.

Statistically, false-positive and false-negative rates of any test are determined by the sensitivity and specificity of the test and by the prevalence of the condition being tested for in the population. Because of the low prevalence of perinatal mortality (approximately 20 in 1000 pregnancies), the false-negative rate of any test will be very low and the false-positive rate will be very high, unless the test is very sensitive and specific. In the case of NSTs and CSTs, the false-positive rate is high and may lead to unnecessary intervention, with associated risks for both mother and baby. At the same time,

Steps in Antepartum Fetal Heart Rate Testing

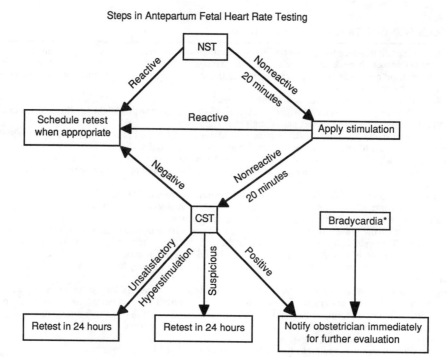

Figure 6.3. Steps in antepartum fetal heart rate testing.* Bradycardia is fetal heart rate of less than 100 beats/minute or a reduction of 40 beats/minute below the baseline for 60 seconds or longer. (Adapted from Scalone R: Determination of fetal status. In Buckley K, Kulb NW (eds): *Handbook of Maternal-Newborn Nursing.* New York, John Wiley & Sons, 1983, p 200.)

the low false-negative rate is statistically more related to the low prevalence of the condition in the population than to the specificity of the test. For this reason, after extensive review of the literature, Thacker and Berkelman of the Centers for Disease Control conclude that "published studies to date do not support use of the oxytocin challenge test or NST as screening tests or as diagnostic tests on which to base clinical intervention" (5, p 136). They encourage further study in randomized trials with large populations to determine if these tests are of clinical benefit.

Again, clinically, with both NSTs and CSTs, false-negative results are rare but false-positive rates are high. For CSTs, false-positives are reported in a range of 8–57%, averaging 30%, and false-positive NSTs are reported to occur in 10–35% of cases (35). False-positive CSTs occur more frequently when normal fetal heart reactivity and acceleration patterns accompany periodic decelerations. If the fetal heart reactivity is poor, there is a high probability of fetal compromise (40). The NST alone is a nonspecific test. Some clinicians believe that the loss of fetal heart rate variability and accel-

erations results from significant fetal acidosis, and they prefer the CST as an earlier measure of fetal jeopardy because it tests uteroplacental sufficiency and fetal response to stress. Because of this significant incidence of false-positive tests, management decisions about high risk pregnancy should incorporate variables other than positive NST or CST results alone (41, p 283).

It is imperative, with any test of placental insufficiency, for the client to be in the semi-Fowler's position, tilted slightly to the left side; her blood pressure should be checked regularly. This is to avoid the supine hypotension syndrome: compression of the vena cava by the uterus, resulting in decreased uterine blood flow. This could not only cause temporary fetal compromise but also a false-positive result, which will not accurately reflect fetal status.

Biophysical Profile

A biophysical profile has been developed based on the theory that multiple assessments of fetal status will provide a more reliable and sensitive evaluation than any one indicator. Five parameters are used together in this scored system of analysis: (1)

Table 6.7.
FETAL BIOPHYSICAL PROFILE[a]

BIOPHYSICAL PARAMETER	NORMAL: SCORE = 2	ABNORMAL: SCORE = 0
Nonstress test	Reactive pattern: At least 3 FHR accelerations of ≥15 BPM and ≥15 seconds' duration, associated with fetal movement in a 20-min period.	Nonreactive pattern: <2 FHR accelerations of ≥15 BPM and 15 seconds' duration associated with fetal movement in 40 min.
Fetal breathing movements	Present: Presence of at least 1 episode of fetal breathing of ≥60 sec duration within a 30-min period of observation.	Absent: Absence of fetal breathing movements or the absence of an episode of fetal breathing movements of ≥60 seconds' duration during a 30-min period of observation.
Gross fetal body movement	Present: Presence of at least 3 discrete episodes of fetal movement within a 30-min period. Simultaneous limb and trunk movements are counted as a single movement.	Decreased: Two or fewer discrete fetal movements in a 30-min period of observation.
Fetal tone	Upper and lower extremities in full flexion. Trunk in position of flexion and head flexed on chest. At least 1 episode of extension of limbs with return to position of flexion and/or extension of spine with return to flexion.	Decreased: Limbs in position of extension or partial flexion. Spine in extension. Fetal movement not followed by return to flexion. Fetal hand open.
Volume of amniotic fluid	Fluid evident throughout the uterine cavity. Largest pocket of fluid greater than 1 cm in vertical diameter.	Decreased: Fluid absent in most areas of uterine cavity. Largest pocket of fluid measure 1 cm or less in vertical axis. Crowding of fetal small parts.

[a]Adapted with permission from Oxorn, H: *Human Labor and Birth*, ed 5. Norwalk, CT, Appleton-Century-Crofts, p 609.

NST; (2) count of fetal breathing movements; (3) count of gross body movements; (4) assessment of fetal body tone; and (5) measure of amniotic fluid volume. Recently, placental grading, an evaluation of placental maturity, has been added as a sixth parameter in some institutions. These physiologic variables are associated with a well-functioning, well-oxygenated fetal central nervous system (43). Since each individual variable may be affected by cyclic variations, simultaneous evaluation of all factors is thought to reduce the possibility of false-positive results.

These five variables are assigned a score of 2 for a normal response or 0 if the normal response is absent. Table 6.7 details the scoring process.

A score of 8–10 correlates well with a normal outcome for the fetus. A score of 0–2 is associated with a high incidence of perinatal mortality. More research is needed to fine tune interpretation of scores 4–6. It is known that a score of 4–6 when oligohydramnios is present warrants immediate intervention.

Radiologic Assessment

The risks of ionizing radiation to the developing fetus have long been established, with mutation and increased risk of malignancy in childhood the most commonly recognized (41, p 230). In addition, techniques requiring the injection of radi-

opaque agents are associated with meconium staining, falsely low estriols, and falsely elevated lecithin/sphingomyelin (L:S) ratios.

With the development of ultrasound, x-ray has been used less frequently in obstetric care. Much of the information sought by x-ray technique can be obtained by a good sonogram. However, x-ray sometimes may be justified in evaluation of the fetus.

A simple x-ray will show the fetal skeleton after about 16 weeks' gestation and will identify the number of fetuses in a multiple pregnancy. Some clinicians have used x-ray to evaluate lower limb ossification in the third trimester as an index of fetal maturity. In late pregnancy a single x-ray may identify gross abnormalities such as anencephaly or confirm a fetal malpresentation, such as transverse lie or breech with head extension.

Amniography is a technique that requires the injection of a radiopaque agent into the amniotic sac. It is used to evaluate abnormalities in AFV or placental location, and it provides a silhouette of the fetus that may suggest certain anomalies. Several hours after the injection of the agent and after the fetus has swallowed a quantity of fluid, the fetal gastrointestinal tract can be visualized in order to determine the presence of anomalies.

Fetography also requires the injection of a special radiopaque agent into the amniotic sac. This agent adheres to the vernix, providing a sharper silhouette of the fetus, and thus is more useful in the diagnosis of some soft tissue anomalies.

Intrauterine Assessment

Although clinical and ultrasonic methods of assessment can provide a great deal of information about the fetus, sometimes it is necessary to enter the uterine cavity to obtain important or timely data about the baby's condition.

Amniocentesis

Amniocentesis is the most common and best studied of the intrauterine procedures. It is done at different times during pregnancy for various reasons. In early pregnancy (before 20 weeks' gestation) it is used to determine fetal genetic normalcy; in the late third trimester it provides data on fetal maturity or well-being. Generally, the procedure is done under direct ultrasound visualization of the uterine contents to reduce the risk of trauma to the baby or placenta.

Once the entry site through the abdominal wall is determined, the skin is washed with an antiseptic solution, and the area is infiltrated with local anesthetic. A 20- to 22-gauge 4-inch needle is inserted through the abdominal wall into the uterus, and amniotic fluid is aspirated; this specimen is then centrifuged into two fractions: a cellular portion used for chromosomal and enzyme studies and a supernatant used for biochemical analyses. After the procedure, the client should be monitored for cramping or contractions, and the fetal heart also should be monitored if appropriate.

The risks of amniocentesis include trauma to the fetus, cord, placenta, or maternal organs; intrauterine infection; abortion; or premature labor. The National Institutes of Child Health and Human Development (NICCHD) established an Amniocentesis Registry in 1971 to undertake a prospective evaluation of the risks of midtrimester amniocentesis; to date, there has been no evidence of increased rates of fetal loss, perinatal problems, birth defects, or neonatal complications. Long-term follow-up has not revealed differences in infant growth, development, or behavior at 1 year of age (15). However, a study in Britain (43) did indicate a slightly higher fetal loss and an increase in neonatal respiratory difficulties and orthopedic problems in the amniocentesis group. In general, however, the NICCHD concluded that the overall accuracy of diagnosis with midtrimester amniocentesis is greater than 99.4%, and the overall risk of fetal loss is less than 0.5% in the United States (1–2% in the United Kingdom studies).

Third trimester amniocentesis has not been studied as extensively, but the NICCHD task force on amniocentesis concluded that serious adverse consequences are extremely uncommon, although fetal hemorrhage and premature labor may occur. Therefore, it is imperative that mother and fetus be monitored carefully after the procedure. In all cases of amniocentesis, the unsensitized RH-negative mother should receive RhoGAM due to the possibility of fetomaternal transfusion. Bloody contamination of amniotic fluid during the procedure may alter the results of some of the biochemical tests (see next section).

The benefits of amniocentesis are clear: it is indispensable in the prenatal diagnosis of certain congenital defects and in the management of some high risk conditions, such as Rh isoimmunization. It is certainly indicated when preterm delivery of the infant is being considered.

Fetoscopy

Fetoscopy allows direct visualization of the fetus and placenta. This procedure generally is done in the second trimester and requires ultrasound confirmation of fetal and placental location to choose an entry site. The abdominal skin is washed with an antiseptic solution, and local anesthesia is given. The abdominal and uterine walls are incised and a cannula inserted into the amniotic cavity. A narrow instrument is then inserted through the cannula, allowing small areas of the fetus to be visualized; the extremities, genitalia, or facies can be examined for defects. Skin biopsy may be done, and fetal blood samples can be obtained from the umbilical cord or, preferably, from the large placental blood vessels in order to diagnose hemoglobin abnormalities such as sickle cell anemia or fetal infections (e.g., rubella) (44).

Risks of this procedure are similar to but greater than those associated with amniocentesis. Miscarriage may occur in 5–10% of pregnancies (3–5% in centers that have more experience), and a 9–10% prematurity rate has been reported (17). Since the procedure still is considered "applied research," it must be performed by experienced clinicians in well-equipped institutions. Ultrasound and amniocentesis may provide much of the same information, but fetoscopy will be of benefit in certain situations (such as dermatologic or hematologic abnormalities) when diagnosis is otherwise unobtainable but necessary. A major future application of fetoscopy undoubtedly will be fetal surgery and therapy.

Chorionic Villi Sampling

Chorionic villi sampling (CVS) is a relatively new procedure under research in the United States, although it has been used for several years in certain European countries. Performed under ultrasound visualization in early gestation (8–12 weeks, after fetal organogenesis is complete), the procedure is used to detect chromosomal abnormalities in the fetus. It requires the insertion of a cannula through the vagina and cervix and into the uterus. A sample of the chorionic villi is removed by gentle suction for analysis. The accuracy of CVS seems similar to that of amniocentesis except in the case of neural tube defects. Since this tissue is of fetal origin, results can be obtained in 2 weeks rather than the 3–4 weeks required for amniocentesis. Thus, diagnosis of certain congenital anomalies can be made at a much earlier point in pregnancy than with traditional amniocentesis. Therapeutic termination of pregancy, if required, may be done at an earlier point in gestation with lower risk. Preliminary reports suggest that the fetal loss after CVS is somewhat higher than with amniocentesis; however, since the procedure is done in the first trimester, the possibility exists that some of these losses would have terminated spontaneously even without CVS, so the true rates of pregnancy loss may be lower.

LABORATORY ASSESSMENT

Amniotic Fluid

Chromosomal analysis for detection of genetic abnormality or hereditary disease requires cultivation of amniotic fluid cells by tissue culture methods. Fetal sex and chromosomes can be identified with a sufficient number of growing cells. Genetic abnormalities such as chromosomal aberrations and x-linked or autosomal disorders then can be identified. Approximately 75 inborn errors of metabolism are detectable in this way (see Chapter 25). Such procedures generally require 2–4 weeks before results are available. Blood or bacterial contamination of the amniotic fluid sample may inhibit the growth of the cells.

Biochemical constituents of the amniotic fluid can be detected and measured in the laboratory.

Alpha Fetoprotein

Alpha fetoprotein (AFP) is the major circulating protein of the early human fetus; it is synthesized by the yolk sac and fetal liver. Peak levels occur at about 13 weeks of gestation and then decrease with advancing gestational age. Elevated AFP levels are associated with open neural tube and other congenital defects (e.g., congenital nephrosis, esophageal atresia, Turner syndrome, Potter syndrome, and exomphalos). Proper evaluation of AFP levels requires precise dating of the pregnancy since most false-positives are due to incorrectly interpreted gestational age (45) (see chapter 25).

Bilirubin

Bilirubin is detectable in amniotic fluid. Its level should fall progressively in the latter half of a pregnancy uncomplicated by Rh isoimmunization. Bilirubin concentration is measured by spectrophotometric analysis. Disappearance of bilirubin peak at OD (optical density) 450 is considered evidence of fetal maturity, but the major use of bilirubin analysis is in evaluating fetal hemolytic disease (see Chapter 29).

Creatinine

Creatinine concentration in the amniotic fluid rises in the latter half of pregnancy. Near term, it increases rapidly because of expanding fetal muscle mass and maturing kidneys. A level of 2.0 mg/dl in the fluid is probable evidence of maturity. Alterations in maternal serum creatinine will be reflected in the fetal sample and may affect correct interpretation.

Pulmonary Indices

Pulmonary indices are the best measure of fetal maturity. Cells in the maturing fetal lung produce surfactant, or surface active phospholipids, essential for the maintenance of effective respiration after birth. These can be measured to give an indication of fetal readiness for extrauterine life.

1. Crucial components of surfactant (lecithin and phosphatidylglycerol) can be identified and measured in the amniotic fluid. Concentration of lecithin in relation to another lipid, sphingomyelin, is lower in early pregnancy, rising to roughly equal at about 30–34 weeks. After 34 weeks the lecithin/sphingomyelin (L:S) ratio increases as surfactant is produced. When the L:S ratio is ≥2.0:1, the fetal lungs are probably mature and the risk of respiratory distress syndrome (RDS) is slight, unless the mother has diabetes (46). False-positive and false-negative L:S ratios have been reported, but the true incidence is unclear. L:S ratios ≥2.0 associated with neonatal RDS may be due to laboratory error, maternal diabetes, or any event that causes the infant to be compromised seriously at birth. L:S ratios <2.0 associated with pulmonary maturity may occur because the time interval between testing and delivery allowed for maturation of the fetal lungs (47).

2. The shake test is based on the ability of surfactant to produce stable foam when mixed with ethanol. A sample of amniotic fluid and ethanol is shaken vigorously for 15 seconds and then left upright for a period of time. If the ring of bubbles on the fluid surface remains intact for 15 minutes, the test is positive and the risk of RDS is presumed very low (48). However, a false-negative result is common: the ring of foam does not persist for 15 minutes even when the lungs are mature. The L:S ratio is considered more reliable. Both the L:S ratio and the shake test can be contaminated by blood or meconium, causing a false-negative result.

3. Phosphatidylglycerol enhances the surface active properties of lecithin, and its presence in the amniotic fluid sample is presumed to indicate pulmonary maturity and minimal risk of RDS (49, 50). In addition, the detection of phosphatidylglycerol is apparently not hampered by the presence of blood or meconium. A rapid slide test (Amniostat-FLM) detects the presence of phosphatidylglycerol.

Thromboplastic Activity

Thromboplastic activity of the amniotic fluid (TAAF) increases with gestational age, possibly as thromboplastins are liberated from degenerating desquamated fetal cells as the fetus matures (51). TAAF decelerates rapidly after 40 weeks' gestation. TAAF is measured by mixing amniotic fluid with normal plasma and noting the time required for clotting to occur. Studies indicate that in a gestation of 43 weeks or longer, TAAF is less than 45 seconds; pregnancies of 42 weeks or less show TAAF ranging from 45–60 seconds. Proponents recommend that any pregnancy with a TAAF of less than 45 seconds be regarded as postmature and at high risk (52, 53).

Meconium

The presence of meconium in the amniotic fluid when postmaturity is suspected is suggestive of perinatal risk. Most authorities agree that the benefit of this sole finding does not outweigh the risks of amniocentesis (54). When amniotic fluid samples are needed for other biochemical tests, however, this finding will complement the picture. If found, it requires full evaluation.

Maternal Blood and Urine

Alpha Fetoprotein

AFP can be detected in maternal blood as well as in amniotic fluid. Attempts have been made to correlate serum levels of AFP with fetal well-being, but its most important application is as a screening tool to detect congenital defects. As with amniotic fluid AFP levels, correct interpretation is dependent on precise dating of the pregnancy (see Chapter 26).

Estriol

Estriol determination was once a common measure of fetal well-being and placental function. Estriol (E3), the principal estrogen originating in the placenta, is derived from the metabolism of estrone (E1) and estradiol (E2). In the first half of pregnancy, the estrogen precursors originate primarily in the maternal adrenal glands; the fetal adrenals begin to contribute estrogen precursors in the second half of pregnancy. By term about 60% of these precursors are of fetal origin (55). The estriol produced in the fetoplacental unit enters maternal circulation as free or unconjugated E3; most of it is then conjugated in the maternal liver. Levels of E3 should increase during pregnancy until term, with a sharp rise at about 35–36 weeks. Unconjugated E3 is thought to be a better measure of changes in placental function; total E3 levels will be dependent on maternal conjugation, hepatic function, and renal clearance (56).

Estriols can be measured in a single specimen of plasma or in a 24-hour urine collection. Interpretation of serum estriols may be affected by normal fluctuations or diurnal variations in blood levels; 24-hour urine estriols may be difficult to obtain. True levels will be affected by kidney function or other conditions that affect excretion; 24-hour specimens also should have creatinine measurements to ensure reliability of the specimen. Creatinine excretion should exceed 1 g in 24 hours. If less creatinine is present, the specimen should be suspected of containing less than a 24-hour collection. Both serum and urine estriols will be altered by changes in levels of placental precursors. For example, maternal ingestion of corticosteroids or certain fetal anomalies that depress adrenal secretion will lower estriol. Certain antibiotics (ampicillin, neomycin) will lower estriol levels by altering the intestinal flora, resulting in a decreased reabsorption of estriol conjugates into the circulation.

Interpretation of results depends on laboratory standards and analysis. In general, a fall of >50% in a single specimen or a 35–40% drop from the mean of three previous serum measurements is considered significant. A 24-hour urine specimen at term usually will contain ≥12 mg; 4 mg or less is associated with severe fetal compromise.

There is some disagreement as to the reliability of low estriol levels in predicting fetal compromise (55). Only one prospective controlled study has evaluated the usefulness of estriol determinations and found that the use of estriols had little or no effect on reducing perinatal morbidity (57).

Thus, if estriols are used at all, management decisions still will be based on a wider clinical picture. High estriol levels generally are reassuring.

Human Chorionic Gonadotropin

Human chorionic gonadotropin (HCG) is produced by the syncytiotrophoblast. Levels peak in maternal serum and urine at 60–80 days' gestation. The beta subunit of HCG (bHCG) can be detected in maternal serum as early as 10 days after fertilization.

HCG primarily is useful in pregnancy testing; serial quantitative measurements also are used to diagnose certain abnormal conditions such as threatened or missed abortion, hydatidiform mole, or ectopic pregnancy. Studies have correlated the appearance of the gestational sac on ultrasound with bHCG levels of 6000–6500 mIU/ml. If serum levels are higher but no gestational sac is seen, there is a strong probability of ectopic pregnancy. Levels that are dramatically high at a given gestational age are associated with multiple gestation, erythroblastosis fetalis, and hydatidiform mole. If a gestational sac is seen but serum levels are lower than expected, a threatened or missed abortion should be considered (58). Several studies have demonstated the usefulness and accuracy of quantitative bHCG measurements in dating pregnancy because the rapid rise in HCG in the first 60 days of pregnancy apparently has minimal individual variation (59).

Others

Other constituents of maternal serum that have been used in evaluating pregnancy include oxytocinase and placental phosphatase, enzymes originating in the syncytiotrophoblast. Theoretically, the ability of the placenta to oxygenate and nourish the fetus should be reflected in the normal synthesis and release of these enzymes (60). Their usefulness, however, has not been clearly established.

REFERENCES

1. Coleman C: Fetal movement counts: an assessment tool. *J Nurse-Midwifery* 26(1):15, 1981.
2. Sadovsky E, Polishuk W: Fetal movement in utero: nature, assessment, prognostic value, timing of delivery. *Obstet Gynecol* 50:49, 1977.
3. Pearson J: Fetal movements: a new approach to antenatal care. *Nurs Mirror* 144:49, 1977.
4. Neldam S: Fetal movements: A comparison between maternal assessment and registration by means of dynamic ultrasound. *Dan Med Bull* 29:197, 1982.
5. Thacker SB, Berkelman RL: Assessing the diagnostic accuracy and efficacy of selected antepartum fetal surveillance techniques. *Obstet Gynecol Survey* 41:121–141, 1986.
6. Quaranta R: Symphyseal-fundal height in the prediction of IUGR. *Br J Obstet Gynecol* 88:115, 1981.
7. Westin B: The gravidogram and prediction of intrauterine growth retardation. *Acta Obstet Gynecol Scand* 56:273, 1977.
8. Belizan J: Diagnosis of intrauterine growth retardation by measurement of uterine height. *Am J Obstet Gynecol* 131(6):643, 1978.
9. Bowe E: Amnioscopy and fetal blood sampling. In Spellacy W (ed): *Management of High Risk Pregnancy*. Baltimore, University Park Press, 1976, p 227.
10. Bowe E: Amnioscopy. *Clin Obstet Gynecol* 12(2):527, 1969.
11. Roversi G, Canussio M: Importance of amnioscopy. *J Perinatal Med* 6(2):109, 1978.
12. Saling E: Amnioscopy. *Clin Obstet Gynecol* 9(2):472, 1966.
13. Anderson F: Gestational age assessment I. *Am J Obstet Gynecol* 139(2):173, 1981.
14. Anderson F: Gestational age assessment II. *Am J Obstet Gynecol* 140(7):770, 1981.
15. Griffith C: Basic physics. In Sabbagha R (ed): *Diagnostic Ultrasound in Obstetrics and Gynecology*. Hagerstown, MD, Harper & Row, 1980.
16. Romero R, Jeanty P, Hobbins J: Diagnostic ultrasound in the first trimester of pregnancy. *Clin Obstet Gynecol* 27(2):286, 1984.
17. *Antenatal Diagnosis. Report of a Consensus Development Conference National Institutes of Health Publication #79-1973*. Washington, DC, U.S. Government Printing Office, 1979.
18. NIH Consensus Development Panel: The use of diagnostic ultrasound imaging in pregnancy. Report of a conference at NIH, February 1984. Reprinted in *J Nurse-Midwifery* 29(4):235, 1984.
19. Kremkau F: Safety and long term effects of ultrasound. *Clin Obstet Gynecol* 27(2):269, 1984.
20. Fletcher J, Evans M: Maternal bonding and ultrasound. *N Engl J Med* 308(7):392, 1983.
21. Petrucha R, Golde S, Platt L: Use of ultrasound in prediction of fetal pulmonary maturity. *Am J Obstet Gynecol* 144(8):931, 1982.
22. Sabbagha R, Hughey M: Standardization of sonar cephalometry and gestational age. *Obstet Gynecol* 52:402, 1978.
23. Sabbagha R: Growth-adjusted sonographic age. *Obstet Gynecol* 51:383, 1978.
24. O'Brien G: Assessment of gestational age in second trimester by real-time ultrasound measurement of femur length. *Am J Obstet Gynecol* 139:540, 1981.
25. Chervenak F, Jeanty P, Hobbins J: Current status of fetal age and growth assessment. *Clin Obstet Gynecol* 10(3):424, 1983.
26. Campbell S, Dewhurst C: Diagnosis of small for dates fetus by serial ultrasound cephalometry. *Lancet* ii:1002, 1971.

27. Campbell S, Thoms A: Ultrasound measurement of fetal head to abdomen ratio in assessment of growth retardation. *Br J Obstet Gynecol* 84:165, 1977.
28. Hadlock F: Sonographic detection of abnormal fetal growth patterns. *Clin Obstet Gynecol* 27(2):342, 1984.
29. Manning F, Hill L, Platt L: Qualitative amniotic fluid volume determination by ultrasound. *Am J Obstet Gynecol* 139:254, 1981.
30. Crowley P: Nonqualitative estimation of amniotic fluid volume in prolonged pregnancy. *J Perinatal Med* 8:249, 1980.
31. Chamberlain P, Manning F: Ultrasound evaluation of amniotic fluid volume. *Am J Obstet Gynecol* 150(3):245, 1984.
32. Gottesfield K: Clinical role of placental imaging. *Clin Obstet Gynecol* 27(2):327, 1984.
33. Grannum P: Ultrasound examination of the placenta. *Clin Obstet Gynecol* 10(3):464, 1983.
34. Grannum P, Berkowitz R, Hobbins J: Ultrasonic changes in the maturing placenta and their relation to fetal maturity. *Am J Obstet Gynecol* 133:915, 1979.
35. Harman C, Manning F: Correlation of ultrasonic placental grading and fetal pulmonary maturation. *Am J Obstet Gynecol* 143(8):941, 1982.
36. Oki E: A protocol for a nipple stimulation contraction stress test. *Contemp Obstet Gynecol* 22(4):157, 1983.
37. Huddleston J, Sutcliff G, Robinson D: Contraction stress test by intermittent nipple stimulation. *Obstet Gynecol* 63(5):669, 1984.
38. Lenke R, Nemes J: Use of nipple stimulation to obtain a contraction stress test. *Obstet Gynecol* 63(3):345, 1984.
39. Viegas O, Arulkunaran S, et al.: Nipple stimulation in late pregnancy causing uterine hyperstimulation. *Br J Obstet Gynecol* 91(4):364, 1984.
40. Freeman R, Garite T: *Fetal Heart Rate Monitoring*. Baltimore, Williams & Wilkins, 1981, p 145.
41. Pritchard J, MacDonald P: *Williams Obstetrics*, ed 17. New York, Appleton-Century-Crofts, 1984.
42. Manning F, Platt L, Sipos L: Antepartum fetal evaluation: development of a fetal biophysical profile. *Am J Obstet Gynecol* 136(6):787.
43. Working Party on Amniocentesis: Report to the MRS. *Br J Obstet Gynecol* 85 (Suppl):2, 1978.
44. Rodeck C: Fetoscopy and fetal blood sampling. In Wald N (ed): *Antenatal and Neonatal Screening*. London, Oxford University Press, 1984, p 457.
45. Chard T: Monitoring of the high risk pregnancy by alpha fetoprotein. In Spellacy W (ed): *Management of High Risk Pregnancy*. Baltimore, University Park Press, 1976, p 83.
46. Gluck L: Diagnosis of the respiratory distress syndrome by amniocentesis. *J Obstet Gynecol* 109:440, 1971.
47. Farrell P, Zachman R: Pulmonary surfactant in respiratory distress syndrome. In Farrell P, Avery M (eds): *Hyaline Membrane Disease. Am Rev Resp Dis* 3:657, 1975.
48. Clemens J: Assessment of risk of RDS by a rapid test for surfactant in amniotic fluid. *N Engl J Med* 286:1077, 1972.
49. Hallman M: Absence of phosphatidylglycerol in the respiratory distress syndrome in newborns. *Pediatr Res* 11:714, 1977.
50. Hallman M: Phosphatidylinositol and phosphatidylglycerol in amniotic fluid: indices of lung maturity. *Am J Obstet Gynecol* 125:613, 1976.
51. Hastwell G: Accelerated clotting time: an amniotic fluid thromboplastic activity index of fetal maturity. *Am J Obstet Gynecol* 131(6):650, 1978.
52. Yaffe H, Hay-am E, Sadovsky E: Thromboplastic activity of amniotic fluid in term and postmature gestation. *Obstet Gynecol* 57(4):490, 1981.
53. Yaffe H, Elder A, Hornshtein E: Thromboplastic activity in amniotic fluid during pregnancy. *Obstet Gynecol* 50:454, 1977.
54. Green J, Paul R: Value of amniocentesis in prolonged pregnancy. *Obstet Gynecol* 51(3): 293, 1978.
55. Tulchinsky D: Value of estrogens in high risk pregnancy. In Spellacy W (ed): *Management of High Risk Pregnancy*. Baltimore, University Park Press, 1976, p 29.
56. Distler W: Estriol in pregnancy. *Am J Obstet Gynecol* 130(4):424, 1978.
57. Duenholter J, Whalley P, MacDonald P: Analysis of utility of plasma estrogen measurements in determining delivery time of gravidas with a fetus considered at risk. *Am J Obstet Gynecol* 125:889, 1976.
58. Kadar N: Discriminatory HCG zone: its use in evaluation of ectopic pregnancy. *Obstet Gynecol* 58(2):156, 1981.
59. Lagrew D, Wilson E, Fried A: Accuracy of serum HCG concentrations and ultrasonic fetal measurements. *Am J Obstet Gynecol* 149:165, 1985.
60. Hensleigh P: Enzymatic assessment of the high risk pregnancy: oxytocinase and placental phosphatase. In Spellacy W (ed): *Management of High Risk Pregnancy*. Baltimore, University Park Press, 1976, p 49.

Section II: Selected Health Problems

Chapter 7
Disorders of the Immune System

Kathleen Buckley, C.N.M., M.S.N.

INTRODUCTION

Immunity is the mechanism that provides specific protection against a particular foreign microorganism or molecular entity. It is characterized by two major factors: (1) the ability to differentiate the body's own cell structure (self) from that which is foreign (nonself) and (2) the ability to inactivate or destroy foreign microorganisms or molecular entity matter (1, p 115).

The ability to inactivate or destroy foreign microorganisms is due to the body's ability to create and to activate specific protein substances (i.e., antibodies). One way in which antibodies are classified is according to their destructive capabilities (1, p 116):

1. Precipitants render a foreign substance insoluble;
2. Opsonins increase the ability of leukocytes to ingest bacteria;
3. Antitoxins counteract bacterial toxins;
4. Agglutinins cause clumping of foreign cells; and
5. Lysins dissolve cells.

The lymphoreticular system is responsible for producing the human immune response. Important organs and systems of the lymphoreticular system include the bone marrow, spleen, thymus, lymph nodes, tonsils, and various groups of lymphocytes and macrophages. The immune system originates in the bone marrow stem cells, which produce potential immunocompetent cells. These cells, then, are transported to and mature in specific microenvironments in the gastrointestinal tract or the thymus (2, p 288).

Functional Divisions of the Immune System

Two major forms or divisions of the immune system have been identified: humoral and cellular.

Humoral immunity is mediated by B-cell lymphocytes. B lymphocytes are so named because they were first discovered in the bursa of Fabricius in birds. This designation still stands because the analogous human organ or system has yet to be identified. However, it is thought that the human B cells probably mature in the lymphoid tissue of the gastrointestinal tract (3, p 81). These cells play an active role in the inflammatory response and are the first line of defense against foreign substances or antigens. They act by secreting specific proteins called immunoglobulins, and they attach to foreign substances circulating in serum and exocrine or extravascular fluid. Important human immunoglobulins are IgG, IgM, and IgA (4). Their properties and functions are detailed in Table 7.1.

After the body has been exposed to an antigen, B-cell immunoglobulin *primary* response begins immediately. Specific immunoglobulins—principally IgM—appear within 48–72 hours. A *secondary* response—principally IgG—begins 24–48 hours after antigen contact and lasts much longer.

Another feature of the humoral response is its ability to activate complement. Complement is a complex series of enzymes found in the serum. In the presence of immunoglobulins, these enzymes are activated and become able to fix or cement the invading antigen to a particular antibody (2, p 309).

61

Table 7.1.
PROPERTIES OF SPECIFIC IMMUNOGLOBULINS[a]

PROPERTY	IMMUNOGLOBULINS		
	IgG	IgM	IgA
1. Physiochemical percent of immunoglobulin in normal adult serum	82%	7%	10%
2. Principal site found	Serum; extravascular fluids	Serum	Serum; exocrine fluids (e.g., breast milk, mucin, saliva, tears)
3. Complement fixation	Yes	Yes	No
4. Crosses placenta	Yes	No	No
5. Principal functions	Agglutination; detoxification lysis; enhanced phagocytosis	Agglutination; lysis; enhanced phagocytosis	Protection of mucosal surfaces

[a]Adapted from Mahoney E, Flynn J: *Handbook of Medical-Surgical Nursing.* New York, John Wiley and Sons, pp 115–119.

This action futher ensures dissolution of the antigen.

The other dimension of the immune system is cellular immunity. Cellular immunity is based on the function of T cells. T cells are so named because they mature in the thymus (1, pp 116–117). These cells are responsible for initiating response to nonself cells found in organs or systems. Thus, they mediate defense against neoplastic growth and are responsible for rejection of transplanted organs. T cells also play a large role in the chronic, progressive diseases discussed in this chapter because an immune system that is damaged and unable to distinguish self from nonself may direct its powerful capacities to destroy its own body's organs (5, p 475).

Disorders of the Immune System

Disorders of the immune system can be classified into four categories (2, p 315):

1. Decreased immune response system (e.g., AIDS; DiGeorge syndrome—absence of neonatal thymus resulting in absence of T-cell response; infantile sex-linked agammaglobulinemia—grossly depressed B-cell production).
2. Hypergammopathies—overproduction in response to inappropriate antigen stimulation (e.g., multiple myeloma).
3. Hypersensitivity—allergy (e.g., hemolytic disease of the newborn, transfusion reactions, glomerulonephritis, tuberculin reaction).
4. Autoimmunity—inability to distinguish self from nonself (e.g., rheumatoid arthritis, lupus erythematosus).

Antinuclear Antibodies

In autoimmune disease the body's immune system perceives portions of its own cell nuclei as foreign. The immune system produces specific antibodies against the nuclei, and these are designated as antinuclear antibodies (ANA).

ANA are found in the serum of patients with viral disease, chronic hepatic disease, and autoimmune disease. Levels of ANA tend to be highest in the autoimmune diseases. The highest titers are seen with systemic lupus erythematosus with levels rising as high as 1:256 (2, p 315).

Changes in the Immune System during Pregnancy

Pregnancy has been described as an immune suppressed state. It has been documented that T-cell function is inhibited and that the number of B cells produced is decreased (5, p 475).

Besides B-cell decrement, evidence points to further decreased effectiveness of the humoral response:

1. Suppressed bactericidal potential;
2. Decreased ability to lyse or fix cells (e.g., complement fixation); and
3. Decreased response to antigens, possibly mediated by a pregnancy-related glycoprotein (e.g., PZP or pregnancy zone protein).

Although all of these mechanisms are poorly understood, it is not hard to imagine that the suppression of the immune system during pregnancy constitutes a protective milieu for the fetus—a truly nonself being. Furthermore, the overall suppressed immune response is thought to decrease the inflammatory response, which may account for the improvement noted in some autoimmune diseases during pregnancy (6, p 265). It would also seem likely that decreased immune function might play a role in increasing the rate of infection during

Table 7.2.
DRUGS USED TO TREAT RHEUMATOID ARTHRITIS DURING PREGNANCY

DRUG USED	DOSE	MATERNAL SIDE EFFECTS	FETAL SIDE EFFECTS
Salicylates	3.6–4.0 g p.o. per day to achieve 20 mg/100 ml blood level	Salicylism; gastrointestinal irritation; anemia, prematurity, prenatal/postpartum hemorrhage due to prostaglandin inhibition	Withdrawal syndrome; decreased platelet function causing hemorrhage; increased intracranial hemorrhage in premature or low birth weight babies; increased prenatal mortality
Gold	50 mg i.m. per week for 20 weeks then decrease to maintain effects	Pruritic skin rash; bone marrow suppression; immune system nephritis; colitis; lung toxicity; hepatotoxicity	No known side effects; poor placental transfer
Corticosteroids, Intra-articular	5–20 mg, intra-articular, depending on size of joint	Minimal systemic absorption—none noted	Minimal systemic absorption—none noted

[a]Adapted from Burrow G, Ferris, T. *Medical Complications in Pregnancy*. Philadelphia, WB Saunders, 1982, pp 474–497.

pregnancy, particularly those infections in the susceptible genitourinary tract. Although this hypothesis seems logical, research to support it is scanty.

However, it is interesting to note that the dual suppression of the immune system brought about by the normal changes in pregnancy and the pathological changes of increased psychological stress has been postulated as a cause of preterm labor (see Chapter 28).

Physical and emotional stress are thought to be implicated in the initiation and exacerbation of many chronic diseases, and they may somehow alter the immune system. The synergistic effects of pregnancy and stress on the immune system and on the incidence of infection and preterm labor, as well as the role of chronic stress in the cause of autoimmune diseases, will be the focus of intensive future research.

RHEUMATOID ARTHRITIS

Definition

Rheumatoid arthritis is a chronic systemic disease occurring in joint cavity bursae and tendon sheaths (e.g., the synovium). It is three times more common in women than men. Onset usually occurs between ages 25–45 (3, p 97). Thus, it can be expected to be seen in women of childbearing age.

The disease follows a progressive, destructive course (1, p 586):

1. Inflammation of the joints, bursae, and tendon sheaths.

2. Development of an inflammatory exudate overlying synovial cells.
3. Further swelling because of the process described in #2 causes distention of joints and stretching of capsule and collateral ligaments.
4. Finally, destruction of the protective synovial membrane leads to bone and joint destruction and deformity. Normal joint motion is impaired and ultimately destroyed.

Etiology

Although the etiology is unknown, there is strong evidence to support impairment of the autoimmune system as the causative factor. Studies have demonstrated a specific impaired T-cell response—delayed hypersensitive skin test reaction. The B-cell immune response also is implicated in the synovial inflammatory process. Quantities of IgG have been found in synovial fluid and sera of patients with rheumatoid arthritis. IgG, combining with complement fixation factors in the synovium, may be the cause of the rheumatoid inflammatory reaction (1, p 586).

Other postulated etiologies include viral, bacterial, or genetic factors.

Signs and Symptoms

The patient typically presents with the complaint of symmetrical joint pain, tenderness, and stiffness, swelling, and redness of the involved joints. Usually, this is accompanied by morning stiffness, early afternoon fatigue, anorexia, weight loss, low grade fever, and systemic malaise. The disease is characterized by cyclic acute exacerbations and remissions.

TABLE 7.3.
DRUGS USED TO TREAT RHEUMATOID ARTHRITIS INTRACONCEPTUALLY[a]

DRUG USED	DOSE	MATERNAL SIDE EFFECTS	FETAL SIDE EFFECTS
Azathioprine	Varies—1 mg/kg/day	Gastrointestinal irritation; bone marrow suppression; predisposition to infection and cancer thrombocytopenia	Unknown, maybe teratogenic
Indomethacin	25 mg b.i.d., increased weekly until dose is 150–200 mg/day	Gastrointestinal irritation; corneal deposits, retinal changes; headache; toxic hepatitis; aplastic anemia; psychic disturbance; hypertension; prolonged pregnancy and/or labor	Phocomelia; Penal agenesis; meconium staining; oligohydramnios; hemorrhage; newborn pulmonary hypertension
Ibuprofen	900–1600 mg p.o./day	Headache; gastrointestinal irritation; visual changes; prolonged pregnancy and/or labor	Unknown; unstudied and not recommended
Hydrochloroquine	200 mg b.i.d. for 6 months; decrease to 200 mg q.d.	Gastrointestinal upset; rash; headache; retinal changes, blindness	Chromosome damage; blindness
Corticosteroids (prednisone), systemic	Range: 1 mg to 200 mg p.o., i.m., or i.v./day depending on severity of disease	Gastrointestinal ulceration; osteoporosis; psychologic disturbances; diabetes mellitus; cataracts; hypokalemia; hypertension	Adrenal suppression leading to hypogonadism and/or masculinization of female fetus; cataracts
Penicillamine	250 mg p.o. daily to increase to 500 mg to 750 mg	Same side effects as gold	Unknown
Cyclophosphamide	Individually determined	Chromosome abnormality; bone marrow depression; gastrointestinal irritation; hemorrhagic cystitis; predisposition to infection and cancer	Congenital defects with use in first trimester; possible chromosome abnormality

[a]Adapted from Burrow G, Ferris, T. *Medical Complications in Pregnancy*. Philadelphia, WB Saunders, 1982, pp 474–497.

Deformities of the joints in the hand may be seen. The skin covering the hand may be thin, pale, smooth, and shiny. Nails are rough and brittle, and the intrinsic muscles of the hand may be wasted (1, p 586).

If the disease is advanced, gross local distortion of joints, dislocation, or muscle wasting and/or contracture may be present in the hands, wrists, knees, ankles, shoulders, or spine.

A common finding is the rheumatoid nodule that histologically is an area of necrosis surrounded by immune system elements. These usually are seen on the forearm but may also be present internally on the heart, lungs, or sclera (5, p 477).

Diagnosis

Diagnosis is based on history and physical examination that reveals the above signs and symptoms, as well as selected laboratory testing. Labora-

tory findings suggestive of rheumatoid arthritis include (2, p 542):

1. Increased white blood cell count, indicative of inflammation;
2. Normocytic, normochromic anemia due to chronic disease process;
3. Hypergammaglobulinemia;
4. Increased erythrocyte sedimentation rate (ESR) indicative of inflammation;
5. Presence of a disease-specific immunoglobulin complex—the rheumatoid factor; and
6. Abnormal synovial fluid—poor viscosity due to inflammatory reaction.

Arthroscopy and/or x-ray confirm the diagnosis by demonstrating narrowing of joint space, damaged articular cartilage, and bony erosion.

Maternal and Fetal Outcome

Rheumatoid arthritis does not affect the physiologic process of conception or pregnancy (7). Pregnant women who have the disease may experience remission owing to suppressed immune system inflammatory process. However, the prognosis of this chronic disease—progressive disability and pain—may be emotionally devastating to the woman and her family. Anxiety, stress, and depression are common and understandable reactions.

During the postpartum period, patients who experienced remission during pregnancy are likely to develop exacerbations. A small number of women will experience onset of rheumatoid arthritis after parturition (5, p 476, 7). It is not known whether onset is related to a rebound effect in immune system elements or is merely coincidental.

Medical Management

Treatment consists of measures to avert pain, control inflammation, maximize function, and prevent as much damage as possible. A team effort to achieve these treatment goals is essential. Treatment modalities include family education/support, drug therapy, surgical intervention, physical therapy, and occupational therapy (2, pp 543–546).

Evaluation of the patient's personality and her reaction to the disease is an important initial step in preparation for parenting and in involving the patient in her long-term care. Family evaluation also is important since significant others will be involved in the patient's and her baby's ongoing daily care. Individual family counseling may be indicated.

Drug therapy is aimed at controlling or decreasing inflammation and thus reducing joint damage. During pregnancy, salicylate is the drug of choice (5, p 483). However, use of salicylates during pregnancy to decrease joint inflammation may result in maternal gastrointestinal irritation, as well as anemia or prenatal/postpartum hemorrhage. The fetus, too, is at risk for hemorrhage due to decreased platelet count. Preterm or low birth weight infants are more likely to have intracranial hemorrhage (5, p 476). Because gold is a very large molecule and does not cross the placenta, it is used for patients unresponsive to salicylate. Small amounts of corticosteroids can be injected into an affected joint to decrease inflammation (5, 483).

Other commonly used drugs like azathioprine, indomethacin, ibuprofen, penicillamine, or cyclophosphamide are not used during pregnancy because of the synergistic reaction between pregnancy and maternal side effects, as well as the teratogenic fetal side effects. (5, p 483). Tables 7.2 and 7.3 detail maternal and fetal side effects of drugs used to treat rheumatoid arthritis during pregnancy and interconceptually.

Surgical intervention may improve the patient's joint mobility or alleviate pain. However, due to anesthetic risks to mother and fetus, surgery is a last resort. Procedures include the following (1, p 587):

1. Osteotomies to correct deformities;
2. Arthrodesis to stabilize a joint;
3. Arthroplasties to improve motion; and
4. Synovectomy to relieve pain.

Passive and active range of motion are necessary to preserve joint function and to prevent contractures. Thus, physiotherapy should be begun as soon as the diagnosis is confirmed. A daily exercise program should be developed, and the patient and her family should be involved. Exercise should be performed within the limits of pain and the severity of the disease. However, exercise should be tempered with rest and immobilization of acutely inflamed joints.

The patient should be helped to maintain and maximize activities of daily living. She should be referred to an occupational therapist in order to assess and to correct individual deficits.

NURSING MANAGEMENT

Nursing management specific for a patient with *rheumatoid arthritis*:

☐ Discuss the effects of rheumatoid arthritis during pregnancy and on plans for parenting/family life with the patient and her family.

☐ Promote patient comfort:
— Medications (e.g., salicylates, gold);
— Exercise; and
— Rest.

☐ Teach self-help efforts to reduce pain:
— Hot tub baths;
— Heating pad;
— Warm clothing.

☐ Teach the patient/family the impact of drug therapy on pregnancy:

NURSING MANAGEMENT

— Acceptable drugs (e.g., salicylates, gold, local cortisone injections) and

— Side effects (e.g., maternal gastritis, potential for postpartum hemorrhage)

☐ Work with patient to develop modifications in daily activities to compensate for physical changes of pregnancy and arthritis.

☐ Teach the patient and significant other to avoid skin breakdown.

— Frequent position changes (use of trapeze, when necessary);

— Backrubs;

— Use of special mattress and/or sheep skins; and

— Foam elbow and heel guards.

☐ Be prepared to provide emotional support to the patient exhibiting depression and to make referrals as necessary.

☐ Ensure that the patient is referred to a visiting nurse service for evaluation of home environment, her ability to perform activities of daily living, and continued assessment of psychological status.

☐ During labor and the postpartum period, position the patient carefully, taking care to protect affected joints.

☐ In the postpartum period observe for postpartum hemorrhage (for those patients taking high dose salicylates).

☐ Help the patient and significant others prepare for care of the infant. Consider referral for homemakers/home health aide services.

Nursing diagnoses most frequently associated with *rheumatoid arthritis*:

☐ Pain.

☐ Knowledge deficit regarding etiology, disease process, treatment, and expected outcome.

☐ Impaired physical mobility.

☐ Self-care deficit: feeding, bathing/hygiene, dressing/grooming, toileting.

☐ Disturbance in body image, self-esteem.

LUPUS ERYTHEMATOSUS

Definition

Systemic lupus erythematosus (SLE) is an inflammatory disease that involves chronic, progressive, and destructive biochemical and structural changes in the skin, joints, kidneys, nervous system, and/or mucous membranes (3, p 661). However, it can involve any other organ, and multiple organ involvement is common. Women may be affected as much as ten times more than males—with the peak incidence between 30 and 40 years of age. Overall, it occurs in approximately 1 out of every 800 people—making it a fairly common disease during pregnancy. Black women are thought to have a higher incidence (1 per 250) (6, p 260).

Etiology

SLE has been termed the "classic" autoimmune connective tissue disease. Although the etiology is unknown, the inability to distinguish "self" from "nonself" as evidenced by extremely high levels of antibodies attacking the body's cells and proteins clearly indicates a deficit in an immunologic system (3, p 660).

Genetic factors are also to be taken into account. Family history of SLE makes the development more likely, although research is still anecdotal and exact correlations are unknown.

Certain drugs may also produce a syndrome closely resembling SLE. Drugs implicated are hydralazine, isoniazed, procainamide, quinidine, dilantin, phenobarbital and oral contraceptives. Drug-induced SLE is usually relieved by discontinuation of the causative medication (5, p 481).

Signs and Symptoms

Since SLE may affect any body system, clinical manifestations are confusingly diverse. As with rheumatoid arthritis, the patient will experience periods of remission and exacerbation. Periods of physical and/or emotional stress typically precede exacerbation. Common complaints that bring the patient to the health care team include weight loss, joint pain, skin rash, and/or pulmonic pain associated with pleural effusion (5, p 481).

The skin frequently is affected. A symmetrical, erythematous rash may appear on the face, neck, and/or extremities, particularly the back of the fingers, palms, and/or elbows. Approximately 15% will develop the facial "butterfly" rash characteristic of SLE. The rash will be aggravated by exposure to sunlight. Hair loss and baldness are common, and the loss will be accelerated by the use of sprays and dyes (8, p 161).

Alteration in mental status runs the gamut, from nonorganic depression to acute organic brain

Table 7.4.
DIAGNOSTIC STUDIES AND FINDINGS INDICATING SYSTEMIC LUPUS ERYTHEMATOSUS[a]

TEST	FINDINGS INDICATING POSSIBLE SLE
LE cell reaction (LE prep)	Positive
ANA	Positive, titer high ($\geq$1:80 = disease; $\geq$1:160 = exacerbation)
Complete blood count	Decreased white blood cells; decreased red blood cells (anemia); decreased platelets
Serology	Positive (false)
Blood urea nitrogen	Elevated
Urinalysis	Proteinuria; hematuria; casts
Chest x-ray	Pleural effusion or cardiomegaly

[a]Adapted from Tucker S, et al.: *Patient Care Standards*. St. Louis, Mosby, 1988, p 477.

syndrome. Overall, 18% of patients will exhibit some symptoms, including grand mal seizures (16%) or ascending mixed motor-sensory loss (10%). The etiology of these alterations is multifactorial and could be the result of the disease itself on the neural system, drug therapy (specifically corticosteroids), or psychologic reaction to the diagnosis/prognosis of chronic disease (8, p 161).

The American Rheumatism Association states that if a client presents with any four of the fourteen signs and symptoms listed below, a diagnosis of SLE is highly likely (9):

1. Facial erythema (butterfly rash)
2. Skin lesions
3. Raynaud's phenomenon
4. Alopecia
5. Skin photosensitivity
6. Oral or nasopharyngeal ulceration
7. Arthritis without deformity
8. Positive LE preparation
9. Chronic false-positive serologic test for syphilis
10. Profuse proteinuria (greater than 3.5 g/day)
11. Cellular urinary casts
12. Pleurisy or pericarditis
13. Psychosis or convulsions
14. Hemolytic anemia, leukopenia, or thrombocytopenia

Diagnosis

Because of the many organs that may be involved, diagnosis is difficult. SLE may mimic cardiac or renal disease in 50% of patients (2, p 560).

Diagnosis is based on finding at least four of the significant signs and symptoms as well as other laboratory findings (Table 7.4). The detection of ANA with titers $\geq$1:80 and with a specific immunoflorescent rim pattern is diagnostic (2, p 315).

It should be noted that SLE should be considered as a differential diagnosis in the evaluation of toxemia-like symptoms, especially in older black women.

Maternal and Fetal Outcome

Maternal fertility rates are unaffected. However, pregnancy does not seem to exert a beneficial effect as with rheumatoid arthritis. Maternal complications mainly revolve around deteriorating renal, cardiac, or neural function. Hypertension and other toxemia-like symptoms (including seizures) are the primary manifestations of SLE exacerbation during pregnancy.

Fetal outcome is jeopardized. It is postulated that immune complexes deposited on the trophoblast basement membrane of the fetal kidney may be implicated in perinatal morbidity and mortality (8, p 163). The three main areas of morbidity and mortality include the following (6, p 264):

1. Forty percent risk of spontaneous abortion between 12–14 weeks' gestation;
2. Increased risk of preterm delivery associated with deteriorating maternal renal status; and
3. Neonatal lupus syndrome, consisting of congenital heart block and transplacental passage of antibodies producing an Rh-like disease, resulting in fetal anemia, leukopenia, and thrombocytopenia.

Fetal exposure to corticosteroids and immunosuppressants has not produced congenital anomalies as might have been expected. Infants who survive will have positive titers of ANA through passive placental transfer until 2–3 months of age, but the ANA have not proven pathogenic (8, p 163).

Medical Management

Prior to conception, it is desirable that the disease be in remission and that drug therapy be kept to a minimum. The patient and her significant others should have the opportunity to discuss the effects of pregnancy on herself and her fetus. Some patients with severe cardiac or renal manifestations of SLE will not be able to accommodate the physiologic demands of pregnancy. Patients with a current diagnosis of carditis, congestive heart failure, diastolic hypertension, excessive proteinuria (3 g/ 24 hours), or diffuse, proliferative histologic renal changes should be discouraged from attempting pregnancy, because it would be life threatening (8, p 163). Psychological support for the patient and her family are crucial in the decision-making process.

Following conception the patient should be monitored closely for development of neurologic, cardiac, or renal signs and symptoms of SLE. Management should involve both the internist and the obstetrician. Since physical and emotional stress are associated with increased incidence of exacerbation, every effort should be made to support the client, and need for counseling or psychiatric referral should be evaluated actively. The patient should be instructed regarding periodic daily rest and avoidance of physical exertion, and she should also be instructed to seek medical care at the first sign of infection.

Since the most common manifestation of SLE involves the renal system, the patient should be monitored carefully for nephrotic, toxemia-like symptoms (10) (see Chapter 17). Specifically, weekly evaluation of serum creatinine and urinary microscopic examination provide a basis for evaluation of renal function. Monitoring of blood pressure should include determination of mean arterial pressure and the rollover test (see Chapter 13). Because they are indicative of progressing renal failure, diastolic hypertension, elevated creatinine ($\geq$2 mg/ 100 ml) and excessive proteinuria are associated with poor maternal and fetal prognosis (8, pp 160– 165).

Presence of renal, neurologic, or cardiac signs and symptoms denoting progressive deterioration should call for vigorous treatment with high dose corticosteroids. Concurrent use of immunosuppressants has not proven beneficial, and their use in pregnancy is controversial. Antimalarial or cytotoxic drugs, which are thought to be beneficial in SLE treatment, are contraindicated in pregnancy (8, pp 160–165).

The fetus should be monitored closely with serial ultrasound and biophysical profile. Deteriorating maternal status may necessitate preterm cesarean section.

If maternal status is stable, vaginal delivery can be anticipated. Corticosteroid coverage should be continued during labor and delivery. The fetus should be monitored continuously, with heart rate and rhythm carefully assessed because of the possibility of fetal heart block.

Perhaps because of the physical and emotional stress of labor and delivery, postpartum SLE exacerbations are to be expected, and these may be severe. Aggressive management should include not only high dose drug therapy but also hemodialysis if indicated (11). These same severe reactions also can occur after spontaneous or voluntary abortion.

When the patient has achieved postpartum remission, the importance of birth control should be stressed. Because oral contraceptives carry with them the risk of drug-induced SLE, barrier methods should be advised.

Whether or not the mother should breastfeed is controversial (8, p 169). Some authorities feel that the physiologic processes involved are too stressful or that maternal medications will be transferred to the infant. Others feel that mothers on low doses of medication can breastfeed safely if the newborn can be closely monitored and that the process promotes confidence in mothering, which will decrease anxiety or stress.

NURSING MANAGEMENT

Priorities for care of a patient with *SLE*:
☐ Discuss the effects of SLE during pregnancy with the patient and her family.
☐ Teach health-promoting behaviors:
  — Skin care (e.g., clean lesions with mild soap, avoid sun exposure, use sunscreens, avoid hair sprays and coloring products)
  — Nutrition (e.g., special diets as indicated by cardiac and renal status; otherwise, balanced, nutritious meals)
  — Balance between activity and rest

☐ Teach patient/family factors that precipitate/ indicate exacerbation:
  — Fever
  — Cough
  — Rash
  — Infection
  — Increased joint pain
☐ Review implications of drug therapy for SLE and pregnancy

Nursing diagnoses most frequently associated with *SLE*:
☐ Anxiety/fear
☐ Ineffective individual coping

NURSING MANAGEMENT

- ☐ Knowledge deficit regarding etiology, disease process, treatment and expected outcome
- ☐ Disturbance in body image, self-esteem
- ☐ Altered maternal tissue perfusion

- ☐ Altered tissue perfusion
- ☐ Knowledge deficit regarding medication regimen.

WOMEN AND AIDS

Definition

AIDS (Acquired Immune Deficiency Syndrome) is a disease complex caused by the human immunodeficiency virus (HIV) that leads to massive irreversible collapse of the immune system—and subsequent development of progressive infections or cancers that, over time, prove fatal.

In 1981, the first five cases of AIDS in the U.S. were officially reported to Centers for Disease Control. By 1991, it is estimated that over 270,000 cases of AIDS will be diagnosed with a pool of 1 to 2 million HIV-infected persons. AIDS has been found in all 50 states, the District of Columbia, and the 4 U.S. territories. Over half of all cases have occurred in New York and California. There is no cure for AIDS, and one-half of victims do not survive for more than 18 months after diagnosis (12, pp 1016–1017).

In 1981, there were no reported cases of women with AIDS in the U.S. Today women comprise 7% of known cases. This is in sharp contrast to other countries such as South Africa where 40 to 50% of cases reported are women—perhaps a chilling projection of future epidemiology (13, p 32).

The following statistics detail the profile of women and AIDS in the United States today (13, p 32):

1) 51% are Black, 20% Latino, 28% White.
2) 52% are intravenous drug users (IVDUs).
3) 27% are non IVDUs infected by a male partner—usually an IVDU.
4) 78% are women of childbearing age.

Women who are HIV-positive, regardless of ethnicity, culture, or income, must struggle through unique and sometimes insurmountable obstacles (13, p 34):

1) Extreme isolation—needed community and peer support of other infected women has not been developed.
2) Grief for loss of health, body image, sexuality, and childbearing potential.

3) Lack of insurance to pay for health care and inability to access human services such as housing, child care, or mental health services.
4) The burden of making decisions about initiation, continuation, and termination of pregnancy.
5) Diagnosis first being confirmed at birth of an infected infant.
6) The agony of caring for her infected child and watching him die.
7) Dealing with the stigma that "all women with AIDS are prostitutes."
8) The societal norm that men do not have to bear responsibility for control of sex or conception.

Etiology

AIDS is the result of a continuum of ever more severe illnesses caused by the human immunodeficiency virus (HIV). Different researchers have given different names to this virus: human T-lymphotropic virus, type III (HTLV-III); lymphadenopathy-associated virus (LAV); or AIDS-related virus (ARV).

HIV preferentially infects specific T-cells (T4) and the glial cells in the brain. T4 cells produce chemicals that regulate the functions of other lymphocytes, including monocytes and B cells. As T-cells are destroyed and replaced by HIV, the immune system is destroyed, and viral or bacterial pathogens that are normally harmless overwhelm the body's failing defenses.

However, in the beginning of the disease process, not all HIV-positive individuals have significant damage to the immune system. For example, the great majority of the HIV-positive population in the United States still have normal T4 levels. What causes HIV to move from a parasitic to a pathogenic state is still unknown.

HIV is transmitted by penetrative sexual contact; inoculation with contaminated blood products, needles, or syringes; and by mother to infant in utero, during the birth process, or possibly when breastfeeding. Low levels of HIV are also present in other body fluids, i.e., saliva, tears, urine, and sweat. However, nonsexual transmission from these fluids has not been documented. Thus, it is assumed that the transmission is dose-related.

Because the rectal lining is easily damaged, anal intercourse has been a risk factor for many HIV-positive gay men. Usually heterosexual transmission is from a bisexual or IVDU man to an uninfected woman, although the reverse is possible. Women are at risk for HIV infection if they (14, p 3):

○   Have used IV drugs.
○   Have engaged in prostitution.
○   Have had sexual partners who are infected or are at risk for infection because they are bisexual or are IV-drug abusers or hemophiliacs.
○   Are living in communities or were born in countries where there is a known or suspected high prevalence of infection among women, i.e., Central Africa.
○   Received a transfusion before blood was being screened for HIV antibody but after HIV infection occurred in the United States (e.g., between 1978 and 1985).

Signs and Symptoms

At first, signs and symptoms may be absent. The onset of symptoms of HIV infection ranges from 6 months to several years, and one or more usually persist throughout the course of the disease after onset of symptoms, even in the absence of any acute opportunistic infection. They include (14, p 9):

—extreme tiredness, sometimes combined with headache, dizziness or lightheadedness;
—continued fever or profuse night sweats;
—weight loss of more than 10 lbs. that is not due to dieting or increased physical activity;
—swollen glands in the neck, armpit, or groin;
—purple or discolored growths on the skin or the mucous membranes (inside the mouth, anus, or nasal passages);
—heavy continual dry cough that is not from smoking or that has lasted too long to be a cold or flu;
—continuing bouts of diarrhea;
—thrush, coating the tongue or the throat which may be accompanied by sore throat or dysphagia;
—unexplained bleeding from any body opening or from growths on the skin or mucous membranes; bruising more easily than usual;
—progressive shortness of breath.

In addition, 30% of HIV-positive individuals experience neurologic symptoms including demen-

tia, peripheral neuropathy, seizures, hemiparesis, cognitive and sensory deficits, and coma.

Diagnosis

There is no diagnostic test to determine whether a person has AIDS or will develop AIDS in the future.

There are tests that do determine presence of HIV antibodies. A test for HIV antibody is considered positive when a sequence of tests starting with a repeatedly reactive enzyme immunoassay (EIA) and including additional more specific assay, such as a Western blot, are consistently reactive (15, pp 1–5).

AIDS is diagnosed when an HIV-positive individual develops a life-threatening opportunistic infection. Principle infections include pneumocystis carinii pneumonia (PCP), toxoplasmosis, leukoencephalopathy, crytococcal meningitis, Candida esophagitis, chronic herpes, cytomegalovirus (CMV), and/or disseminated bacterial infections. Other conditions associated with AIDS are Kaposi's sarcoma, Burkett lymphoma, or a primary lymphoma of the central nervous system.

To make diagnosis more complex, researchers have not been able to verify a relationship between levels of antibody titers and either degree of infectivity or disease development.

The Centers for Disease Control have classified diagnosis into the following categories (16, pp 1–10):

1)   Asymptomatic HIV infection
    ○   HIV antibodies present
    ○   Immune system normal
    ○   No signs or symptoms present
2)   Primary HIV infection
    ○   HIV antibodies present
    ○   Elevated erythocyte sedimentation rate
    ○   Mononucleosis-like symptoms with or without meningitis
    ○   Rash
    ○   Abdominal cramps, diarrhea
3)   Persistent   generalized   lymphadenopathy (PGL)
    ○   HIV antibodies present
    ○   Immune system comprised (e.g., fewer T4 cells, low T4:T8 ratio)
    ○   Lymph node enlargement of 1 cm or more at two or more sites, persisting for more than 3 months, in absence of other illness to explain PGL

4) AIDS-related complex (ARC)
    o   Presence of two well-defined symptoms
        (see Signs and Symptoms) of immu-
        nodeficiency combined with two labora-
        tory test abnormalities
5) AIDS
    o   Presence of any life-threatening opportu-
        nistic infections or cancer.

Maternal Fetal Outcome

AIDS is a progressive fatal disease. At the present time there is no cure. Overall, the mortality
rate approaches 70% 2 years after diagnosis. Mortality varies by ethnicity and sex. Mortality in adults
is higher among women than men and among
blacks and Hispanics than whites—a bleak future
for HIV-positive minority women. A child born to
an HIV-positive mother runs a 30 to 50% chance of
infection. An infected child is likely to die or be severely ill by age 2.

Medical Management

There are no drugs available to cure the disease. Treatment is specific to the specific opportunistic infection(s) identified. Many of the drugs
used in treatment are both toxic to the mother and
potentially teratogenic to the fetus. However, given
the catastrophic nature of these infections, the benefits of treatment outweigh the risks.

Concerns of Health Care Workers

Research related to risk to health care workers
acquiring HIV in health care settings—even for
those with documented percutaneous or mucous
membrane exposure to blood or body fluids—
seems, so far, to be very low (e.g., 1%). Pregnant
health care workers are more at risk for contracting
potentially teratogenic superinfections (e.g., CMV,
toxoplasmosis) than for contracting AIDS.

The Centers for Disease Control recommends
the following universal precautions (17, pp 1–13):

1. All health care workers should routinely use
    appropriate barrier precautions to prevent skin
    and mucous-membrane exposure when con-
    tact with blood or other body fluids of any pa-
    tient is anticipated. Gloves should be worn for
    touching blood or other body fluids, mucous
    membranes, or nonintact skin of all patients,
    for handling items or surfaces soiled with
    blood or other body fluids, and for performing
    venipuncture and other vascular access proce-
    dures. Gloves should be changed after contact

with each patient. Masks and protective
eyewear or face shields should be worn during
procedures that are likely to generate droplets
of blood or other body fluids to prevent exposure of mucous membranes of mouth, nose,
and eyes. Gowns or aprons should be worn
during procedures that are likely to generate
splashes of blood or other body fluids.

2. Hands and other skin surfaces should be
    washed immediately and thoroughly if con-
    taminated with blood or other body fluids.
    Hands should be washed immediately after
    gloves are removed.
3. All health care workers should take precau-
    tions to prevent injuries caused by needles,
    scalpels, and other sharp instruments or de-
    vices during procedures; when cleaning used
    instruments; during disposal of used needles;
    and when handling sharp instruments after
    procedures. To prevent needlestick injuries,
    needles should not be recapped, purposely bro-
    ken or bent by hand, removed from disposable
    syringes, or otherwise manipulated by hand.
    After they are used, disposable syringes and
    needles, scalpel blades, and other sharp items
    should be placed in puncture-resistant con-
    tainers for disposal; the puncture-resistant
    container should be located as close as practi-
    cal to the use area. Large-bore reusable need-
    les should be placed in a puncture-resistant
    container for transport to the reprocessing
    area.
4. Although saliva has not been implicated in
    HIV transmission, to minimize the need for
    emergency mouth-to-mouth resuscitation,
    mouthpieces, resuscitation bags, or other ven-
    tilation devices should be available for use in
    areas in which the need for resuscitation is
    predictable.
5. Health care workers who have exudative le-
    sions or weeping dermatitis should refrain
    from all direct patient care and from handling
    patient care equipment until the condition is
    resolved.
6. Pregnant health care workers are not known
    to be at greater risk of contacting HIV infec-
    tion than health care workers who are not
    pregnant; however, if a health care worker de-
    velops HIV infection during pregnancy, the in-
    fant is at risk of infection resulting from pre-
    natal transmission. Because of this risk,
    pregnant health care workers should be espe-
    cially familiar with and strictly adhere to pre-
    cautions to minimize the risk of HIV transmis-
    sion.

Invasive Procedure Precautions

An invasive procedure is defined as surgical entry into tissues, cavities, or organs or repair of major traumatic injuries (a) in an operating or delivery room, emergency department, or outpatient setting, including physicians' and dentists' offices; (b) cardiac catheterization and angiographic procedures; (c) a vaginal or cesarean delivery or other invasive obstetric procedure during which bleeding may occur; or (d) the manipulation, cutting, or removal of any oral or perioral tissues, including tooth structure, during which bleeding occurs or the potential for bleeding exists. The universal blood and body fluids precautions listed above, combined with the precautions listed below, should be the minimum precautions for all such invasive procedures.

1. All health care workers who participate in invasive procedures must routinely use appropriate barrier precautions to prevent skin and mucous-membrane contact with blood and other body fluids of all patients. Gloves and surgical masks must be worn for all invasive procedures. Protective eyewear or face shields should be worn for procedures that commonly result in the generation of droplets, splashing of blood or other body fluids, or the generation of bone chips. Gowns or aprons made of materials that provide an effective barrier should be worn during invasive procedures that are likely to result in the splashing of blood or other body fluids. All health care workers who perform or assist in vaginal or cesarean deliveries should wear gloves and gowns when handling the placenta or the infant until blood and amniotic fluid have been removed from the infant's skin and should wear gloves during postdelivery care of the umbilical cord.

2. If a glove is torn or a needlestick or other injury occurs, the glove should be removed, and a new glove should be used as promptly as patient safety permits; the needle or instrument involved in the incident should also be removed from the sterile field.

NURSING MANAGEMENT

Nursing management specific for patients with AIDS:

1. Teach all women precautions to reduce the risk of contracting or spreading AIDS, including;
    — Refraining from sexual contact with any person whose past history and current health status are unknown.
    — Refraining from sexual intercourse with multiple partners or with persons who have had multiple partners.
    — Avoiding abuse of intravenous drugs.
    — Not sharing needles, syringes, toothbrushes, razors, or other personal items with HIV-at-risk or HIV-positive individuals.
    — Using a condom during sexual intercourse if HIV status of partner is positive or unknown (or if partner is at high risk).
2. Screen all pregnant women for risk status and offer HIV testing and counseling, as appropriate.

3. Ensure that HIV-positive pregnant women have comprehensive care, including case management of both health and human service needs.
4. Ensure that all health workers, laboratory personnel who are working with HIV-positive pregnant women, follow recommended safety precautions to minimize exposure to AIDs, hepatitis B virus, and other infectious diseases.

Nursing diagnoses most frequently associated with AIDS:

☐ Grief
☐ Knowledge deficit regarding etiology, disease process, treatment, and expected outcome
☐ Disturbance in body image, self-esteem
☐ Anxiety/fear
☐ Spiritual distress
☐ Ineffective individual coping
☐ Altered nutrition: less than body requirements
☐ Potential for trauma related to seizures

REFERENCES

1. Mahoney E, Flynn J: *Handbook of Medical-Surgical Nursing*. New York, John Wiley and Sons, 1983.

2. Nursing Reference Library *Diagnostics*. Springhouse, PA, Springhouse Corporation, 1986.

3. Miller B, Keone C: *Encyclopedia and Dictionary of Medicine, Nursing and Allied Health*. Philadelphia, Saunders, 1983.

4. Phipps W, et al.: *Medical Surgical Nursing*. St. Louis, Mosby, 1982.

5. Yrowitz M, Gladman D: Rheumatic Diseases. In Burrow G, Ferris T: *Medical Complications of Pregnancy*. Philadelphia, Saunders, 1982.

6. deSwiet M: *Medical Disorders of Pregnancy*. Boston, Blackwell Scientific Publications, 1984.

7. Vorner M, et al: Pregnancy in patients with systemic lupus erythematosis. *Am J Obstet Gynecol* 145:1025–1040, 1983.

8. Slaughter L: Effects of SLE on pregnancy. *Contemp. OB/GYN* 17: 161–174, (1981)

9. Cohen A, et al: Preliminary criteria for classification of SLE *Bull Rheum Dis* 21: 643, 1972.

10. Burkett, G. Lupus nephropathy and pregnancy. *Clin Obstet Gynecol* 28: 310–323, 1983.

11. Gimonsky M, et al: Pregnancy outcome in women with systemic lupus erythematosus. *Obstet Gynecol* 63 (5): 686–92, 1984.

12. AIDS continuing education. Am J Nurs 86(9): 1016–1028.

13. *Report of the Surgeon General's Workshop on Children with HIV Infections and Their Families*. Washington, DC, United States Department of Health and Human Resources, April 1987.

14. AIDS—100 Questions and Answers *NY State Dep Health* March 1: 1986.

15. Public Health Service guidelines for counseling and antibody testing to prevent HIV infection and AIDS. *MMWR* 1–5.

16. Classification system for human T-lymphotic virus type III/lymphadenopathy-associated virus infections. *MMWR* 35:1–10.

17. Recommendations for prevention of HIV transmission in health care settings. *MMWR* 36:1–13.

Chapter 8
Hematologic Disorders
Kathleen Buckley, C.N.M., M.S.N.

INTRODUCTION

Hemodynamic Changes in Pregnancy

Pregnancy is accompanied by dynamic changes in the hematopoietic system. A hypervolemic state develops as total blood volume increases an average of 30–40%. However, the actual increase varies from woman to woman and may even double in some individuals. The increase in amount usually averages between 1.5 and 2.1 liters. Expansion begins as early as 6 weeks' gestation, peaks at 32–34 weeks, slightly decreases at term, and returns to nonpregnant status by 3–6 weeks postpartum (1).

Although total blood volume, including plasma and red blood cell volume, increases, the rate of increase of each component is not parallel. Plasma volume begins expansion in the first trimester and peaks at 28 weeks' gestation. It is thought that placental lactogen stimulates aldosterone secretion and causes an increase of approximately 50%. The red blood cell volume will increase by 25% (300–350 ml). This increase lags behind, beginning as early as 12 weeks' gestation and reaching the widest gap at approximately 28 weeks' gestation, resulting in a relative disproportion of the ratio of plasma volume to total red cell volume. This disproportion produces a two- to four-point drop in hematocrit and has been termed "physiologic anemia" (2, p 63). This is a misnomer, because the drop in hematocrit/hemoglobin is not indicative of disease but rather of a normal physiologic process. The hypervolemic state in pregnancy is thought to be protective in that it serves the following three functions (3, p 191):

1. Meeting the increased blood volume demands of the enlarging uterus;
2. Promoting maternal and fetal oxygenation by preventing impaired venous return in the supine and erect positions; and
3. Safeguarding the mother from blood loss at birth.

ANEMIA

Definition

Anemia is a reduction below normal in the quantity of hemoglobin. This alteration in the hematologic system interferes with the nutritional needs of the body's cells and decreases the oxygen-carrying capacity of the blood. Anemia is not a disease. Rather, it is a symptom of underlying pathology (4, p 351, 5, p 50).

Etiology

Anemias are classified according to their etiology and can be either acquired or inherited (3, p 562). Acquired anemias are caused by dietary deficiencies in iron, folic acid, or other nutrients. They may also result from blood loss or infection. Inherited anemias are genetically determined and result from one of the following (6, p 60):

1. Abnormal structure of the hemoglobin chain of the hemoglobin molecule;
2. Reduced rate of production of the globulin chain; or
3. Enzyme abnormalities of the red blood cell.

74

Signs and Symptoms

The signs and symptoms of anemia result from the following physiologic changes (7, p 696):

1. Reduced oxygen-carrying capacity of the blood;
2. The concurrent manifestations of the underlying cause of the anemia; and
3. Decreased cardiovascular and pulmonary compensation capacity.

Mild anemias developing over a long period of time tend to produce few symptoms, and those that do occur are vague (e.g., fatigue, irritability, and a loss of a sense of well-being). Moderate to severe anemias that develop quickly will produce many signs and symptoms that relate not only to the anemia but also the underlying causative factors. These include pallor of the skin, mucous membranes, and conjunctiva; tachycardia; dyspnea; headache; depression; nausea/vomiting; weight loss; abdominal pain; fever; jaundice; edema; diaphoresis; paresthesias; and a cold feeling (7, p 696). Common signs and symptoms of both acquired and inherited anemias are given in detail in Table 8.1.

Diagnosis

In order to ensure an accurate diagnosis of the underlying causative pathology, a thorough health history, physical examination, and battery of laboratory tests should be employed. Table 8.1 also details possible findings of the health history and physical examination in acquired and inherited anemias.

Tests Used to Diagnose Anemia

Red Cell (Erythrocyte) Indices

This portion of the complete blood count is particularly important in pinpointing the diagnosis of anemia. Indices include (4, p 14, 5, p 50):

1. Mean corpuscular volume (MCV)—average red blood cell size—cells may be normal (normocytic), small (microcytic), or large (macrocytic).
2. Mean corpuscular hemoglobin (MCH)—average amount of hemoglobin in a red blood cell—cell may appear normal (normochromic), pale (hypochromic), or hyperemic (hyperchromic) depending on the amount of hemoglobin/cell.
3. Mean corpuscular hemoglobin concentration (MCHC)—concentration of hemoglobin in 100 ml of packed red cells.

Low MCV and MCH indicate a microcytic, hypochromic anemia such as that caused by iron deficiency or thalassemia. Macrocytic, hypochromic indices characterize folic acid anemia. Normochromic, normocytic cells with a decreased MCHC typically are seen in cases of acute hemorrhage because anemia is a result of the sudden decrease of hemoglobin volume rather than an alteration in cell structure or color. Table 8.2 lists common findings of red cell indices in varying diagnoses (4, p 14).

Other Tests

Other tests needed in order to evaluate the type of anemia present are (4, pp 14–25):

1. Serum iron—measures the amount of plasma iron bound to the glycoprotein transferrin. It is the amount available for distribution to body compartments for storage and synthesis.
2. Total iron binding capacity (TIBC)—measures the amount of iron that would be circulating in plasma if transferrin would be completely saturated with iron. During pregnancy, the TIBC normally is elevated.
3. Hemoglobin electrophoresis—measures amounts of normal and abnormal hemoglobin. Abnormal hemoglobins detected by this test include A, A_2, S, and C.
4. Glucose-6-Phosphate Dehydrogenase—detects presence of this particular enzyme deficit.
5. Stool for ova and parasites—detects presence of parasites which cause nutritional deficit in the host and chronic gastrointestinal bleeding.

Normal values of significant laboratory tests of the hematologic system are listed in Table 8.3.

Types of Anemias

Acquired

Iron Deficiency

Because of the monthly loss of iron stores through menstruation, many women begin pregnancy with minimal iron stores. Iron deficiency anemia accounts for approximately 95% of all the anemias in pregnancy, and as many as 60% of all pregnant women will become anemic, depending on the geographic and socioeconomic groups evaluated. Before full-blown anemia develops, the body will attempt to compensate by using up iron stores in the liver, spleen, and bone marrow and then by decreasing serum iron and increasing the iron binding capacity. If these measures fail, anemia occurs. It should be noted that the fetus is able to capture adequate iron stores throughout this process (2, p 63).

Table 8.1.

COMMON FINDINGS IN ACQUIRED AND INHERITED ANEMIAS[a]

	ACQUIRED ANEMIAS	HEREDITARY HEMOGLOBINOPATHIES
<Subjective>		
Family origin	Worldwide	Africa, Mediterranean, Eastern hemisphere
Family health history	Anemia; cultural practices related to poor nutrition	Hemoglobinopathy; family members with joint pain or crises
Psychosocial	Poverty, adolescent food fads, listless, poor attention span, irritable	Variable
Nutrition	Diet deficient in sources of protein, iron, folate, vitamins, and/or calories	Fava beans trigger anemia in G-6-PD deficiency
Pica	Clay, starch, ice, salt cravings, and others; cultural variations	May experience pica
Medications	Noncompliance with iron, vitamin, and folate therapies	Degree of compliance
Systems review of past and current complaints		
Musculoskeletal	Weakness, chronic fatigue	Joint and muscle pain
Integumentary	History of bleeding or bruising, paresthesias	Sensitivity to cold
Optical	Visual disturbances	May have visual disturbances if severe
Gastrointestinal	History of nausea, vomiting, heartburn, epigastric pain, diarrhea, dark or bloody stools, gastrointestinal surgery	Right upper quadrant pain, eructation, flatulence, abdominal and epigastric pain or tenderness
Urinary tract	Dysuria, hematuria, frequency in excess of normal pregnancy, urgency, history of repeated urinary tract infections	History of repeated urinary tract infections, dysuria, frequency, urgency, cloudy, dark or bloody urine, flank pain
Cardiorespiratory	Palpitations, shortness of breath, chest pain	Chest pain, dyspnea, history of respiratory infections
Reproductive	History of heavy or abnormal menstrual bleeding, or bleeding during pregnancy	History of infertility, spontaneous abortions, stillbirths, or low birth weight
<Objective>		
Musculoskeletal system		Long, thin extremities and digits; edema of hand or foot
Integumentary system	Pallor of conjunctiva, skin, mucous membranes, nail beds; bruising	Pallor, jaundice, leg and ankle ulcerations, edema
Gastrointestinal system	Stomatitis, parasites	Rebound tenderness of abdomen; enlarged liver and spleen
Cardiorespiratory system	Tachycardia, heart murmur, fever	Tachycardia, cardiomegaly, silent areas in lungs, rales, ronchi in pneumonia or pneumonitis
Urinary system		Costovertebral angle tenderness on palpation or percussion, hematuria, suprapubic pain on palpation
Reproductive system	Possible measurement small for gestational age	Intrauterine growth retardation, decreased or absent fetal heart rate or movements (signs of fetal distress or demise)

[a]Adapted from Dewees C: Hematologic disorders in pregnancy. *Nurs Clin N Am* 17:59, 1982, pp 57–67.

Signs and symptoms of iron deficiency anemia are vague, including fatigue, anorexia, and depression. It is not unusual to note pale conjunctiva and mucous membranes. A grade II systolic cardiac murmur often accompanies iron deficiency anemia.

Diagnosis is based on laboratory findings. Serum iron levels will be decreased, and the number of newly developing red cells (reticulocytes) will be low. Classically, the mature red cells are small (microcytic) and pale (hypochromic). Thus, all

Table 8.2.

COMPARATIVE RED CELL INDICES

TEST	NORMAL	IRON DEFICIENCY ANEMIA	FOLIC ACID ANEMIA	HEMOGLOBINOPATHY	ACUTE HEMORRHAGE
MCV	84–95	Decreased	Increased	Decreased	Normal
MCH	26–32	Decreased	Decreased	Decreased	Normal
MCHC	30–36%	Decreased	Normal	Decreased	Decreased

Table 8.3.

HEMATOLOGIC CHANGES DURING PREGNANCY[a]

VALUES	NONPREGNANT	PREGNANT
Complete blood count		
Hemoglobin, g/100 ml	12–16	10–14
Hematocrit, %	37–47	32–42
Red cell volume, ml	1600	1900
Plasma volume, ml	2400	3700
Red blood cell indices	Normal	Normal
Erythropoietic system		
Serum iron, μg	75–150	65–120
Total iron binding capacity, μg	250–450	300–500
Iron saturation, %	30–40	15–30
Vitamin B_{12}, folic acid, ascorbic acid	Normal	Moderate decrease

[a]Adapted from Ziegal E, Cranley M: *Obstetric Nursing*. New York, MacMillan, 1984, p 719.

three indices—MCH, MCV, and MCHC—will be decreased (8, p 39).

Anemia resulting from iron deficiency is not a significant cause of maternal/fetal morbidity and mortality. However, an anemic woman is more prone to infection and to exhibit delayed healing time in the postpartum period. More intangible symptoms, such as fatigue or lassitude, affect her ability to maintain a desired life-style and to relate to significant others. The fetus is fairly well protected by the physiologic mechanism that spares fetal iron stores at the expense of maternal stores.

At the beginning of pregnancy, laboratory data should establish baseline hematopoietic data and ensure that the clinician is able to distinguish iron deficiency from normal physiologic hemodilution. However, routine prophylactic iron supplementation is recommended by many authorities (300 mg/day), especially in the second half of pregnancy when iron stores can be depleted severely.

Although the classic clinical definition of anemia is a hematocrit of <30 mg, many clinicians begin to treat iron deficiency (as diagnosed by decreased MCH and MCV) beginning at a hematocrit of 34 mg. Treatment consists of diet counseling and iron supplementation (300 mg/day). One 300-mg iron compound tablet should contain about 60 mg of elemental iron; approximtely 6 mg (10%) can be absorbed. If the hematocrit falls below 30%, some authors recommend tripling the dose of iron (300 mg three times a day). With severe iron deficiency anemia (<30 mg), most clinicians—even without diagnostic justification—will also prescribe folic acid supplementation. Those experienced with iron deficiency treatment feel that the extra folate supplementation does improve the results. If the patient is compliant, simple iron deficiency should respond to therapy by the end of 4 weeks, and laboratory indices should be reevaluated at that time. Even if the anemia is corrected, iron therapy should be continued.

Folic Acid Deficiency

One of the B complex vitamins, folic acid, is fundamental in both cell growth and division. Need for folic acid during pregnancy is increased to meet the demands of the growing fetus, the placenta, the enlarged uterus, and the maternal red blood cell expansion. Folic acid requirements also are increased in the following nonnutritional conditions (2, p 64):

1. Twin pregnancy
2. Acute infectious processes
3. Malabsorption syndromes, such as sprue
4. Use of anticonvulsant drugs like diphenylhydantoin
5. Hemoglobinopathies
6. Alcoholic cirrhosis

The red blood cells are macrocytic; therefore, the MCV will be elevated. The MCH and MCHC may be within normal levels or, in the face of a mixed iron/folic acid deficiency, may be decreased. Serum folate levels will be below 5 mg/ml.

Symptoms include glossitis, anorexia, dyspepsia, flatulence, and diarrhea. A careful dietary history will reveal inadequate intake of folic acid sources such as green, leafy vegetables.

Folic acid deficiency does not have a major deleterious effect on maternal or fetal outcome. However, as an indicator of overall poor nutrition, it is crucial to identify and to treat. Treatment consists of diet counseling and folic acid supplementation (1 mg/day). Since most prenatal vitamins already contain 1 mg of folic acid, the patient actually is ingesting at least 2 mg daily. Women at special nonnutritional risk for folic acid deficiency may be given prophylactic supplementation up to as much as 5 mg/day (9).

Other

Chronic blood loss during pregnancy sometimes is overlooked in the differential diagnosis of anemia. However, with the hyperemic state of the mucous membranes and the possible development of epulis, bleeding from nasal passages or gums may be both progressive and severe. Bleeding hemorrhoids or intestinal parasites are sources of gastrointestinal blood loss. A careful evaluation always should include investigation of these possible etiologies of anemia. Signs, symptoms, and diagnostic laboratory findings are the same as for iron deficiency anemia. Chronic blood loss causes an iron deficiency anemia. Maternal and fetal outcome depend on the magnitude of blood loss.

Chronic disease often predisposes to a specific type of anemia, because the disease process can affect the life span of the red blood cell and/or may cause a decreased production of reticulocytes. Diseases implicated in producing anemia include (6, p 60):

1. Neoplasms
2. Chronic liver disease
3. Collagen diseases, rheumatoid arthritis, and systemic lupus erythematosus (SLE)
4. Kidney disease or removal of the kidney
5. Tuberculosis
6. Bronchiectasis
7. Bacterial endocarditis

Severity of signs and symptoms usually will parallel activity of the underlying disease. Laboratory studies will reveal slightly decreased hemoglobin (<9 mg/100 ml) and reds cells that are normocytic and normochromic. Reticulocyte production may be decreased or may result in abnormally shaped cells. Maternal and fetal outcome are dependent more on the course of the underlying disease than on the anemia. Presence of the above laboratory findings should alert the caregiver to investigate the possibility of an underlying chronic disease process.

Hypochromic, microcytic anemias resulting from blood loss, chronic disease, or infection should be treated as iron deficiency anemias. Identification and treatment of the underlying cause and amelioration of the condition produce the best possible response.

Inherited

Glucose-6-Phosphate Dehydrogenase

Glucose-6-phosphate dehydrogenase (G-6-PD) is an enzyme necessary for the oxidation of glucose-6-phosphate—an intermediate in carbohydrate metabolism. Hereditary deficiency of the enzyme in red blood cells can lead to hemolysis when a particular food—e.g., fava beans—and/or a wide variety of drugs are ingested (5, p 299) (Table 8.4). The disease occurs primarily in the black population but also in Greeks, Sardinians, and Sephardic Jews. It is a sex-linked recessive disorder; thus, more men (13%) are likely to be affected than women (3%). However, 20% of women in the susceptible populations will be carriers (6, p 62 and 243).

Signs and symptoms are those of any inherited hemoglobinopathy. The severity will depend on the degree of the deficiency and the amount of food/drug ingested. Diagnosis is confirmed by a special blood test positive for G-6-PD deficiency. The anemia will be normocytic and normochromic because the quantity of red blood cells is reduced through hemolysis but the quality is unaffected.

Generally, the disease is associated with higher frequency of coronary heart disease and cholelithiasis. During pregnancy, women with G-6-PD deficiency are more prone to urinary tract infection. Women with G-6-PD deficiency in the presence of some other disease, such as diabetes mellitus or pneumonia, have an increased risk of significant morbidity and mortality. Generally, no significant fetal risks are present. However, maternal hypoxia resulting from a severe crisis episode could have a major deleterious impact on fetal health.

The crucial element in treatment is to ensure that the client understands the importance of avoiding foods and drugs that may produce a hemolytic reaction. She should be given a written list of every substance that is implicated and urged to:

1. Review it before she takes any medication and
2. Show it to every physician prescribing medication.

Iron and folic acid supplements may be prescribed routinely or if laboratory studies indicate anemia.

Urinary cultures should be done more frequently (once per trimester) to screen for urinary tract infection. Signs and symptoms of urinary tract infection should be evaluated at each prenatal visit.

Thalassemia: Alpha Thalassemia Major, Beta Thalassemia Major, Beta Thalassemia Minor

The thalassemias are the most common genetic disorder of the blood. They are most prevalent in persons of central African, Mediterranean, or Asian descent.

Thalassemia is an autosomal recessive genetic disorder. It results in the reduction or absence of the alpha- or beta-globin chain in the hemoglobin

Table 8.4.

DRUGS CAUSING HEMOLYTIC REACTION IN CLIENTS WITH GLUCOSE-6-PHOSPHATE DEHYDROGENASE DEFICIENCY[a]

NITROFURANS	ANTIMALARIALS	ANTIPYRETICS AND ANALGESICS	SULFONAMIDES	OTHERS
Furaltadone (Altafur)	Pamaquine	Acetanilid	N-2-acetylsulfanil-	Acetyphenylhydrazine
Furazolidone	Pentaquine	Acetophenetidin	amide	Chloramphenicol
(Furoxone)	Primaquine	(phenacetin,	Salicylsulfapyridine	Chloroquine
Pitrofurantoin	phosphate	Empirin)	(Azulfidine)	hydrochloride
(Furadantin)	Quinacrine	Acetylsalicylic acid	Sulfacetamide sodium	Dimercaprol (BAL)
Nitrofurazone	hydrochloride	Aminopyrine	(Sulamyd)	Fava beans
(Furacin)	(Atabrine)	Antipyrine	Sulfamethoxypyrid-	Methylene blue
	Quinidine	Para-aminosalicylic	azine (Kynex,	Halidixic acid
	Quinine	acid	Midicel)	(NegGram)
	Quinocide		Sulfanilamide	Naphthalene (moth
			Sulfapyridine	balls, moth spray)
			Sulfisoxazole	Phenylhydrazine
			(Gantrisin)	Probenecid
				Tolbutamide
				(Orinase)
				Vitamin K (water
				soluble)

[a]Reprinted with permission from Buckley K, Kulb N: *Handbook of Maternal-Newborn Nursing.* New York, John Wiley and Sons, 1983, p 361.

molecule. Diagnosis of the specific type of thalassemia is confirmed by hemoglobin electrophoresis, which will show high levels of the abnormal hemoglobin A2 or F. Another important general diagnostic indicator is the presence of "target" cells in the red cell morphology section of the complete blood count. These are red blood cells that have dark centers encircled by pale rings. Targets cells are so characteristic of the thalassemias that they constitute a presumptive diagnosis (4, p 311).

During pregnancy, persons with the absence of two or three of the alpha chains (alpha thalassemia) will show signs and symptoms of severe hemolytic anemia. Although pregnancy severely stresses these poorly developed hematologic systems, a normal outcome for mother and fetus can be expected, although the fetus will inherit some form of the disorder. One exception is the fetus with no alpha-globin chain. The fetus without all four alpha-globin chains will have no chance of survival; preterm labor will ensue, and a grossly hydropic dead or dying infant will be delivered (8, p 51).

Women with alpha thalassemia routinely should be referred for genetic counseling. If they elect to carry the pregnancy, major risks include increased incidence of toxemia and severe anemia. Throughout the pregnancy, biweekly or weekly evaluation should be ongoing to detect any signs of toxemia (see Chapter 13). Iron and folate supplementation are vital throughout the entire pregnancy. Because the bone marrow will be so severely stressed to create red blood cells by both the severe

anemia and the demands of pregnancy, some authorities recommend 5 mg of folic acid daily. Parenteral iron should never be given due to the possiblity of exogenous hemosiderosis.

Beta thalassemia major (also called Cooley's anemia) is the homozygous form of the disease in which the affected individual inherits a defective beta-globin chain from each parent. It is an extremely rare condition. Availability of regular transfusion prolongs life only into the teens or early twenties. Thus, pregnancy in affected women is rare and probably fatal for both mother and fetus due to the negative synergistic affect of pregnancy and the anemia on maternal status.

Beta thalassemia minor is the heterozygous form of the disease in which the affected individual inherits one defective beta-globin chain. These persons may have only a mild anemia with no other sequelae. In fact, the diagnosis may only be confirmed during the pregnancy. A good outcome for the pregnant woman can be expected. However, the fetus runs the risk of inheriting the disease, either the major or minor variation, depending on its parentage (8, p 51).

Use of oral iron in patients with beta thalassemia minor is controversial because of the possibility of hemosiderosis. Parenteral iron is contraindicated. Blood transfusion is suggested to achieve an adequate hemoglobin for delivery or during pregnancy if the patient becomes symptomatic. The father of the baby should be evaluated for the trait. If he has the trait or is unavailable for testing, further genetic studies should be done to determine whether or not the fetus has beta thalassemia major. Since beta thalassemia major presents such a poor prognosis, the parents may elect to terminate the pregnancy.

Sickle Cell Disease

Sickle cell disease (SS) is an inherited chronic disease that results from abnormal hemoglobin synthesis. About 12% of the American black population carries the sickle cell gene. However, only about 1 in 500 American blacks actually will have the homozygous form and experience the devastating effects. Although SS is found almost exclusively in the black population, it is also present in some other populations (e.g., Greeks, Italians, Spaniards, French, Turks, North Africans, Middle Eastern Nationals, and Asian Indians) (5, p 362).

The disease is due to the homozygous inheritance of hemoglobin S, which substitutes valine for glutamic acid in position 6 of the beta chain (5, p 362). In SS red blood cells characteristically are rigid and crescent shaped. When a sickling phenomenon occurs (due to lack of oxygen), the poorly developed hemoglobin molecules collect into rigid crystals and distort the cell into this crescent shape. This results in red blood cell fragility and destruction. Smaller blood vessels can be occluded or infarcted by the clumped crescent-shaped cells. With reoxygenation, some of the process will be reversed, but repeated episodes decrease the cells' ability to return to normal, and more cells will retain the crescent shape after each hypoxic episode.

Symptoms are caused by destruction of red blood cells. This results in hemolytic anemia and occlusion/infarction of blood vessels by the abnormally shaped cells. Infarction of blood vessels leads to thrombosis, embolism, and eventually destruction of function at a cellular level in major organs such as the lung, kidney, liver, and spleen. Severity of symptoms will vary, and those with the most severe symptoms may not outlive childhood. Symptoms are acute during periods of hypoxia. Such periods include infection (especially pulmonary), dehydration, trauma, strenuous physical activity/emotional stress, air travel, high altitudes, tight, restrictive clothing, or excesses of heat or cold (10, p. 363).

Symptoms in crisis include:

1. Pain in the extremities, chest, abdomen, or back and ulceration and edema of the extremities because of vasoocclusion and infarction.
2. Pallor, weakness, dyspnea, and jaundice owing to hemolytic anemia.

3. Progressive renal disease with bacteriuria and inability to concentrate urine; renal failure because of kidney cell damage.
4. Headache, paralysis, stroke, blindness, convulsions, and other neurologic disturbances because of cerebral thrombosis.
5. Nausea, vomiting, and severe abdominal pain and distention owing to liver and spleen involvement.
6. Bone and joint pain owing to vasoocclusion and infarction of the marrow itself.

SS definitely increases the risks in pregnancy for both mother and fetus, and the outcome always is in doubt. Since pregnancy places such stress on the hematologic system, pregnancy itself constitutes a crisis, and episodes of severe symptomatology occur more often. Infections occur more frequently than in normal pregnancy, and these precipitate even more crises.

In order to decrease the severity of the disease and pregnancy-related exacerbations, transfusion is the treatment of choice. Whether the treatment should be prophylactic or palliative is most controversial. While some evidence points to decreased prenatal mortality with prophylactic transfusion, the treatment carries serious risks: (1) hemosiderosis, (2) development of immune response to blood products, and (3) transmission of hepatitis, AIDs, etc., with the serum.

One suggested protocol for prophylactic transfusion is as follows (10, p 363):

1. Perform a partial exchange transfusion at 28 weeks' gestation in order to:
   a. Obtain a hematocrit value of 35%.
   b. Obtain a normal hemoglobin (A1) concentration of 40%.
2. Repeat the partial exchange transfusion when:
   a. A crisis occurs.
   b. Normal hemoglobin drops below 20%.
   c. At 36–38 weeks' gestation in preparation for delivery.

Others transfuse only if the hematocrit falls below 25%, or a crisis occurs (11).

Patients should receive iron therapy only if laboratory values indicate iron deficiencies. As with other hemoglobinopathies, folic acid should be given in order to assist bone marrow production of red blood cells.

Meticulous attention should be paid to monitoring cardiac, renal, and liver function (see Chapters 9, 12, and 17).

Development of toxemia should be anticipated in the majority of patients. Thus, the patient carefully should be taught to report immediately any signs or symptoms, and clinical manifestations of the disease should be looked for at each visit. Urinary tract infection and pneumonitis are common. Any infection should be treated vigorously.

SS crises that do occur in pregnancy may be very severe and may result in cerebral, pulmonary, or bone marrow infarction. Congestive heart failure may ensue as the anemia becomes pronounced because of not only repeated crises but also the physiologic hemodilution of pregnancy. Toxemia is associated with renal damage. Acute crises in the first or second trimester are associated with increased maternal and fetal morbidity and mortality. Interruption of the pregnancy should be discussed with the patient. Acute crisis in the third trimester may necessitate emergency cesarean section.

A crisis is managed aggressively with exchange transfusions, oxygen, intravenous therapy, and sedation. Acidosis, infection, and congestive heart failure should be treated and anticoagulation therapy initiated in order to prevent embolism. The fetus should be monitored continuously. Fetal distress necessitates emergency cesarean section if viability is probable (2, p 67).

Some authorities recommend cesarean section at 36 weeks in order to avoid the maternal physical stress of labor and to remove the fetus from a suboptimal environment. If cesarean section is anticipated, exchange transfusion is suggested before delivery. General anesthesia should be avoided at all costs due to the possibility of hypoxia and further crisis. Postpartum hemorrhage may occur, and the resulting hypoxia could result in a crisis.

No matter how stable the maternal health appears, the fetal health is always poor owing to placental infarction during the sickling process. Intrauterine growth retardation and placental insufficiency are to be expected. Evaluation of fetal status, including biophysical profile, should begin as soon as it is feasible.

The infant may inherit the homogenous form of the disease, depending on the genetic makeup of the parents. Even if the disease is inherited, the newborn generally will not show signs or symptoms at birth. Hypoxia will begin to cause crisis only after fetal hemoglobin has been replaced by adult hemoglobin S. However, affected infants always should be kept warm and well oxygenated (12).

Sickle Cell Trait

Sickle cell trait (AS) is the condition of being heterozygous for hemoglobin S. It occurs in about 8% of the black population. AS is associated with an increased incidence of anemia. However, because of the chronicity of the disease, reported symptoms of anemia usually are absent. Crisis states occur only as the result of *extreme* hypoxia. Diagnosis is suspected with a positive sickle preparation test and confirmed by hemoglobin electrophoresis.

During pregnancy, women with AS have an increased incidence of bacteriuria. If urinary tract infection is undiagnosed or untreated, pyelonephritis may ensue. Etiology for the increased incidence of bacteriuria is unknown. However, increased susceptibility to infection or subclinical renal damage as trait sequelae are postulated etiologies.

Pregnant women with AS may develop a crisis during anesthesia unless carefully oxygenated. However, risks are much lower than with the homozygous form of the disease (12).

Fetal outcome is not jeopardized, unless both of the parents have the trait. The fetus has a 25% chance of inheriting the homozygous form of the disease.

Routine iron and folic acid supplementation usually are prescribed. Careful evaluation of urinary tract infection signs and symptoms and urinary microscopic examination should be done at each visit. A urine culture should be done once each trimester in order to assess for the presence of bacteriuria and to treat before pyelonephritis develops.

NURSING MANAGEMENT

Nursing care specific for a patient with *anemia*:

☐ Screen all pregnant women on an ongoing basis for signs and symptoms of anemia: (e.g., fatigue, malaise, headache, sore tongue, skin pallor, pale mucous membranes/nail beds, loss of appetite, nausea, vomiting, and/or pica).

☐ Teach all pregnant patients the importance of taking iron and vitamin supplements including appropriate timing of medication (e.g., iron to be taken between meals with glass of orange juice to maximize absorption).

☐ Teach patients to avoid constipation secondary to iron therapy by drinking 8 glasses of water/day, including the natural laxative prunes or

NURSING MANAGEMENT

prune juice in diet, increasing fiber, and daily exercise.

☐ Be aware that many "unexplained" anemias are due to epistaxis, bleeding gums, intestinal parasites, or bleeding hemorrhoids, and include evaluation of these conditions in ongoing patient evaluation.

☐ Instruct patients with G-6-PD deficiency about foods and drugs thay may not use, and provide them with a list of contraindicated items to carry with them at all times.

☐ Refer couples with the thalassemias or sickle cell disease for genetic screening, as ordered.

☐ Screen all patients with G-6-PD deficiency and sickle cell trait for urinary tract infection, at least once each trimester.

☐ During the postpartum period, make every effort to minimize blood loss (see Chapter 42).

☐ Upon postpartum discharge of an anemic patient, ensure that orders are written for iron and vitamin supplementation, as appropriate.

Nursing diagnoses most frequently associated with *anemia*:

☐ Grieving related to potential/actual loss of infant or birth of an imperfect child.

☐ Anticipatory grieving related to actual/perceived threat to self.

☐ Spiritual distress.

☐ Pain.

☐ Knowledge deficit regarding etiology, disease process, treatment and expected outcome.

☐ Potential for infection.

☐ Knowledge deficit regarding medication regimen.

☐ Altered nutrition: less than body requirements.

☐ Impaired tissue integrity.

COAGULOPATHIES

Introduction

Pregnancy is termed a hypercoagulation state. Specifically, platelets, fibrinogen, and clotting factor VIII are increased significantly during pregnancy. Other components of the coagulation system are increased moderately. Etiology is unknown, but some experts believe that chronic microhemorrhage occurs in the placental vascular bed throughout pregnancy and triggers increased production of clotting elements. Whatever the cause, the mechanism is protective in that it helps the prevention of postpartum hemorrhage. At the same time, it sets the stage for increased incidence of phlebitis and thromboembolism.

Disseminated Intravascular Coagulation

Definition

Disseminated intravascular coagulation (DIC) represents a series of pathological events characterized by increased thrombin formation, increased utilization of platelets and coagulation factors, formation of thrombi in microcirculation, and rebound activation of the clotting factors. Paradoxically, DIC ultimately produces hemorrhage because of consumption and finally exhaustion of the body's supply of prothrombin; platelets; coagulation factors V, VIII, and X; and fibrinogen (2, p 336). Clotting in the microcirculation interferes with oxygen-

ation and nutrition of cells and results in ischemia and death of tissues and cells of the heart, brain, kidney, liver, and other vital organs. It is not a disease but an intermediate mechanism in a number of obstetric, surgical, hemolytic, and neoplastic disorders, all of which activate—in various ways—the coagulation sequence. It also is referred to as consumptive coagulopathy or defibrination syndrome (5, p 337).

Etiology

As has been stated, DIC is a complication of a wide variety of diseases that in some manner activate the coagulation cascade mechanism. Three specific mechanisms activate the abnormal clotting of DIC (10, p 375, 13, p 36):

1. Massive or prolonged spillage of tissue thromboplastin into the blood, triggering the extrinsic coagulation sequence. Obstetric complications that can increase tissue thrombin release include abruptio placentae, hydatidiform mole, retained dead fetus, or chorioamnionitis.

2. Destruction of vascular endothelium, triggering the intrinsic pathway. Obstetric complications involved include amniotic fluid embolism, eclampsia, and intraamniotic injection of hyperosmolar urea or hypertonic saline.

3. Damage to blood cells, triggering the intrinsic pathway. Chorioamnionitis or septic abortion specifically caused by gram-negative endotoxins would initiate the intrinsic pathway directly by converting factor XII to factor XIIa.

Table 8.5.
CAUSES OF DISSEMINATED INTRAVASCULAR COAGULATION[a]

EVENTS THAT INITIATE DIC	SPECIFIC CLINICAL CONDITIONS
1. Massive, prolonged, or widespread spillage of tissue thromboplastin into the blood	1. Abruptio placentae 2. Extensive surgery 3. Severe tissue injury, especially crush injuries 4. Neoplastic diseases, such as leukemia or cancer of the prostate, lung, colon, breast, or stomach 5. Shock syndromes 6. Burn injuries 7. Venomous snake bites of the pit viper type 8. Hydatidiform mole 9. Retained dead fetus 10. Brain injuries (traumatic and/or surgical) 11. Endotoxins (released from gram-negative bacteria)
2. Extensive alteration or destruction of the vascular endothelium	1. Prolonged cardiopulmonary bypass 2. Amniotic fluid emboli 3. Heat stroke 4. Malignant hyperthermia 5. Anoxia 6. Shock syndromes 7. Adult respiratory distress syndrome (ARDS) 8. Eclampsia 9. Endotoxins
3. Damage to the blood cells	1. Malaria 2. Sickle cell disease 3. Transfusion reactions 4. Burn injuries 5. Hemolysis of RBCs 6. Endotoxins

[a]Reprinted with permission from Darovic G: Disseminated intravascular coagulation. *Critical Care Nursing* November/December: 40, 1982.

An extensive list of obstetric and nonobstetric causes of DIC is given in Table 8.5. Because DIC is an underlying complication of such serious diseases, the survival rate for patients who develop DIC often is less than 50% (2, p 76).

The most frequent obstetric cause is abruptio placentae, occurring in as many as a third of cases of abruption—usually within 8 hours of onset of symptoms (see Chapter 31) (2, p 43).

Signs and Symptoms

The clinical symptomatology depends on a number of factors, including the patient's overall general health, the underlying causative condition, and the manner in which DIC occurs (e.g., acute or chronic).

In some conditions such as cancer or retained dead fetus, the pathologic process of DIC is prolonged over a period of time. Utilization and regeneration of blood coagulation components reach a subnormal balance. Generalized, less obvious, and sometimes easily missed signs and symptoms include sweating, cold and mottled fingers and toes, petechiae, easy bruising, recurrent minor episodes of bleeding, or thrombophlebitis.

When massive thromboplastin is released, extensive destruction of vascular endothelium and/or widespread destruction of red blood cells occur; symptoms are acute, abrupt, and severe. These include (2, p 77):

1. Dyspnea, cyanosis, increased respiratory rate
2. Pain and swelling of joints
3. Bleeding from mucous membranes throughout the body and trauma sites
4. Nausea, vomiting, severe abdominal pain
5. Flank/back pain, hematuria, anuria
6. Congestive heart failure
7. Restlessness, confusion, anxiety, convulsions, coma
8. Shock

Patients with DIC often present with a shock-like syndrome. The mechanism by which DIC produces shock is detailed in Figure 8.1. Unfortunately, lack of circulation because of the hemorrhage reactivates the pathologic process of DIC, and a deadly feedback mechanism is stimulated after which the symptoms worsen.

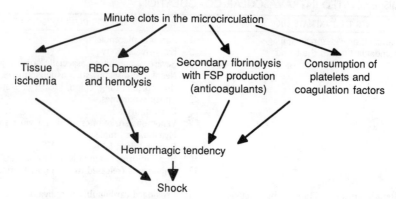

Figure 8.1. Mechanisms by which DIC produces shock. (Adapted from Darovic G: Disseminated intravascular coagulation. *Critical Care Nursing.* November/December: 39, 1982.)

Diagnosis

Diagnosis is confirmed by hematologic laboratory tests showing prolonged thrombin time, prothrombin time, and partial thromboplastin time; decreased platelet count; and elevated fibrin split products. It is important to keep in mind the pregnancy-induced changes in the coagulation system when evaluating laboratory tests. Table 8.6 lists these tests, their pregnant and nonpregnant values, and the expected findings in DIC.

Coagulation factors will be depressed—particularly factors V, VIII, and X. Increased serum bilirubin or creatinine indicates renal damage, and increased lactic dehydrogenase (LDH) indicates tissue damage. High levels of endogenous protamine sulfate differentiates DIC from heparin overdose in those patients receiving heparin. Laboratory baseline data are obtained and updated hourly or as the condition warrants. A gross evaluation of clotting time is usually done while waiting for the initial results to be reported. A 15-ml tube of blood is drawn and inverted gently four or five times. If no clot forms with 12 minutes or if the clot is not solid and dissolves within 1 hour, clotting defects are present. This test tube usually is taped to the head of the patient's bed while awaiting more definitive diagnostic levels but should be removed when the diagnosis is confirmed (7, p 706).

Table 8.6.
LABORATORY BLOOD TESTS[a]

TEST	COAGULATION PARAMETERS MEASURED	NONPREGNANT VALUES	PREGNANT VALUES	RESULTS IN DIC
Platelets	Platelets	150,000–400,000/ mm^3	Normal	Reduced
Fibrin split products	Action of plasmin on fibrin or fibrinogen	—	Usually absent	Present (positive)
Fibrinogen	Fibrinogen	200–400 mg/100 ml	300–500 mg/100 ml	Usually depressed
Prothrombin time	Extrinsic and common pathways	11–13 seconds	Shortened	Usually prolonged
Partial thromboplastin time	Intrinsic and common pathways	40–60 seconds	Shortened	Usually prolonged
Activated partial prothrombin time	Intrinsic and common pathways	25–45 seconds	Shortened	Usually prolonged
Clotting time	Intrinsic and common pathways	6–12 minutes	Normal	Normal
Thrombin time	Rate of fibrin conversion	12–18 seconds	Shortened	Usually prolonged
Euglobulin lysis time	Rate of fibrinolysis	—	Normal	Usually shortened
Ethanol or gelatin tests	Presence of fibrin split products	—	Fibrin monomer absent	Fibrin monomer present

[a]Adapted from Mayberry L, Forte A: Pregnancy related DIC. *MCN* 10:171, 1985.

Table 8.7.
BLOOD COMPONENTS TO PROMOTE HEMOSTASIS[a]

BLOOD COMPONENTS	FACTORS PRESENT	NURSING CONSIDERATIONS
Fresh whole blood	All factors	Use immediately (within 3–4 hours of collection) to retain all clotting factors. The advantage of using fresh whole blood is the presence of all blood factors. The disadvantage may be insufficient time for complete screening checks for AIDS, viral hepatitis, blood grouping, and cross-matching procedures. Therefore careful monitoring before, during, and after administration for transfusion reactions and signs of infection are essential.
Fresh frozen plasma	All factors except platelets	Use within 30 minutes to minimize rapid deterioration of coagulation factors caused by thawing. Side effects include allergic reactions, chills, fever, and circulatory overload. Risk of infection.
Platelets	Platelets	Infuse as quickly as possible (storage limited to between 48 and 72 hours). Must be infused at room temperature (usually stored at room temperature). Transfusion risks include urticaria, chills, fever, infection, and immunization to red blood cell antigens.
Cryoprecipitate	Fibrinogen factor VIII, factor XIII	Infuse as quickly as possible (can only be used for 6 hours after thawing). Risk of infection and allergic and febrile reactions.

[a]Adapted from Mayberry L, Forte A: Pregnancy related DIC. *MCN* 10:168, 1985.

Maternal and Fetal Outcome

Maternal and fetal outcome are severely jeopardized. Degree of risk depends on underlying causative factors and rapidity of onset. If the fetus dies in utero, maternal risk is increased further.

In cases of abruption complicated by DIC, maternal mortality is approximately 3%. Fetal mortality rises above 50%, with many deaths occurring before the mother has time to reach the hospital (4).

Medical Management

Management revolves around slowing hemorrhage while prohibiting excessive microclotting at the same time. Restoring the delicate balance of coagulation and fibrinolysis can pose a major challenge. The following principles govern the medical management of DIC (4, p 48):

1. Correction of the causative factor. This is the most important consideration. Evacuation of the fetus and placenta from the uterus is the treatment of choice in DIC caused by abruption, retained fetal demise, septic abortion, and hypertonic saline pregnancy termination. Coagulation levels are reported to return to normal within 24 hours without the necessity for any further treatment.
2. Interruption of the coagulation cascade. Heparin can be used to interrupt the cascade mechanism specifically because it prevents clot formation, sparing coagulation factors, and

retards the rebound activation of the fibrinolytic systems. Its use in both DIC management and in pregnancy is controversial. In obstetric causes of DIC, heparin usually is used only to stabilize blood volume until the uterus can be evacuated. Since heparin is metabolized by the liver and excreted by the kidney, patients with hepatic or renal damage—and this includes eclamptic patients—should receive heparin only with extremely careful monitoring of organ function and drug level.

3. Deactivation of the fibrinolytic system. If obstetric therapy fails and severe hypofibrinogenemia persists after the uterus has been emptied, use of an antifibrinolytic agent (epsilon aminocaproic acid—EACA or Amecar) sometimes is recommended. Use is controversial because while it will slow bleeding, it may also prevent lysis of pathologic clots that are causing necrosis in vital organs.
4. Replacement of blood components. Platelets, fibrinogen, and/or coagulation factors can be replaced carefully after evaluation. During pregnancy, expanded blood volume and hypercoagulation decrease the need for replacement. Usually, replacement of clotting factors is titrated with heparin therapy in order to minimize pathologic microclotting. Table 8.7 lists coagulation factors available from various blood components and the nursing management involved in their administration.

NURSING MANAGEMENT

Nursing care specific for a patient with *DIC*:

☐ Be aware of obstetric conditions that predispose toward DIC (e.g., abruptio placentae, hydatidiform mole, retained dead fetus, chorioamnionitis, septic abortion, toxemia, amniotic fluid embolus, or other embolus.

☐ Screen all at-risk patients for signs and symptoms of DIC (e.g., petechiae, oozing from intravenous or venipuncture site, bruising, hemorrhage from incision(s) or uterus in the postpartum period, hematuria or guaiac positive stools).

☐ If DIC is diagnosed:

— Monitor vital signs every 15 minutes;

— Observe for new sites of hemorrhage in all body systems and report changes immediately;

— Stay with the patient, provide emotional support, and ensure that the bedside manner of the team and the care provided is calm, quiet, and nonstressful.

☐ Protect the patient from further bruising/bleeding by:

— Performing gentle mouth care;

— Avoiding tape on the skin, when possible;

— Padding the side rails;

— Turning carefully and gently;

— Providing gentle skin care;

— Applying pressure for 5 minutes at intramuscular injection sites.

Nursing diagnoses most frequently associated with *DIC*:

☐ Grieving related to potential/actual loss of infant or birth of an imperfect child.

☐ Anticipatory grieving related to actual/perceived threat to self.

☐ Fluid volume deficit.

☐ Altered maternal tissue perfusion.

☐ Knowledge deficit regarding etiology, disease process, treatment, and expected outcome.

☐ Impaired gas exchange.

☐ Anxiety/fear.

☐ Pain.

Von Willebrand's Disease

Definition

Von Willebrand's Disease is an autosomal dominant trait characterized by prolonged bleeding time. It is associated with epistaxis; menorrhagia; and hemorrhage after trauma, surgery, tooth extraction, or during the postpartum period. It is also called pseudohemophilia or angiohemophilia (14, p 39). Although it accounts for only 10% of all inherited coagulopathies, it is the most clinically significant coagulation disorder in women and the most frequently encountered in obstetrics (5, p 1210).

Etiology

Von Willebrand's disease results from a deficiency of coagulation factor VIII.

Signs and Symptoms

Mucous membrane bleeding is one of the most prominent signs. Tooth extraction may cause major hemorrhage. Incidence of menorrhagia and postpartum hemorrhage makes this disorder uniquely significant for women (2, p 71).

Diagnosis

Diagnosis is confirmed if factor VIII is deficient and bleeding time is *prolonged*. It should be noted that this disease is the only coagulopathy characterized by a prolonged bleeding time. In order to further differentiate it from the other factor

VIII disease—hemophilia—a factor VIII antigen test can be performed. In persons with hemophilia, the antigen activity will be normal; in persons with von Willebrand's disease, absent or deficient levels will be shown (2, p 71).

Because of the normal increase in factor VIII during pregnancy, it is difficult to make a firm diagnosis of the disorder. Levels will not return to nonpregnant levels until 6 weeks postpartum (4, p 61).

Maternal and Fetal Outcome

Pregnancy course usually is benign. Since factor VIII normally is increased during pregnancy, those women with tendency toward hemorrhage actually may experience some diminution of symptoms. However, patients do have an increased risk of bleeding from spontaneous or voluntary abortion early in pregnancy because the physiologic increase in factor VIII has not yet occurred. Women with the disease may begin pregnancy with an iron deficiency anemia due to chronic blood loss. The major maternal risk is postpartum hemorrhage. Fetal outcome is not affected by maternal disease, but the fetus does have the potential to inherit the disease. (8, p 88).

Medical Management

If the patient is known to have the disease, levels of factor VIII should be monitored. In preparation for delivery, these should be maintained at least at 50% of normal, by transfusion if necessary. Factor VIII is not tranfused directly because it may lack certain elements specific to coagulation factor stimulation; but, rather, three units of fresh frozen plasma or six units of cryoprecipitate give a maximum amount of factor VIII in its most useful form. For patients who fail to respond to this, massive therapy doses of cryoprecipitate (15–30 units of cryoprecipitate) are indicated.

However, even patients with very low levels of factor VIII may not bleed after delivery. Since the course is so variable during pregnancy, a detailed history of the result of trauma, surgery, menstruation, and childbirth are better predictors of current tendency toward hemorrhage and the need for replacement therapy than the level of factor VIII (8, p 88).

Even though pregnancy course is said to be benign, special emphasis should be placed on optimizing hematologic status. The presence and etiology of anemia should be assessed and rigorous treatment initiated. Careful evaluation of bleeding tendencies should be ongoing, with particular emphasis on bleeding from pores, gums, or hemorrhoids. If emergency tooth extraction becomes necessary during pregnancy, preparation should be the same as for delivery, and the patient should be hospitalized. Dental work should be done with extreme care in a hospital setting, and the dentist/oral sur-geon must be made aware of the underlying pathology.

If the patient desires a therapeutic termination of pregnancy or is aborting spontaneously in the first or early second trimester, major hemorrhage should be anticipated, the patient admitted to the hospital, and factor VIII levels boosted to at least 50% of normal. Preterm labor also carries similar risks of hemorrhage because normal physiologic elevations of factor VIII are proportional to gestational age and are highest only at term.

If levels of 50% of normal are achieved prior to delivery, bleeding from the uterus, episiotomy, or lacerations should be within normal limits. Cesarean section can be performed safely. The levels should be maintained for at least 5 days after normal delivery or any surgical procedures (i.e., episiotomy, repair of laceration), as well as cesarean section.

Fetal outcome is not affected by maternal disease. However, the fetus may inherit the disease. It will be important to assess this prior to delivery in order to be prepared to prevent or to treat newborn hemorrhage. Paternal and maternal genetic studies and amniocentesis should be done. If the fetus is a disease carrier, at birth vitamin K should be administered immediately and suctioning of the oral and nasal passages done with extreme caution. Signs and symptoms of hemorrhage and shock should be assessed carefully.

NURSING MANAGEMENT

Nursing care specific for a patient with *von Willebrand's disease:*

- ☐ Educate the patient regarding the following:
  - — Importance of regular dental care by a qualified oral surgeon;
  - — Dangers of tooth extraction (have the patient report signs and symptoms of tooth pain to oral surgeon immediately); and
  - — Routine dental care and hygiene (e.g., use soft toothbrush); avoidance of foods (e.g., apples, corn) that may traumatize gums.
- ☐ Assess for anemia; ensure that appropriate treatment is maintained.
- ☐ Monitor uterine bleeding carefully if patient has first trimester spontaneous or therapeutic abortion, observing for severe hemorrhage.

- ☐ Observe patient for hemorrhage (e.g., bleeding gums, bleeding hemorrhoids, etc.).
- ☐ Monitor uterine bleeding, episiotomy site, and/or cesarean section incision during the postpartum period, carefully observing for severe hemorrhage.

Nursing diagnoses most frequently associated with *von Willebrand's disease:*

- ☐ Anticipatory grieving related to actual/perceived threat to self.
- ☐ Grieving related to potential/actual loss of infant or birth of an imperfect child.
- ☐ Knowledge deficit regarding etiology, disease process, treatment, and expected outcome.
- ☐ Fluid volume deficit.
- ☐ Altered maternal tissue perfusion.

REFERENCES

1. Ziegal E, Cranley M: *Obstetric Nursing*. New York, Macmillan, 1984, p 14.

2. Burrow G, Ferris T: *Medical Complications of Pregnancy*, ed 2. Philadelphia, WB Saunders, 1982, p 63.

3. Pritchard J, MacDonald PC, Gant NF: *Williams Obstetrics*, ed 17. Norwalk, CT, Appleton-Century-Crofts, 1985, p 391.

4. Nursing Reference Library: *Diagnostics*. Springhouse, PA, Springhouse Corporation, 1986, p 351.

5. Miller B, Keane C: *Encyclopedia and Dictionary of Medicine Nursing and Allied Health*. Philadelphia, WB Saunders, 1983, p 50.

6. Dewees C: Hematologic disorders in pregnancy. *Nurs Clin* 17:57–67, 1982.

7. Mahoney E, Flynn J: *Handbook of Medical-Surgical Nursing*. New York, John Wiley and Sons, 1983, p 696.

8. de Swiet M: *Medical Disorders of Pregnancy*. Boston, Blackwell Scientific Publications, 1984, p 39.

9. Tucker S, et al.: *Patient Care Standards*. St. Louis, Mosby, 1984, p 124.

10. Doenges M, et al.: *Nursing Care Plans*. Philadelphia, FA Davis, 1984, p 363.

11. Arias F: *High Risk Pregnancy and Delivery*. St. Louis, Mosby, 1984, p 235.

12. Friedman E: *Obstetrical Decision Making*. St. Louis, Mosby, 1982, p 76.

13. Darovic G: Disseminated intravascular coagulation. *Critical Care Nursing* November/December: 36–43, 1982.

Chapter 9
Cardiac Disorders
Nancy W. Kulb, C.N.M., M.S.

INTRODUCTION

Physiology

Normal pregnancy requires major adaptations in the maternal cardiovascular system. A cardiac disease that prevents these normal changes from occurring or prevents the heart from responding normally to these changes can prove life threatening for the mother and her fetus.

The uteroplacental circulation acts much like a large arteriovenous fistula, requiring an increase in both blood volume and cardiac output. Blood volume progressively increases during the pregnancy, with approximately a 40–50% increase when it peaks near term. Cardiac output at rest (measured in the left lateral position) begins to increase appreciably in the first trimester and remains elevated throughout the pregnancy. It is, of course, elevated even more with physical activity. Overall, the average increase in cardiac output in pregnancy is about 50% (1). In late pregnancy, the supine position inhibits normal cardiac output because the weight of the gravid uterus compresses the vena cava, thus preventing venous return to the heart. A change from the supine to the left lateral recumbent position increases cardiac output 22% (2, p 195).

Cardiac output is increased further during labor and the immediate postpartum period. There is approximately a 15% increase early in the first stage, 30% late in the first stage, and a 45% increase during the second stage. Superimposed on this is a 15–20% increase in cardiac output with each uterine contraction. In the immediate postpartum period, the decrease in size of the venous capacitance beds with minimal blood loss and relief of pressure on the vena cava results in a relative autotransfusion. Cardiac output is increased approximately 65% 5 minutes after delivery, decreasing to 40% 1 hour after delivery (3).

During pregnancy the resting pulse rate increases 10–15 beats/minute. The stroke volume also increases. Cardiac volume increases approximately 75 ml, or slightly more than 10%, probably both from dilatation and hypertrophy. Left ventricular wall mass and end-diastolic cardiac dimensions also increase (2, p 194). Normal changes in blood pressure are discussed in Chapter 13.

The position of the heart changes during pregnancy. As the diaphragm is pushed upward progressively by the expanding uterus, the heart is displaced upwards and to the left. It is rotated on its long axis, thus moving the apex laterally, and it is positioned somewhat closer to the anterior chest wall. The extent of these changes is determined by the size and position of the uterus, configuration of the abdomen and thorax, and strength of the abdominal muscles (2, p 194).

Some heart sound changes that are abnormal in a nonpregnant person are common and normal during pregnancy (2, p 193):

1. An exaggerated split of the first heart sound.
2. A loud, easily heard third sound that develops in up to 80% of women at some time during the pregnancy and parallels the increase in cardiac output (4, pp 161–167).
3. A systolic murmur that is heard in up to 90% of gravidas but disappears soon after delivery. The murmur is intensified by inspiration in some women and by expiration in others.
4. A transient, soft diastolic murmur that is heard in up to 19% of pregnant women. (Some experts disagree that a diastolic murmur is normal, stating that it is always pathological but that a third heart sound with its vibrations

89

Table 9.1.

SYMPTOMS SUGGESTIVE OF CARDIAC DISEASE[a]

COMMON WITH PREGNANCY	ABNORMAL WITH PREGNANCY (REQUIRE FURTHER INVESTIGATION)
Fatigue	Severe fatigue
Dyspnea	Orthopnea or nocturnal dyspnea
Chest pain	Increasing chest pain
Palpitations	—
Syncope	Recurrent syncope
Peripheral edema	—
Increased neck veins	Increase persists during entire cardiac cycle
Systolic murmur	Systolic murmur grade >3/6, all systolic murmur, hemoptysis, pulmonary rales

[a]Adapted from Veille JC: Sounding the value of maternal-fetal echocardiography, *Contemp. OB/GYN* 24:94, 1984.

could easily be mistaken for a diastolic murmur [4, p 162].)

5. A continuous murmur, heard in 10% of patients, particularly in the third trimester. It is thought to actually result from increased blood flow through the breast vasculature.

Diagnosis of Cardiac Disease

The diagnosis of cardiac disease is much more difficult in the pregnant woman because normal maternal adaptations to pregnancy result in signs and symptoms that would otherwise be indicative of heart disease. It is equally important that cardiac disease not be overlooked or overdiagnosed. Table 9.1 lists symptoms that are common in normal pregnant women and those that require further investigation. At least 50% of cardiac disease diagnosed during pregnancy was not suspected prior to pregnancy (5).

When obtaining the initial medical history, the care provider should question all pregnant women about a history of rheumatic fever, cardiac disease, or a heart murmur prior to pregnancy. Dyspnea, dependent edema, and decreased tolerance for physical activity are symptoms that often occur in normal pregnancy, but a history of them prior to pregnancy would raise suspicion of cardiac disease (4, p 161).

As noted above, heart sounds may change with pregnancy. A normal systolic murmur should be no greater than grade 2/6, should be heard best on the left sternal border, should have no thrill, and should not radiate to the axilla (4, p 161).

A chest x-ray may be used to detect cardiomegaly, selective chamber enlargement, and pulmonary overcirculation. Its interpretation, however, especially in the diagnosis of cardiomegaly, must take into consideration the normal changes in the position of the heart that make it appear larger and the normal increase in cardiac volume. Chest x-ray is contraindicated in the first trimester. It may be done later in pregnancy with the abdomen shielded, but interpretation becomes increasingly difficult. Therefore, if a chest x-ray done prior to pregnancy is available, it may be the most beneficial for diagnosis (4, p 162).

The electrocardiogram (ECG) is essentially normal during pregnancy, except for a slight deviation of the electrial axis to the left because of the change in the position of the heart. It is useful for detecting ventricular hypertrophy and atrial enlargement (4, p 162).

Echocardiography is an ultrasound examination of the heart and usually is performed with a simultaneous ECG. It can be used to aid in the diagnosis of mitral valve prolapse, mitral stenosis, hypertrophic cardiomyopathy, and aortic valve disease (4, p 162).

Burwell and Metcalf (6) in 1958 stated that any one of the following conditions confirms heart disease:

1. Diastolic, presystolic, or continuous cardiac murmur.
2. Unequivocal cardiac enlargement.
3. Loud, harsh systolic murmur (especially if associated with a thrill).
4. Severe arrhythmia.

Severe cardiac disease without one of the above findings is rare. Once the obstetrical team detects an abnormality, referral to a cardiologist often is required for specific diagnosis and collaborative management.

Incidence

The incidence of heart disease in pregnancy is estimated to be 1–2% (7, pp 353–357). It used to be that rheumatic heart disease (RHD) was the leading cause, but the incidence of RHD has been declining in the United States and Western Europe over the past 50 years. With better medical management and surgical techniques, more women with congenital heart disease are surviving and conceiving, thus comprising a greater proportion of the obstetrical population with heart disease.

Table 9.2.
FUNCTIONAL CLASSIFICATION OF HEART DISEASE[a]

Class I: Uncompromised. Patients with cardiac disease and no limitation of physical activity. Patients in this class do not have symptoms of cardiac insufficiency, nor do they experience anginal pain.
Class II: Slightly compromised. Patients with cardiac disease and slight limitation of physical activity. These patients are comfortable at rest, but if ordinary physical activity is undertaken, discomfort results in the form of excessive fatigue, palpitations, dyspnea, or anginal pain.
Class III: Markedly compromised. Patients with cardiac disease and marked limitation of physical activity. These patients are comfortable at rest, but less than ordinary activity causes discomfort in the form of excessive fatigue, palpitations, dyspnea, or anginal pain.
Class IV: Patients with cardiac disease and inability to perform any physical activity without discomfort. Symptoms of cardiac insufficiency or of the anginal syndrome may occur even at rest, and if any physical activity is undertaken, discomfort is increased.

[a]From Pritchard JA, MacDonald PC, Gant NF: *Williams Obstetrics*, ed 17. Norwalk, Ct. Appleton-Century-Crofts, 1985, p 590. Adapted from New York Heart Association, Inc: *Diseases of the Heart and Blood Vessels—Nomenclature and Criteria for Diagnosis*, ed 6. Boston, Little, Brown, and Co, 1964.

Maternal and Fetal Outcome

The prognosis for both the patient with heart disease and her fetus depends upon the functional capacity of the heart; the likelihood of developing other complications that will also increase the cardiac workload; the quality of medical care; and the psychologic and socioeconomic capabilities of the patient, her family, and perhaps the community, if prolonged hospitalization is required (2, p 589).

Heart disease is the number one nonobstetric cause of maternal death in the United States (8). With severe disease the maternal mortality rate is 2%, and the perinatal mortality rate is up to 50%. (Although they comprise only 15% of patients with heart disease in pregnancy, women with Class III or IV disease represent 85% of maternal deaths [9]. Table 9.2 gives functional classifications of heart disease.) Two-thirds of all maternal deaths occur during labor and delivery and the postpartum period.

It has been suggested that pregnancy somehow has a deleterious effect on heart disease, causing an acceleration of deterioration and resulting in an earlier death. Chesley, in 1980 (10) did not confirm this in investigating women with rheumatic heart disease.

If maternal hypoxia is severe, the fetus will be affected adversely. There is an increased incidence of spontaneous abortion, preterm delivery, and fetal death in women with heart disease. Whittemore et al. found 36% fetal wastage; if maternal hypoxia was so severe as to cause maternal polycythemia, with a hematocrit >65%, fetal wastage was essentially 100% (11). In addition, offspring of women with congenital heart disease have a six times greater incidence of structural cardiac anomalies than children of normal women (12).

Classification of Heart Disease

A very useful system for functional classification of heart disease was developed by the New York Heart Association in 1964 (Table 9.2). This classification system is based on function—not diagnosis. Different individuals with the same diagnosis may be in different functional classifications, and individuals with various diagnoses will be in each functional classification. During pregnancy, it is quite possible for the patient's classification to change.

The following section of this chapter will deal with management of cardiac disease in pregnancy according to functional classifications.

MANAGEMENT OF CARDIAC DISEASE IN PREGNANCY

Specific management depends upon the functional capacity of the heart. For all pregnant women with heart disease, it is important to prevent conditions that will increase cardiac workload—e.g., excess weight gain, abnormal fluid retention, or anemia, which results in a compensatory increase in cardiac output. Therefore, the patient needs specific nutritional counseling regarding expected weight gain in pregnancy, limiting sodium intake to 1 g daily (by elimination of high sodium foods and table salt), high iron foods, and iron and vitamin supplementation.

Since anxiety will also increase the cardiac workload, it, too, must be prevented or alleviated as much as possible. The patient will need a great deal of emotional support during the pregnancy, particularly if the diagnosis of heart disease is first made during pregnancy or if the prognosis for herself or her baby is poor. She may be required to stop working and go on disability leave early in the pregnancy. Inability to perform usual household duties may require the services of a homemaker. Prolonged hospitalization and/or expensive diagnostic and treatment procedures may create a financial burden for the patient and her family. Therefore, referral should be made, as necessary, to psychiatrists, social workers, clergy, public assistance programs, or other professionals. The continued understanding and support of the entire medical team throughout the pregnancy, labor, delivery, and the postpartum period are essential.

Every attempt should be made to prevent and adequately treat pregnancy-induced hypertension, because it causes an increase in cardiac workload commensurate with the increase in blood pressure (2, p 590). Hypotension can severely limit oxygenation, especially in women with septal defects, patent ductus arteriosus (PDA), or other right-to-left shunts.

Vaginal delivery usually is preferred since the cardiac condition is a relative contraindication to surgery, and even cesarean section cannot prevent the tremendous increase in cardiac workload required during late pregnancy and the postpartum period. Analgesia to prevent anxiety during labor is very important. Usually, regional anesthesia is used, with precautions to prevent maternal hypotension. The patient is placed in the left lateral or semirecumbent position to enhance uteroplacental blood flow. Continuous monitoring of maternal and fetal heart rate and maternal central venous pressure often is useful. Forceps may be used to shorten the second stage and prevent hemodynamic changes associated with the Valsalva maneuver. Third and fourth stage blood loss is kept to a minimum by prompt delivery of the placenta, oxytocin administration, and bimanual compression when necessary. Drugs that may adversely affect cardiac status (e.g., scopolamine, ergonovine, methylergonovine) are avoided (4, p 166).

Management of Class I and II Cardiac Disease

The focus of management of class I and II disease is on prevention and early recognition of deteriorating cardiac status. Although symptoms are minor, it must be remembered that 15% of maternal deaths owing to heart disease are among women who initially are classified as class I or II. Therefore, intensive surveillance during pregnancy is mandatory.

The patient must have adequate rest to minimize cardiac demand, and she must understand that it is an important part of her care. It may be helpful to "prescribe" a specific routine—e.g., 10 hours of rest each night, and one-half hour of rest after each meal.

Since infection can lead to cardiac failure, the patient should be counseled to avoid people with upper respiratory infections or crowds. Pneumococcal and influenza vaccines may be indicated. Personal hygiene measures should be taught and reinforced. The patient should be advised to report any signs or symptoms of infection at once.

Frequent prenatal visits (every 1–2 weeks) are required and should include measurment of vital capacity. Vital capacity is the total amount of air that can be moved into or out of the lungs (i.e., the total lung capacity minus the residual volume that cannot be moved). It is measured with a spirometer. The patient inhales as much as possible and then exhales as much as possible into the spirometer. The volume is compared to that expected of a person of the same age, sex, or height. The average vital capacity in a pregnant woman is 3310 ml, a negligible increase over the nonpregnant value (2, p 196). A sudden decrease in vital capacity may indicate cardiac failure.

The physician must constantly screen for signs and symptoms of deteriorating status. Persistent rales (i.e., rales that do not clear after two or three deep breaths) at the base of the lungs may indicate congestive heart failure. Tachycardia and progressive edema may also indicate deteriorating cardiac status. The patient should be questioned at each visit (and taught to report between visits) any decrease in ability to carry out normal activities, increased dyspnea, orthopnea, excessive or unusual coughing, or hemoptysis.

The patient may be hospitalized prior to delivery if her condition requires it. Vaginal delivery is planned unless a cesarean section is necessary for an obstetric indication. For a primigravida, epidural anesthesia is usually used. For a multipara for whom an easy vaginal delivery is anticipated, analgesics may be sufficient. Vital signs (particularly pulse and respirations) are taken every 15 minutes in the first stage of labor and every 10 minutes in the second stage. A pulse greater than 100 or respirations greater than 24, especially with associated dyspnea, should be regarded as cardiac embarrassment or decompensation that could progress to cardiac failure (inability to pump sufficient blood to meet the needs of the body).

If signs of cardiac embarrassment occur, medical treatment to stabilize the cardiac status is required—not cesarean section, which will prove to be a further stress on the heart. At full dilation, however, immediate forceps delivery is indicated. Morphine sulfate should be given intravenously in a sufficient dose to alleviate anxiety and concomitantly to decrease the respiratory rate and voluntary muscle activity in the second stage. Oxygen should be given to improve oxygenation. Intermittent positive pressure breathing (IPPB) may be required if there is evidence of pulmonary edema. Diuretics are given to decrease the venous return to the heart, thereby decreasing the pulmonary and left atrial blood pressure and therefore, reducing pulmonary congestion. Furosemide (50–100 mg) is the drug usually used (Table 9.3). Antihypertensives should be given to decrease cardiac afterload if the patient is hypertensive. If she is hypotensive, the cause must be identified and treated. The goal is for the hematocrit to be within normal limits and urinary output to be adequate.

Table 9.3.
DRUGS COMMONLY USED IN TREATMENT OF HEART DISEASE[a]

DRUG	ABILITY TO CROSS PLACENTA	SECRETION IN BREAST MILK	ADVERSE EFFECT ON FETUS OR NEONATE WHEN USED IN USUAL DOSES
Digoxin	Yes	Yes	None, if maternal levels do not exceed therapeutic range.
Furosemide	Yes	Yes	No adequate studies in humans. In animals, increased incidence of abortion, fetal death, and anomalies.
Heparin	No	No	Stillbirths (12.5%) and prematurity (20%). Mechanism of this effect not understood.
Hydralazine	[b]	[b]	Fetal anomalies reported, but considered the drug of choice in treatment of hypertension during labor and delivery.
Quinidine sulfate	[b]	[b]	None reported to date.
Phenytoin	[b]	Yes	10–30% incidence of multiple anomalies, neonatal hemorrhage.
Procainamide	Yes	[b]	Has potential of accumulating in the fetus where it is much more slowly eliminated. Should be used with caution.
Propranolol	Yes	Yes	Postnatal bradycardia, hypoglycemia, impaired fetal responsiveness to anoxia. Reports on safety during lactation are conflicting.
Thiazide diuretics	Yes	Yes	Neonatal jaundice, electrolyte and water depletion, thrombocytopenia. Should be avoided during lactation.
Warfarin	Yes	Yes	Facial and skeletal anomalies, mental retardation, blindness, and deafness. Avoid during lactation, although some data suggest only a small amount passes into milk.

[a]Adapted from Arditi LI: Heart disease. In Caplan RM (ed): *Principles of Obstetrics.* Baltimore, Williams & Wilkins, 1982, p 165.
[b]no published information available.

After delivery, the patient still must be observed carefully, even if she had no problems during pregnancy or the delivery, since cardiac output increases even more immediately postpartum. Postpartum hemorrhage, infection, and thromboembolism can all precipitate crises and must be prevented if possible or immediately recognized and treated vigorously. There is no contraindication to breastfeeding as long as there was no cardiac embarrassment in pregnancy, labor, delivery, or postpartum to date. Counseling regarding contraception is very important for cardiac patients. If the patient desires bilateral tubal ligation, it should not be done until the patient is stable: ambulating well with no fever or anemia (2, p 592).

Management of Class III Cardiac Disease

From the physician's point of view, women with class III disease probably should not get pregnant. Without adequate preventive treatment, one-third of these women will have cardiac decompensation during the pregnancy. Some women with class III disease truly desire pregnancy and are willing to undertake the risk and strictly comply with management. Therefore, early in the pregnancy, the patient and her family should be fully counseled regarding the risks of pregnancy, the extent of treatment (which may require hospitalization for the duration of the pregnancy), and the alternative of therapeutic abortion. Since the mother's life expectancy is somewhat decreased, she and her family must take into consideration the somber possibility that the child will be left motherless at a young age.

Treatment includes strict bedrest, preferably in the hospital, for the entire pregnancy. Medical treatment of the cardiac condition will depend upon the specific diagnosis and functional response to pregnancy. Vaginal delivery is preferred since the cardiac condition is in itself a contraindication to cesarean section. With good medical and obstetrical care and strict compliance on the part of the patient, the maternal death rate has been demonstrated to be only slightly greater than that in the general obstetric population (13).

Management of Class IV Cardiac Disease

With class IV disease, the patient is in cardiac decompensation. Without correction there is a very high fetal and maternal mortality rate. The treatment is the same as for cardiac failure. These patients should be strongly advised against becoming pregnant and counseled regarding therapeutic abortion, when medically stable, if already pregnant.

CARDIAC COMPLICATIONS

There are certain cardiac complications that may arise from a variety of different diagnoses. This section reviews these major cardiac complications.

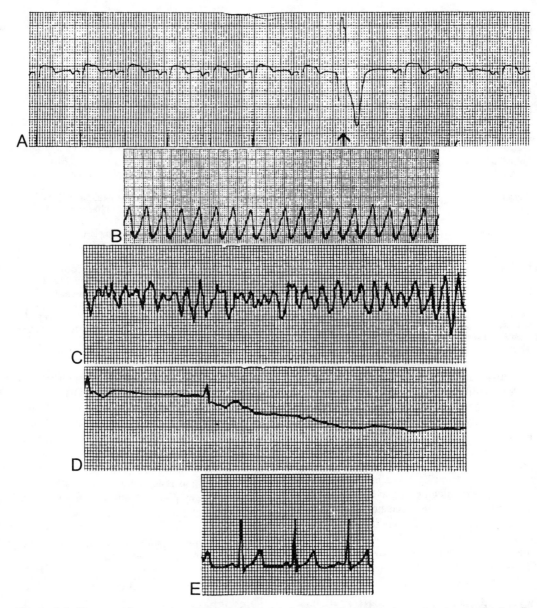

Figure 9.1. Electrocardiogram appearance of selected arrhythmias. **A**, Premature ventricular contraction. **B**, Ventricular tachycardia. **C**, Ventricular fibrillation. **D**, Asystole. **E**, Electromechanical dissociation (normal sinus rhythm in absence of pulse or respirations).

Congestive Heart Failure

Diagnosis of congestive heart failure is made more difficult since edema, apparent cardiomegaly, and rales at the base of the lungs can be quite normal in pregnancy. However, once the diagnosis is evident, management consists of digitalization, salt restriction, and, if necessary, the judicious use of diuretics (see Table 9.3). Diuretics must be used with caution since they can cause hyponatremia and hypotension. Potassium replacement should accompany diuretic use to prevent hypokalemia. Diuretics may cause water and electolyte depletion in the fetus (4, pp 163-164).

Cyanotic Heart Disease

Cyanotic heart disease usually is the result of a congenital anomaly. If the anomaly is corrected prior to pregnancy with no major residual effects, a fairly normal pregnancy, labor, and delivery can be expected. However, if the defect is uncorrected (as when the diagnosis is not made until pregnancy), there is a poor prognosis for both mother and baby. There is a poorer prognosis with pulmonary hypertension associated with cyanotic heart disease.

There is a progressively higher risk of spontaneous abortion or low birth weight with increasing degrees of maternal polycythemia (2, p 594).

Arrhythmias

There is an increased incidence of paroxysmal atrial tachycardia during pregnancy. Atrial or ventricular premature beats (Fig. 9.1) or ventricular bigeminy are not necessarily due to heart disease. Tachyarrhythmias are more common during pregnancy than bradyarrhythmias. They can be treated with digoxin if necessary. Digoxin does cross the placenta, but there is no known harm to the fetus. Successful outcomes have been reported in pregnancies complicated by bradyarrhythmias, including complete heart block. Pacemakers can be implanted with no greater risk than in a nonpregnant individual. Dysarrhythmias may be treated with selected drugs, such as quinidine and procainamide, but propranolol should be avoided if possible because of the potential for intrauterine growth retardation and neonatal sequelae (see Table 9.3) (4, p 163). Countershock conversion is not contraindicated in pregnancy. It may be lifesaving for the mother, and there is no evidence of adverse effects on the fetus.

Cardiac Tamponade

Cardiac tamponade results from effusion of fluid (resulting from pericarditis or injury to the heart or great vessels) into the pericardial sac. It decreases the ability of the heart to fill properly, resulting in decreased cardiac output, decreased arterial blood pressure, and decreased tissue perfusion. Treatment consists of emergency pericardiocentesis and supportive therapy (14).

Cardiac Surgery

Cardiovascular surgery is best performed, of course, when the patient is not pregnant. During pregnancy, it is reserved for those few patients who do not respond adequately to conservative medical management (e.g., diet, rest, reassurance, medications). Whenever surgery is considered, its risks must be weighed against the risk of continuing the pregnancy without surgery. Alternatively, therapeutic abortion should be discussed with the patient and her family.

Usually, open heart surgery for correction of congenital defects is not required during pregnancy. However, there are reports in the literature of successful correction of the following conditions during pregnancy (8, p 118): pulmonic stenosis, atrial and ventricular septal defects, coarctation of the aorta, PDA, and tetralogy of Fallot. If possible, surgery should be performed between 12 and 14 weeks of gestation—i.e., after the first trimester when embryogenesis is complete but before the peak cardiac demands of pregnancy.

Early reports of cardiopulmonary bypass in pregnant patients are difficult to evaluate because of the variable equipment, flow rates, perfusion times, and gestational ages. However, the reported perinatal death rates were high. More recently, cardiopulmonary bypass has been done with concurrent electronic fetal monitoring. During the procedure, fetal bradycardia (60–100 beats/minute) has always been evident. After intrinsic circulation has been restored, there has been fetal tachycardia. It is possible that the fetal hypoxia was due to stasis of blood in the placental intervillous space because of the nonpulsatile blood flow. High flow rates are recommended to attempt to maintain fetal oxygenation as much as possible when cardiopulmonary bypass is required (8, p 118).

Bacterial Endocarditis

Bacterial endocarditis may be acute or chronic. In the obstetrical population, most often it is associated with intravenous drug abuse. It can result in maternal death due to valvular incompetence or emboli to the brain. Treatment consists of prosthetic valve replacement and antibiotic therapy (2, p 595).

Women with endocardial damage, organic heart murmurs, valvar prostheses, mitral valve prolapse, and aortal anomalies, such as PDA and coarctation of the aorta, are at risk for subacute bacterial endocarditis (SBE). There is little research to document that prophylactic antibiotics at the time of delivery or surgery prevent SBE, but since the cost and risk are minimal, it is recommended. Prophylaxis is directed against *Streptococcus faecalis*. It should be given in labor 30 minutes to 1 hour prior to delivery and should continue for 24–48 hours after. Suggested protocols follow (2, p 595, 4, p 164):

1. Aqueous penicillin G, 2 million units, and gentamycin or tobramycin, 1.5 mg/kg every 8 hours intravenously, *or*
2. Ampicillin, 1 g intramuscularly or intravenously, and gentamycin, 1.5 mg/kg, or streptomycin, 1 g intramuscularly, every 8 hours.
3. For patients allergic to penicillin, vancomycin, 1 g.

During pregnancy, patients with a history of rheumatic fever or RHD may also be given benzathine penicillin G, 1.2 million units intramuscularly each month for prophylaxis.

Cardiac Arrest

Cardiac arrest during pregnancy may occur after eclamptic seizure, amniotic fluid embolism, hemorrhagic or septic shock, myocardial infarction, cardiac tamponade, pulmonary embolism, or anesthesia. The risk is increased in patients with cardiac or hypertensive disease, or endocrine, pulmonary, or collagen-vascular disease (15). Fortu-

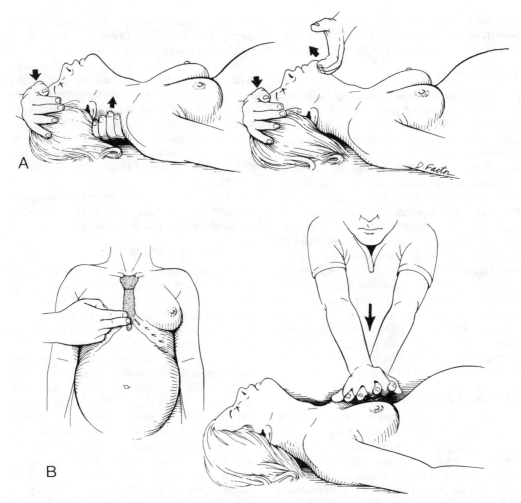

Figure 9.2. A, The first step in CPR is to open the airway for mouth-to-mouth resuscitation by tilting the head back and lifting the neck forward (*left*). Pull the chin farther forward with the tips of the fingers, if necessary (*right*). **B,** In performing external chest compression, position the hands on top of one another, on the lower half of the sternum, above the xiphoid process. Keep fingers off the chest and shoulders over the hands. (From Songster GS, Clark SL: Cardiac arrest in pregnancy—what to do. *Contemp OB/Gyn* 27: 141–143, 1985.)

nately, pregnant women in cardiac arrest are younger and tend to have fewer medical problems than the usual victim of cardiac arrest; thus, they usually respond well to treatment.

Cardiac arrest is characterized by the inability to detect a peripheral or cardiac pulse. Usually, an ECG will show ventricular fibrillation, but occasionally it may show electromechanical dissociation or asystole (Fig. 9.1). All will result in death without treatment.

The initial treatment of cardiac arrest is cardiopulmonary resuscitation (Table 9.4 and Fig. 9.2). The person who discovers that the patient is in arrest is obligated to begin CPR, call for help, and continue CPR until relieved by a more experienced person or until the patient is pronounced dead by a physician. The most experienced person present should direct the entire resuscitation procedure.

One person should be appointed to document procedures, medications, events, and times.

While CPR is progressing, a wedge should be placed under the patient's right hip to displace the uterus and alleviate compression of the vena cava. One hundred percent oxygen should be administered, an intravenous infusion should be started if one is not already in place, and cardiac monitoring leads should be attached to the patient (15, p 143).

If ventricular fibrillation is seen on the cardiac monitor, countershock should be used as needed. The patient should be intubated since that is the best way to deliver oxygen and prevent aspiration. An experienced person should perform the intubation. Drugs may be used as necessary. Any concern regarding adverse effects on the fetus are irrelevant (15, p 146). Table 9.5 gives protocols for resuscitation of the various arrhythmias resulting in cardiac arrest.

Table 9.4.
TECHNIQUE OF CARDIOPULMONARY RESUSCITATION[a]

1. Upon finding a patient who is unconscious, without detectable pulse or respirations, attempt to arrouse the patient: shake her, call out her name.
2. Call for help.
3. If she is on a cardiac monitor and is having ventricular tachycardia, give her a precordial thump (sharp blow to the midsternum). Otherwise, begin CPR.
4. Feel, look, and listen for spontaneous respirations. If there are none, position the patient on her back on a flat, firm surface. (Placing a wedge under the right hip will displace the uterus off the vena cava but should only be done when it will not delay or interrupt CPR).
5. Open the patient's airway by tilting the head back and lifting the lower jaw forward.
6. Pinch the patient's nose, place your mouth over the patient's mouth, and give four deep breaths in rapid succession.
7. Check for a carotid pulse. If none is detectable, begin chest compression.
8. Chest compression is done by kneeling beside the patient, placing one hand on top of the other on the sternum, and keeping your fingers off the patient's chest. Your shoulders should be directly over your hands. The sternum is depressed 4–5 cm with each compression, with compression time equal to relaxation time.
9. When CPR is done by one person, compressions are at the rate of 80/minute. After each 15 compressions, two respirations are given.
10. When CPR is done by two people, one is responsible for chest compression and the other for ventilation. The rate of compressions is 60/minute, with one inflation after each five compressions.
11. When equipment and personnel are available, bag-and-mask ventilation is substituted for mouth-to-mouth respiration. Intubation is done as soon as possible since that is the best way to deliver oxygen and prevent aspiration.
12. CPR is continued until spontaneous respirations return or the physician pronounces the patient dead. It should not be interrupted longer than 30 seconds to check patient response or to perform other procedures (e.g., intubation).

[a]Adapted from Songster GS, Clark SL: Cardiac arrest in pregnancy—what to do. *Contemp OB/GYN* 27:141–143, 1985.

Once the patient is resuscitated successfully, she should be moved to the intensive care unit where she can be observed closely. She is at high risk for a repeat cardiac arrest soon after successful resuscitation. Neurologic status, fluid and electrolyte balance, acid-base balance, and renal and liver function all should be assessed, with an awareness that normal laboratory values of many tests are altered during pregnancy. Cardiac enzymes, a chest x-ray, and a 12-lead ECG can be used to assess cardiac status.

The condition of the fetus should be monitored. Often, the fetus will recover from hypoxia quickly once the mother is resuscitated. If the fetus is dead, delivery should be postponed until the mother is stable. If the fetus is alive but compromised, the gestational age and condition of both mother and fetus should be weighed in reaching a decision about timing and route of delivery (15, p 155)

MANAGEMENT OF SPECIFIC CARDIAC DISEASES DURING PREGNANCY

Rheumatic Fever/Rheumatic Heart Disease

Rheumatic fever is a systemic inflammatory disease. It usually occurs about two weeks after an episode of pharyngitis caused by β-hemolytic streptococcus. It is not the result of direct bacterial invasion of the tissue but is rather a hypersensitivity immune reaction. Only a small part of the population is susceptible to it.

The clinical course of the disease varies. Some patients with RHD cannot recall ever having had rheumatic fever. It is likely that many of these had mild fever, transient arthralgia, a fleeting rash, and/or malaise—symptoms too mild and nonspecific to require diagnosis at the time (7, p 354).

A classic case of rheumatic fever is characterized by high fever with tachycardia. There is arthritis in the larger joints, which may shift from joint to joint.

Less commonly, the patient may experience a rash of flat red patches on the trunk and extremities that appear and disappear within a few hours. Occasionally, the central nervous system is affected, resulting in chorea (incoordination, ataxia, weakness). Cardiac manifestations may include carditis with cardiomegaly; valvulitis with a pathological murmur; acute pericarditis with chest pain and a friction rub; and congestive heart failure. Blood tests reveal leukocytosis, C-reactive protein, an elevated sedimentation rate, and rising serum antistreptolysin O titers. Diagnosis, even in the presence of symptoms, often is not conclusive (7, p 354).

Rheumatic fever causes a specific inflammatory lesion, called the Aschoff body, located among the subendocardial muscle bundles. There also may be diffuse interstitial myocarditis, swelling and inflammatory infiltration of valves, small platelet-fibrin nodules along the valvular lines of closure, and fibrinous pericarditis (7, pp 353–354).

The disease is self-limited, subsiding in 8–12 weeks. Fever and arthritis respond to aspirin. Penicillin may be required for treatment of streptococcal pharyngitis.

Table 9.5.

PROTOCOLS FOR LETHAL DYSRHYTHMIAS[a]

VENTRICULAR FIBRILLATION	ASYSTOLE
Defibrillate at 200–300 J. Repeat if ineffective.	Intubate and ventilate with oxygen. Give epinephrine, 0.5–1.0 mg i.v. Repeat every 5 minutes. Give sodium bicarbonate, 1 mEq/kg (75–100 mg). Repeat with half the dose every 10 minutes as needed.
Intubate and ventilate with oxygen. Give epinephrine, 0.5–1.0 mg i.v. Repeat every 5 minutes. Give sodium bicarbonate, 1 mEq/kg (75–100 mg). Repeat with half the dose every 10 minutes as needed.	Give atropine, 1.0 mg i.v.
Defibrillate at 360 J; repeat.	Give calcium chloride 10% solution, 5 ml i.v. Repeat every 10 minutes.
Give bretylium tosylate (Bretylol). 5 mg/kg i.v. (350–500 mg).	Give isoproterenol (Isuprel) infusion, 2–20 μg/minute.
Defibrillate at 360 J; repeat.	Arrange for pacemaker placement.
Give bretylium, 10 mg/kg i.v. (750–1000 mg).	
Defibrillate at 360 J; repeat.	*Electromechanical dissociation*
After the maximum dose of bretylium, or as an alternative, one may give lidocaine hydrochloride (Xylocaine) or procainamide hydrochloride (Pronestyl) as an adjunct to defibrillation.	Intubate and ventilate with oxygen. Give epinephrine, 0.5–1.0 mg i.v. Repeat every 5 minutes. Give sodium bicarbonate, 1 mEq/kg (75–100 mEq). Repeat half the dose every 10 minutes as needed.
Give 1 mg/kg of lidocaine as an initial bolus, and follow after 10 minutes by 0.5 mg/kg. This may be repeated until a total dose of 225 mg is reached, and followed by maintenance infusion at 2–4 mg/minute.	Give calcium chloride, 10% solution i.v. 5 ml. Repeat every 10 minutes.
Give 100 mg of procainamide over 5 minutes, repeated every 5 minutes. Stop bolus dosage on noting hypotension, suppression of dysrhythmia, a 50% increase in width of the QRS complex, or on reaching a total dose of 1 g. Maintenance is 1–4 mg/minute.	Give isoproterenol infusion. 2–20 μg/min.
	Consider hypovolemia, tension pneumothorax, and cardiac tamponade as possible causes, and treat appropriately.

[a]From Songster GS, Clark SL: Cardiac arrest in pregnancy—what to do. *Contemp OB/GYN* 27:141–155, 1986.

The disease usually occurs between the ages of 6 and 16, but it may occur earlier or later. Some patients have recurring disease, whereas others seem to have it only once. The only lasting consequence is valvular deformity, known as RHD. Although the incidence has decreased over the past 50 years, still over one million Americans have RHD (7, p 353).

The effects of rheumatic fever on cardiac status may be quite variable. The most common lesion is mitral stenosis (see below). Recurrent disease increases the incidence and severity of cardiac sequelae. Some patients have minor defects that remain unchanged for years. Others have slowly progressive disease that first becomes symptomatic in middle age. Others, especially those with recurrent rheumatic fever, have severe disease by adolescence (7, p 356).

Mitral Stenosis and Valvotomy

Mitral stenosis is the most common rheumatic valvular lesion seen in pregnancy. Significant stenosis may cause progressive dyspnea beginning as early as the third month. Orthopnea, atrial fibrillation, and pulmonary edema can occur (7, p 471).

Cardiac output will decrease if diastolic filling time is inadequate. Therefore, tachycardia (which may result from pain or anxiety) can result in decreased cardiac output, hypotension, pulmonary edema, and maternal and fetal compromise. Epidural anesthesia may be used during labor to prevent pain and apprehension, but it cannot prevent the postpartum fluid shifts that may severely tax the compromised heart.

With pulmonary edema, very careful diuresis may be attempted with the aid of hemodynamic monitoring with a pulmonary artery catheter (Fig. 9.3). If pulmonary hypertension is present, hypotension must be avoided or the decreased venous return to the heart could result in cardiovascular collapse and even death.

Management of patients with mitral stenosis depends upon the functional capacity of the patient. Patients with severe stenosis should preferably have valvotomy or valve replacement before contemplating pregnancy. However, successful valvotomy has been documented during pregnancy.

Valvotomy is a palliative procedure rather than corrective. The benefits are of limited duration, since the condition usually progresses at the same rate as before surgery. The surgery during pregnancy should not be considered unless the patient's condition is deteriorating in spite of strict in-hospital management, and it is clear that valvotomy will alleviate it. The optimal time for the procedure is between 12 and 24 weeks' gestation, after embryogenesis is complete and the risk of spontaneous abortion is decreased, but before the peak cardiac demands of pregnancy. Alternatively, surgery may be delayed until after 28 weeks' gestation when the chance of fetal survival is fairly good. A cesarean section then can be performed, followed by cardiac surgery. If an open heart procedure is required, the fetus will not be exposed to the risks of cardiopulmonary bypass (8, p 118).

Patients with uncorrected mitral stenosis are admitted at term for induction. A pulmonary artery

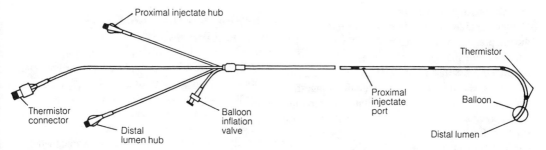

Figure 9.3. Swan-Ganz elements. The pulmonary artery catheter (Swan-Ganz catheter) is inserted into the internal jugular vein with the tip (distal lumen) terminating in the pulmonary artery and the other lumen placed in the right atrium or superior vena cava. This catheter can give information about cardiac output and pressures where the lumina are placed. It is particularly useful in management of severe preeclampsia with oliguria or pulmonary edema; pulmonary edema of unknown cause; septic or cardiogenic shock; hypovolemic shock in the presence of cardiac disease; or labor and delivery in the presence of valvular heart disease or pulmonary hypertension. (Picture from and text adapted from Clark SL, Phelan JP: OB uses for the pulmonary artery catheter, *Contemp OB/GYN* 24:172–185, 1984.)

catheter (Swan-Ganz catheter) is placed prior to induction to permit hemodynamic monitoring (Fig. 9.3). The patient is given oxygen, epidural anesthesia, and an intravenous infusion of D_5W to run at 30–40 ml/hour. The mother is placed in the left lateral position to promote normal circulatory status. Prophylactic antibiotics are given to prevent SBE. Vaginal delivery is the route of choice (1, p 132).

Valve Replacement

Successful pregnancy can occur after implantation of a prosthesis to replace a severely defective mitral or aortic valve. Successful replacements also have been reported *during* pregnancy (2, p 593).

Maternal complications during a pregnancy following valve replacement may include thrombosis, thromboembolism, hemorrhage, deterioration in cardiac function, and death. Since there is approximately a one-in-three risk of pregnancy wastage, patients should be counseled after their cardiac surgery about the risks of pregnancy and offered effective contraception. Once pregnant, the option of therapeutic abortion should be discussed.

Continuous anticoagulant therapy is given after valve replacement (except in special circumstances such as some implantations of porcine valves) to prevent emboli. The selection of the anticoagulant to use is controversial. Warfarin sodium crosses the placenta. It is teratogenic and may cause hemorrhage and death in the fetus or newborn. On the other hand, heparin does not cross the placenta. But it also has the potential to cause hemorrhage and requires frequent subcutaneous administration (which the patient can be taught to perform). Prolonged use can cause bone demineralization. The use of heparin during pregnancy is associated with a 12% incidence of stillbirth and 20% incidence of preterm delivery, and the effectiveness of low doses of heparin has not been established. Hall et al. (16) conclude that the risks are similar; therefore, warfarin should be used since its

effectiveness has been established and it can be administered by mouth. Others suggest a combination approach: heparin in the first trimester, then warfarin until 3 weeks before term, when heparin is used again (4, p 165). Heparin is discontinued just before delivery. Protamine sulfate can be used to counteract heparin and thus prevent hemorrhage if it is still effective at the time of delivery. The day after delivery, warfarin is resumed unless the patient is breastfeeding. The nursing patient again is placed on heparin.

Contraceptive counseling is necessary because of the high maternal and fetal risk of pregnancy after a valve replacement. Oral contraceptives are contraindicated because of the risk of thrombosis. Sterilization should be considered.

Congenital Heart Disease

When congenital heart defects are corrected prior to pregnancy, with no major residual effects, a basically normal pregnancy, labor, delivery, and postpartum course can be expected. The major congenital anomalies that are seen in pregnant women are atrial septal defect, PDA, ventricular septal defect, pulmonary stenosis, and coarctation of the aorta. In this section PDA and coarctation of the aorta are discussed.

Patent Ductus Arteriosus

PDA often is associated with normal pregnancy outcome. However, if the systemic blood pressure falls, blood flow may reverse, going from the pulmonary artery to the aorta, resulting in cyanosis. A sudden drop in blood pressure may result in maternal death. It is therefore crucial to avoid systemic hypotension if at all possible. Measures to avoid hypotension with conduction anesthesia (see Chapter 38) and to prevent or immediately and adequately treat hemorrhage are required. Ligation of a PDA during pregnancy is fairly simple and results in dramatic improvement (2, p 594).

Coarctation of the Aorta

Fortunately, coarctation of the aorta is rare during pregnancy. It is manifested clinically by hypertension in the upper extremities and normal or low blood pressure in the lower extremities. Complications during pregnancy include congestive heart failure (which often necessitates termination of the pregnancy), bacterial endocarditis, and aortic rupture. Rupture of the aorta is most likely to occur late in pregnancy, during labor (especially with increased pressure from the Valsalva maneuver in second stage), or in the early postpartum period (2, p 595). The preferred method of delivery is controversial. Some say cesarean section is preferred to prevent aortic rupture, while others state there is no proven benefit to cesarean over vaginal delivery.

Correction of coarctation of the aorta can be performed during pregnancy but not without great risk to the fetus. All of the collateral vessels must be clamped at some time during the procedure, and this may result in severe fetal hypoxia.

Coronary Artery Disease

Fortunately, coronary artery disease during pregnancy is quite rare. Pregnancy following myocardial infarction should be discouraged, especially if angiography demonstrates severe cardiac damage.

When myocardial infarction occurs during pregnancy, the initial treatment to stabilize the patient is the same as in the nonpregnant patient. Labor and delivery require intensive fetal and maternal monitoring: pulmonary artery catheter for hemodynamic monitoring (Fig. 9.3), blood pressure measurements through an arterial line, a continuous ECG, frequent measurements of cardiac output, and internal fetal monitoring. Epidural anesthesia usually is given (without a fluid load prior to administration) to relieve pain and inhibit second stage pushing.

Other Cardiac Diseases

Peripartal Myopathy

Peripartal myopathy is a syndrome characterized by congestive heart failure with cardiomegaly, pulmonary congestion, and ECG evidence of nonspecific cardiac damage. Usually, it occurs in older (over 30 years old), black, multiparous patients. Most commonly it occurs in the postpartum period, but it can occur earlier. It is controversial whether this myopathy is a distinct clinical entity.

After a patient has experienced peripartal myopathy once, future pregnancy should be strongly discouraged because of the high maternal mortality in subsequent pregnancy (4, p 166). If cardiomegaly and the other symptoms clear quickly and completely after pregnancy, a subsequent pregnancy has a greater chance of a successful outcome (2, p 594).

Mitral Valve Prolapse

Mitral valve prolapse is a relatively common problem, thought to occur in 5–10% of young women. The diagnosis is suspected when there is an apical systolic murmur with a midsystolic click and is confirmed by echocardiogram. It is considered a risk factor for SBE; thus, antibiotic prophylaxis should be given at delivery. Otherwise, it presents no problem in pregnancy, except a greater risk of pulmonary edema when β-mimetic drugs are given for prevention of preterm labor.

Marfan Syndrome

Marfan syndrome is a rare genetic disorder of the connective tissue. Death from Marfan syndrome usually is due to valvar insufficiency, congestive heart failure, or a dissecting aneurysm. Because of the high risk in pregnancy complicated by Marfan syndrome, termination of pregnancy is recommended. Cesarean section is not especially helpful since it does not prevent the great stress on the aorta prior to labor or in the immediate postpartum period (2, pp 595, 622).

NURSING MANAGEMENT

Nursing care specific for a patient with cardiac disease:
- ☐ Be alert to signs/symptoms of cardiac disease in all patients, differentiating them from normal discomforts of pregnancy.
- ☐ Assist in the diagnostic workup for cardiac disease.
- ☐ Ensure that the patient and family are aware of the impact of pregnancy and cardiac disease on maternal/fetal outcome; explore options (e.g., therapeutic abortion) if indicated.
- ☐ Explain and encourage compliance with management plan:
  - Normal weight gain;
  - Sodium restriction (e.g., avoid salty foods, avoid adding salt at the table);
  - Use of iron and vitamin supplements;
  - Balanced activity and rest (e.g., schedule 10 hours of sleep at night and a 30-minute rest period after each meal and activity); and
  - Avoidance of crowds or people with communicable diseases.
- ☐ Provide appropriate referrals to assist the patient in complying with management (e.g., home health services, disability, financial assistance, visiting nurse).

NURSING MANAGEMENT

☐ Teach the patient to report signs/symptoms of infection; screen for infection at each prenatal visit; and administer vaccines as ordered.

☐ Teach signs/symptoms of deteriorating cardiac status and how to report them; screen for deteriorating status at each prenatal visit (e.g., dyspnea, orthopnea, coughing, hemoptysis, decreased tolerance for usual activities).

☐ Offer sterilization counseling, as appropriate.

☐ Assist the patient in the management of pain and anxiety during labor to minimize cardiac stress (e.g., stay with the patient, provide comfort measures, administer analgesics as ordered).

☐ Anticipate forceps delivery; be prepared for an emergency cesarean section (see Chapter 40).

☐ Prepare for cardiac emergency:
 — Check that all equipment, drugs, and personnel necessary for resuscitation are readily available, and
 — Be prepared to initiate cardiopulmonary resuscitation.

☐ Be familiar with the procedures and equipment the patient may require before assuming a nursing responsibility for a patient who is seriously ill (collaboration with colleagues in intensive or cardiac care units may be required).

☐ Continue to closely monitor maternal status after delivery since cardiac workload is great.

☐ Provide counseling regarding cardiac condition and prognosis for future pregnancies.

☐ Provide contraceptive counseling; appropriately encourage its use.

Nursing diagnoses most frequently associated with *cardiac disease*:

☐ Grieving related to potential/actual loss of infant or birth of an imperfect child.

☐ Anticipatory grieving related to actual/perceived threat to self.

☐ Spiritual distress.

☐ Self-care deficit.

☐ Anxiety/fear.

☐ Pain.

☐ Disturbance in body image, self-esteem.

☐ Knowledge deficit regarding etiology, disease process, treatment, and expected outcome.

☐ Knowledge deficit regarding medication regimen.

☐ Potential for infection.

☐ Excess fluid volume.

☐ Altered maternal tissue perfusion.

☐ Altered fetal cardiac and cerebral tissue perfusion.

REFERENCES

1. Clark SL: How labor and delivery influence mitral stenosis. *Contemp OB/GYN* 27:127–132, 1986.
2. Pritchard JA, MacDonald PC, Gant NF: *Williams Obstetrics*, ed 17. Norwalk, CT, Appleton-Century-Crofts, 1985.
3. Clark SL, Phelan JP: Ob uses for the pulmonary artery catheter. *Contemp OB/GYN* 24:172–185, 1984.
4. Arditi LI: Heart disease. In Caplan RM (ed): *Principles of Obstetrics*. Baltimore, Williams & Wilkins, 1982.
5. Buckley KA: Antepartum deviations. In Buckley KA, Kulb NW (eds): *Handbook of Maternal-Newborn Nursing*. New York, John Wiley and Sons, 1983, p 372.
6. Burwell CS, Metcalfe J: *Heart Disease and Pregnancy*. Boston, Little, Brown, and Co, 1958.
7. Stapleton JF: *Essentials of Clinical Cardiology*. Philadelphia, FA Davis, 1983.
8. Ueland K: Cardiovascular surgery and the ob patient. *Contemp OB/GYN* 24:117–120, 1984.
9. Cavanagh D: Medical emergencies in obstetrics. In Cavanagh D, Woods RE, O'Connor TCF (eds): *Obstetric Emergencies*. Hagerstown, MD, Harper and Row, 1978, p 359.
10. Chesley LC: Severe rheumatic cardiac disease and pregnancy: the ultimate prognosis. *Am J Obstet Gynecol* 136:552, 1980.
11. Whittemore R, Wright MR, Leonard MF, Johnson M: Results of pregnancy in women with congenital heart defects. *Pediatr Res* 14:452, 1980.
12. Veille JC: Sounding the value of maternal-fetal echocardiography. *Contemp OB/GYN* 24:92–102, 1984.
13. Gorenberg H, Chesley LC: Rheumatic heart disease in pregnancy: the remote prognosis in patients with "functionally severe" disease. *Ann Intern Med* 49:278, 1958.
14. Cavanagh D: Shock. In Cavanagh D, Woods RE, O'Connor TCF (eds): *Obstetric Emergencies*. Hagerstown, MD, Harper and Row, 1978, pp 25–64.
15. Songster GS, Clark SL: Cardiac arrest in pregnancy– what to do. *Contemp OB/GYN* 27:141–155, 1986.
16. Hall JG, Pauli RM, Wilson KM: Maternal and fetal sequelae of anticoagulation during pregnancy. *Am J Med* 68:122–140, 1980.

Chapter 10
Disorders of the Endocrine System
Nancy W. Kulb, C.N.M., M.S.

INTRODUCTION

The body processes affected by hormones are metabolism, growth and development, activity of other endocrine glands, development and functioning of the reproductive organs, development of personality, ability of the body to cope with stress, and resistance to disease.

Endocrine disorders often are familial. Generally, symptoms result from excessive, insufficient, or inappropriate hormone secretion. Sometimes the failure is in an abnormal response by target tissue. Often, the symptoms of disease are subtle and occur slowly; the patient may not even be aware of the changes.

The menstrual cycle is regulated by hormones and their influence on target tissue. Thus, many disorders of the hypothalamus, pituitary, or ovary result in infertility. This chapter emphasizes the endocrine disorders that most often occur concomitantly with pregnancy: thyroid disorders and diabetes mellitus. Other disorders that rarely occur during pregnancy also are discussed briefly.

THYROID DISORDERS

Introduction

The thyroid gland is a shield-shaped organ located in the anterior part of the neck. Its function is to synthesize and release the three thyroid hormones:

1. Thyroxine (T_4), which regulates body metabolism; aids in regulation of growth and develop-

ment; and is involved in the metabolism of protein, carbohydrates, and fat.
2. Triiodothyronine (T_3), which regulates vitamin requirements and assists in resistance to infection.
3. Thyrocalcitonin, which regulates serum calcium and phosphorous (1).

The synthesis and release of the thyroid hormones are governed by thyroid-stimulating hormone (TSH), also called thyrotropin. TSH is released by the thyrotropic cells in the anterior pituitary. Secretion of TSH is regulated by thyrotropin-releasing hormone (TRH) from the hypothalamus. A negative feedback loop regulates thyroid hormone synthesis and release.

Most of the T_3 and T_4 circulating in the plasma is bound to protein and is physiologically inert. The free (unbound) T_3 and T_4 are physiologically active—they can cross cell membranes and interact with the intracellular receptor sites. Thus, the free hormone level reflects thyroid status. An indirect measure of the free hormone level is the free T_4 index.

T_3 is three to four times more potent in metabolic effect than T_4. Only 20% of circulating T_3 is secreted directly by the thyroid; 80% results from peripheral conversion of T_4 to T_3, which occurs primarily in the liver and kidneys. T_3 is *not* converted back to T_4.

Normal Thyroid Function in Pregnancy

In general, the thyroid functions normally during pregnancy. However, there are some normal alterations during pregnancy (see Table 10.1):

Table 10.1.
CHANGES IN THYROID FUNCTION VALUES DURING PREGNANCY[a,b]

TEST	SUBSTANCE MEASURED	NORMAL VALUE	VALUE IN PREGNANCY	COMMENT
Radioimmunoassay	TSH	10 μU/ml	No change	Increased in primary hypothyroidism
	T_4	4.5–12.5 μg/100 ml	Increased by 2–4 μg/100 ml	Elevation from normal range is secondary to the increase in thyroxine-binding globulin levels
	T_3	90–190 ng/100 ml	Increased by 20–50 ng/100 ml	Elevation from normal range is secondary to the increase in thyroxine-binding globulin levels
RT_3U	Resin uptake of T_3	25–35%	20–25%	Indirect test of protein binding, *not* a measurement of T_3
Hemagglutination	Thyroid autoantibodies			
	Thyroglobulin	None	None	May be present in subacute and Hashimoto's thyroiditis and Graves' disease
	Microsomal (MSA)	None	None	
Uptake of ^{131}I by thyroid gland		10–25% at 24 hours	THIS TEST IS CONTRAINDICATED IN PREGNANCY	

[a]Adapted from Creasy R, Resnick R: *Maternal-Fetal Medicine, Principles and Practice*. Philadelphia, WB Saunders, 1984.
[b]Normal values must be determined for each laboratory in which the test is performed.

1. Serum concentration of total T_4 is elevated beginning early in the first trimester and persisting until 6–12 weeks postpartum. Whereas the normal plasma T_4 level in the nonpregnant euthyroid patient is 5–12 μg/dl, in pregnancy it is 9–16 μg/dl (2, p 202).

2. Serum T_3 levels also are increased throughout pregnancy.

3. The high estrogen state of pregnancy stimulates both increased production of T_4-binding proteins (especially α-globulin), and resin T_3 uptake, a measure of unsaturated T_4-binding sites, in the hypothyroid range in spite of the increase in T_4. Whereas the normal nonpregnant level for T_4-binding globulins is 3.6 mg/dl, it rises to 7.1 mg/dl in the first trimester and 9.0 mg/dl in the second and third trimesters (3). Thus, although both T_3 and T_4 are increased during pregnancy, the unbound (i.e., physiologically active) level is not increased significantly.

4. TSH has been reported to be normal throughout pregnancy, or slightly higher during the first trimester. Recent evidence suggests that TSH may even be slightly lower in early pregnancy because human chorionic gonadotropin (HCG), which is present in high levels in early pregnancy, may mildly stimulate thyroid activity. However, TSH generally remains within normal limits throughout the pregnancy.

5. The radioiodine thyroid uptake is increased because of thyroid stimulation and lowered serum iodine during pregnancy. This test generally is contraindicated during pregnancy.

Small amounts of T_3 and T_4 may cross the placenta, the amount depending upon the gestational age, but TSH does not. TRH does cross the placenta. A thyrotropic substance from the placenta has been found by several investigators, but its role in stimulating the thyroid gland is not clear (2, p 203).

During pregnancy, the basal metabolic rate is increased up to 25%, primarily because of the metabolism of the products of conception. There is normally a diffuse enlargement of the thyroid gland (as much as two- to three-fold increase in size) because of hyperplasia of thyroid tissue and increased vascularity. Serum iodine level is decreased because of the increased glomerular filtration rate, which allows urinary loss. Women with marginal dietary intake may develop goiter as the thyroid enlarges to compensate for the lower serum iodine level. This problem rarely occurs in the United States (4, pp 187–188).

The fetal thyroid does not begin to produce thyroid hormone until 10–12 weeks of fetal life. Before that time, the mother must provide any thy-

Table 10.2.
CAUSES OF HYPERTHYROIDISM[a]

Graves' disease
Silent thyroiditis
Subacute thyroiditis
Other thyroiditis
Toxic multinodular goiter
Toxic adenoma
Excessive TSH production
Extremely high βHCG levels (i.e., with hydatidiform
    mole, choriocarcinoma—very rare)
Drug-induced (e.g., iodine)

[a]Adapted from Mendel AM, Fitzgerald PA: The spectrum of autoimmune thyroid disease. *Contemp OB/GYN* 21:149, 1983.

roid hormone that is required for fetal growth and development (4, p 192).

HYPERTHYROIDISM

Definition

Hyperthyroidism is the hypermetabolic state characterized by excessive thyroid hormone activity. It occurs in approximately 0.2% of pregnancies (5). Table 10.2 lists the causes of hyperthyroidism. Table 10.3 lists the clinical signs and symptoms of hyperthyroidism in nonpregnant individuals. Determining the significance of some signs and symptoms is made more difficult during pregnancy because of some of the normal changes of pregnancy (2, p 604):

1. Heat intolerance because of increased cutaneous blood flow.
2. Modest tachycardia.
3. Increased plasma T_4 level and increased thyroid uptake of radioiodine.

Table 10.4.
SIGNS AND SYMPTOMS OF
HYPERTHYROIDISM SPECIFIC TO
PREGNANCY[a]

Tachycardia (greater than normal for pregnancy)
Tachycardia while sleeping
Thyroid enlargement
Exophthalmos
Failure to gain weight normally

[a]Adapted from Cunningham FG, MacDonald PC, Gant NF: *Williams Obstetrics*, ed 18. Norwalk, CT, Appleton and Lange, 1989, p 823.

Signs and Symptoms

Signs and symptoms that are significant for hyperthyroidism in pregnancy are listed in Table 10.4. Usually, the plasma T_4 is markedly increased without the decrease in resin T_3 uptake that characterizes normal pregnancy.

Maternal and Fetal Outcome

It has been reported that fertility is impaired in patients with hyperthyroidism, but if the disease is mild to moderate and appropriately treated, fertility is not necessarily decreased. There is a slight increase in neonatal mortality and a significant increase in low birth weight. The maternal course often improves during pregnancy, possibly because of suppression of the immune system, but relapses may occur during the postpartum period.

Medical Management

Initially, hyperthyroidism may require hospitalization until it is controlled. During pregnancy, it can almost always be treated effectively medi-

Table 10.3.
SIGNS AND SYMPTOMS OF HYPERTHYROIDISM[a]

SYMPTOMS	SIGNS	NONTHYROID LABORATORY ABNORMALITIES
Weight loss	Tachycardia	Anemia
Fatigue	Eyelid retraction or lid lag	Granulocytopenia
Weakness	Tremor	Increased serum calcium
Heat intolerance	Warm, smooth, moist skin	Increased alkaline phosphatase
Palpitations	Fine hair	Increased ferritin
Anxiety	Restlessness	Decreased catecholamines
Increased appetite	Wide pulse pressure	
Increased perspiration	Hyperreflexia	
Dyspnea	Heart failure	
Diarrhea	Soft, fragile nails	
Menstrual irregularities		
Emotional lability		
Insomnia		

[a]Adapted from Mendel CM, Fitzgerald PA: The spectrum of autoimmune thyroid disease. *Contemp OB/GYN* 21:148, 1983.

cally. Subtotal thyroidectomy is indicated only if drug therapy is ineffective. If surgery must be done, it is preferable to do it during the second trimester—after embryogenesis is complete and before there is danger of preterm delivery resulting from the stress of surgery. Thyrotoxicosis must be controlled prior to surgery.

The drug of choice during pregnancy is propylthiouracil (PTU). It acts in the thyroid gland by decreasing synthesis of thyroid hormones and, peripherally, by inhibiting the conversion of T_4 to T_3. It has the advantage of a short half-life, making dose adjustment easier. PTU crosses the placenta slowly, but it can cause fetal hypothyroidism and goiter. Therefore, the goal in management is to titrate the dose to the minimal amount required to achieve minimal symptoms and the T_4 at or just above the upper range of normal for pregnancy (2, p 605, 6). A common dose is 100 mg PTU three times daily initially. It may be possible to decrease it after control is achieved to less than 100 mg a day. Breastfeeding while taking PTU probably is contraindicated, although only a very small amount is detectable in breast milk.

Radioactive iodine, used to treat hyperthyroidism in nonpregnant patients, is contraindicated during pregnancy. Its action is to destroy thyroid tissue, which is therapeutic for hyperthyroid patients but destructive to the fetal thyroid. Propranolol, which is used in nonpregnant patients to decrease pulse and cardiac workload as well as control neuromuscular symptoms, is not used in pregnancy except in emergencies (see Thyroid Storm section). The practice of administering L-thyroxine along with PTU, which was once popular, is no longer accepted since it does not cross the placenta to help keep the fetus euthyroid; it may mask remission of hyperthyroidism; and it may require an increase in the dose of PTU required for control (6).

This chapter will discuss only the hyperthyroid disorders most significant for pregnant patients, as well as thyroid storm.

GRAVES' DISEASE

Definition

Graves' disease, also called toxic diffuse goiter, is an autoimmune disorder resulting in hyperthyroidism. It is eight times more prevalent in women than men, and peak incidence is in the reproductive years—20–40 years old. It occurs in about 1:2000 pregnancies.

Etiology

Graves' disease is caused by a deficiency of certain suppressor T lymphocytes. Lack of these suppressor T lymphocytes allows other destructive lymphocytes to attack the thyroid and plasma cells to produce antibodies against the thyroid's receptor for TSH, resulting in thyroid stimulation. Its onset may be preceded by emotional trauma or metabolic stress. Pregnancy certainly is a time of metabolic stress and can contribute to emotional trauma. It occurs in genetically susceptible individuals and often coexists with other autoimmune disorders.

Signs and Symptoms

The signs and symptoms of Graves' disease include those of hyperthyroidism: weight loss, fatigue, tremor, a fixed "stare," heat intolerance, thin hair, warm moist palms, tachycardia, palpitations, etc. The thyroid gland is soft and diffusely enlarged up to three to four times its normal size. It may actually encroach on the trachea or esophagus. A bruit may be heard over the thyroid because of the increased vascularity. Exophthalmos is common. The T_3, T_4, and free thyroid hormone indices are elevated above normal for pregnancy.

Diagnosis

Diagnosis is made more difficult in pregnancy because of normal changes that overlap the symptoms of hyperthyroidism. The clinical picture, along with elevated T_3 and free thyroid index, usually is sufficient for diagnosis. Further tests usually are not required and some are contraindicated in pregnancy.

Maternal and Fetal Outcome

With Graves' disease, fertility is decreased and the rate of spontaneous abortion is increased significantly. The fetus may be born with symptoms of thyrotoxicosis (e.g., goiter or exophthalmos). Presumably, this is because the thyroid-stimulating immunoglobulins cross the placenta, thus causing fetal hyperthyroidism. Fetal tachycardia is a clue that the fetus is hyperthyroid.

Because of PTU treatment, the baby may be born in a hypothyroid state. Even when the baby is born in a euthyroid state to a mother treated with PTU, it may become hyperthyroid after a few days. PTU that crossed the placenta to the baby prior to delivery is metabolized within a few days. The thyroid-stimulating immunoglobulins that also crossed the placenta may not be metabolized for several weeks. In the interim, the baby may require antithyroid medication. The baby also has the risk imposed by the medications or surgery necessary to control maternal hyperthyroidism.

The mother's prognosis is good if PTU controls the hyperthyroidism. Since treatment modalities are limited during pregnancy, she may have the risk of surgery (rarely required by nonpregnant patients) if the disease cannot be controlled medically. Usually, however, Graves' disease is less severe during pregnancy because of the normal suppression of the immune system (see Chapter 7). Exacerbation may occur in the postpartum period.

Medical Management

The treatment of choice in pregnancy is PTU, given in a dose sufficient to maintain the mother in a slightly hyperthyroid state (i.e., with minimal symptoms and T_3 and T_4 at or just above the normal limits for pregnancy). The initial dose usually is 100 mg three times daily or less. Clinical response occurs within 3–4 weeks. After that time, the dose may be reduced gradually to 25–50 mg every 6–8 hours. During the third trimester, it may be possible to withdraw the medications because of the normal suppression of immunologic activity during pregnancy.

If PTU does not control the hyperthyroidism, subtotal thyroidectomy in the second trimester may be required. Because thyrotoxicosis must be under control prior to surgery, preparation with propranolol may be necessary. After surgery, thyroid storm (see below) may occur. Twenty percent of patients become hypothyroid transiently and require treatment with L-thyroxine (6, p 205). Hypoparathyroidism, due to inadvertent removal of the parathyroid glands, laryngeal nerve paralysis, and anesthetic complications also are risks.

THYROID STORM

Definition

Thyroid storm, also called thyrotoxic crisis, is a life-threatening emergency in which the symptoms of hyperthyroidism are exaggerated. Fortunately, it is quite rare in pregnancy.

Etiology

The pathogenesis of thyroid storm is not clear. It usually occurs in hyperthyroid patients (those with Graves' disease or multinodular goiter) who are not being treated at all or are not being treated adequately. Usually, thyroid storm is precipitated by some other condition (e.g., infection, trauma, surgical emergency, or labor). Rarely, it may be the first clinical manifestation of hyperthyroidism. There is no correlation between severity of clinical symptoms and the circulating levels of thyroid hormones (7).

Signs and Symptoms

The signs and symptoms primarily are exaggerated signs and symptoms of hyperthyroidism: fever as high as 106°F; warm, flushed skin; severe dehydration; central nervous system alterations, which may range from disorientation to psychosis to coma; cardiac symptoms, such as tachycardia, atrial fibrillation, and congestive heart failure; and gastrointestinal disturbances, such as diarrhea, vomiting, abdominal pain, or jaundice. If it is not treated promptly and adequately, severe shock may ensue.

Diagnosis

The diagnosis of thyroid storm is based upon clinical symptoms and laboratory evidence of hyperthyroidism. The T_3 and T_4 levels may be in the same range as uncomplicated hyperthyroidism, but their free hormone indices and radioiodine uptake are elevated. Severe illness can block peripheral conversion of T_4 to T_3, so the T_3 may even be as low as normal for a euthyroid patient.

Diagnostic efforts should be directed toward identifying the illness that precipitated thyroid storm. Cultures, a complete blood count, urinalysis, serum electrolyte and biochemical profiles, chest x-ray, and electrocardiogram may be indicated, along with other tests dictated by the patient's clinical picture.

Maternal and Fetal Outcome

Mortality from thyroid storm ranges from 10–50%. Death usually is the result of infection or cardiac complications. Fetal loss is correspondingly high. Outcome depends upon the precipitating condition as well as the promptness and adequacy of treatment.

Medical Management

Because the disorder is life-threatening, aggressive management begins as soon as the diagnosis is suspected. Transfer to an intensive care unit generally is required. Treatment is directed toward treating the precipitating illness, decreasing thyroid hormone concentrations, blocking the peripheral effects of circulating thyroid hormones, and controlling the symptoms of thyroid storm.

Treatment of the precipitating illness may include administration of broad-spectrum antibiotics until culture reports are available; digitalization, diuretics, and administration of oxygen; maintenance of fluid and electrolyte balance (large volumes of intra-

Table 10.5.
CAUSES OF HYPOTHYROIDISM[a]

WITH GOITER	WITHOUT GOITER
Hashimoto's disease	Postablative (i.e., surgery,
Iodine deficiency	radioactive iodine
Genetic defects	therapy)
Drug-induced (e.g.,	Pituitary/hypothalamic
iodine, PTU, lithium)	insufficiency[b] (e.g.,
Infiltration of thyroid—	destructive tumors,
rare (lymphoma,	postpartum pituitary
amyloid, sarcoid)	necrosis)
Impaired peripheral	Thyroid dysgenesis
sensitivity to thyroid	
hormone—rare	

[a]Adapted from Mendel MC, Fitzgerald PA: The spectrum of autoimmune thyroid disease. *Contemp OB/GYN* 21:147, 1983.
[b]The only disorder not associated with an elevated TSH.

venous fluids may be required to maintain normal blood pressure and urine output because of the excessive loss through perspiration); and antipyretic measures, such as cooling blankets, tepid water and alcohol sponge baths, and acetaminophen. Salicylates are contraindicated because they interfere with the binding of T_3 and T_4 to thyroxine-binding globulins, thus increasing the physiologically active free T_3 and T_4. Supportive care is given for pulmonary edema, hypoxia, or other associated conditions.

PTU is administered to decrease thyroid hormone concentrations; 300–600 mg is given by mouth initially (or by nasogastric tube if the patient cannot swallow), followed by 150–300 mg every 6 hours. After 4 days, the dose can be decreased gradually to maintenance levels. Iodide is given in the form of Lugol's solution, potassium iodide, or sodium iodide, beginning 1 hour after the initial dose of PTU. Iodides have an acute effect of inhibiting thyroid hormone secretion but should be given for no more than a few days.

Propranolol usually is not given during pregnancy because it can cause intrauterine growth retardation, neonatal bradycardia, hypoglycemia, and impaired responsiveness to asphyxia during labor and birth. However, in the treatment of thyroid storm, the benefits outweigh the risks. Propranolol causes peripheral blockage of β-adrenergic thyroid receptors, thus inhibiting the effects of the circulating thyroid hormones. It also inhibits conversion of T_4 to T_3, and it is especially effective in controlling tachycardia and psychomotor symptoms. The usual dose is 1 mg/minute intravenously up to 10 mg until the heart rate is under control. The subsequent dose is 20–40 mg every 4–6 hours by nasogastric tube, titrated to keep the pulse rate just over 90. After 7–10 days, the propranolol can be tapered off.

Corticosteroids also may be given to inhibit peripheral conversion of T_4 to T_3. Suggested regimens are 200–300 mg hydrocortisone intravenously in three to four divided doses daily or 2 mg dexamethasone intravenously every 6 hours (7).

HYPOTHYROIDISM

Definition, Etiology, Signs and Symptoms

Hypothyroidism is the hypometabolic condition characterized by insufficient thyroid hormone activity. The causes are multiple and are listed in Table 10.5. 80% of adults with hypothyroidism are women. Signs and symptoms are listed in Table 10.6.

Diagnosis

The diagnosis of hypothyroidism during pregnancy is based upon clinical presentation (although a pregnant woman rarely presents with full-blown obvious symptoms), lack of the increase in total T_4 and/or T_3 that normally occurs during pregnancy, and an increased level of TSH. Supporting evidence for the diagnosis of hypothyroidism may include the presence of antithyroid antibodies or a history of thyroidectomy or radioiodine therapy for treatment of hyperthyroidism.

Maternal and Fetal Outcome

With overt hypothyroidism the patient often is infertile. When pregnancy occurs, there is a significantly higher risk of spontaneous abortion than normal, and the stillbirth rate is doubled. With appropriate treatment, babies that survive usually are healthy and without sequelae. Since TSH does not cross the placenta, the fetus is not stimulated to hyperthyroidism. The neonate should be evaluated for hypothyroidism since it may have become accustomed to exogenous thyroid hormone in utero. Some authorities recommend prophylactic treatment for hypothyroidism (2, p 606). Maternal treatment during pregnancy must prevent the T_4 from falling into the hypothyroid range since that could cause impairment of the baby's mental and fine motor development. The degree of developmental retardation depends on the degree of thyroid deficiency and the time of onset during fetal life. Undifferentiated developmental retardation has been reported at 8 months of age in offspring of hypothyroid patients (4, p 196). If hypothyroidism is severe or is a result of maternal treatment with radioactive iodine during the pregnancy, the baby could have cretinism or congenital myxedema, characterized by lack of physical and mental development.

Table 10.6.
SIGNS AND SYMPTOMS OF HYPOTHYROIDISM[a]

SYMPTOMS	SIGNS	NONTHYROID LABORATORY ABNORMALITIES
Weakness	Bradycardia	Anemia (iron deficiency, folic acid
Lethargy	Slow relaxation phase of reflexes	deficiency, pernicious anemia)
Weight gain	Nonpitting generalized edema	Decreased sodium
Dry skin	Dry, scaly, cool skin	Elevated cholesterol
Hair loss	Coarse hair, alopecia	Elevated SGOT
Hoarseness	Large tongue	Elevated LDH
Cold intolerance	Heart failure	Elevated CPK
Constipation	Slow movements	Decreased glucose
Decreased sweating	Slow speech	Pleural or pericardial effusion
Diminished hearing, taste	Hypothermia	Increased pCO_2
Paresthesias	Ataxia	Increased prolactin
Psychiatric disorders	Hypertension	Elevated central spinal fluid protein
Arthralgia	Sallow complexion	
Menstrual irregularities	Increased sensitivity to narcotics, barbiturates, and anesthetics	
	Bladder atony	

[a]Adapted from Mendel CM, Fitzgerald PA: The spectrum of autoimmune thyroid disease. *Contemp OB/GYN* 21:143, 1983.

Medical Management

Treatment consists of replacement of thyroid hormone with L-thyroxine (Synthroid). The usual dose is in the range of 0.15–0.2 mg/day, but it is titrated to a dose that will keep the T_4 in the normal range. During pregnancy, the T_4 should be monitored monthly to ensure that it is within the normal range to prevent adverse fetal effects.

Women who were being treated for hypothyroidism prior to pregnancy should continue the medication throughout the pregnancy. A slight increase in the dose may be required because of the increased thyroxine-binding globulin during pregnancy. The dose should be altered according to serum T_4 concentration.

SILENT THYROIDITIS

Silent thyroiditis, also called lymphocytic thyroiditis, is a subacute disease. It is self-limited, lasting several months, and occurs most often in the postpartum period. It is characterized by mild hyperthyroidism, followed by transient hypothyroidism. Complete recovery usually occurs within 5–10 months, but long-term follow-up studies demonstrate that these patients have a greater incidence of goiter, antithyroid antibodies, and hypothyroidism. During pregnancy the autoimmune thyroiditis is ameliorated, only to intensify after delivery. Similar episodes may develop after subsequent pregnancies.

NURSING MANAGEMENT

Nursing care specific for a patient with
thyroid disease:

☐ Observe all patients for signs/symptoms of hypo/hyperthyroidism, differentiating them from normal physiological changes of pregnancy; assist with diagnostic tests.

☐ Educate patient regarding the following:
   — Signs/symptoms of spontaneous abortion and how to report them and
   — Medication(s) (e.g., dose, route, timing, therapeutic effect, potential adverse maternal/fetal effects).

☐ Comfort measures for hyperthyroidism:
   — Maintain cool environmental temperature;
   — Wear lightweight clothing;

   — Bathe frequently, as needed, for excessive perspiration;
   — Avoid gastric stimulants (e.g., bulky, spicy food);
   — Maintain calm environment (subdued lighting, no loud noise, limited visitors); and
   — Maintain high calorie, high protein diet, with up to six meals daily.

☐ Comfort measures for hypothyroidism:
   — Maintain warm environmental temperature;
   — Wear warm clothing; and
   — Maintain diet high in fluids/fiber to combat constipation.

NURSING MANAGEMENT

☐ Monitor effectiveness of medical treatment (e.g., laboratory values, maternal symptoms, fetal heart rate).

☐ Assess hypothyroid patient's ability to carry out activities of daily living, refer the patient to a homemaker service, if necessary.

☐ Communicate to the pediatric staff at delivery the patient's diagnosis and treatment so they can manage the baby appropriately.

☐ For the patient requiring surgery:
   — Provide routine preoperative and postoperative teaching and care; monitor fetal heart rate throughout.
   — Observe for signs/symptoms of complications after surgery:
      * Hypocalcemia (e.g., muscular spasm or twitching, low serum calcium levels resulting from inadvertent removal of parathyroid glands);
      * Laryngeal nerve paralysis (e.g., hoarseness, voice changes);
      * Thyroid storm;
      * Hypothyroidism; and
      * Alteration in cardiac or respiratory status.
   — Maintain hydration/nutrition status with oral and intravenous fluids until soft foods are tolerated (1–2 days after surgery).
   — Support patient's head and neck when moving.

☐ For the patient with thyroid storm:
   — Be prepared to transfer the patient to the intensive care unit.

   — Monitor cardiac and respiratory status; fluid and electrolyte balance; and fetal heart rate.
   — Administer medications as ordered.
   — Assist with diagnostic tests as needed.
   — Provide nursing care specific for the precipitating illness.
   — Provide antipyretic measures as needed:
      * Acetaminophen;
      * Cooling blanket;
      * Sponge bath with tepid water and alcohol; and
      * Thermally cool environment.
   — Provide comfort measures:
      * Clean dry clothes and sheets for patient with profuse perspiration and
      * Eye care.
   — Recognize psychiatric manifestations of the disease; institute measures to ensure patient's safety; maintain calm environment.

Nursing diagnoses most frequently associated with *hyper/hypothyroidism*:

☐ Anxiety/fear.

☐ Knowledge deficit regarding etiology, disease process, and expected outcome.

☐ Altered nutrition: less than body requirements.

☐ Altered nutrition: more than body requirements.

☐ Disturbance in body image, self-esteem.

☐ Altered maternal tissue perfusion.

☐ Altered fetal cardiac and cerebral tissue perfusion.

DIABETES MELLITUS

Definition

Diabetes mellitus (DM) is a chronic disease resulting from a relative or absolute lack of insulin, which is required for carbohydrate metabolism. Long term, it causes degenerative changes in the vascular system. The incidence in the general population is 5%, up significantly in recent decades, probably because of both genetic and environmental (possibly viral) factors (2, p 598). Before insulin became available for treatment, diabetics rarely conceived—as many as 50% were amenorrheic (8). Among those who conceived, maternal mortality was 30% and fetal loss was 65% (9), a picture that has changed drastically in recent years. Since diabetics reproduce successfully

now, it is possible that the genetic factor will increase, thus increasing the prevalence in the general population and in pregnant women. It is estimated that DM is now present in 2–3% of pregnant women; 90% of these have gestational diabetes (10).

Several classification systems for DM currently are available. Table 10.7 gives the White classification. Table 10.8 gives the classification proposed by the National Diabetes Data Group in 1979.

Overt DM, also called fasting hyperglycemia, corresponds to White's classes B–T. The diagnosis requires the fasting hyperglycemia to occur on two or more occasions, with plasma glucose ≥105 mg/dl in a pregnant patient. Abnormal glucose tolerance, also called chemical or latent DM, corresponds to White's class A. This entity is character-

Table 10.7.

WHITE'S CLASSIFICATION OF DIABETES IN PREGNANT WOMEN (1978)[a]

A	Chemical diabetes
B	Maturity onset (age over 20 years), duration under 10 years, no vascular lesions
C_1	Age 10–19 years at onset
C_2	10–19 years' duration
D_1	Under age 10 years at onset
D_2	Over 20 years' duration
D_3	Benign retinopathy
D_4	Calcified vessels of legs
D_5	Hypertension
E	No longer sought
F	Nephropathy
G	Many failures
H	Cardiomyopathy
R	Proliferating retinopathy
T	Renal transplant

[a]From Pritchard JA, MacDonald PC, Gant NF: *Williams Obstetrics*, ed 17. Norwalk, CT, Appleton-Century-Crofts, 1985, p 599.

ized by a normal fasting glucose level but an abnormal glucose tolerance test (see Diagnosis).

Etiology

Insulin deficiency may be caused by damage to β cells in the pancreas, inactivation of insulin by antibodies, or increased insulin requirements, as in obesity or pregnancy. It was once thought to be a single disease entity with gradations of severity. Now it is believed that the etiology and pathogenesis may be heterogenous. Approximately 90% of cases are spontaneous in onset. About 80% of type I cases are associated with circulating antibodies to islet cells. Approximately 80% of type II cases have no circulating antibodies (4, p 42). In 5–10% of cases, DM is secondary to some other identifiable factor: pancreatic disease, ingestion of certain drugs, hypersecretion of

Table 10.8.

NATIONAL DIABETES DATA GROUP CLASSIFICATION OF DIABETES MELLITUS

A. Insulin-dependent type (type I)
B. Noninsulin-dependent type (type II)
   1. Nonobese
   2. Obese
C. Other types (secondary diabetes)
   1. Pancreatic disease
   2. Hormonally induced
   3. Chemically induced
   4. Insulin receptor abnormalities
   5. Certain genetic syndromes
   6. Others
D. Impaired glucose tolerance (subclinical diabetes)
E. Gestational diabetes (pregnancy-induced glucose intolerance)

hormones antagonistic to insulin, or a genetic syndrome characterized by hyperglycemia.

Pregnancy is said to be diabetogenic. The following section discusses normal carbohydrate metabolism in pregnancy as well as factors that serve to increase the insulin requirement of the pregnant woman. If the pancreas cannot meet the increased demand for insulin, DM will result.

Pathophysiology of Diabetes Mellitus in Pregnancy

Most of the fuel requirements of the fetus are met by glucose. Glucose is used as a precursor for the synthesis of fat and glycogen, as well as for energy. The movement of glucose across the placenta is by facilitated diffusion (i.e., there is a net transfer of glucose from mother to baby). Amino acids are transported actively from mother to baby. Thus, the pregnant woman normally has a lower plasma level of both glucose and amino acids. By 15 weeks' gestation, the plasma fasting glucose level (after a normal 12–14 hour overnight fast) is 15–20 mg/dl lower than in the nonpregnant patient. With longer periods of fasting, the glucose levels may drop even lower—to 40–45 mg/dl. Blood levels of ketones after an overnight fast are two to four times higher in a normal pregnant patient than a nonpregnant patient. Thus, she is more prone to metabolic acidosis. Ketones may be used by the fetus for fuel if glucose is not available, but some research indicates that this may have an adverse effect on fetal neurological development. Glucosuria is not uncommon in the normal pregnant woman owing to the decreased renal threshold.

Insulin is a pancreatic hormone that promotes passage of glucose into muscle and adipose tissue cells, thus lowering the blood glucose level. When glucose is not present in sufficient amounts or insulin is not present to get the glucose into the cells to be used for energy, the body is required to get energy from oxidation of fats and protein. Negative nitrogen balance and ketosis may result. When insulin deficiency is the cause, blood glucose levels rise far above their normal limits. Eventually, extracellular dehydration, acidosis, and hyperlipemia may occur.

Insulin is secreted in response to carbohydrate intake. In a nonpregnant person, the plasma insulin level increases twofold to tenfold after carbohydrate stimulation. Glucose is taken up by many tissues, facilitated by insulin; especially important is the liver, where much of the glucose is stored as glycogen and triglycerides until needed for energy later. Therefore, glucose levels in a normal nonpregnant person fluctuate only 30–40 mg/dl in spite of intermittent intake.

There have been conflicting reports about whether fasting insulin levels are greater than, less

Table 10.9.
SCREENING CRITERIA FOR DIABETES
MELLITUS IN PREGNANT WOMEN

Previous macrosomic infant (> 4000 g)
Previous unexplained stillbirth
Poor obstetric outcome
Polyhydramnios (past or present)
Excessive weight gain or obese
Congenital anomalies in offspring
Hypertension
Recurrent infections, including recurrent vaginal
    monilial infections
Recurrent glucosuria
Age >35

than, or the same as normal during pregnancy. The secretion of insulin in response to carbohydrate intake is greater than in the nonpregnant patient. However, there is decreased sensitivity to insulin. Liver uptake of glucose is decreased even in the presence of insulin; in fact, tissue sensitivity to insulin may be reduced up to 80% in normal pregnancy (4, p 40). Insulin does not cross the placenta. Thus, food intake results in hyperinsulinemia and hyperglycemia.

The reasons for the resistance to insulin in pregnancy are not completely clear. Insulinase, a placental enzyme, slightly accelerates degradation of insulin. Human placental lactogen opposes insulin and promotes lipolysis, which provides free fatty acids for the mother to use as fuel instead of glucose. Estrogen acts as an antagonist to insulin but does not inhibit its secretion. Progesterone causes an increase in glucose-stimulated insulin secretion. There may be a postreceptor mechanism that also contributes to insulin resistance (4, p 41).

The pancreas normally undergoes both hyperplasia and hypertrophy during pregnancy. It is primarily the insulin-producing β cells in the islets of Langerhans that are affected. Fetal insulin does not cross the placenta to help supply the maternal need. When the pancreas cannot keep up with the increased insulin demand of pregnancy, DM will occur. For a patient who was diabetic prior to pregnancy, the insulin requirements will be increased.

Signs and Symptoms

The signs and symptoms of DM vary from none to shock or even coma. The classic symptoms of polydipsia, polyphagia, and polyuria are obscured by normal changes of pregnancy. Symptoms of advanced disease, such as retinopathy, neuropathies, or vascular disease in the lower extremities, are not common during pregnancy. Glucosuria, a sign in nonpregnant patients, is not a reliable sign of DM during pregnancy; it may merely reflect the lowered renal threshold during pregnancy. However, glucosuria should be

noted, and, especially if it is repetitive, the patient should be tested for DM. Factors that may indicate DM in pregnancy are listed in Table 10.9.

Diagnosis

Diagnosis of DM in pregnancy is based upon circulating glucose levels. Overt DM (White's class B–T) is diagnosed when fasting plasma glucose is ≥105 mg/dl (≥140 mg/dl for a nonpregnant patient) on two or more occasions.

Diagnosis of class A DM requires a glucose tolerance test (GTT). The oral GTT is preferred over the intravenous GTT because it more closely approximates normal carbohydrate metabolism (results depend upon the balance between absorption of glucose from the intestine versus glucose uptake by the tissues and renal excretion), and it stimulates the release of hormones from the intestines that in turn stimulate the β cells in the islets of Langerhans to secrete insulin. During pregnancy, results of the oral GTT may be altered by the increased variability in the rate of glucose absorption from the intestine. Some pregnant women have nausea and vomiting from the glucose load, thus invalidating the test. The intravenous GTT is reserved for those patients who are unable to tolerate the oral glucose solution.

The oral GTT requires advance preparation. For three days before the test the patient should consume 150–200 g of carbohydrates. The patient begins fasting the night before the test. After a fast of 8–14 hours, blood is drawn. The patient then is given a 50% solution of 100 g glucose to drink within 5 minutes. Otherwise, she continues to fast until the test is completed. Blood is drawn at 1, 2, and 3 hours after the glucose load. The upper limits of normal for glucose levels in a GTT may vary slightly among laboratories, but a sample of normal limits is given in Table 10.10. The diagnosis of class A DM requires that two or more levels exceed the limit of normal. Overt DM technically requires fasting hyperglycemia on two or more occasions. So if the fasting level is elevated, subsequent fasting levels should be monitored to determine whether overt DM is present. It should be noted that plasma glucose levels are approximately 15% higher than blood glucose levels.

Many practitioners now use a 1-hour glucose challenge test (GCT) as a screening test for DM. It may be used on all pregnant women or only on those with certain risk factors (e.g., over age 25 or presence of a factor associated with DM such as those listed in Table 10.9). The GCT requires no advance preparation, such as fasting. The patient drinks a 50-g glucose solution, and 1 hour later her blood is drawn. A plasma glucose level ≥135 mg/dl

Table 10.10.

UPPER LIMITS OF NORMAL, PLASMA GLUCOSE
LEVELS FOR GLUCOSE TOLERANCE TEST

Fasting	105 mg/dl
1 hour	190 mg/dl
2 hours	165 mg/dl
3 hours	135 mg/dl

warrants a GTT for diagnosis. With strong suspicion of DM, the GCT may be bypassed and the GTT done initially to avoid delay in diagnosis.

The usual time for performing the GCT is at 26–28 weeks, when the diabetogenic effect of pregnancy is maximal but while there is still time for diagnosis and treatment before the critical last few weeks of pregnancy. With strong suspicion of DM, however, a GCT or GTT may be done early in the pregnancy to avoid delay in diagnosis. If negative, the test can be repeated at 26–28 weeks.

Glycosylated hemoglobin (Hgb A_{1c}) is a blood test that reflects overall glucose status during the 4–6 week period prior to the test. It is not a diagnostic test for DM. The results correlate with the degree of metabolic control rather than with the class of DM. The Hgb A_{1c} level may be useful at the time of the first prenatal visit in evaluating metabolic control prior to that point in pregnancy. It may also be checked occasionally during the pregnancy to confirm that periodic tests of glucose levels reflect overall glucose status (i.e., that the patient has not modified her dietary intake in anticipation of the periodic glucose tests).

Maternal and Fetal Outcome

Most pregnant women with DM in pregnancy have gestational DM; 10–15% of these will develop overt DM over the course of the pregnancy. After delivery, glucose tolerance returns to normal in 98% of gestational diabetics; the remaining 2% continue to have abnormal glucose tolerance. However, long-term follow-up reveals that 60% of women with gestational diabetes develop overt DM within 16 years (11). For women with overt disease, there is controversy over whether pregnancy accelerates microangiopathic or neuropathic complications of DM (4, p. 66, 12). Often, during the first half of pregnancy, insulin requirements decrease because of nausea and vomiting and the transfer of glucose to the fetus. During the second half of pregnancy, insulin requirements often increase markedly (averge 186%) (13) as the diabetogenic effect of pregnancy develops. In spite of the increase in insulin requirements, metabolic control is not difficult to achieve. "Brittle" diabetics (i.e., those with wide, unpredictable swings in glucose levels) become

more predictable and thus easier to control during pregnancy. Diabetogenic ketoacidosis or hypoglycemic coma may occur during pregnancy. These disorders are described in Table 10.11.

Maternal and fetal/neonatal prognosis depend to a great extent upon control of the DM and the degree of cardiovascular or renal disease resulting from DM. Several complications of pregnancy are more common in diabetic patients, and they increase the maternal and fetal risks accordingly. These are listed in Table 10.12.

Maternal mortality is negligible except in patients with ischemic heart disease. The rates of infertility and spontaneous abortion are not increased significantly. The overall risk of perinatal death increases with severity of DM and is reported to be 3.6–4.6% in patients with overt DM—two to three times greater than in the general population (2, p. 602). It is thought that the dramatic decline in perinatal death that has occurred in recent years is probably due to the trend toward tighter metabolic control during pregnancy, improved techniques for fetal assessment, and improved neonatal care.

Currently, the entity responsible for more perinatal death than any other is congenital anomalies. Animal studies have indicated that severe fetal hyperglycemia during the period of embryogenesis is teratogenic. In humans the major anomalies seen are those of the heart, nervous system, and skeletal system. It is thought that most of these develop before 7 weeks' gestation—at a time when the patient may not even realize she is pregnant. Indeed, women with elevated glycosylated hemoglobin early in gestation have a higher incidence of anomalous offspring (14). It is hypothesized that tight metabolic control from the time of conception (or even prior to conception) will be necessary to prevent congenital anomalies resulting from DM.

Macrosomia is thought to occur in the patient with hyperglycemia and no vascular compromise, because fetal hyperglycemia stimulates the production of fetal hyperinsulinemia. Together, the hyperglycemia and hyperinsulinemia stimulate the synthesis of glycogen, lipids, and protein, resulting in large fetal size. The macrosomic infant has increased length and organ size (particularly the liver) as well as weight. The brain and skull size, however, are not increased.

Intrauterine growth retardation occurs more often in class D–T DM, presumably because maternal vasculopathy interferes with fetal nutrition.

Respiratory distress syndrome is less prevalent now among infants of diabetic mothers but still occurs in 3–11% (five to six times more often than in babies of the same gestational age in the general

Table 10.11.

DIABETIC COMA VERSUS HYPOGLYCEMIC COMA

	KETOACIDOSIS (DIABETIC COMA)	HYPOGLYCEMIA PROGRESSING TO HYPOGLYCEMIC COMA
Definition	Excessive accumulation of ketone bodies resulting in acidosis	Inadequate blood glucose level
Causative factors	Too little insulin because of increased need, omitted dose of insulin, or inadequate dose of insulin; may be precipitated by infection.	Overdose of insulin; decreased food intake (e.g., skipped meal); increased exercise without compensatory intake of carbohydrate; nausea and vomiting
Symptoms	Polyuria, polydipsia, nausea and vomiting, dehydration (dry mucous membranes, warm flushed skin), hypotension, shock, oliguria progressing to anuria, abdominal pain, Kussmaul's respirations, odor of acetone on breath, weakness, paralysis, paresthesias, coma	Headache; weakness; irritability; poor muscular coordination; apprehension; diaphoresis; pallor; bradycardia, shallow respirations; visual disturbances; memory loss, confusion, hallucinations; seizures—generalized or focal
Diagnosis	Based on clinical symptomatology and laboratory studies demonstrating hyperglycemia and ketonemia greater than normal for pregnancy	Based on clinical symptomatology and laboratory studies demonstrating hypoglycemia
Treatment	Administer insulin (continuous i.v., 2–6 units/hour); restore blood volume with hypotonic fluids; correct fluid and electrolyte imbalance; administer sodium bicarbonate to treat acidosis if necessary; correct precipitating factors	If mild, give orange juice or other sugar solution by mouth; if severe, administer 50% glucose solution i.v., 20–50 ml, followed by oral fluids with high levels of carbohydrate; administer glucagon; administer epinephrine
Perinatal outcome	Perinatal mortality greater than 50%	Possible intellectual impairment

obstetric population). Tighter metabolic control and fetal assessment techniques have made it possible to wait until term or near term to deliver most babies of diabetic mothers. In the past the risks of preterm delivery were weighed against the increasing risk of intrauterine fetal death after 36 weeks' gestation, and the decision usually was made to deliver the patient at approximately 36 weeks. Now, with good metabolic control and reassuring tests of fetal status, it is often possible to wait until the lecithin:sphingomyelin (L:S) ratio is >2.0. In nondiabetic patients, an L:S ratio of 2:0 indicates fetal ma-

turity; in diabetic patients, one study showed an 18% risk of respiratory distress syndrome even with a "mature" L:S ratio (15). Thus, the added information of phosphatidylglycerol (PG) is useful for determining lung maturity (see Chapter 6).

Hypoglycemia (<30 mg/dl in term babies and <20 mg/dl in preterm babies) occurs in 20–30% of infants of diabetic mothers. The incidence can be minimized by appropriate glucose and insulin administration in labor. Presumably, hypoglycemia results from high endogenous insulin levels that persist after glucose is metabolized. Neonatal glu-

Table 10.12.

COMPLICATIONS OF PREGNANCY ASSOCIATED WITH DIABETES MELLITUS

1. Hypertension in approximately 12–13%[a] with a fourfold increase in preeclampsia/eclampsia.
2. Maternal infections, with increases in both frequency and severity. Monilial vaginitis is common. Pyelonephritis occurs in 1.5–12%.
3. Polyhydramnios in 6–25%.
4. Systemic generalized edema in 10–22%.
5. Macrosomia (especially in DM classes A–C), resulting in an increased incidence of labor dysfunction, traumatic delivery and operative delivery, and birth injuries.
6. Postpartum hemorrhage, resulting primarily from overdistention of the uterus due to polyhydramnios and/or macrosomia.
7. Intrauterine growth retardation, particularly in class D–T DM.
8. Intrauterine fetal death in 1–4% (twice the rate in the general population).
9. Congenital anomalies in 6–12% (three to four times the rate in the general population).
10. Prematurity, owing to uterine overdistention or medically indicated termination of pregnancy.
11. Neonatal hypoglycemia in 20–60%, hypocalcemia in 8–22%, hyperbilirubinemia in 15–20%.
12. Neonatal respiratory distress syndrome in 3–11%.

[a]Percentages from Burrow and Ferris (4).

cose levels are easily monitored and can be treated readily.

The infant of the diabetic mother, because of positive family history, is predisposed to develop DM later in life.

Medical Management

Excellent care of the diabetic gravida contributes significantly to a favorable prognosis for both mother and baby. This care requires a team approach, including obstetrician, internist, nutritionist, nurse, social worker, and pediatrician.

The first step in management is diagnosis of the problem. The practitioner must be aware of the factors suggesting that a patient may have DM—especially her obstetrical and family history and her weight status. Appropriate screening should be done to identify patients with DM as soon as possible. Patients with established DM prior to pregnancy should be counseled preconceptionally, if possible, about the importance of strict metabolic control at the time of conception and throughout the pregnancy.

Once DM is identified, tight metabolic control through diet and exogenous insulin administration is the priority. The goal is euglycemia. Hospitalization usually is required until a diet and insulin regime can be established for the individual patient. Frequent prenatal visits are required to monitor her status subsequently.

The diet of the diabetic gravida is very important. Although weight loss might be a long-term goal for the overweight woman, it is contraindicated in pregnancy because ketosis may adversely affect neurological development of the fetus. Therefore, the goal is normal pregnancy weight gain. Regularity of food intake is crucial—both in timing and content of meals and snacks. Alterations in food intake patterns require alterations in insulin dose and/or timing. Generally, the woman's intake should be 30–35 kcal/kg of actual body weight. Of these calories 35–45% should be complex carbohydrates (approximately the proportion of carbohydrates in a normal diet). Concentrated sweets should be avoided, however, since they can cause large swings in plasma glucose levels. A woman with glucosuria may need to increase her carbohydrate intake to compensate for renal loss. The remainder of the calories are made up of protein— approximately 125 g/day—and fats—approximately 60–80 g/day. A diet high in fiber may assist in maintaining a steady blood sugar level.

Class A diabetics usually are managed by diet alone; 35 kcal/kg/day is the rule. Fasting and postprandial blood sugars should be checked periodically to identify the 10–15% of class A diabetics who de-

velop overt DM over the course of the pregnancy. Some practitioners are now giving NPH insulin to class A diabetics beginning before 34 weeks' gestation to decrease macrosomia and its associated complications (e.g., operative delivery, birth trauma). This practice has not been demonstrated to decrease perinatal morbidity and mortality (4, p 52).

Insulin dosage is adjusted, as needed, based on frequent monitoring of blood glucose levels. Blood testing equipment that can be used at home is now available for the highly motivated patient. Ideally, blood glucose should be monitored four times daily—a fasting level in the morning before breakfast and then 2 hours after each meal. Urine should be checked daily for ketones. The goal is to maintain plasma glucose at <120 mg/dl without ketonuria (4, p 52). Insulin usually is given in one to two subcutaneous injections daily as a mixture of NPH (intermediate-acting) and regular (short-acting) insulin. A portable pump that delivers insulin continuously currently is being used by some patients.

Oral hypoglycemic agents are contraindicated during pregnancy. Their effectiveness in pregnancy has not been demonstrated. Tolbutamide in large doses has caused teratogenesis in animals. It may also cause serious hypoglycemia in the neonate (2, p 603).

Insulin requirements often decrease in the first half of pregnancy but may jump to two to four times the prepregnancy requirement in the second half. Frequent monitoring of blood glucose will allow the necessary adjustments to be made while maintaining good control. Occasional Hgb A_{1c} levels may be taken to confirm that periodic blood sugar tests are an accurate reflection of the patient's status (i.e., that she has not altered her usual diet in preparation for the blood test).

Precise knowledge of gestational age becomes critical in the management of the diabetic gravida as she approaches term. Therefore, an early sonogram may be warranted along with careful documentation of all the historical and physical parameters for assessing gestational age: last normal menstrual period, regularity of cycles, uterine size in early pregnancy and pattern of growth, date of quickening, and date the fetal heart is first heard with a stethoscope.

Since infections tend to be more frequent and more severe in diabetic women and since they rapidly can lead to ketoacidosis, the patient should be encouraged to report immediately any signs or symptoms of infection, even if mild. Periodic screening for urinary tract infection may be warranted. Nausea and vomiting also must be reported since compensatory alterations in insulin dosage may be required.

Timing of delivery is very important in the management of the diabetic gravida since the risks of prematurity must be weighed against the increasing risk of intrauterine fetal death after 36 weeks. Intensive fetal monitoring is required, beginning at 28–35 weeks (depending upon the individual's clinical presentation). Usually, the nonstress test (NST) is used to assess fetal status, but it is usually done at least twice weekly. A contraction stress test (CST) is done if the NST is nonreactive. Serum or urine estriols done three to seven times a week may be used to monitor fetal status but are less popular now than they once were because results may be misleading. Sonograms also may be used to assess fetal macrosomia, amniotic fluid volume, or a complete biophysical profile. Amniocentesis may be done near term (37–38 weeks) to perform an L:S ratio to assess fetal lung maturity. The decision should be made to deliver the patient when she has gross polyhydramnios, severe hypertension, evidence of fetal distress, or is near term when there is evidence of fetal maturity.

The intensive fetal monitoring and need for tight metabolic control may require hospitalization from 34–36 weeks' gestation until delivery. The motivated, compliant patient who can monitor blood glucose levels at home, come in frequently for tests of fetal status, and has telephone access to a perinatologist at any time may be managed successfully on an outpatient basis.

When the decision is made to deliver the patient, induction of labor may be attempted. The reported cesarean section rates are very high, however, ranging from 55–81% (2, p 604). Reasons for the high rate of operative delivery include fetopelvic disproportion, dysfunctional labor, unsuccessful induction, unripe cervix discouraging attempt at induction, or other obstetrical indications.

During labor, glucose control must be maintained to prevent excessive neonatal hypoglycemia. This must be done despite the increased glucose requirement for the energy for the work of labor and the lack of oral intake. One suggested protocol is to withhold oral intake and subcutaneous insulin on the morning of labor. An intravenous infusion is begun, with 5% dextrose given at the rate of 125 cc/hour by constant infusion pump. Ten units of regular insulin is added to each liter of the dextrose solution, resulting in administration of 1.25 units/hour. The plasma glucose and plasma ketone levels should be checked frequently during labor. The insulin dose should be increased if the plasma glucose is >100 mg/dl and decreased if it is <60 mg/dl. The usual dose in labor is 0–1.5 units/hour (4, p 55). Alternatively, intravenous glucose solution may be given with 10 units of regular insulin subcutaneously.

When cesarean section is planned, oral intake and insulin are withheld the morning of the surgery. The surgery should be performed at about breakfast time. The patient can be given saline solution intravenously until the baby is delivered. A glucose solution then may be given.

Postpartum insulin requirements may fluctuate for a few days; therefore, frequent glucose monitoring is required. Often, insulin requirements decrease dramatically postpartum, even below prepregnancy levels, especially in the postoperative patient who is not allowed oral intake. Such a patient may require an intravenous infusion containing both glucose and insulin until oral intake in resumed. Insulin requirements gradually increase to prepregnant levels by 4–6 weeks postpartum.

Breastfeeding is not contraindicated for the diabetic patient, but metabolic control may require a regular pattern of feeding rather than an "on-demand" schedule.

The postpartum patient must be observed for signs and symptoms of infection. She should be treated adequately and promptly if they occur, since infection can lead to ketoacidosis and insulin resistance.

The patient should be counseled about the available methods of birth control. There is an increased risk of pelvic inflammatory disease in diabetics using the intrauterine contraceptive device. Oral contraceptives may not only intensify the diabetes but also potentiate the vasculopathy associated with DM. Therefore, barrier methods should be recommended as a reversible method. The patient should be counseled about the option of sterilization when she has completed childbearing.

NURSING MANAGEMENT

Nursing care specific for a patient with
diabetes mellitus:
☐ Counsel patients with established DM preconceptionally, if possible, regarding the impor-
tance of strict metabolic control prior to conception and throughout pregnancy.
☐ Assist in the diagnosis of DM:
— Observe all patients for risk factors and signs/symptoms of DM.

NURSING MANAGEMENT

— Ensure that appropriate patients are screened at 26–28 weeks' gestation (or sooner if indicated) with a GCT.

— Provide appropriate information for the patient scheduled for a GTT:

  * Consume a high carbohydrate (200 g) diet for 3 days before the test;

  * Begin fasting at 10:00 P.M. the night before the test for an 8:00 A.M. test);

  * Drink the glucose solution within a 5-minute period of time; and

  * Consume no other food or beverage until the test is completed.

☐ Educate the patient regarding diet:

— Need for regular intake, both in content and timing of meals and snacks;

— Avoidance of intake of concentrated sweets;

— Goal of normal, but not excessive, weight gain;

— Specific dietary requirements (e.g., total caloric intake and percentage to be derived from protein, fat, and carbohydrate at each meal/snack); and

— Use of American Diabetes Association exchange lists to simplify meal planning.

☐ Educate the patient regarding insulin.

— Dose, route, timing, and technique for self-administration of insulin (whether by subcutaneous injection or constant infusion pump);

— Physiologic effect of insulin;

— Relationship between dietary intake, exercise, and insulin requirements; and

— Need to notify physician promptly if dietary intake is altered or the patient becomes ill.

☐ Educate the patient regarding glucose monitoring:

— Importance of glucose monitoring;

— Use of home blood glucose monitoring equipment; (how to record results and significance of results); or

— Reporting to clinic or office frequently for blood glucose checks.

☐ Teach the patient to report signs/symptoms of infection; obtain periodic urine cultures to screen for asymptomatic bacteriuria.

☐ Teach the patient the need for frequent prenatal visits.

☐ Monitor maternal/fetal status at prenatal visits:

— Assist in the documentation of gestational age throughout pregnancy (see Chapter 6);

— Assess urine for glucose/ketones at each visit;

— Observe for complications associated with DM (e.g., hypertension, polyhydramnios, infection); and

— Assist in tests of fetal status (e.g., NSTs, biophysical profile in last 2–3 months of pregnancy).

☐ Administer glucose solutions and subcutaneous or intravenous insulin, as ordered, during labor; assist with blood glucose monitoring.

☐ Assist with oxytocin induction of labor as required (see Chapter 37).

☐ Use continuous electronic fetal monitoring.

☐ Be prepared for emergency cesarean section and neonatal resuscitation; alert pediatrician to attend delivery.

☐ Continue frequent monitoring of blood glucose after delivery since levels may swing markedly; administer glucose solutions and insulin, as ordered.

☐ Encourage breastfeeding, but teach the need for following a schedule rather than feeding on demand.

☐ Educate patient regarding contraception, including specific risks to diabetics of oral contraceptives and intrauterine devices.

☐ Teach the overt diabetic the expected changes in insulin requirements in the first few weeks postpartum; refer the patient to the internist for follow-up.

☐ Teach the gestational diabetic the need to be tested for DM at the 4–6 week postpartum checkup and periodically thereafter, since many will develop DM; encourage her to maintain optimum weight to prevent/postpone onset of DM.

Nursing diagnoses most frequently associated with *diabetes mellitus*:

☐ Anxiety/fear.

☐ Grieving related to potential/actual loss of infant or birth of an imperfect child.

☐ Altered nutrition: less than body requirements.

☐ Altered nutrition: more than body requirements.

☐ Potential altered parenting.

☐ Disturbance in body image, self-esteem.

☐ Alterer maternal tissue perfusion.

☐ Altered fetal cardiac and cerebral tissue perfusion.

PITUITARY DISORDERS

In general, normal pituitary function is required for pregnancy to occur. There are rare circumstances, however, in which pituitary disorders occur concomitantly with pregnancy.

In recent years there has been an increasing incidence of prolactinomas owing to the use of bromocriptine to induce ovulation. The degree of risk is unclear. Successful pregnancies have been reported, with postpartum regression of the tumor. However, the patient should be followed closely with monthly visual field examinations. Alterations of visual field, headaches, blurred vision, or funduscopic changes may require treatment with bromocriptine or transsphenoidal hypophysectomy.

Sheehan's syndrome—pituitary necrosis—results in consecutive failure of secretion of gonadotropins, growth hormone, thyroid-stimulating hormone, and adrenocorticotropic hormone (ACTH). It would seem that pregnancy with Sheehan's syndrome would be impossible, but it does occur. Treatment consists of replacement of adrenal corticosteroids and thyroid hormone. Chapter 43 discusses the development of this disorder after blood loss at delivery.

Diabetes insipidus is rare coexisting with pregnancy, occurring in approximately 1:100,000 cases. There is no impairment of fertility, and pregnancy progresses normally with adequate treatment with the synthetic analog of vasopressin. Vasopressin may stimulate uterine contractions, but there are no consistent reports of an increased incidence of spontaneous abortion or preterm labor with its use. There have been a few inconsistent reports of impaired labor with diabetes insipidus, thought to result from decreased levels of endogenous oxytocin.

ADRENAL DISORDERS

Addison's Disease

Addison's disease—adrenocortical insufficiency—may result from obstruction of the adrenal glands, inadequate pituitary secretion of ACTH, or inadequate steroid replacement. Symptoms include weakness, fatigue, increased pigmentation, hypoglycemia, and nervousness—all of which may occur in normal pregnancy. Weight loss and persistent nausea and vomiting are significant symptoms during pregnancy. Diagnosis may be difficult but is based on the clinical presentation and the lack of the normal rise in plasma cortisol concentration after cosyntropin infusion. Treatment consists of steroid replacement (cortisone acetate and 9-alpha-fluoro-hydrocortisone). The amount of replacement needed during pregnancy is often the same or less than that needed prior to pregnancy, except in times of stress such as labor and delivery or surgery, when the dose should be increased. During labor, hydration should be maintained with normal saline. After delivery, any factors contributing to physiological stress (e.g., hemorrhage, bacterial infection) should be treated promptly and vigorously. There is an increased incidence of low birth weight, thought to result from fetal hypoglycemia. The newborn infant may need steroid and glucose therapy if adrenal activity at birth is suppressed.

Pheochromocytoma

Pheochromocytoma is caused by a tumor that usually is located in the adrenal medulla (but may be located in other chromaffin tissue) that secretes epinephrine and norepinephrine. It is rare in pregnancy but significant in that many of it signs and symptoms are the same as those of preeclampsia/eclampsia, from which it must be differentiated. Symptoms include severe hypertension, severe headaches, profuse sweating, palpitations, nausea and vomiting, blurred vision, vertigo, termulousness, seizures, generalized weakness, and physical signs of hyperthyroidism (e.g., tachycardia, lid lag, fine tremor). X-ray studies may be required to make the diagnosis and are justified in view of the potentially poor outcome. Maternal mortality is approximately 50%, usually due to pulmonary edema, cerebral hemorrhage, and cardiovascular collapse. Fetal mortality is correspondingly high. Treatment is surgical removal of the tumor. Near term, the hypertension may be controlled with antihypertensives while cesarean section and tumor resection are performed.

PARATHYROID DISORDERS

Hyperparathyroidism

Hyperparathyroidism is a chronic disease, more common in women than men, that is characterized by excessive parathyroid hormone and elevated serum calcium concentration. Usually, it is caused by a parathyroid adenoma. Symptoms may be vague, resulting in delayed diagnosis, but include muscular weakness and increased nausea and vomiting during pregnancy. If serum calcium levels are very high, renal calculi may occur. Decreased serum phosphate levels and phosphaturia may occur. Since serum calcium levels normally are lower during pregnancy, diagnosis is more difficult, but a serum calcium level greater than 9.5 mg/dl is considered abnormal. Treatment is surgical removal of the adenoma. If there is renal insufficiency, termination of pregnancy may be required. A normal maternal course in labor and delivery can usually be anticipated. Hyperparathyroid crisis is a risk during the postpartum period. Perinatal outcome is poor. There is an increased rate of spontaneous abortion and stillbirths, and neonatal death occurs in approximately 20%. Intrauterine growth retardation also is more common. More than half the newborns experience neonatal tetany 5–14 days after delivery because of hypocalcemia. Calcium may be given to the neonate prophylactically to prevent tetany.

Hypoparathyroidism

Hypoparathyroidism is a deficiency in parathyroid hormone resulting in significant hypocalcemia. Usually, it is caused by inadvertent removal of the parathyroid glands or disruption of the blood supply to them during thyroid surgery. It may also result from an autoimmune disease or recessive inheritance. Symptoms include numbness, tingling, muscle cramps, tetany, seizures, weakness, fatigue, psychiatric manifestations, or, less commonly, laryngeal stridor or convulsions. The diagnosis is based on increased serum phosphate, decreased serum calcium, and decreased parathyroid hormone. Treatment during pregnancy consists of supplementation with 2 g elemental calcium daily and vitamin D to enhance absorption and retention of calcium. During labor, a calcium gluconate infusion may be required to maintain normal serum calcium levels. If adequately treated, hypoparathyroidism causes no adverse fetal or maternal sequelae. If not treated adequately, the normal decrease in serum calcium in pregnancy may increase maternal symptoms. The newborn may have hyperparathyroidism at birth that resolves within about 4 months. The baby may have hypoparathyroidism if he inherits the recessive genetic disease. Breastfeeding is contraindicated because breastmilk contains 400 mg calcium/liter—a loss that is difficult to replace.

REFERENCES

1. Camuñas C: Altered endocrine and metabolic functioning. In Mahoney EA, Flynn JP (eds): *Handbook of Medical-Surgical Nursing*. New York, John Wiley and Sons, 1983, pp 727–787.
2. Pritchard JA, MacDonald PC, Gant NF: *Williams Obstetrics*, ed 17. Norwalk, CT, Appleton-Century-Crofts, 1985.
3. Mulaisho C, Utiger RD: Serum thyroxine-binding globulin: determination by competitive ligand-binding assay in thyroid disease and pregnancy. *Acta Endocrinol* 85:314, 1977.
4. Burrow, GN, Ferris TF: *Medical Complications During Pregnancy*, ed 2. Philadelphia, WB Saunders, 1982, pp 187–188.
5. Niswander KR, Gordon M, Berendes HW: *The Women and Their Pregnancies*. Philadelphia, WB Saunders, 1972.
6. Witter FR: Treating thyroid disease during pregnancy. *Contemp OB/GYN* 23:203–208, 1984.
7. Singer PA, Mestman JH: Thyroid storm need not be lethal. *Contemp OB/GYN* 22:135–146, 1983.
8. Williams JW: The limitations and possibilities of prenatal care. *JAMA* 64:95, 1915.
9. Queenan JT, Gadov EC: Polyhydramnios: chronic versus acute. *Am J Obstet Gynecol* 108:349, 1970.
10. US Department of Health and Human Services: *Public Health Guidelines for Enhancing Diabetes Control through Maternal and Child Health Programs*. Atlanta, Centers for Disease Control, 1986, p 1.
11. O'Sullivan JB: Establishing criteria for gestational diabetes. *Diabetes Care* 3:437, 1980.
12. Freinkel N, Dooley SL, Metzger BE: Care of the pregnant woman with insulin-dependent diabetes mellitus. *N Engl J Med* 313:96–101, 1985.
13. Coustan DR, Berkowitz RL, Hobbins JC: Tight metabolic control of overt diabetes in pregnancy. *Am J Med* 68:845, 1980.
14. Miller E, Hare JW, Cloherty JP, Dunn PJ, Gleason RE, Soeldner S, Kitzmiller JL: Elevated maternal hemoglobin A in early pregnancy and major congenital anomalies in infants of diabetic mothers. *N Engl J Med* 304:1331, 1981.
15. Mueller-Heubach E, Caritis SN, Edelstone DI, Turner JH: Lecithin/sphingomyelin ratio in amniotic fluid and its value for the prediction of neonatal respiratory distress syndrome in pregnant diabetic women. *Am J Obstet Gynecol* 130:28, 1978.

Chapter 11
Gastrointestinal System Disorders
Nancy W. Kulb, C.N.M., M.S.

INTRODUCTION

The gastrointestinal system undergoes many dramatic changes during pregnancy. These changes contribute to several of the common discomforts of pregnancy, and at times they delay or obscure the diagnosis of gastrointestinal disease. Common gastrointestinal discomforts of pregnancy, along with relief measures, are listed in Table 11.1.

In the mouth there is increased edema and vascularity of the gums. Consequently, many pregnant women experience bleeding of the gums with minor trauma, such as tooth brushing. A very vascular, localized swelling of the interdental papillae, called epulis, may cause profuse bleeding and may even require surgery but will regress postpartum. Pregnant women are more prone to gingivitis and are somewhat more likely to have dental caries. Their saliva is slightly more acidic than normal (1). Women with nausea and vomiting tend to produce more saliva than normal—some to the extent of ptyalism—while others have less saliva than normal.

The lower sphincter of the esophagus has less tone during pregnancy, allowing reflux of gastric contents into the lower esophagus. As pregnancy progresses, the stomach is displaced upward in the abdomen, and its capacity may be decreased somewhat. Gastric acidity tends to decrease slightly during pregnancy (1). Normal gastric motility is slowed; therefore, normal gastric emptying time is prolonged.

The normal placement of the intestines in the abdomen is altered progressively during pregnancy because of displacement and pressure by the growing uterus. The motility of the intestines also is de-

creased during pregnancy, probably as a result of the effect of progesterone in relaxing smooth muscle. More water and electrolytes are absorbed from the intestines during pregnancy (1). These factors, in addition to pressure on the intestines from the growing uterus, contribute to constipation during pregnancy. Constipation, along with increased pressure on pelvic veins and the smooth muscle relaxation from progesterone, contributes to the common problem of hemorrhoids during pregnancy.

Nausea and vomiting are common discomforts of early pregnancy, but the cause is not really known (see the next section, Hyperemesis Gravidarum). Since nausea and vomiting also are frequent symptoms of gastrointestinal disease, they must never be dismissed casually. The diagnosis of "morning sickness" can be made only if other pathology is ruled out. Nausea and vomiting that occur in the second half of pregnancy, that are severe or protracted, or that are associated with other symptoms of pathology (e.g., abdominal pain, weight loss) must be evaluated carefully (Table 11.2).

HYPEREMESIS GRAVIDARUM

Definition

Literally, hyperemesis gravidarum means "excessive vomiting of the pregnant woman." Clinically, it is nausea and vomiting so severe as to interfere with nutrition and to cause systemic effects, such as fluid and electrolyte imbalances and meta-

Table II.I.

COMMON GASTROINTESTINAL DISCOMFORTS OF PREGNANCY[a]

DISCOMFORT	RELIEF MEASURES

Bleeding gums	1. Discuss dental care and hygiene measures:
	  a. Brush teeth very gently with a *soft* brush.
	  b. Avoid eating foods that traumatize the gums (e.g., apples, corn on the cob).
	  c. Use dental floss or Water Pic regularly.
	  d. Have regular dental cleaning done by dental hygienist or dentist.
	2. Reassure the patient that this condition will regress after delivery.
	3. Explain the cause of the discomfort.

Constipation	1. Evaluate the patient's diet and advise the following measures as necessary:
	  a. Increase fluid intake to eight glasses of water daily.
	  b. Add sources of roughage and fiber to the diet (e.g., bran, whole grain breads, fruit, celery, lettuce).
	  c. Add a natural laxative (e.g., prunes or prune juice) to the diet daily.
	2. Encourage daily exercise, such as walking.
	3. Discuss bowel habits and advise the following, as appropriate:
	  a. Establish a regular time of day for having a bowel movement.
	  b. Provide for privacy and a sufficient uninterrupted time for having the bowel movement.
	  c. Never ignore the "urge" to have a bowel movement. Warm liquids (water or herb tea) may stimulate the sensation.
	4. Evaluate iron therapy. A modified iron supplement like Ferro-Sequels, which contains a stool softener, may be effective.
	5. Ensure that mild laxatives, stool softeners, and/or suppositories are used only when natural methods have proven ineffective.
	6. Explain to the patient the possible causes of the discomfort.

Flatulence	1. Suggest avoidance of gas-forming foods (e.g., cabbage, beans, onions). 2. Explore the patient's activities of daily living. A sedentary life-style may contribute to flatulence. Encourage some form of exercise and frequent position changes. 3. Explain relief measures for constipation. 4. Explain the cause of the discomfort.

Heartburn	1. Evaluate the diet and make the following suggestions as appropriate:
	  a. Eat six small meals daily, spread over short time periods, rather than three large meals, which may overload the stomach.
	  b. Drink a small glass of milk between meals and at bedtime. (Note: milk often provides symptomatic relief, although it may also cause a rebound in gastric acidity. The calcium in milk stimulates acidity, although the fat in whole milk tends to counteract acidity.).
	  c. Avoid spicy, greasy, fatty foods.
	  d. Avoid orange juice, tomato juice, tomato paste, chocolate, and cigarette smoking because they decrease esophageal sphincter tone.
	  e. Avoid large meals before bedtime.
	2. Advise the patient to avoid wearing clothing with a tight waistband.
	3. Suggest that she sleep with her head on two pillows to allow gravity to enhance esophageal functioning.
	4. Advise her to avoid bending forward, heavy lifting, or straining at stool.
	5. Teach the patient about any antacids that are ordered, including dose, route, timing, side effects, and expected therapeutic effect.
	6. Teach the patient to avoid Rolaids and Alka-Seltzer because of their high sodium content.
	7. Explain the possible causes of the discomfort.

Hemorrhoids	1. Explain the relief measures of constipation. 2. Suggest using chilled witch hazel compresses to reduce the size and relieve the discomfort of hemorrhoids. 3. Urge avoidance of long periods of sitting or standing. 4. For moderate to severe hemorrhoids, teach the client to elevate her hips and lower extremities several times a day and at night. 5. Suggest the use of topical anesthetics, such as Anusol. 6. Teach the client to replace internal hemorrhoids after each bowel movement. 7. Explain the possible causes of the discomfort.
Morning sickness	1. Recommend the following dietary modifications:

Table 11.1.
(Continued)

	a. Take an adequate amount of vitamin B complex daily. (Prenatal vitamins provide 100% of the requirements. Liver and other organ meats are important food sources of all B vitamins.) b. Eat three or four dry crackers before sitting up in bed in the morning. c. Restrict fat in the diet. d. Avoid greasy, fatty, and spicy foods. e. Eat six small meals rather than three large meals daily. f. Have a bedtime snack. 2. Advise the patient to rise from bed slowly in the morning to minimize orthostatic vascular changes. In addition, she should plan her morning so that she does not have to rush. 3. Reassure her about the limited nature of the discomfort. 4. Explain the possible causes of the discomfort.
Ptyalism	1. Advise the patient to use astringent mouthwashes and to suck on hard candies frequently during the day. 2. Reassure her about the limited nature of the discomfort.

[a]Adapted from Buckley K, Kulb NW. *Handbook of Maternal Newborn Nursing*, New York, John Wiley and Sons, 1983, pp 163–181.

bolic derangement. The incidence of hyperemesis gravidarum, especially severe cases, has been decreasing over the last two to three decades, probably because of prompt recognition and adequate treatment. Currently, about 3.5 out of 1000 pregnant women will have it (2, p 259).

Etiology

The cause of hyperemesis gravidarum is unknown. It is known that it always starts as the "normal" nausea and vomiting of pregnancy, but then continues and increases in severity. Theories of its etiology include hormonal changes of early pregnancy, especially high levels of human chorionic gonadotropin (HCG) or estrogen; decreased gastric motility; emotional/psychological factors, such as

Table 11.2.
CAUSES OF NAUSEA AND VOMITING DURING PREGNANCY[a]

SECONDARY TO PREGNANCY	NOT SECONDARY TO PREGNANCY
Simple nausea and vomiting in pregnancy	Acute gastroenteritis
Hyperemesis gravidarum	Cholecystitis, cholangitis, and biliary obstruction
Hydatidiform mole	Hepatitis
Multiple gestation	Pancreatitis
Reflux vomiting of late pregnancy	Peptic ulcer
Hydramnios	Intestinal obstruction
Preeclampsia	Pyelonephritis
Labor	Uremia
Pica	Diabetic ketoacidosis
Ptyalism	Appendicitis
	Peritonitis
	Twisted ovarian cyst
	Increased intracranial pressure

[a]Adapted from Midwinter A: Vomiting in pregnancy. *Practitioner* January, 743, 1971.

changes or anticipated changes in one's self-concept and relationships as a result of pregnancy or parenting; neurosis; disturbed sexual adjustment; immune response to tiny fragments of chorionic villi that enter the maternal bloodstream; or immune response to the "foreign" products of conception. It is thought that hyperemesis occurs more often in primigravidae than in multiparae; in multiparae with a history of hyperemesis in a previous pregnancy or poor pregnancy outcome; in highly sensitive or neurotic women; and in asthmatics (3). Hyperemesis may occur in association with molar pregnancy or multiple gestation.

Signs and Symptoms

Hyperemesis starts as simple nausea and vomiting of pregnancy. As it becomes more severe, the woman is unable to retain any solids or liquids. Rapidly, she becomes dehydrated, exhibiting a low grade fever (up to 101°F, 38.3°C), rapid pulse rate (up to 110), dry skin, poor skin turgor, decreased urine output, increased specific gravity, and sometimes thirst. She appears listless and weak, her eyes are dull, her lips may be cracked and sore, and her tongue may be coated or raw. She may lose as much as 5–10% of her body weight. She may be constipated as a result of starvation and dehydration. As the disease progresses, she may experience jaundice, resulting from necrotic liver changes, and polyneuritis, resulting from vitamin deficiency. Blood tests may reveal an increase in nonprotein nitrogen, urea, and uric acid, with a decrease in potassium and a moderate decrease in chlorides. The breath may smell of acetone, and both acetone and diacetic acid may be found in the highly concentrated urine. Hyperemesis can progress to the point of confusion, coma, or hepatic or renal failure, but that is quite rare.

Diagnosis

The diagnosis is made after the exclusion of other causes of severe nausea and vomiting, such as gastroenteritis, cholecystitis, hepatitis, peptic ulcers, pyelonephritis, and central nervous system disorders. Because hyperemesis gravidarum may be associated with molar pregnancy and multiple gestation, the woman should be evaluated for both of those complications (see Chapters 31 and 33).

Maternal and Fetal Outcome

The prognosis for both the woman with hyperemesis and her fetus is good. Rapid improvement in the woman's condition can be expected soon after treatment is begun (4). Occasionally, a patient may relapse soon after hospital discharge, lending support to the psychosocial theories of the etiology of hyperemesis. It has been demonstrated that women with moderate nausea and vomiting during pregnancy are less likely to have spontaneous abortion or premature labor, suggesting that a favorable pregnancy outcome can be anticipated (5, p 323).

Medical Management

The medical management of hyperemesis gravidarum begins with hospitalization, which serves to remove the woman from her potentially stressful home environment while providing her a place to rest. Visitation during hospitalization may be limited, depending upon the degree to which the family environment is felt to contribute to the individual's symptoms. Laboratory studies to rule out other pathology and to determine the degree of fluid/electrolyte and acid/base imbalance should be done. The woman is placed on bedrest. Oral foods and fluids are withheld for 24 hours or until vomiting has stopped. Intravenous fluids are given, with the goal of correcting fluid/electrolyte and acid/base imbalance. Three liters of fluid or more will be needed in the first 24 hours. A glucose solution will provide calories for energy. Electrolyte imbalance should be corrected with appropriate additions of sodium, chloride, and potassium. Acidosis may be treated with bicarbonate. Vitamin supplements may be added to intravenous fluids or may be given intramuscularly or subcutaneously. Parenteral antiemetics, such as promethazine (Phenergan), prochlorperazine (Compazine), or vitamin B$_6$ may be given (2, p 260, 6). A sedative may be ordered to promote rest. An enema or rectal suppository may be ordered to relieve constipation. Assistance with psychosocial problems may be provided by a psychiatrist or other appropriate professional. Family members should be included in therapy, as appropriate.

As the woman improves, after the first 24 hours and after vomiting has stopped, light oral feedings may begin. Meals should be small, every 2–3 hours, with liquids taken between meals.

If the woman does not improve after 24 hours of treatment, tube feedings may be required to prevent further deterioration in her nutritional status. Termination of pregnancy is rarely required, but therapeutic abortion may be necessary if the woman has jaundice, delirium, or other cerebral symptoms; tachycardia of 130 beats per minute or more; fever of 38.3°C or more in spite of adequate hydration; or retinal hemorrhage (3, p 206).

NURSING MANAGEMENT

Nursing care specific for a patient with hyperemesis gravidarum:

☐ Assist in prevention of hyperemesis by:
- Identifying women with psychosocial problems and making appropriate referrals, and
- Teaching prevention/relief measures for nausea/vomiting in pregnancy.

☐ Provide a positive environment for a patient hospitalized with hyperemesis:
- Place in private room if possible;
- Restrict visitors as needed, and encourage family to call the nurse for a report on progress;
- Convey warmth and concern; and

- Reassure the patient that a rapid improvement is expected.

☐ Provide appropriate intake to maintain hydration/nutrition status:
- Withhold oral intake for the first 24 hours or until vomiting ceases.
- Administer intravenous fluids (glucose and/or electrolyte solutions) as ordered.
- Administer vitamin supplements as ordered.
- Administer tube feedings as necessary.
- Provide oral feedings when patient is able to tolerate them:
  * Begin with carbohydrates (e.g., dry cereal, toast, crackers);

NURSING MANAGEMENT

* Serve food in small amounts every 2–3 hours;
* Serve liquids about 100 cc at a time between meals;
* Ensure that food is properly served (e.g., attractive setting, hot foods hot, cold foods cold);
* Encourage patient not to let stomach become completely empty as that may increase vomiting; and
* Allow patient to choose foods, if possible.

☐ Monitor the effectiveness of treatment plan:
— Inform the physician immediately of changes in mental or neurological status, fever, or tachycardia, as alterations in management may be required.
— Weigh the patient on admission and daily thereafter.
— Monitor serum electrolytes and the acid/base balance.

☐ Assist the patient with hypotension with ambulation.

☐ Provide comfort measures:
— Provide mouth care (e.g, mouthwash, toothbrushing);
— Eliminate stimuli that may increase nausea (e.g., do not discuss food in her pres-ence, keep emesis basin out of sight, keep room airy and free of kitchen or other odors); and
— Administer antiemetics or sedatives as ordered.

☐ Investigate factors that may contribute to hyperemesis gravidarum (e.g., dietary habits, relationships, feelings, fears):
— Use problem-solving techniques as appropriate and
— Make appropriate referrals (e.g., psychologist, nutritionist, visiting nurse).

☐ Educate patient regarding the following:
— Self-care after hospital discharge (e.g., diet, activity) and
— Pregnancy, labor, delivery, parenting; refer to preparation for childbirth classes.

Nursing diagnoses most frequently associated with *hyperemesis gravidarum*:

☐ Ineffective individual coping.
☐ Potential altered parenting.
☐ Disturbance in body image, self-esteem.
☐ Knowledge deficit regarding etiology, disease process, treatment, and expected outcome.
☐ Altered nutrition: less than body requirements.
☐ Anxiety/fear.

HIATAL HERNIA

Definition

Hiatal hernia is the protrusion of the upper part of the stomach through the esophageal hiatus of the diaphragm and into the chest. Estimates of the incidence during pregnancy vary tremendously, from about 10–70% (7). Hiatal hernias often resolve during the postpartum period, but they remain in approximately one-third of patients.

Etiology

The etiology of hiatal hernia during pregnancy is not known. It is thought that it may result from the intermittent but long-term increase in intraabdominal pressure that is characteristic of pregnancy. It is three times more common in multiparae than in primigravidae (5), but among primigravidae it is more common in older women (7a, p 30). Obesity also may be a predisposing factor.

Signs and Symptoms

The most common symptom of hiatal hernia is severe, persistent heartburn. Since heartburn owing to gastric reflux is a common discomfort of the third trimester of pregnancy, it may be difficult to differentiate it from hernia. Patients with hiatal hernia may also experience nausea and vomiting persisting into the latter part of pregnancy, epigastric pain, or hematemesis. Peptic esophagitis and rupture of the esophagus resulting in mediastinitis have been reported (8, p 2).

Diagnosis

The diagnosis of hiatal hernia during pregnancy is quite difficult, since radiography is contraindicated and procedures requiring analgesia/anesthesia are to be avoided if possible. Since the medical management during pregnancy is essentially the same as that for heartburn, the diagnosis of hiatal hernia often is not crucial and is often delayed to determine whether symptoms persist postpartum. Clinically, the diagnosis is suggested by heartburn unrelieved by antacids, aggravated by a recumbent or leaning forward position, or accompanied by nausea and vomiting, epigastric pain, or other symptoms.

Maternal and Fetal Outcome

The prognosis for both mother and baby is good. Symptoms of hiatal hernia resolve in most patients during the postpartum period, persisting in only 36% (8, p 2). Those patients with persisting symptoms will be able to pursue further diagnosis, medical treatment, or surgery if necessary. Unless severe symptoms interfere with the mother's nutritional status or require early delivery, the outcome for the fetus can be expected to be good.

Medical Management

Medical management of hiatal hernia during pregnancy primarily is symptomatic. Anatacids are prescribed ½ to 1 hour after each meal and at bedtime. At times, the frequency of antacid therapy may need to be increased. Patients are instructed to sit up after meals, to avoid the recumbent position, and to avoid leaning forward. Occasionally, induction of labor may be required because of severe symptoms or threatened perforation of the esophagus (indicated by severe epigastric pain or hematemesis) (8, p 3). During labor, special care to avoid gastric reflux is indicated, especially if general anesthesia is anticipated. Oral intake should be curtailed, except for antacids every 4 hours.

NURSING MANAGEMENT

Nursing care specific for a patient with *hiatal hernia*:
- ☐ Educate patient regarding the following:
  - — Comfort/nutritional measures to prevent/relieve heartburn;
  - — Danger signs and how to report them (e.g., severe chest or abdominal pain, hematemesis);
- ☐ Restrict oral intake during labor except for antacids every 4 hours.

- ☐ Encourage the patient to seek further diagnosis and treatment if symptoms persist postpartum.

Nursing diagnoses most frequently associated with *hiatal hernia*:
- ☐ Knowledge deficit regarding etiology, disease process, treatment, and expected outcome.
- ☐ Knowledge deficit regarding medication regimen.
- ☐ Pain.
- ☐ Altered nutrition: less than body requirements.

ACUTE APPENDICITIS

Definition

Appendicitis is the inflammation of the appendix. It is most common between the ages of 5 and 50. During pregnancy, the incidence has been reported to range from 0.38–1.41 per 1000 pregnant women, with a slightly greater frequency in the second trimester (9).

Etiology

The etiology of appendicitis is poorly understood. Predisposing factors are those that favor intestinal obstruction or infection: diet low in fiber, hard fecal masses, parasitic infection. Apparently, obstruction causes pressure on the epithelial lining of the appendix, resulting in ulceration and bacterial invasion. If the appendix ruptures, the inflammation quickly spreads throughout the abdomen.

Signs and Symptoms

Signs and symptoms of appendicitis in the pregnant woman may present a challenge in diagnosis. In nonpregnant patients initially there is generalized or periumbilical pain that later localizes in the right lower quadrant, at McBurney's point. After the third month of pregnancy, the point of maximal tenderness in appendicitis shifts (Fig. 11.1) because the location of the appendix moves up and rotates horizontally on its base (9). In the third trimester as many as 80% of patients may *not* have pain if the appendix is not in contact with the parietal peritoneum (9). Because of distention of the abdominal wall, it may not be possible to elicit rebound tenderness or muscle guarding. Anorexia, almost always present in the nonpregnant patient with appendicitis, may not be present in the pregnant woman or may be dismissed as insignificant since many pregnant women have a poor appetite. Nausea and vomiting are common with appen-

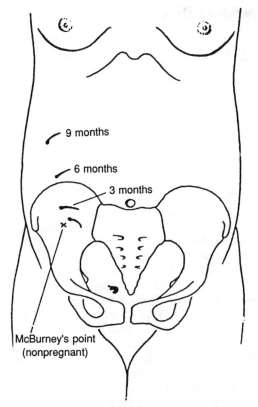

Figure 11.1. Location of maximal tenderness of appendicitis as pregnancy advances. (From Beischer NA, Mackay EV: Obstetrics and the Newborn: For Midwives and Medical Students. Sydney, Australia, Saunders, 1976, p 206.)

dicitis but are also considered normal in the first trimester of pregnancy.

Diagnosis

Laboratory tests must be interpreted in the light of normal values for the pregnant woman. Since leukocytosis (up to 16,000 WBCs/μl is normal in pregnancy, the complete blood count may be of little help in diagnosis (although a WBC >20,000/μl suggests perforation) (10). WBCs in urine may result from the inflamed appendix being positioned next to the ureter,

but it must be remembered that the presence of WBCs without bacteriuria is not uncommon in the pregnant patient.

Therefore, the diagnosis of appendicitis in pregnancy primarily is clinical. The accuracy of diagnosis at the time of surgery is 67–72%, similar to the accuracy in nonpregnant patients of 75% (9). Pelvic and rectal exams are important parts of the clinical evaluation of women presenting with symptoms of appendicitis. The differential diagnosis for pregnant women includes a long list: ruptured ectopic pregnancy, cholecystitis, twisted ovarian cyst, degenerating myoma, ruptured corpus luteum, ruptured dermoid cyst, premature labor, placental abruption, pneumonia, renal cholic, or pyelonephritis (9).

Maternal and Fetal Outcome

The maternal and fetal outcome depend upon the severity of the appendicitis. Primarily, mortality is a result of delaying surgery. The maternal mortality for umcomplicated appendicitis is 0.1%, but after perforation it rises to 4% (9). Fetal complications generally result from abortion or premature labor. The overall fetal death rate is 8.5%, but with peritonitis, gangrene, or infarction, it may be as high as 35–70% (9). Concern for fetal exposure to the hazards of surgery and anesthesia is overridden quickly by the extreme risk of delay.

Medical Management

The management of acute appendicitis is always appendectomy as soon as the diagnosis is made.

For uncomplicated appendicitis, no prophylactic antibiotics are required. If gangrene or perforation has occurred, aminoglycosides, penicillins, and/or clindamycin may be begun prior to surgery. Generally, it is not recommended that a cesarean section be performed at the same time as the appendectomy, but if it must be done simultaneously for obstetric reasons and if the appendix is gangrenous or perforated, some experts believe that a hysterectomy should also be performed to reduce maternal morbidity.

NURSING MANAGEMENT

Nursing care specific for a patient with
appendicitis:

☐ Avoid abdominal stimulation (e.g., unnecessary abdominal palpation, heat to abdomen, laxatives, enema) when appendicitis is suspected.

☐ Avoid administration of analgesics until the diagnosis is made to avoid masking clinical signs/symptoms; subsequently administer analgesics as ordered.

☐ Place patient in Fowler's position to minimize spread of infection if rupture should occur.

NURSING MANAGEMENT

☐ Provide routine preoperative and postoperative care if surgery is required; monitor fetal status throughout.

☐ Administer antibiotics as ordered.

Nursing diagnoses most frequently associated with *appendicitis*:

☐ Grieving related to potential/actual loss of infant or birth of an imperfect child.

☐ Anticipatory grieving related to actual/perceived threat to self.

☐ Pain.

☐ Knowledge deficit regarding etiology, disease process, treatment, and expected outcome.

☐ Anxiety/fear.

☐ Impaired tissue integrity.

PEPTIC ULCER

Definition

A peptic ulcer is an open sore or lesion of the stomach (gastric ulcer) or duodenum (duodenal ulcer). It occurs in approximately 5% of the population but is rare in women of childbearing age (9).

Etiology

The pathogenesis of gastric ulcer is largely unknown. It was once believed that diet and emotional stress were the major etiological factors, but now it is believed that physiological factors play a more important role. It is known that increased levels of hydrochloric acid (HCl) and pepsin play a role either in initiation or maintenance of peptic ulcer. People prone to peptic ulcer may have a greater than normal number of parietal cells, the HCl-secreting cells of the stomach; greater responsiveness of the parietal cells to food, gastrin, or histamine; and greater responsiveness to nerve stimulation resulting in increased gastrin secretion (9). The role of gastric pepsin in ulcer formation is unclear. People with type O blood have a slightly higher incidence of ulcer. Genetic factors may be involved, and stress and emotions may play a part, but the mechanism is not clear. Peptic ulcer in young women frequently is associated with excessive aspirin intake (11). On the other hand, prostaglandins may have a protective effect on the lining of the stomach.

Signs and Symptoms

Peptic ulcer is characterized by moderate to severe pain well localized in the midepigastric region. The pain is intermittent, lasting 15–60 minutes, occurring several times daily, when the stomach is empty. It is described as burning, boring, or pressing pain and is relieved by food or antacids. The pain is made worse by coffee, alcohol, or aspirin. Nausea and vomiting are rare, but hematemesis or melena may occur if there is bleeding at the base of the ulcer.

Diagnosis

Physical examination is of little benefit in establishing the diagnosis. Occasionally, there may be midepigastric tenderness. Some experts believe that the classical history of burning epigastric pain when the stomach is empty and that is relieved by eating is sufficient to establish an empirical diagnosis of peptic ulcer. They will treat the patient with antacids and will do further diagnostic studies only if the treatment is not successful. Other experts believe that endoscopy should be performed immediately to confirm the diagnosis and to rule out cancer or duodenitis. Since endoscopy can be performed without premedication, it can be done with minimal hazard during pregnancy.

Maternal and Fetal Outcome

Fortunately, during pregnancy, peptic ulcer usually is not a serious problem: 44% of peptic ulcer patients become totally asymptomatic during pregnancy, 44% improve markedly, and only 12% remain the same or become worse. Thus many ulcer patients look forward to the relief provided by pregnancy (9). The reasons for the improvement are not fully understood, but it is thought that progesterone, which is produced in large amounts during pregnancy, decreases gastric acid production and increases the production of protective gastric mucus. Also, in the latter part of pregnancy, the placenta secretes plasma histaminase, which inactivates histamine and blocks the acid-producing effect of the parietal cells (9). The possible serious sequelae of peptic ulcer are perforation, gastrointestinal bleeding, and obstruction because of edema or fibrosis. The effects of peptic ulcer on the fetus are minimal, unless serious complications compromise the health of the mother.

Medical Management

The management of peptic ulcer has changed in recent years. Ulcers tend to heal regardless of management—treatment merely assists and speeds up the process (11). Some physicians no longer rec-

Table 11.3.
MEDICATIONS USED IN TREATING PEPTIC ULCER

MEDICATION	DOSE, ROUTE, TIMING	ACTION	MATERNAL AND FETAL SIDE EFFECTS
Aluminum hydroxide[a]	Generally, 80 mEq 1 hour after meals, every 1–2 hours thereafter, and a double dose at bedtime. Follow directions for each medication.	Antacid. Slow onset of action. Not potent.	Phosphate depletion. May absorb some medications, thus hindering assimilation. May cause constipation. Considered safe to use in pregnancy except in patients with renal disease or hypersensitivity.
Calcium carbonate[a]	As above.	Antacid. Potent effects.	Acid rebound, mild alkali syndrome, or hypercalcemia may occur. May cause constipation.
Magnesium hydroxide[a]	As above.	Antacid. Slow, prolonged action.	Poorly absorbed. May act as a laxative. Serum magnesium may increase, especially in patients in renal insufficiency. Considered safe to use in pregnancy except in patients with renal disease or hypersensitivity.
Sodium bicarbonate	As above.	Antacid.	May cause fluid retention because of the sodium content, so should not be used in patients with hypertension or heart disease.
Propantheline bromide (Pro-Banthine)	15 mg p.o. taken 30 minutes before meals and 30 mg q.h.s.	Anticholinergic. Inhibits gastrointestinal motility and decreases secretion of gastric acid. Inhibits action of acetylcholine.	Should not be used in the first trimester of pregnancy if at all. Studies have not been conducted concerning effects in pregnancy. Potential side effects include dry mouth, blurred vision, mydriasis, urinary retention, tachycardia, headache, nervousness, confusion, drowsiness, nausea, vomiting, constipation.
Cimetidine (Tagamet)	300 mg q.i.d. p.o. during exacerbation. Maintenance therapy is 400 mg p.o. q.h.s.	Histamine analog. Inhibits basal secretion of gastric acid as well as secretion stimulated by histamine, caffeine, insulin, and food.	There is a low rate of significant side effects, but maternal side effects may include increased plasma creatinine, gynecomastia, mental confusion, leukopenia, possible agranulocytosis; Rarely, headache, diarrhea, dizziness, somnolence, rash, arthralgia. It crosses the placental barrier in experimental animals, but fetal effects are unknown. Therefore it is *not* recommended in pregnant women.
Sucralfate (Carafate)	1 g p.o. q.i.d., 1 hour before meals.	Basic sulfated aluminum salt of sucrose. In the presence of gastric acid, it turns into a viscous substance that adheres to the ulcer, protecting it from acid. It inhibits action of pepsin and may absorb bile salts.	Effects on the fetus are not known, so it is *not* recommended in pregnancy at this time. However, very little is absorbed, and no side effects are known.

[a]These preparations are rarely used individually but are commonly found in combination antacids.

ommend any modifications in the diet, other than elimination of particularly irritating foods, such as coffee or alcohol. Others believe that some patients may feel better with bland, frequent, small meals. The primary treatment during pregnancy is antacids. There is not enough known about fetal ef-

fects of other medications commonly used to treat peptic ulcer to recommend them (Table 11.3).

The treatment of gastrointestinal bleeding or perforation is surgical repair. The fetal mortality with those complications is much less with surgery than with nonsurgical, medical treatment. Gastrointestinal obstruction resulting from peptic ulcer is treated with nasogastric suction for at least 72 hours. If it is unsuccessful, a surgical procedure to provide drainage may be necessary. If surgery is re- quired during the third trimester, a cesarean sec- tion may be performed first to provide better visual- ization and to prevent the fetal distress that may result from hypotension during surgery (12).

NURSING MANAGEMENT

Nursing care specific for a patient with peptic ulcer:

☐ Teach the patient to note the relationship be- tween life-style behaviors/specific foods (e.g., aspirin, smoking, coffee, alcohol) and onset of epigastric discomfort to avoid aggravating be- haviors/foods.

☐ Assist patient to evaluate life-style, stress man- agement, and coping mechanisms.

☐ Educate patient regarding the following:

— Dietary measures that *may* provide relief:

 * Small, frequent, bland meals and
 * Ingestion of milk (note: milk may pro- vide relief initially, although it may cause a rebound in gastric acidity).

— Medications (e.g., dose, route, timing, po- tential side effects, expected therapeutic effect).

— Danger signs of complications:

 * Hemorrhage: vomiting blood, tarry stools, faintness, dizziness, thirst, apprehension, restlessness, dyspnea;
 * Pyloric obstruction: epigastric full- ness, pain, projectile vomiting, dehy- dration, weight loss, aversion to food, and
 * Perforation: sudden, sharp, abdomi- nal pain; tender, board-like abdo-

men; rapid, shallow respirations; profuse perspiration; referred shoul- der pain.

☐ Evaluate the following if the patient has signs/ symptoms of complications:

— Vital signs, including fetal heart tones;
— Hemoglobin, hematocrit;
— Intake and output; and
— Color and amount of emesis/stool.

☐ Provide routine preoperative and postoperative care if surgery becomes necessary, monitoring fetal status throughout.

☐ If nasogastric suctioning is required:

— Note color and amount of aspirate and
— Ensure proper positioning, taping, and lubrication of tube.

Nursing diagnoses most frequently associated with peptic ulcer:

☐ Ineffective individual coping.
☐ Anxiety/fear.
☐ Pain.
☐ Knowledge deficit regarding etiology, disease process, treatment, and expected outcome.
☐ Knowledge deficit regarding medication regi- men.
☐ Fluid volume deficit.

REFERENCES

1. Martin C: Physiological changes during pregnancy. In Quilligan EJ (ed): *Fetal and Maternal Medicine*. New York, Wiley, 1980, p 166.
2. Dobbins JW, Spiro HM: Gastrointestinal complica- tions. In Burrow GN, Ferris TF (eds): *Medical Com- plications During Pregnancy*. Philadelphia, WB Saunders, 1982.
3. Beischer NA, Mackay EV: *Obstetrics and the New- born: For Midwives and Medical Students*. Sydney, Australia, WB Saunders, 1976, p 206.
4. Clausen JP, Flook MH, Ford B: *Maternity Nursing Today*, ed 2. New York, McGraw-Hill, 1977, p 736.
5. Pritchard JA, MacDonald PC: *Williams Obstetrics*, ed 16. East Norwalk, CT, Appleton-Century-Crofts, 1980.
6. Fabro S: Treating nausea and vomiting in preg- nancy. *Contemp OB/GYN* 21:24, 1983.

7. Bonica JJ: *Principles and Practice of Obstetric Anal- gesia and Anesthesia*. Philadelphia, FA Davis, 1967, p 676.
8. Hart DM: Heartburn in pregnancy. *J Int Med Res* 6 (Suppl 1): 2, 1978.
9. DeVore GR: Nonobstetric abdominal pain in preg- nancy: what's the cause? *Contemp OB/GYN* 22:64– 86, 1983.
10. Beal JM: How to diagnose the acute abdomen. *Con- temp OB/GYN* (Update on General Surgery Supple- ment) 21:13–30, 1983.
11. Spiro HM: Duodenal ulcer—is the battle won? *Con- temp OB/GYN* (Update on General Medicine Supple- ment) 23:87–100, 1984.
12. DeVore GR: How to treat nonobstetric abdominal pain in pregnancy. *Contemp OB/GYN* 22:47–58, 1983.

Chapter 12
Hepatic Disorders of Pregnancy
Nola Geraghty Snyder, R.N., M.S.N.

INTRODUCTION

The changes induced by pregnancy sometimes can make diagnosis of liver disease difficult. It is helpful to know that most of the normal changes in the liver's function are more likely to occur toward the end of gestation and resolve following delivery.

Anatomic changes: The liver does not enlarge during pregnancy. In fact, it is difficult to palpate the liver late in gestation due to displacement by the enlarged uterus.

Histological changes: Nonspecific histological changes include variation in size and shape of hepatocytes and increases in cellular glycogen and fat (1, p 278, 2, p 1561). Hepatocytes are one of three major cell types in the liver and are those most responsible for metabolic activity (2, p 1561).

Physiological changes: Physiological changes of the liver are related to changes in the cardiovascular system. There is an increase of 40% in blood volume and cardiac output that reaches its peak in the late second or early third trimester. Hepatic blood flow does not increase, resulting in a net reduction in proportion of the cardiac output going to the liver. This factor may be responsible for a reduced capacity of the liver to clear various substances from the blood toward the end of gestation.

Functional changes: The most significant effects of pregnancy on the liver are on its function. There is decreased serum protein concentration, particularly albumin, in pregnancy that can be explained partially by increased blood volume. The estrogens of pregnancy stimulate increased production of ceruloplasmin, fibrinogen, and several clotting factors (2, p 1561). Despite these increases in clotting factors, the prothrobin time remains normal.

Lipid metabolism increases progressively during pregnancy. Not only the estrogenic hormonal effects that reduce lipoprotein lipase activity but also the increased triglyceride synthesis results in increased serum lipids (1, p 280). Cholesterol concentration is up to double the normal nonpregnant value, reaching its maximum at about 8 months' gestation. The increase in cholesterol actually is beneficial during pregnancy because it is a precursor for progesterone production. However, the increase in serum cholesterol can complicate diagnosis of cholestatis.

Liver enzyme alteration is evident during pregnancy. Most notably, the alkaline phosphatase increases slowly beginning in the seventh month, to levels that would be considered abnormal in the nonpregnant patient. It will decrease to normal within 20 days postpartum. An enzyme indicator of cholestatis, the γ-glutamyl-transpeptidase (GGTP) normally is increased in the latter third of pregnancy and therefore is of little diagnostic value in pregnancy. Serum lactic dehydrogenase (LDH) and ornithine transcarbamylase also increase in the third trimester. The serum glutamic oxaloacetic transaminase (SGOT) and glutamic pyruvic transaminase (SGPT) are changed only slightly in pregnancy, which makes them more useful laboratory indicators of liver damage (2, p 1563).

Decreased excretory function of the liver in pregnancy can be demonstrated by increased bromsulphalein (BSP) retention in the last month of gestation. There is a two-fold increase in BSP retention and a 27% decrease in excretory rate. Bilirubin may be elevated slightly in some normal pregnancies. However, an elevated serum bilirubin should be considered as presumptive evidence of liver disease (1, p 279).

Table 12.1.

CHANGES IN LIVER FUNCTION INDICES DURING PREGNANCY

INCREASED	SLIGHT INCREASE	DECREASED	NO CHANGE
Ceruloplasmin	Bilirubin	Serum albumin	Prothrombin
Transferrin	BSP retention	Serum protein	time
Fibrinogen	LDH	Albumin: globulin ratio	SGOT
Prothrombin		Serum cholinesterase	SGPT
Factor VII			
Factor VIII			
Factor X			
Cholesterol			
Triglycerides			
GGTP			
Alkaline phosphatase			

It is important to recognize the changes in liver function tests that accompany pregnancy when determining the presence of liver disease. Use of multiple indicators, history, and clinical findings are essential for accurate diagnosis. A summary of these changes can be found in Table 12.1. When liver pathology accompanies pregnancy, additional changes in liver function tests will be evident.

ACUTE FATTY LIVER OF PREGNANCY

Definition

Acute fatty liver of pregnancy is a rare and often fatal complication involving progressive destruction of hepatic cells. It occurs primarily in primigravidas during the third trimester.

Etiology

The etiology is unknown. However, oral or intravenous tetracycline has been implicated in some fatty liver development, especially with decreased renal function. Researchers now are exploring similarities between acute fatty liver and Reye's syndrome (3).

Signs and Symptoms

Symptoms begin abruptly, usually after 36 weeks' gestation. Symptoms include severe nausea and vomiting, tachycardia, epigastric pain, jaundice, and lethargy. There may be signs and symptoms of preeclampsia (hypertension, edema, proteinuria) just before or concurrent with the onset of the disorder. Liver failure may occur and may lead to hepatic coma. Encephalopathy as well as renal failure and hematemesis may ensue. Disseminated intravascular coagulation (DIC) has been reported and may be implicated as a cause of death (4).

Diagnosis

Diagnosis is based on clinical signs and symptoms and laboratory findings. Laboratory findings include leukocytosis and elevated levels of alkaline phosphatase, blood urea nitrogen, bilirubin, prothrombin time, transaminases, and serum ammonia. Fibrinogen is low and hypoglycemia is common. Clinically, the disorder resembles hepatitis, but, histologically, there is fatty infiltration without inflammation. The characteristic histological changes are documented by liver biopsy. Fatty changes also may be found in the kidney, brain, pancreas, and bone marrow.

Maternal and Fetal Outcome

The maternal death rate in this severe disorder is 75%. The perinatal death rate is correspondingly high (3). Women who survive will improve after delivery. There are no long-term effects on mother or baby if they survive (1, p 286). There does not appear to be an increased incidence of the disease in subsequent pregnancies of women who survive.

Medical Management

Limited experience with this rare disorder makes medical management problematic. Dialysis equipment should be available, and the patient should be in an intensive care setting. The ultimate treatment is delivery (5). Cesarean section has the advantage of minimizing deterioration of liver function but carries with it the risk of hemorrhage in a patient with the potential for DIC. Delayed recovery from cesarean section may occur because of hypoproteinemia and ascites.

Conservative treatment consists of efforts to correct hyperammonemia, hypoglycemia, renal failure, acidosis, and hemorrhage.

NURSING MANAGEMENT

Nursing care specific for a patient with *acute fatty liver of pregnancy*:

☐ Be aware of signs/symptoms of the disease and associated disorders (e.g., preeclampsia, DIC).

☐ Be prepared to provide intensive care; collaborate with intensive care nursing colleagues as needed to provide optimum care for mother and baby.

☐ Provide emotional support for patient/family. Coordinate efforts of medical, obstetric, and pediatric team to effect delivery at the optimum time.

Nursing diagnoses most frequently associated with *acute fatty liver of pregnancy*:

☐ Grieving related to potential/actual loss of infant or birth of an imperfect child.

☐ Anticipatory grieving related to actual/perceived threat to self.

☐ Pain.

☐ Knowledge deficit regarding etiology, disease process, treatment, and expected outcome.

☐ Anxiety/fear.

☐ Fluid volume deficit.

CHOLECYSTITIS

Definition

Cholecystitis is an inflammation of the gallbladder secondary to obstruction by gallstones.

Etiology

The cause of cholecystitis is development of gallstones. Gallstones are formed when the gallbladder smooth muscle is hypoactive, and incomplete emptying of the gallbladder occurs. The residual bile solidifies into stones, causing both mechanical irritation and infection (6, p 76).

Signs and Symptoms

Symptoms include severe epigastric or right upper quadrant (RUQ) pain that may radiate to the back or right shoulder, nausea, vomiting, fatty food intolerance, and fever. Patients will have tenderness upon palpation in the area of the liver. Fever is present during acute cholecystitis only. Blockage of the common bile duct leads to jaundice and symptoms of pruritus. Coagulation defects have been reported (7).

Diagnosis

Diagnosis is made by evaluation of symptoms, history of previous acute episodes of gallbladder disease, and visualization of the stones with ultrasound and/or cholecystogram. Ultrasound examination can be used to determine the presence and location of stones and is preferred during pregnancy to avoid the hazards of radiation. A cholecystogram may be obtained after oral ingestion of a contrast medium or after injection of an iodinated contrast medium directly into the bile duct. Because of risk to both the mother and fetus, direct injection cholecystogram rarely is used in pregnancy. Oral cholecystogram is the most common diagnostic tool in the general population. However, in pregnancy, because of the risks of fetal irradiation, it may be used only in the third trimester. Laboratory findings indicative of cholecystitis include increased white blood cell count, BSP retention, and elevated liver enzymes. The differential diagnosis will include pancreatitis, perforated ulcer, right kidney disease, intestinal obstruction, and myocardial infarction (7).

Maternal and Fetal Outcome

As with any surgery during pregnancy, maternal outcome may be compromised if cholecystectomy is necessary. Also, surgery itself may result in spontaneous abortion or preterm delivery. There is no adverse effect on maternal or fetal outcome if surgery is not required.

Medical Management

Medical management should consist of conservative treatment, if possible, primarily to avoid surgery during pregnancy. Approximately 75% of patients with local cholecystitis will have remission of symptoms in 1–4 days. When symptoms are local, the patient can be treated at home with bedrest, analgesics, and a low fat diet. When systemic disease is present, as evidenced by fever and/or altered liver function tests, the patient is hospitalized and given intravenous hydration and antibiotics. The presence of severe systemic symptoms may be indicative of the need for surgical treatment. If cholecystitis occurs early in pregnancy, it is recommended that surgery be delayed until the second trimester in order to decrease the risk of fetal loss and to operate at a time when the uterus is not large enough to impinge on the gallbladder. Delay of surgery until postpartum is best, if possible, to reduce anesthetic risk to mother and fetus, as well as the risk of premature delivery (6, p 78).

Operative and postoperative care is the same as for nonpregnant patients. The need for fetal eval-

uation and possibly tocolysis will be the only postoperative difference in care.

NURSING MANAGEMENT

Nursing care specific for a patient with cholecystitis:
- [ ] Be aware of signs/symptoms of cholecystitis.
- [ ] Teach the patient to consume a low fat diet; teach her to read food labels to determine fat content of foods.
- [ ] For patients who require surgery:
  - — Provide routine preoperative and postoperative teaching (e.g., coughing, deep breathing, ambulation);

- — Monitor fetal status; and
- — Monitor uterus for contractions; be prepared to administer tocolytics.

Nursing diagnoses most frequently associated with cholecystitis:
- [ ] Pain.
- [ ] Knowledge deficit regarding etiology, disease process, treatment, and expected outcome.
- [ ] Knowledge deficit regarding medication regimen.

CIRRHOSIS

Definition

Cirrhosis is a chronic disease resulting in destruction of liver cells, followed by cell regeneration with an increase in connective tissue. The increased connective tissue and decreased functional cell mass cause impaired liver function and obstruction of venous and sinusoidal channels, resulting in portal hypertension.

The three major types of cirrhosis are portal (Laënnec's), biliary, and postnecrotic (8). Portal cirrhosis is the most common type during pregnancy and is emphasized in this chapter.

Etiology

Portal cirrhosis results from alcoholism. Biliary cirrhosis is caused by direct obstruction, resulting from the back-up of bile into the liver. It occurs more commonly in older women (40–60 years old). Postnecrotic cirrhosis usually occurs after an acute viral or toxic hepatitis, but it may also be present without any history of hepatitis (8).

Signs/Symptoms and Diagnosis

The signs/symptoms and differential diagnosis for the three types of cirrhosis are presented in Table 12.2.

Maternal and Fetal Outcome

The sequelae of portal cirrhosis are more severe in the pregnant woman (9). These include the expected coagulopathies, anemia, malnutrition, and jaundice, but also, during pregnancy, one-fifth

of cirrhotic patients will progress to ascites or liver failure. The prognosis is even worse if these symptoms develop early in the first trimester. Bleeding from esophageal varices may occur and become life-threatening. This is aggravated by reflux esophagitis of pregnancy and increased portal pressure secondary to increased intraabdominal pressure from an enlarged uterus.

The increase in blood volume from pregnancy also increases the incidence of portal hypertension. Portal hypertension may also occur in the second stage of labor due to elevated venous pressure associated with maternal expulsive efforts. Ascites, if present, may mechanically prevent the fetus from assuming a longitudinal lie and/or the presenting part from engagement. Abnormal decreased clotting factors may predispose to postpartum hemorrhage.

The fetus is at risk. Fetal alcohol syndrome, prematurity, intrauterine growth retardation, anoxia, meconium staining, and death are associated with maternal ingestion of alcohol.

Medical Management

Medical management depends upon the severity of the disease and number of weeks' gestation. General management consists of treatment with corticosteroids, but these should be kept at the lowest possible level. When this therapy fails, use of azathioprine, an immunosuppressant, may be instituted. This drug has not been proven safe in human pregnancy, but the risk to benefit ratio must be weighed. A high protein diet supplemented with fat-soluble vitamins K, A, and D, as well as calcium,

Table 12.2.
LAËNNEC'S, POSTNECROTIC, AND BILIARY CIRRHOSIS[a]

LAËNNEC'S	POSTNECROTIC	BILIARY
<Symptoms>		
Insidious onset of anorexia, fatigue, and weakness. Abdominal pain from hepatomegaly, gastritis, or pancreatitis. Vomiting with or without hematemesis. Gradual jaundice and ascites. Symptoms of alcohol withdrawal or overdose. Fever, dehydration, and coma.	Malaise, weakness, anorexia, jaundice, low grade fever, spider angioma, ascites, and peripheral edema.	Early: pruritus, jaundice, dark urine, and pale stools. Later: cutaneous xanthoma, symptoms of cholestasis, and ascites.
<Complications>		
Bleeding from esophageal varices, sudden onset of ascites, hepatic encephalopathy and coma, signs of hepatic carcinoma, portal hypertension, anemia, and malnutrition.	Hepatic coma and bleeding from esophageal varices.	Bleeding.
<Diagnosis>		
Health history and physical examinations, firm and enlarged liver.	Health history and physical examinations, very tender and shrunken liver; splenomegaly (mild or massive); endocrine disorders (absence of axillary and pubic hair).	Health history and physical examination, firm and enlarged liver and splenomegaly.
<Laboratory Data>		
Serum levels: increased conjugated bilirubin, increased transaminase, variable alkaline phosphatase, decreased potassium, increased uric acid, and anemia.	Serum levels: same as for Laënnec's cirrhosis; may mimic biliary cirrhosis.	Serum levels: same as for cholestasis; rising or decreased serum bilirubin.
Liver biopsy: bile stasis and parenchymal cells that are distended with fat droplets contain hyaline-eosinophilic cytoplasmic inclusions and are infiltrated with inflammatory cells.	Liver scan: macronodular liver.	

[a]Reprinted with permission from Mahoney E, Flynn J: *Handbook of Medical-Surgical Nursing.* New York, John Wiley and Sons, 1983, p 723.

should be encouraged to treat malnutrition. All drugs metabolized in the liver should be avoided, and the patient must abstain from alcohol. Liver function tests and fetal well-being must be monitored frequently in the prenatal period. During labor, ascites may need to be removed by paracentesis. Delivery should be by forceps, and pushing may need to be avoided entirely because increased pressure can cause varices to bleed. A compression balloon tube may be inserted to treat bleeding esophageal varies. Collaboration with a gastroenterologist may be needed in the treatment of varices and evaluation for possible surgery (9). Portocaval shunting is possible during pregnancy if bleeding occurs in those patients with portal hypertension.

NURSING MANAGEMENT

Nursing care specific for a patient with
cirrhosis:

☐ Emphasize to patient/family the need to abstain from alcohol; refer to Alcoholics Anonymous or other treatment program as appropriate.

☐ Encourage the patient to consume a high protein diet, with supplements of vitamins A, D, and K and calcium, as needed.

☐ Monitor the patient for signs/symptoms of complications (e.g., ascites, liver failure, hemorrhage from esophageal varices); be prepared to assist with treatment (e.g., paracentesis, insertion of a compression balloon).

☐ Monitor uterine growth during pregnancy for signs/symptoms of intrauterine growth retardation.

NURSING MANAGEMENT

- ☐ Teach patient signs/symptoms of preterm labor and how to report them; evaluate symptoms promptly.
- ☐ Monitor fetal status during labor.
- ☐ Teach patient to avoid pushing in labor; prepare for a forceps delivery.
- ☐ Request pediatrician to attend delivery; prepare for neonatal resuscitation.

Nursing diagnoses most frequently associated with cirrhosis:

- ☐ Grieving related to potential/actual loss of infant or birth of an imperfect child.
- ☐ Anticipatory grieving related to actual/perceived threat to self.

- ☐ Ineffective individual coping.
- ☐ Potential altered parenting.
- ☐ Pain.
- ☐ Knowledge deficit regarding etiology, disease process, treatment, and expected outcome.
- ☐ Knowledge deficit regarding medication regimen.
- ☐ Fluid volume deficit.
- ☐ Altered nutrition: less than body requirements.
- ☐ Altered fetal cardiac and cerebral tissue perfusion.
- ☐ Altered maternal tissue perfusion.

HEPATITIS

Definition

Viral hepatitis is the most common cause of jaundice during pregnancy. There are three forms of the disease: hepatitis A, hepatitis B, and non-A non-B hepatitis. They all have similar clinical presentations. Table 12.3 contrasts types A and B.

Hepatitis A

Hepatitis A is transmitted primarily by the fecal-oral route, with an incubation period of 15–40 days. It also may be transmitted by other secretions, contaminated food or water, or shellfish. Symptoms are flu-like, with malaise, fatigue, anorexia, nausea, myalgia, pruritus, fever, and RUQ pain (10). The symptoms occur rapidly and last 10–15 days. They diminish gradually, and the patient does not become a carrier. Laboratory findings include a great elevation in SGOT and SGPT. Diagnosis depends on clinical data and identification of hepatitis A antibody (1, p 290).

Maternal-fetal risks are small. There is a somewhat increased incidence of preterm labor when the disease occurs in the early third trimester of pregnancy. There is also a very small risk of transplacental transmission to the fetus.

Medical management consists of supportive care, enteric precautions, and immunization of close contacts of the patient with immunoglobulin.

Hepatitis B

The incidence of hepatitis B has increased approximately fivefold since the 1970s. Hepatitis B is primarily transmitted through inoculation with blood or blood products—making intravenous users at special risk. This disease is also sexually transmitted. Other at risk groups are detailed in Table 12.4. As

Table 12.3.
COMPARISON OF TYPE A AND TYPE B HEPATITIS[a]

	TYPE A	TYPE B
Causative factor	Infectious hepatitis virus	Serum hepatitis virus
Mode of transmission	· Oral, fecal, or respiratory route · Blood, serum, or plasma transfusion from an infected person · Contaminated food (particularly milk and shellfish), polluted water are implicated · Contaminated syringes and needles	· Parenteral route · Blood or blood component transfusions from an infected person · Contaminated needles and syringes · Skin puncture with contaminated medical instruments · Mucosal transmission: dental instruments or venereal contact
Incubation	3–7 weeks	6 weeks to 6 months
Incidence	· Worldwide prevalence · Higher during fall and winter months · Higher among children and young adults	· Worldwide prevalence · Higher among recipients of blood and blood products (e.g., surgical, dialysis clients)

[a]Adapted from *American Journal of Nursing*, 1985 Nursing Review Boards, Nurseco, 1984, p 295.

Table 12.4.
WOMEN AT HIGHEST RISK TO BE EXPOSED TO HEPATITIS B AND/OR TO BE A HEPATITIS B CARRIER[a]

Health care workers: nurse, physician, medical technologist, dental hygienist, dentist (due to exposure to blood)
Asians, Pacific Islanders, Native Alaskans, Haitians, Africans (due to epidemic/endemic exposure in country of origin and refugee camps)
Intravenous drug abusers (due to contact with contaminated needles)
Those with active disease or history of hepatitis (may be a chronic carrier)
Those with a history of venereal disease
Those rejected as blood donors (due to possible previous detection of HBs Ag)
Those who work or receive treatment in a renal dialysis unit, including spouses of men on dialysis (due to frequent exposure to blood)
Employees and residents in an institution for the retarded (due to hygiene practices and biting and breaking of skin)
Those living with hepatitis patients or carriers
Recipients of multiple blood transfusions (due to receiving donated blood)
Acute and chronic liver disease patients

[a]Reprinted from public domain. Centers for Disease Control: Recommendations for protection against viral hepatitis. *Morbidity and Mortality Weekly Report* 34, 1985.

many as one million Americans are chronic carriers. The disease is caused by the hepatitis B virus. There is some evidence to support the fact that the resulting liver damage is caused not by the disease itself but by the immune system reaction to the antigen.

The clinical presentation is similar to hepatitis A. However, fever occurs less often and skin rash more often. Symptoms increase with age. Thus, children may experience no symptoms, while almost everyone over 30 will be symptomatic. SGOT and SGPT will be elevated. Diagnosis is confirmed by presence of serum hepatitis B antigen (HBs Ag) and serum hepatitis B antibody (anti-HBe and anti-HBc). Table 12.5 details the significance of these tests.

Pregnancy does not affect the maternal course of the disease. Complication rates are the same as for nonpregnant women. Fulminating liver failure occurs in about 1% of cases and carries an 80–90% mortality rate. Approximately 5–10% of infected women become chronic carriers. Carrier status usually is not reversible. One-third of carriers develop chronic hepatitis. Carriers are at high risk of developing hepatocellular cancer, because hepatitis B virus is a potent human carcinogen.

During pregnancy, the fetus is not at risk. Hepatitis B is not associated with malformation or intrauterine growth retardation. Risk develops at birth when the fetus comes in contact with maternal serum.

If the pregnant women is positive for both HBs AG and HBe Ag at delivery, the baby is at grave risk. The following statistics reveal the impact on neonatal health status:

1. 70–90% of newborns become infected with hepatitis B virus through exposure to maternal serum during delivery.

2. 90% of newborns become hepatitis B carriers.
3. 25% of carriers die of cirrhosis or liver cancer before adulthood.

Medical management should first and foremost be aimed at identification of the disease. The Centers for Disease Control now recommends screening all pregnant women for hepatitis B in order to ensure prompt treatment of the newborn within the first 12 hours after birth (Table 12.5).

Management is the same in pregnancy as in nonpregnant patients: supportive care (i.e., rest and adequate fluid and nutritional intake). Liver function tests should be monitored carefully in order to assess the extent of liver damage.

A woman who is identified as a carrier should be educated about the impact of carrier status on herself, on her fetus, and on her significant other. Special notification of the labor and delivery unit to expect a hepatitis B patient should be sent well in advance of the patients' due date.

Evaluation of close contacts for presence of the virus is advised. Immunization of close contacts with hepatitis immune globin (HBIG) should be considered for all close contacts who test negative.

During labor and delivery and in the postpartum period, the hospital staff should observe the following precautions:

1. Immediately dispose of needles in a container in the patients' room; do not recap, bend, or break.
2. Wear gloves when handling blood or blood-stained peripads, bed liners, bed linens, etc.
3. Dispose of contaminated items in labeled containers.

Table 12.5.

SERODIAGNOSIS OF ACUTE VIRAL HEPATITIS[a]

TEST RESULTS				INTERPRETATION
HBe Ag	HBs Ag	Anti-HBc IgM	Anti-HAV IgM	
−[b]	−	−	+	Recent acute hepatitis A infection
+	+	+	−	Acute hepatitis B infection
+	+	−	−	Early acute hepatitis B infection or chronic hepatitis B
+	−	+	−	Confirms acute or recent infection with hepatitis B virus
−	−	−	−	Possible non-A non-B hepatitis infection, other viral infection, or liver toxin
+	+	+	+	Recent probable hepatitis A infection and superimposed acute hepatitis B infection: uncommon profile

[a]Adapted from Nursing Reference Library: *Diagnostics*. Springhouse, PA, Springhouse Corporation, 1986, p 334.
[b]−, negative; +, positive.

4. Ensure that *all* staff members practice meticulous handwashing techniques, using a bactericidal solution after patient contact.
5. Use the double glove technique during cesarean section.

At birth, measures to prevent neonatal infection should include efforts to remove maternal blood from the newborn immediately. The newborn nasopharynx should be suctioned vigorously, the stomach aspirated, and the infant thoroughly bathed before 12 hours of age. HBIG should be given as soon as possible after birth. Follow-up serial immunizations should continue until the infant is 15 months old (Table 12.6). Any parturient woman who has not been screened during pregnancy should be assumed to be positive, and prophylactic treatment of the newborn should be initi-

ated. At the present time, there is even discussion of including hepatitis B immunization as a routine procedure for all infants in the United States.

Obstetric health care givers are at a high risk of developing hepatitis B infection due to exposure to blood during patient care. Exposure to blood is the greatest risk factor.

The National Centers for Disease Control recommend a hepatitis B vaccine for all health care workers in high risk areas (Table 12.4). Although the vaccine is completely ineffective for treating established carriers, it is 92% effective against contracting the disease.

Non-A Non-B Hepatitis

Non-A non-B hepatitis describes forms of the disease that have no immunological markers as A and B do. Thirty to forty percent of sporadic hepati-

Table 12.6.

HEPATITIS B PROPHYLAXIS FOR INFANTS OF HBs Ag MOTHERS[a]

AGE	RECOMMENDED TREATMENT BY CENTERS FOR DISEASE CONTROL	RATIONALE
As soon as possible; within 12 hours of birth	Hepatitis B immune globulin—HBIG (0.5 ml i.m.)	Give baby antibodies (passive immunity) to immediately protect baby from infection with hepatitis virus in mother's blood and body fluids.
As soon as possible; within 12 hours of birth or up to 7 days	Hepatitis B vaccine (0.5 ml i.m.) at a different site	Active immunity—challenge infant's immune system to begin hepatitis B antibody production.
1 month	Hepatitis B vaccine (0.5 ml i.m.)	Active immunity—second of three vaccines for basic hepatitis B immunization.
6 months	Hepatitis B surface antigen test	If positive, baby is already carrying HBs Ag—therapeutic failure. Do not give third immunization. Do not repeat tests at 12 months. If negative (no HBs Ag present), continue immunization.
	Hepatitis B vaccine (0.5 ml i.m.)	
12–15 months	Hepatitis B surface antigen test	If positive, chronic carrier state has developed—therapeutic failure.
	Hepatitis B surface antibody test	If positive, active immunity has developed—therapeutic success.

[a]Adapted from Centers for Disease Control: Recommendations for protection against viral hepatitis. *Morbidity and Mortality Weekly Report* 34, 1985.

tis is attributed to this form. Usually, there is a long incubation period. Clinically, the illness presents and is treated as other forms of hepatitis in preg-

nant and nonpregnant patients. The fetus usually is not affected.

NURSING MANAGEMENT

Nursing care specific for a patient with *hepatitis:*

☐ Screen all patients for hepatitis.

☐ Teach all patients modes of transmission of hepatitis (e.g., sexual contact, sharing needles); refer to drug treatment program as necessary.

☐ Encourage adequate rest and diet.

☐ To prevent spread of hepatitis B:
   — Utilize isolation precautions, and
   — Encourage all obstetric health care workers in high risk areas to receive the hepatitis B vaccine.

☐ Prevent infection of the neonate:
   — Remove maternal blood from the newborn immediately;
   — Vigorously suction nasopharynx and aspirate stomach;

   — Bathe the baby thoroughly when stable (before 12 hours of age); and
   — Administer HBIG as ordered.

☐ Encourage evaluation and immunization with HBIG, if appropriate, of sexual partner(s), family members, or other close contacts.

Nursing diagnoses most frequently associated with *hepatitis:*

☐ Impaired skin integrity.

☐ Ineffective individual coping.

☐ Potential altered parenting.

☐ Pain.

☐ Knowledge deficit regarding etiology, disease process, treatment, and expected outcome.

☐ Altered nutrition: less than body requirements.

CHOLESTASIS

Definition

Intrahepatic cholestasis of pregnancy, also called recurrent jaundice of pregnancy or pruritus gravidarum, is the second most common cause of jaundice in pregnancy after hepatitis. Pruritus gravidarum is discussed in Chapter 18. This chapter briefly discusses the hepatic aspects of the disease.

Signs and Symptoms

The syndrome is characterized by mild jaundice and pruritus that disappear after delivery. Pruritus may begin anywhere between 6 and 38 weeks of gestation, but most often it starts in the third trimester. It involves the trunk, palms, and soles of the feet. Itching can be severe, especially at night, which may lead to symptoms of fatigue and insomnia (2, p 1568). Mild jaundice usually follows these symptoms in 1–2 weeks. Dark urine, clay-colored stools, nausea, anorexia, and epigastric pain have been documented in some instances. The liver is rarely enlarged or tender (11).

Diagnosis

Diagnosis is based on clinical and laboratory findings. Liver biopsy may be needed to differentiate cholestasis from hepatitis, acute fatty liver, biliary tract disease, and cholestasis drug reactions. A history of the symptoms in previous pregnancies or while taking oral contraceptives may be indicative of cholestasis of pregnancy since it tends to recur. Laboratory findings of a serum bilirubin below 5 mg/dl, with serum bile acids concurrently increased 10–100 times, are strongly suggestive of cholestasis. Alkaline phosphatase normally is increased in pregnancy and may be further elevated 7–10 times the normal level. It can also remain within normal pregnancy values. BSP retention of 10–25% always is observed. The serum transaminases also are elevated but usually no more than 250 Sigma Units. There are few histological changes evident. Occasionally, binucleate cells or increased nuclear size is observed on biopsy (12).

Maternal and Fetal Outcome

Maternal implications are related to the discomfort of pruritus. Occasionally, coagulation abnormalities from impaired vitamin K absorption are found. These can, in turn, increase the risk of postpartum hemorrhage. The risk of recurrence of cholestasis in future pregnancies must be considered (12).

The fetus is at risk for an increased incidence of preterm labor (33–87%). This has not been found in every study, and the incidence is proportional to the severity of maternal disease (1, p 283).

Medical Management

Medical management primarily is aimed at diagnosis, ruling out other hepatic disorders. Relief of pruritus by reducing skin bile acids can be achieved by giving cholestyramine resin. Side effects are minimal but may include nausea, anorexia, and constipation. Due to the effect of cholestasis on vitamin K absorption, the patient's clotting profile should be evaluated and parenteral vitamin K given near term. Women should be counseled to avoid oral contraceptives.

NURSING MANAGEMENT

Nursing management specific for a patient with *cholestasis*:
- ☐ Be aware of symptoms of cholestasis; differentiate from normal pruritus in pregnancy.
- ☐ Teach comfort measures for pruritus:
  - — A daily bath with use of one-half cup of baking soda, corn starch, or Aveeno oatmeal powder;
  - — Cut fingernails short and avoid scratching as much as possible.
- ☐ Monitor blood clotting profile during pregnancy; administer vitamin K as ordered.
- ☐ Teach patient signs/symptoms of preterm labor and how to report them.

- ☐ Teach patient to avoid oral contraceptives.

Nursing diagnoses most frequently associated with *cholestasis*:
- ☐ Impaired skin integrity.
- ☐ Grieving related to potential/actual loss of infant or birth of an imperfect child.
- ☐ Pain.
- ☐ Knowledge deficit regarding etiology, disease process, treatment, and expected outcome.
- ☐ Knowledge deficit regarding medication regimen.
- ☐ Fluid volume deficit.
- ☐ Altered nutrition: less than body requirements.

BUDD-CHIARI SYNDROME

Budd-Chiari syndrome is an uncommon disease characterized by hepatic vein occlusion, sometimes associated with pregnancy or oral contraceptive use. The etiology of this hypercoagulable state is not known. Onset may be sudden or insidious. In pregnancy the symptoms begin close to term. Symptoms include vomiting, jaundice, fever, and abdominal pain and distention. Diagnosis is made by liver biopsy. Usually, there are no fetal effects (4).

CHOLELITHIASIS

The development of gallstones occurs in 10% of the adult population, particularly women. Pregnancy may contribute to development of gallstones by the action of progesterone on the smooth muscle of the gallbladder, leading to biliary stasis, atony of the gallbladder, and increased cholesterol (1, p 296). Thus, cholelithiasis is common during pregnancy.

DRUG-INDUCED LIVER DISORDERS

Any drug that causes liver disorders in nonpregnant women certainly will have effects during pregnancy. Drug-induced liver disease is difficult to diagnose since liver function tests are not specific. Diagnosis is made by history, clinical signs, and by exclusion. A summary of liver-toxic drugs is presented in Table 12.7. Several drugs that cause jaundice are of particular interest in pregnancy. Chlorpromazine is used occasionally as an antiemetic in early pregnancy. Tetracycline has been implicated in fatty liver of pregnancy and is contraindicated. Long-term phenytoin therapy has been demonstrated to have cholestatic effects (13).

Fetal effects can be related to maternal sequelae as well as independent teratogenic effects.

Medical management consists of appropriate diagnosis of hepatic symptoms and cessation of the offending drug.

Table 12.7.
HEPATOTOXIC DRUGS

HEPATOCELLULAR DAMAGE	CHOLESTASIS
Isoniazid	Chlorpromazine
Methyldopa	Erythromycin
Acetaminophen	Estrogens
Cimetidine	Phenytoin
Penicillin	
Oxacillin	
Tetracycline	

PREECLAMPSIA/ ECLAMPSIA

The liver becomes involved in preeclampsia as a result of generalized vascular disturbances. Liver function changes are more closely associated with severe preeclampsia if DIC is concomitant (14). The changes most often found are elevations in alkaline phosphatase, SGOT, and bilirubin (see Chapter 13). A life-threatening condition associated with liver involvement in toxemia is hepatic rupture or hemorrhage from a subcapsular hematoma.

Clinical findings of hepatic rupture include shock, abdominal pain, leukocytosis, oliguria, and fever. Ultrasound examination may reveal a hematoma. Rupture is diagnosed by peritoneal aspiration of blood. Treatment consists of surgical control of bleeding and cardiovascular support. All patients with preeclampsia should be evaluated for DIC, which also increases the risk of heptatic rupture due to uncontrollable bleeding. Researchers have also identified a hepatic syndrome that may accompany preeclampsia, characterized by hemolysis, elevated liver enzymes, and low platelet count ("HELLP" syndrome) (15). Nursing care is discussed in Chapter 13.

WILSON'S DISEASE

Wilson's disease is an inherited metabolic disorder resulting from decreased hepatic ability to metabolize copper. It occurs in teens and young adults. Signs and symptoms include tremor, dysphagia, dystonia, excessive salivation, and decreased glomerular filtration rate. A hallmark of Wilson's disease is the presence of Kayser-Fleischer rings, golden-brown discolorations on the cornea. Pregnancy is uncomplicated if the patient is treated. Treatment consists of chelation by 1–2 g/ day of D-penicillamine. Patients also should be in-

formed to avoid copper-rich foods such as shellfish, cocoa, mushrooms, liver, nuts, and organ meats (16).

REFERENCES

1. Fallon HJ: Liver diseases. In Burrow GN, Ferris TF (eds): *Medical Complications during Pregnancy*, ed 2. Philadelphia, WB Saunders, 1982, p 278.
2. Krejs GJ, Haemmerli VP: Jaundice during pregnancy. In Schiff L, Schiff E (eds): *Disease of the Liver*, ed 5. Philadelphia, JB Lippincott, 1982, p 1561.
3. Wenk RE, Gebhardt FC, Bhagavan BS, Lustgarten JA, McCarthy EF: Tetracycline induced fatty liver of pregnancy, including possible pregnancy risk after chronic dermatologic use of tetracycline. *J Reprod Med* 26:135–141, 1981.
4. Varner M, Rinderknecht NK: Acute fatty metamorphosis of pregnancy. *J Reprod Med* 24:177–180, 1980.
5. Ebert EC, Sun MD, Wright SH, Decker JP, Librizzi DO, Bolognese MD, Lipshutz WH: Does early diagnosis and delivery in acute fatty liver of pregnancy lead to improvement in maternal and infant survival? *Dig Dis Sci* 29:453–455, 1984.
6. Madden JL: Surgery of the liver and bile system in pregnancy. In Barber HR, Graber EA (eds): *Surgical Disease in Pregnancy*. Philadelphia, WB Saunders, 1974, p 76.
7. Alpers DH, Isselbacher KJ: Derangements of hepatic metabolism. In Thorn GW, Adams RD, Braunwald E, Isselbacher KJ, Petersdorf RG (eds): *Harrison's Principles of Internal Medicine*, ed 8. New York, McGraw-Hill, 1977, p 1628.
8. Donius MAH: Altered hematopoietic and hepatic functioning. In Mahoney EA, Flynn JP (eds): *Handbook of Medical-Surgical Nursing*. New York, John Wiley and Sons, 1983, p 722.
9. Cheng YS: Pregnancy in liver cirrhosis and/or portal hypertension. *Am J Obstet Gynecol* 128:812–822, 1977.
10. Rogge PT: Gastrointestinal complications. In Niswander KR (ed): *Manual of Obstetrics*. Boston, Little Brown, 1980, p 77.
11. Kreek MJ, Weser E, Sleisenger MH, Jeffries GH: Idiopathic cholestasis of pregnancy. *N Engl J Med* 277:1391–1394, 1967.
12. Sherlock S: The liver in pregnancy. In Sherlock S (ed): *Diseases of the Liver and Biliary System*, ed 6. Oxford, Blackwell Scientific, 1981.
13. Scharsschmidt BF: Bile formation and cholestasis, metabolism and enterohepatic circulation of bile acids and gallstone formation. In Zakim D, Boyer T (eds): *Hepatology: A Textbook of Liver Disease*. Philadelphia, WB Saunders, 1982, p 1147.
14. Killam AP, Dillard SH, Patton RC, Pederson PR: Pregnancy induced hypertension complicated by acute fatty liver disease and disseminated intravas-

cular coagulation. *Am J Obstet Gynecol* 123:823–828, 1975.
15. Weinstein L: Syndrome of hemolysis, elevated liver enzymes and low platelet count: a severe consequence of hypertension in pregnancy. *Am J Obstet Gynecol* 142:159–163, 1982.
16. Gollam JL: Copper metabolism, Wilson's Disease and hepatic toxicosis. In Zakim D, Boyer T (eds): *Hepatology: A Textbook of Liver Disease*. Philadelphia, WB Saunders, 1982, p 1147.

Chapter 13
Hypertension in Pregnancy
Nancy W. Kulb, C.N.M., M.S.

INTRODUCTION

According to Zuspan, hypertensive disease is "the most significant medical complication a pregnant woman encounters in the world today" (1). Hypertension diseases (especially preeclampsia/eclampsia and chronic hypertension with superimposed preeclampsia) are a leading cause of maternal death in the United States today—second only to hemorrhage. Twenty-four percent of maternal deaths are attributed to hypertension (2). Hypertension diseases also are a cause of considerable perinatal morbidity and mortality. Data from the Collaborative Perinatal Project indicated a threefold increase in fetal death from maternal hypertension alone (i.e., without maternal proteinuria) (3). Collectively, these diseases are the most common medical complication of pregnancy; 4–5% of pregnant women have chronic hypertension, and another 4–5% develop pregnancy-induced hypertension (PIH).

Blood Pressure in Normal Pregnancy

Blood pressure (BP) depends upon cardiovascular volume, the size of the blood vessels (i.e., the dilatation or constriction of blood vessels), and the cardiac force propelling the blood through the vessels. During normal pregnancy, there are many changes that affect the BP.

During pregnancy, plasma volume and cardiac output increase about 40% (4). Approximately 80 mEq sodium and 6 liters of water are retained by the woman during pregnancy. Also increased during pregnancy are plasma levels of renin, renin substrate, and angiotensin II, a powerful pressor agent. It would be logical to expect that the increased plasma volume and increased plasma level of angi-

otensin II would result in a higher BP during pregnancy, but that is not the case. Instead, the BP normally drops during the second trimester. It rises again late in the third trimester to near normal (i.e., the nonpregnant level).

The second-trimester drop in BP is due to a decrease in peripheral vascular resistance. The presence of the uteroplacental circulation and vasodilation from progesterone contribute to decreased vascular resistance. However, the primary cause is refractoriness to the effect of pressor agents.

In nonpregnant women pressor responsiveness depends on the plasma concentration of angiotensin II. In pregnant women the concentration of angiotensin II is much less significant than the *response* of smooth muscle in the blood vessels to the angiotensin II that is present (5). Therefore, in normal pregnancy the high plasma levels of angiotensin II do not result in hypertension.

Currently, much research is being conducted to elucidate the physiologic mechanisms responsible for the normal pregnancy refractoriness to pressor agents and the abnormal responsiveness in hypertensive patients. It is known that prostaglandins can affect responsiveness to vasoactive agents, but the relationship is not straightforward. Cyclooxygenase converts arachidonic acid into prostaglandins *or* thromboxane *or* prostacyclin. Thromboxane A_2 is a very potent vasoconstrictor, while prostacyclin is a very potent vasodilator. Both have very short half-lives and are locally active. Both normally increase during pregnancy, in effect, balancing each other out. Women with PIH have altered levels of various prostaglandins, notably a decrease in prostaglandin E_2, which may alter the normal refractoriness to pressor agents.

Clinical Assessment of Blood Pressure

One BP reading is not sufficient for diagnosis of hypertension, since recent activity, position, anxiety, and time of day affect the reading. Indeed, a repeat BP taken within 15 minutes can vary as much as 20–40 mm Hg systolic and 15–30 mm Hg diastolic (6). Therefore, an elevated BP reading must be noted on at least two occasions, at least 6 hours apart, for a diagnosis of hypertension. The proper size BP cuff must be used since a falsely elevated reading will be obtained if a cuff that is too small is used. Some authorities now alternatively define hypertension as a mean arterial pressure (MAP) greater than 106 on two occasions 6 hours or more apart. MAP is determined as follows: diastolic blood pressure + (systolic pressure − diastolic pressure)/3.

Also important is consistency in recording the sound changes heard in taking the BP. The systolic BP is the pressure at which the first sound is heard (Korotkoff's phase I). The diastolic BP is the pressure at which the sound disappears (Korotkoff's phase V). If the sound becomes muffled long before it disappears (Korotkoff's phase IV), both the point at which the sound is muffled and the point at which it disappears should be recorded.

Hypertensive Disorders of Pregnancy

The terminology regarding hypertension in pregnancy is somewhat confusing and misleading. The term "toxemia of pregnancy," which once was applied to any disorder of pregnancy involving hypertension, proteinuria, and edema, implied that the etiology was some toxin in the bloodstream. In truth, there are several disorders that may result in hypertension, proteinuria, and edema. Moreover, the etiology of preeclampsia/eclampsia is not clear, although much is now understood about the pathophysiology.

The term "eclampsia" literally means to "strike forth or suddenly appear" (9). However, the term "preeclampsia" makes clear that it is a progressive disease that can be identified before eclampsia occurs.

The Committee on Terminology of the American College of Obstetricians and Gynecologists has suggested the following classification and definitions of the hypertensive disorders of pregnancy (10):

1. Hypertension: Diastolic blood pressure greater than 90 mm Hg, systolic blood pressure greater than 140 mm Hg, or a rise over the baseline of at least 30 mm Hg systolic and 15 mm Hg diastolic. The elevated blood pressure must be noted on at least two occasions, 6 hours or more apart.
2. Preeclampsia: Development of hypertension with proteinuria and/or edema, induced by pregnancy after 20 weeks' gestation (or perhaps earlier if there are hydatidiform changes in the chorionic villi).
3. Eclampsia: The occurrence of convulsions, not caused by coincidental neurologic disease, in a woman whose condition fulfills criteria for preeclampsia.
4. Chronic hypertensive disease: Persistent hypertension before 20 weeks' gestation (except if hydatidiform changes in chorionic villi are present), or after 6 weeks postpartum, regardless of etiology.
5. Gestational hypertension: Hypertension that develops during the latter half of pregnancy or the first 24 hours postpartum that is not accompanied by any other signs or symptoms of preeclampsia or vascular disease. It disappears by 10 days postpartum.
6. Gestational edema: Generalized accumulation of fluid of greater than 1+ pitting edema after 12 hours of bed rest or a weight gain of at least 5 pounds in a week.
7. Gestational proteinuria: Proteinuria during pregnancy not accompanied by hypertension, edema, renal infection, or other known renal or vascular disease. The existence of this entity is questionable.

Current obstetrical literature often uses the term "pregnancy-induced hypertension" (PIH). Some authors use it to replace the terms "preeclampsia/eclampsia" (11), but, according to *Williams Obstetrics* (8, p 526), PIH includes three entities: (1) preeclampsia, (2) eclampsia, and (3) hypertension alone. In this text an attempt will be made to use the precise terminology; therefore, both preeclampsia/eclampsia and PIH will be used.

Hypertensive diseases of pregnancy may be classified as follows according to Zuspan (12):

I.   PIH (toxemia, preeclampsia/eclampsia, acute hypertension)
II. Chronic hypertensive disease
    A.   Primary (essential, idiopathic)—the most common form of hypertension
    B.   Secondary (related to a known cause)

1. Renal: parenchymal disease such as glomerulonephritis, chronic pyelonephritis, interstitial nephritis, polycystic kidney, renal vascular disease, lupus erythematosus
2. Adrenal gland: cortical—Cushing's disease, hyperaldosteronism; medullary—pheochromocytoma
3. Other: thyrotoxicosis, coarctation of the aorta, etc.

III. Chronic hypertensive disease (any etiology) with superimposed preeclampsia/eclampsia.

IV. Transient hypertension—occurring during labor or the immediate postpartum period.

Although the classification seems straightforward, it is not always easy to diagnose the hypertensive diseases of pregnancy accurately.

This chapter discusses preeclampsia/eclampsia and chronic hypertension, including chronic hypertension complicated by superimposed preeclampsia/eclampsia. Diseases associated with secondary hypertension are discussed in Chapters 10 and 17.

PREECLAMPSIA/ ECLAMPSIA

Definition

Preeclampsia is defined as a BP of $\geq$140/90 mm Hg in a previously normotensive woman or a rise of $\geq$30 mm Hg systolic and $\geq$15 mm Hg diastolic over the baseline on at least two occasions 6 hours apart, occurring in the second half of pregnancy, and accompanied by proteinuria and/or generalized edema.

Mild preeclampsia is defined as relatively mild hypertension and proteinuria and/or edema with no other symptoms. Severe preeclampsia is diagnosed if the BP is $\geq$160/110, if $\geq$5 g protein is excreted in the urine in 24 hours, or if there are symptoms of end-organ ischemia or damage (e.g., severe headache, visual disturbances, epigastric pain, oliguria, renal failure, congestive heart failure). Eclampsia is the same disease process with the appearance of convulsions (13).

The reported incidence of preeclampsia varies widely, depending upon several factors, including accuracy of diagnosis, percentage of primigravidas in the population, and demographic characteristics of the population. However, it occurs in approximately 5–7% overall (6, p 792), with a much higher incidence in primigravidas, especially very young or older primigravidas or women with chronic hypertension. The incidence of eclampsia now is reported to be approximately 1.2–2.6 per 1000 deliveries (9, p 135).

Pathophysiology of Preeclampsia/ Eclampsia

Preeclampsia/eclampsia is a slow, progressive disease. The deviations from normal physiology of pregnancy begin weeks or even months before clinical symptoms appear. Although clinical improvement may occur with treatment, the disease itself does not resolve until after delivery.

The hypertension of preeclampsia/eclampsia is associated with vasoconstriction. Normal pregnant women are relatively refractory to circulating vasopressors. Women destined to become preeclamptic lose that refractoriness in midpregnancy, long before hypertension becomes evident. Eventually, they become more sensitive to pressor agents than nonpregnant women (5, pp 822–823). The precise cause of this altered response is not clear. Some studies show that preeclamptic women, along with smokers and diabetics, produce less prostacyclin—a potent vasodilator—than their normal counterparts (5, pp 828–829). Preeclamptic women also have a decreased level of prostaglandin E_2. It is thought that prostacyclin and/or prostaglandin E_2 may be responsible for the normal refractoriness to pressor agents in pregnancy; therefore, decreased levels in preeclamptic women may be responsible for loss of that refractoriness and, ultimately, for hypertension.

During normal pregnancy, circulating levels of renin, angiotensin II, and aldosterone are increased. With preeclampsia they decrease to near normal nonpregnant levels.

Interestingly, some studies indicate that progesterone is converted to deoxycorticosterone (DOC) more rapidly in women destined to develop preeclampsia. The significance of this finding is not yet clear. It is possible that DOC is produced and metabolized in the kidney, exerting a local effect that alters response to pressor agents.

There is evidence of a decrease in circulating plasma volume occurring 1–4 weeks before clinical symptoms of preeclampsia appear. The decrease does not always occur, however, especially in cases of mild preeclampsia. When it does occur, frequently it is reflected in a relatively high hematocrit (HCT) and intrauterine growth retardation (IUGR) (7, pp 245–247). The lack of normal hypervolemia of pregnancy may be the result of vasoconstriction or generalized edema. The cardiac

Table 13.1.

ALTERATION OF SELECTED LABORATORY TESTS IN THE PRESENCE OF PREECLAMPSIA

LABORATORY TEST	NORMAL PREGNANCY VALUE	CHANGE WITH PREECLAMPSIA
Alkaline phosphatase	20–115 mIU/ml	↑
Bilirubin	<1.2 mg/100 ml	↑
Blood urea nitrogen (BUN)	10 mg/dl	↑
Creatinine	0.9–2.0 mg/dl	↑
Lactic dehydrogenase (LDH)	100–225 mIU/ml	↑
Uric acid	2.2–7.7 mg/100 ml	↑
Prothrombin time (PT)	12–16 seconds	↑
Partial thromboplastin time (PTT)	Normally 35–53 seconds; shorter in pregnancy	↑
Platelets	Usually within normal limits (140,000–340,000)	↓

output usually does not decrease in the patient with preeclampsia, even with a decreased circulating volume; therefore, as the peripheral resistance increases, the BP rises.

Generalized vasospasm contributes to pathological changes throughout the body. In the kidney preeclampsia causes approximately a 20% decrease in renal plasma flow (RPF) and a 25–50% decrease in glomerular filtration rate (GFR). Therefore, normal blood values for blood urea nitrogen (BUN), creatinine, and uric acid may be increased with preeclampsia. The 24-hour creatinine clearance is a fairly accurate indicator of the GFR. Monitoring these values is clinically useful in determining renal effects of preeclampsia. Table 13.1 gives normal values of selected laboratory tests during pregnancy.

Studies of placental blood flow indicate that there is decreased intervillous perfusion in women with preeclampsia. Perfusion remains normal in the first half to two-thirds of pregnancy. It begins to drop 2–4 weeks before hypertension becomes evident. Intervillous perfusion is only 35–50% of normal in women with PIH, regardless of the clinical severity of the disease. With bed rest the clinical picture may improve, but placental perfusion remains compromised, indicating that the fetus remains in jeopardy until delivery (5, p 825).

The cause of the generalized edema of preeclampsia is not clear. It occurs at a time when aldosterone levels are reduced from normal pregnancy levels. The fluid retention first may be noticed because of sudden, excessive weight gain (i.e., more than 2 pounds/week). The electrolyte concentrations are not significantly different from those of normal women unless alterations are induced iatrogenically (e.g., by strict dietary sodium restriction or diuretic therapy).

Proteinuria varies from woman to woman and from hour to hour in the same woman. Usually, it appears after hypertension and edema are evident; therefore, early in the disease it may be minimal or absent. With severe preeclampsia it is usually present and may be as much as 10 g/liter (8). Proteinuria in preeclampsia/eclampsia is caused by glomeruloendotheliosis.

With severe preeclampsia or eclampsia, there may be alterations in tests of liver function, including elevated excretion of bromosulfonphthalein and elevated SGOT and alkaline phosphatase. Hyperbilirubinemia is a rare occurrence. Hemorrhagic necrosis may occur with severe disease but is variable in extent and severity. Very rarely, subscapular hemorrhage in the liver may result in rupture, massive hemorrhage, and, often, death.

After eclamptic convulsions, nonspecific abnormalities of the electroencephalogram may be seen. After death from preeclampsia/eclampsia, the following brain lesions have been seen: edema, hyperemia, focal anemia, thrombosis, and hemorrhage.

It was once thought that disseminated intravascular coagulation (DIC) was a part of the pathological process of preeclampsia/eclampsia. Although it occurs occasionally with severe disease, fibrin levels generally are not very low and fibrin degradation products are not very high, even in eclamptics. There is, however, a decreased platelet count without a change in other coagulation factors, suggesting a microangiopathic thrombocytopenia. This thrombocytopenia may be due to an abnormal interaction between platelets and the vascular epithelium. Whenever thrombocytopenia is present, preeclampsia must be considered severe, regardless of severity of other symptoms. Often, it is accompanied by hemolysis and altered liver function, indicated by an elevated SGOT (5, pp 829–830).

Etiology

The etiology of preeclampsia is unknown, although a great deal is known about the pathophysiology and the impact on target organs. Many theories of etiology have been developed and many predisposing factors have been identified.

Preeclampsia alone (i.e., without chronic hypertension) almost always is a disease of primigravidas. There is some evidence that even abortion in the first pregnancy may be protective against PIH, but that has not been confirmed. When it occurs in multiparas, there is usually some strong predisposing factor that was not present in the first pregnancy (e.g., chronic hypertension, multiple gestation) (14).

Any condition that causes a large placental mass predisposes to preeclampsia. Multiple gestation increases the risk of eclampsia six times. Hydatidiform mole carries with it a 70% incidence of preeclampsia. Indeed, preeclampsia in early pregnancy is one of the diagnostic signs of a mole. Preeclampsia is associated with fetal hydrops (gross edema), which is usually due to Rh isoimmunization, but may result from other conditions. Preeclampsia also is associated with diabetes mellitus. However, because of the renal and vascular changes that occur from diabetes, it is difficult to quantify precisely the risk of associated preeclampsia.

Other factors that predispose to preeclampsia include chronic hypertension, a family history of preeclampsia, and extremes of age. Although most very young pregnant women are primigravidas and many older ones have other predisposing factors, such as chronic hypertension or diabetes mellitus, there is a predisposition to preeclampsia resulting from age alone (14, pp 812–814).

There are a number of other factors that are or have been thought to predispose to preeclampsia, but the relationship is less clear. Polyhydramnios is associated with preeclampsia, but it is not clear whether that association is purely because of multiple gestation, diabetes mellitus, and fetal hydrops that often accompany polyhydramnios. Socioeconomic status has been thought to be a factor, but there are no convincing data to prove it. Dietary deficiencies, especially of protein, have been thought to cause preeclampsia, but this has not been proven. Indeed, some studies show that the incidence of preeclampsia is not related to the level of protein intake and that dietary supplementation does not decrease the incidence (8, p 540). Preeclampsia occurs slightly more often than would be expected with male fetuses, but even so, nearly half of the time it occurs with a female fetus. Other possible predisposing factors include body shape (underweight or short and overweight), black race, city (versus country) residence, illegitimate pregnancy, fetal malformations, time of year (peak incidence

March and April), and geographic distribution (14, pp 815–820).

Because of the effect of pressor agents on the vessels of preeclamptic women, it seems possible that there is some substance in the serum that causes the vasoconstriction. Among proposed theories are (5, p 826):

1. Increased response to vasoconstrictors because of intracellular calcium from a defective calcium-transporting protein or dietary imbalance.
2. Increased serum concentration of catecholamines.
3. Increased serum level of DOC.
4. A parasite (helminth) in the bloodstream.

Signs and Symptoms

The early signs and symptoms of preeclampsia, unfortunately, often are not detected by the patient. Indeed, she may feel quite well. It is because they cannot be detected readily by the patient that so much of prenatal care is directed toward early detection of preeclampsia. It should be noted that although the pathophysiologic process is slow and progressive, the onset of clinical symptoms may be quite abrupt.

Commonly, the patient may experience a sudden, rapid weight gain—as much as 5–6 pounds in a week—reflecting generalized edema. Although this edema frequently is the first clinical sign of preeclampsia, it may occur coincident with or after the onset of hypertension, or it may not occur at all. An elevated BP, ≥140/90 or a rise above baseline of ≥30 mm Hg systolic and ≥15 mm Hg diastolic, usually is seen, although on rare occasions the BP is not elevated significantly. The hypertension may develop prenatally, gradually or suddenly during labor, or even postpartum. Although theoretically the definition of preeclampsia requires that the BP must be elevated on two occasions at least 6 hours apart, frequently it is not prudent to delay treatment that long in order to confirm the diagnosis. Proteinuria is the third classic sign of preeclampsia and is usually the last to develop.

Other clinical signs and symptoms that indicate increasing severity of the disease may include:

1. Headaches, usually frontal or occipital, that are not relieved by analgesics. Headaches may be related to intracranial hemorrhage, cerebral edema, vasoconstriction, or cerebral ischemia.

2. Epigastric pain, which is the result of stretching the hepatic capsule because of hepatic hemorrhage or edema.
3. Visual disturbances, that may range from blurred vision to spots before the eyes to blindness and that result from retinal arteriolar spasm, ischemia, edema, or, rarely, retinal detachment.
4. Hyperreflexia with or without clonus, indicating increasing severity of the disease. Hyperreflexia reflects disease of the upper motor neuron and central nervous system.
5. Rising HCT, reflecting increasing hemoconcentration and hypovolemia.

Atypical PIH may present with modest hypertension but severe abdominal pain, indicating liver involvement.

An eclamptic convulsion typically begins with facial twitching, followed by tonic contraction of the body for 15–20 seconds. There is then a tonic-clonic phase that lasts about a minute, gradually decreasing and ending with the patient in a coma. The coma lasts for a variable length of time. Approximately one-quarter of eclamptic convulsions occur prenatally, one-half intrapartally, and one-quarter postpartally (15). The incidence and severity of eclampsia is not related directly to the BP or to the amount of generalized edema and/or proteinuria.

Diagnosis

Although the diagnosis of preeclampsia seems quite clear, it is not always so clear clinically. The diagnosis of preeclampsia may be applied erroneously to chronic renal disease, chronic hypertension that was not evident in midpregnancy, or latent essential hypertension. Chronic renal disease is not uncommon and is difficult to diagnose clinically during pregnancy. Renal biopsy ruling out chronic renal disease and demonstrating glomeruloendotheliosis, the classic lesion of preeclampsia, is considered diagnostic (although it is not unique to preeclampsia). In studies at the Chicago Lying In Hospital in the 1960s and 1970s, the diagnosis of preeclampsia was confirmed by renal biopsy only 55% of the time (70% of the time if multiparas were excluded). Other renal lesions that were found instead included nephrosclerosis, chronic glomerulonephritis, chronic interstitial nephritis, and chronic pyelonephritis (14, p 811).

The characteristic renal lesion of preeclampsia is glomerular capillary endotheliosis, characterized by swelling of the glomeruli with vacuolization and swelling of the endothelial and mesangial cells. This causes complete or partial occlusion of glomerular capillaries. Also, there are alterations of the juxtaglomerular (JG) cells in the JG apparatus (13, p 843). These renal changes are *not* unique to preeclampsia as was once thought (12, p 857). The characteristic lesions can be diagnosed easily on renal biopsy, but because of the high risk of bleeding that is sometimes severe enough to require nephrectomy, it is indicated rarely in pregnant women.

According to the Committee on Terminology of the American College of Obstetricians and Gynecologists, the clinical diagnosis of preeclampsia requires acute hypertension occurring after 20 weeks gestation, with abnormal edema, proteinuria, or both. Abnormal edema means edema of the hands or face or generalized edema, although generalized edema is quite common in normal pregnancy and cannot be differentiated from the abnormal edema of preeclampsia. Proteinuria is quite common in preeclampsia/eclampsia, although it is a late sign. Indeed, up to 10% of eclamptic women seize *before* proteinuria occurs. However, since the characteristic lesion of preeclampsia is accompanied by proteinuria, the diagnosis is suspect in the absence of proteinuria. The degree of proteinuria gives some evidence of the severity of preeclampsia, but it cannot be used to differentiate preeclampsia from chronic renal disease.

Serum uric acid concentration is high in preeclamptics, increasing with the severity of the disease. Its usefulness for diagnosis is limited, however, since the level normally increases near term, is not very high with mild preeclampsia, and is elevated in normotensive women with small-for-gestational-age babies. Serum creatinine and urea nitrogen also are not diagnostic since their values may be elevated with chronic renal disease. Hepatic studies are used to confirm abnormalities that are suspected clinically, rather than for diagnosis of preeclampsia.

Coagulation abnormalities may occur with preeclampsia but also are not diagnostic. They probably result from endothelial injury, resulting from vasospasm. Thrombin time may be prolonged in some severe preeclamptics/eclamptics, and thrombocytopenia also may be seen. Other laboratory tests that are being studied for their usefulness in the diagnosis and management of preeclampsia include factor VIII, antithrombin III, and serum iron (13, pp 844–849). Table 13.1 summarizes laboratory tests altered by preeclampsia/eclampsia.

Because the key to successful outcome in preeclampsia is early diagnosis and treatment, much effort has gone into finding a reliable predictor of preeclampsia. One such test is based on enhanced sensitivity of women destined to become preeclamptic to angiotensin II. Angiotensin II is administered intravenously, and blood pressure response is monitored. It is not used routinely because the time required for the test and the intravenous route make it cumbersome and impractical to administer. Also, it is more accurate in predicting preeclampsia for a high risk population than for a general population.

Another test sometimes used to predict preeclampsia/eclampsia is the supine pressor test (SPT), also called the rollover test. To administer it, a woman at 28–32 weeks' gestation is placed in the lateral recumbent position. Her BP is monitored until it is stable, usually within 15 minutes. Then, she is rolled over to the supine position, where her BP is taken again. An increase of ≥20 mm Hg in the diastolic BP is considered a positive response.

The original study of the SPT was very promising: 75% of patients with a positive test did get PIH subsequently, while 90% of those with a negative test did not. Efforts to replicate the predictability of the SPT have not succeeded. Although few patients with a negative SPT got PIH later in the pregnancy, only 25–50% of patients with a positive test in subsequent studies had PIH (4, p 91). It is now thought that some of the hypertensive response when a woman is rolled onto her back merely is due to hydrostatics if the BP in the lateral position was taken on the upper arm.

Another test that has been used in an attempt to predict preeclampsia/eclampsia is the mean arterial pressure (MAP).

The BP is taken on the upper arm with the woman in the lateral recumbent position after rest. The proper size cuff must be used, and the fifth sound of Korotkoff is considered the diastolic pressure. An average MAP<90 in the second trimester of pregnancy is quite accurate in predicting that a woman will *not* develop PIH. Of nulliparas with an average MAP≥90 in the second trimester, only one-third developed PIH in one study (16). It is suggested that these women with a MAP≥90 in the second trimester be considered at high risk for PIH and that they be followed by further tests or more frequent BP checks to detect PIH early if it should occur.

Although the diagnosis of preeclampsia/eclampsia is difficult to determine accurately, it is rather academic at times to determine the precise diagnosis. Because PIH is such a serious disease but usually is easily treated, the clinical diagnosis of preeclampsia is made and acted upon when the patient has the onset of hypertension with edema and/or proteinuria in the last half of pregnancy. A definitive diagnosis may not be made until 3–4 months postpartum when the BP has returned to normal.

Maternal and Fetal Outcome

The hypertensive disorders of pregnancy are a leading cause of maternal death. Worldwide, maternal mortality in eclamptics has been reported to range from 0–17% (9, p 135). In the United States it is reported to range from 5–11% (11, p 797). Maternal death usually is from convulsions owing to cerebral hemorrhage, aspiration of gastric contents, or congestive heart failure (13, p 837). Death is a risk whenever the brain, liver, hemopoietic system, and/or renal system are involved in the disease process.

Preeclampsia predisposes to abruptio placentae, acute renal failure, cerebral hemorrhage, disseminated intravascular coagulation, and circulatory collapse. Blood loss at delivery is often twice in eclamptic women what it is in normal patients. Since the blood volume is constricted already, that amount of loss can lead to shock quickly.

Usually, the patient's BP returns to normal within 1–2 days after delivery. Sometimes a mild BP elevation may persist for 6–8 weeks after delivery. Two long-term follow-up studies indicate that chronic hypertension is *not* more likely to occur in women who had eclampsia in the first pregnancy than in the general population (14, p 804). A patient with preeclampsia in the first pregnancy has about a 25–35% chance of having hypertension in a subsequent pregnancy. The risk of recurrence is greater if hypertension persists more than 10 days after delivery, if preeclampsia developed before 36 weeks' gestation, if the average systolic pressure was ≥160 mm Hg during eclampsia, or if the patient is obese (15, p 821).

The risk of spontaneous abortion, prematurity, and abruption in subsequent pregnancies is increased for multiparas with preeclampsia/eclampsia but not for nulliparas (15, p 821). This may be due, at least in part, to other complication(s) coincident with PIH in multiparas.

Perinatal morbidity and mortality also are greatly increased by preeclampsia. Fetal mortality has been reported to range from 10–37% (9, p 135). Ischemia of the uteroplacental vascular bed may cause asphyxia or even fetal death. Long-term decreased placental perfusion may cause IUGR with its attendant increased risk of mortality, cerebral palsy, and other problems (see Chapter 27). Often, early delivery is required for maternal or fetal indications, so prematurity often also contributes to neonatal morbidity and mortality.

It is difficult to distinguish which immediate effects on the newborn are due to the disease process and which are due to MgSO₄ or other drugs used to treat the mother. During labor, decreased variability of the fetal heart rate after the intravenous loading dose of MgSO₄ has been reported in some but not all studies (17). At birth the baby's serum magnesium concentration is the same as that of the mother. The baby may have decreased muscle tone, but usually the Apgar score is not affected much if at all. Within 36–48 hours after birth, the baby's kidneys will excrete the excess magnesium, and blood levels will return to normal.

Medical Management

Since preeclampsia/eclampsia is a progressive disease, the goal of medical treatment is prevention of severe complications through early diagnosis and treatment. Since the cause of the disease is unknown, treatment is directed toward controlling BP and preventing or relieving accompanying symptoms of preeclampsia/eclampsia.

Once preeclampsia is present, the pathological changes persist until delivery, even though the clinical picture may improve with treatment. Therefore, once the fetus is mature, delivery is the treatment of choice.

Mild Preeclampsia

When the fetus is immature, as documented by the L:S ratio, and preeclampsia is mild, often it is possible to gain time for the fetus to mature. Rarely—when the disease is very mild and the mother is very compliant, with excellent family and social support and ready access to the hospital— she may be treated at home. There the patient will be placed on bed rest with urine protein and BP monitored frequently. Frequent trips in to the hospital or clinic will be required to verify her status as well as to perform tests of fetal well-being. The visiting nurse also may monitor the patient's status between clinic visits. It must be emphasized that outpatient treatment is the exception rather than the rule and that many practitioners do not believe it has a place in the treatment of preeclampsia.

When the patient is hospitalized with mild preeclampsia, she is placed on bed rest, with the left lateral position preferred in order to maximize uteroplacental blood flow. Exactly how much bed rest is necessary is unknown, but the patient usually is allowed up for bathroom privileges and for eating, with bed rest the remainder of the time. Some physicians may give phenobarbital, 120–240 mg/day for sedation. Others prefer not to because of the potential for adverse fetal side effects, such as coagulopathies, altered steroid and vitamin D metabolism, hypocalcemia, and neonatal withdrawal.

Because uteroplacental circulation continues to be compromised, fetal surveillance is important. Serial sonograms will detect IUGR or oligohydramnios. Nonstress tests (NSTs) are done biweekly to ensure fetal well-being. In some institutions serial estriols may be done. In general, these tests of fetal status are useful in determining that a fetus is in good health if results are favorable. However, unfavorable results do not necessarily correspond with poor fetal status. The mother's BP, proteinuria, and edema are monitored as well as her subjective complaints (i.e., headaches, visual disturbances, epigastric pain). Deterioration in her status may require delivery, regardless of fetal maturity. Glucocorticoids may be given to enhance fetal lung maturity if the fetus is immature and it is prudent to delay delivery for 24–48 hours. They do not affect maternal BP.

Severe Preeclampsia

When preeclampsia becomes severe, delivery is the definitive treatment. Vaginal delivery is preferred; cesarean section is reserved for patients with obstetric indications. Even in a patient whose cervix seems unfavorable, induction with oxytocin is attempted. The uterus clinically seems more responsive to oxytocin in the presence of preeclampsia, and vaginal delivery often is accomplished (15, p 818). Oxytocin augmentation frequently is required during labor of a patient being treated with MgSO₄ because one of the effects of MgSO₄ is decreased contraction of smooth muscle, including the uterus (see Chapter 28).

Magnesium Sulfate

While awaiting delivery, the cornerstone of treatment of preeclampsia is MgSO₄—given to prevent convulsions and not to treat hypertension. When the diagnosis of preeclampsia is uncertain, it is preferable to overtreat with MgSO₄ and prevent serious sequelae than to undertreat. The anticonvulsant mechanism of MgSO₄ is not understood completely, although it does seem to depress seizure foci in the brain as well as provide peripheral neuromuscular blockade (17, p 163). Because it decreases resistance in the uterine vessels, there may be a transient drop in BP after it is administered, but lowering of the BP is *not* a major effect of MgSO₄. As noted above, it may also decrease amplitude and frequency of uterine contractions.

MgSO₄ may be given either by the intramuscular or intravenous route; both are safe and effective. The intramuscular route has the advantage of simple administration and simpler monitoring for toxic effects. The primary disadvantages are pain at the

Table 13.2.

CLINICAL EFFECTS OF MAGNESIUM LEVELS

EFFECT	BLOOD LEVEL OF MAGNESIUM
Normal	2 mg/dl
Therapeutic effect (for PIH)	4–7 mg/dl
Disappearance of patellar reflex	8–10 mg/dl
Respiratory depression	10–12 mg/dl
Defect in cardiac conduction	>15 mg/dl

injection site; lack of appropriate sites for injection if therapy is prolonged; and slow or unpredictable absorption of the drug, especially in light of the constricted intravascular volume. The intravenous route has the advantages of achieving therapeutic blood levels rapidly, predictable delivery to the bloodstream, and less pain. The intravenous route does require more sophisticated equipment and closer monitoring. It can be stopped immediately if signs of toxicity occur. There is, however, the potential for fluid overload with the intravenous route since the drug is diluted in intravenous fluids (see below). It should not be used in a setting where the equipment or number and skill of personnel are not adequate to administer it properly. Contraindications to the use of MgSO₄ include myasthenia gravis, recent myocardial infarction, and decreased renal function.

When MgSO₄ is given by either route, a loading dose is given in order to saturate body tissues. A 4-g dose is common, but in an obese patient, up to 6 g may be given. The loading dose may be prepared as follows: 8 ml of 50% MgSO₄ is mixed with 12 ml sterile water, for a total volume of 20 ml. It is given slow intravenous push over a period of 5–10 minutes.

Alternatively, 8 ml of 50% MgSO₄ is mixed with 250 ml D₅W and is given intravenous piggyback over 15 minutes. The MgSO₄ must be given quickly enough to achieve optimum blood levels, but too-rapid administration can lead to serious side effects, including apnea and cardiac arrest.

Following the loading dose, 10 g MgSO₄ may be given deep intramuscularly (5 g in each buttock) followed by 5 g every 4 hours; 1–2 ml of 0.5–1% lidocaine may be added to each injection to minimize pain. Before each injection the patient's response to MgSO₄ therapy should be monitored:

1. Deep tendon reflexes should be hypoactive but present.
2. Respirations should be ≥12/minute.
3. Urinary output should be ≥25 ml/hour (or ≥100 ml in 4 hours).

If the above criteria are not met, the MgSO₄ should be withheld (see Table 13.2 on correlation of magnesium levels with clinical effects).

When the intravenous route is chosen for MgSO₄ administration, 1–2 g/hour is given as a maintenance dose via a constant infusion pump. The precise instructions for preparing the intravenous solution, setting up the equipment, and determining the setting that will deliver the desired dose should be written out and followed exactly. Instructions may differ according to the particular infusion pump being used. As an example, 20 g MgSO₄ placed in 1000 ml intravenous fluids and given at the rate of 50 ml/hour will give 1 g/hour. With intravenous MgSO₄ the deep tendon reflexes, respirations, and urinary output should be monitored hourly. In addition, some physicians will monitor serum magnesium levels every 4 hours and alter the dose in order to maintain a therapeutic level. As much as 3 g/hour occasionally may be necessary (17, p 166). The dose will be decreased if the patient is oliguric since magnesium is excreted via the urine and toxic levels can be reached quickly if urine output is below normal.

The antagonist for MgSO₄ is calcium gluconate, which can be given if toxic levels of magnesium are reached; 10 ml of 10% calcium gluconate is given intravenous push over 3–5 minutes. Calcium gluconate always should be readily available when MgSO₄ is used.

MgSO₄ therapy is maintained until 12–24 hours after delivery since there is a chance of convulsions in the early postpartum period. The dose is tapered off over a 2- to 3-hour period.

Antihypertensives

Because MgSO₄ does not have a sustained antihypertensive effect, a dangerously high BP must be controlled with other medications to prevent cardiovascular accident or cerebral edema. Antihypertensive drugs are indicated if the diastolic BP is ≥100 mm Hg. Hydralazine is very effective and is used commonly. It causes reflex tachycardia and increased cardiac output, which may serve to enhance uteroplacental blood flow. Hydralazine, 5 mg, is given intravenous push over 2 minutes. The BP is monitored frequently, at least every 5 minutes for 15 minutes. The goal is to stabilize the diastolic BP between 80 and 100 mm Hg. Too rapid a drop in BP may compromise uteroplacental blood flow and jeopardize the fetus. If a satisfactory lowering of BP is not achieved after one dose of hydralazine, 5 mg boluses may be given every 20–30 minutes, or a constant infusion (100 mg hydralazine in 100 ml normal saline) may be titrated according to the patient's BP to achieve the desired result (18). Diazoxide may be used if hydralazine is not effective. Diuretics should be used *only* if there is pulmonary edema or congestive heart failure. It should be noted that antihypertensive drugs are used only to control BP in severe preeclamptics or eclamptics while awaiting delivery. They are *not* used antepartally for treatment of preeclampsia to "buy time" for the fetus to mature since they do not treat the underlying pathology.

Labor Management

Continuous electronic fetal monitoring is used to assess fetal status. Compromised uteroplacental perfusion increases the risk of fetal distress in labor. Contractions also are monitored electronically to ensure that uterine activity is sufficient to progress toward delivery.

Although intravenous fluid volume may be decreased with preeclampsia, the volume of fluid administered to the patient is restricted to 60–150 ml/hour (unless the patient experiences additional fluid loss from vomiting, diarrhea, or hemorrhage). The preeclamptic patient usually has sufficient fluid available already—it is just maldistributed, with an excess in the extravascular spaces and a relative deficiency intravascularly. Additional intravenous fluids increase the risk of pulmonary and cerebral edema.

During labor and delivery, barbiturates and narcotics should be avoided since they may depress the fetus. Conduction anesthesia also is avoided, because it can cause vasodilatation from splanchnic blockade. This compounds the potential for hypotension already present with the reduced circulatory volume of preeclampsia (9, p 142). Vasopressors and intravenous fluids that are normally given to prevent or relieve the hypotension are contraindicated in the severely preeclamptic or eclamptic patient.

During labor the patient's status is followed by evaluation of the complete blood count, BUN, uric acid, platelet count, SGOT, urine protein checks, and a 24-hour urine for protein and creatinine (19). A Foley catheter may be inserted to monitor urine output precisely. A central venous pressure line or a Swan-Ganz catheter may be inserted to help monitor hemodynamics. Of course, BP is monitored frequently—at least hourly. The patient is questioned frequently about subjective signs and symptoms of serious sequelae of preeclampsia. Respirations, reflexes, and urine output are monitored at least hourly whenever MgSO$_4$ is given.

The patient remains on bed rest throughout labor, preferably in the left lateral position. An attempt is made to keep her environment peaceful and quiet to avoid unnecessary stimulation of the central nervous system (CNS). Siderails of the bed are kept up and padded to prevent injury if the patient convulses. Emotional support of the patient and her family, including teaching regarding the disease, its treatment, and the expected outcome for both mother and baby, is required to allay anxiety.

Emergency drugs and equipment should be readily available. Equipment and personnel should be prepared for emergency cesarean section. The pediatrician should be called to be present for the delivery because of the risks of asphyxia, hypotonia, IUGR and/or prematurity.

Immediate delivery is indicated when signs or symptoms of potentially serious complications occur: CNS disorders (e.g., severe headaches, visual disturbances), oliguria, markedly decreased creatinine clearance, pulmonary edema, epigastric pain, thrombocytopenia, impaired liver function, fetal distress, or severe IUGR (15, p 818).

Eclampsia

Convulsions occur rarely once MgSO$_4$ therapy has begun. When a convulsion does occur, a padded tongue blade or oral airway should be inserted in the patient's mouth to keep her tongue from occluding her airway and to prevent her from biting her tongue. Her head should be turned to the side to prevent aspiration if emesis should occur. The patient's limbs should be restrained sufficiently to avoid injury. MgSO$_4$ is the treatment of choice to control the seizure. If MgSO$_4$ therapy has not been initiated, the 4–6 g loading dose is given over 5–10 minutes. If MgSO$_4$ therapy is in progress, an additional 2–3 g MgSO$_4$ is given intravenous piggyback over 5–10 minutes. Barbiturates and diazepam are not given since they may depress both mother and baby. Hydantoin derivatives are not effective in controlling seizures.

Immediately after a convulsion, a plastic airway is inserted, the airway is suctioned, and the patient is placed in the Trendelenburg position. Oxygen is given as necesary. The stomach may be emptied via a nasogastric tube to prevent aspiration, and intravenous route is started with an appropriate electrolyte solution to maintain fluid balance. A Foley catheter is inserted, and intake and output are monitored hourly. Laboratory tests to monitor the patient's status include a 24-hour urine for protein and creatinine; checks of urine specific gravity and protein at least every 6–8 hours; serial hematocrits; baseline BUN, creatinine, electrolytes, and liver enzymes (if not already obtained); and chest x-ray to rule out aspiration. A constant intravenous infusion of 1–2 g/hour of

MgSO$_4$ is given, and hydralazine is given if needed to control BP (9, pp 141–142).

As soon as appropriate therapy is initiated after the seizure, a decision must be made about how to deliver the patient. Cesarean section is appropriate if the baby is in distress, is very small (<1500 g), or is breech, or if the cervix is not ripe. Otherwise, amniotomy and oxytocin induction or augmentation may be used to hasten vaginal delivery. Labor management is the same for the eclamptic patient as for the severe preeclamptic.

NURSING MANAGEMENT

Nursing care specific for a patient with preclampsia/eclampsia:

- ☐ Counsel all patients prior to conception, if possible, regarding health behaviors that minimize risk of hypertension, e.g., correct dietary deficiencies, attain ideal pregnancy weight, stop smoking, manage stress positively, alter coping style.
- ☐ Take accurate blood pressure readings at each prenatal visit and frequently in labor and the postpartum period:
  - — Use leg cuff for obese patient;
  - — Take blood pressure in same arm, in same position (preferably in left lateral);
- ☐ Record the same sound(s) for the diastolic blood pressure, Karathoff's Phase V (disappearance of sound), or both Phase IV (muffled sound) and Phase V;
  - — Take blood pressure at the same time of day if possible;
  - — Evaluate patient's level of anxiety and recent physical activity when blood pressure is elevated; repeat blood pressure after rest and measures to relieve anxiety.
- ☐ Screen all patients for PIH at each prenatal visit by evaluating blood pressure, edema, proteinuria, and subjective symptoms (e.g., severe headaches, visual disturbances, epigastric pain).
- ☐ Teach importance of bed rest as part of treatment for mild preeclampsia:
  - — Explain rationale for bed rest and expected benefits;
  - — Explain what activity is allowed (e.g., bathroom privileges); assist her to identify times and places where she can rest;
  - — Encourage family/friends to maintain frequent contact and provide activities to prevent boredom while patient is on bed rest.
- ☐ Teach patient importance and rationale of special tests used to assess maternal/fetal status (e.g., sonogram, nonstress test (NST), 24-hour urine blood tests of kidney and liver function). Assist in procedures and obtaining specimens;

teach patient how to collect clean catch urine and 24-hour urine specimens.
- ☐ Administer oxytocin for induction/augmentation, as needed (see Chapter 37).
- ☐ During labor:
  - — Place patient on bed rest in left lateral position;
  - — Monitor fetus by continuous electronic monitoring;
  - — Ensure patent IV for administration of medication and maintenance of fluid balance;
  - — Assist with tests of maternal/fetal status (e.g., serial maternal hematocrits, platelet counts, liver function tests, fetal scalp sampling);
  - — Observe for signs/symptoms of complications (e.g., abruptio placentae, fetal distress, pulmonary edema, renal failure, DIC, increasing severity of preeclampsia/eclampsia).
- ☐ Administer MgSO$_4$ IV or IM, as ordered.
  - — Prepare and administer IV MgSO$_4$ according to instructions for the particular equipment being used;
  - — Evaluate urine output, respirations, and deep tendon reflexes hourly if MgSO$_4$ is given IV, or before each dose, if given IM. Discontinue treatment if respirations are less than 12/minute, urine output is less than 25 ml/hour, or DTRs are absent.
- ☐ Administer antihypertensive (e.g., hydralazine), as ordered. Take blood pressure q 2–3 minutes for the first 15 minutes, then q 5–10 minutes until stable. Repeat after subsequent boluses of medication.
- ☐ Initiate seizure precautions when preeclampsia is present.
  - — Place emergency tray at bedside (including MgSO$_4$, calcium gluconate, padded tongue blade, oxygen equipment);
  - — Pad the side rails of the bed and keep them up;
  - — Minimize CNS stimulation by placing patient in a quiet, dark room.

NURSING MANAGEMENT

☐ Assist with management of seizure (e.g., administer MgSO₄ as ordered, insert airway, turn head to side, gently restrain limbs).

☐ Be prepared for emergency cesarean section.

☐ Alert pediatrician to attend delivery; be prepared for neonatal resuscitation.

☐ Prepare for postpartum hemorrhage; do *not* give ergot preparations, as they are contraindicated in hypertensive patients.

☐ Continue MgSO₄ therapy for 12–24 hours postpartum. Gradually decrease the dose over a period of 2–3 hours.

☐ Monitor patient closely during the postpartum period since convulsions may occur—even for the first time up to 48 hours after delivery.

Nursing diagnoses most frequently associated with *preeclampsia/eclampsia*:

☐ Potential for trauma related to seizures

☐ Excess fluid volume

☐ Grieving related to potential/actual loss of infant or birth of an imperfect child

☐ Anticipatory grieving related to actual/perceived threat to self

☐ Knowledge deficit regarding etiology, disease process, treatment and outcome

☐ Knowledge deficit regarding medication regimen

☐ Altered fetal cardiac and cerebral tissue perfusion

☐ Altered maternal tissue perfusion

☐ Fluid volume deficit

CHRONIC HYPERTENSION

Definition

Hypertension is defined as sustained arterial blood pressure ≥140/90 mm Hg. Chronic hypertension is not induced by the pregnancy; it normally antedates the pregnancy. However, since prepregnancy BPs may not be known for an individual, it may not be *diagnosed* prior to the pregnancy. In some individuals its onset may occur during pregnancy and continue thereafter. Because of the decrease in peripheral vascular resistance that normally occurs during the second trimester of pregnancy, diastolic pressures ≥80 mm Hg during the second trimester should be regarded as suspicious of chronic hypertension.

Chronic hypertension occurs in approximately 4–5% of pregnant women (12, p 854). Its severity, determined by BP readings, is correlated with its effects on the vital organs of the body (Table 13.3).

Etiology

The most common form of chronic hypertension is essential (also called primary or idiopathic) hypertension, with the cause unknown. It is associated with advanced age, overweight, sedentary lifestyle, smoking, stress, and a family history of hypertension.

Secondary hypertension is related to a known cause. It is much less common than primary hypertension. Among the causes are renal disease (e.g., glomerulonephritis, chronic pyelonephritis, polycystic kidney, systemic lupus erythematosus), adre-

nal disease (e.g., pheochromocytoma, Cushing's disease, hyperaldosteronism), thyrotoxicosis, and coarctation of the aorta (12, p 854).

Signs and Symptoms

Primary chronic hypertension is insidious in its onset, with few or no associated symptoms. Often, the patient feels quite well, with an elevated BP noted on a medical visit for an unrelated reason. Signs and symptoms of secondary hypertension are those related to the cause (e.g., acute episodes of vasomotor symptoms may occur with pheochromocytoma or weight loss and enlarged thyroid gland with thyrotoxicosis). The reader is referred to medical texts for a full discussion of signs, symptoms, pathophysiology, and treatment of the specific causes of secondary hypertension.

Diagnosis

The diagnosis of chronic hypertension is made most easily prior to pregnancy. It is based on a persistently elevated BP, preferably taken on several occasions, several days apart, with the patient at rest.

When hypertension is diagnosed, the next step is to attempt to determine the specific cause. A careful history is taken, including family history of hypertension; past medical history of chronic or repeated urinary tract infections, diabetes mellitus, systemic lupus erythematosus, or other associated diseases or previous episodes of elevated BP; and a current history of any associated signs or symptoms. A thorough physical examination is performed, with particular attention to components of the examination that will aid in diagnosis or in as-

Table 13.3.
EFFECTS OF HYPERTENSION ON END ORGANS[a]

SEVERITY	FIRST AND SECOND TRIMESTER DIASTOLIC BP	MAP	THIRD TRIMESTER DIASTOLIC BP	MAP	CARDIAC	FUNDUSCOPIC	RENAL
Mild	80	90	90	95	Normal cardiac size. Normal EKG.	Normal or minimal changes.	Normal (GFR increased 30–50% in pregnancy).
Moderate	90	100	100	105	Left ventricular hypertrophy, with or without cardiac enlargement.	Spastic or sclerotic changes.	GFR equal to normal for nonpregnant woman (therefore decreased for a pregnant woman).
Severe	110	120	110	120	Left ventricular hypertrophy and ischemia. Cardiac enlargement. Some symptoms: e.g., headaches, palpitations.	Above changes and occasional hemorrhages and exudates.	Decreased renal function.
Malignant					Above symptoms and symptoms of cardiac failure. Ischemic pain and/or encephalopathy.	Frank hemorrhages and exudates; papilledema.	Rapidly decreasing renal function, hematuria, proteinuria.

[a]Adapted from Zuspan FP: Chronic hypertension in pregnancy. *Clin Obstet Gynecol* 27:856, 1984.

sessing the effect of hypertension on the end organs (e.g., a funduscopic examination; evaluation of cardiac size; BP of all extremities and BP in various positions; simultaneous palpation of femoral and radial pulses to rule out coarctation of the aorta; and auscultation over renal arteries to listen for the bruit of renal vascular hypertension). Laboratory studies also are performed to rule out specific causes and to assess the effect of hypertension on the organs (e.g., BUN, serum creatinine, creatinine clearance, serum electrolytes, urine catechols, vanillylmandelic acid, electrocardiogram, chest x-ray, ultrasound examination of the kidneys, and intravenous pyelogram in the nonpregnant patient). If no specific cause for the hypertension is found, the diagnosis is primary hypertension (12, pp 862–863).

When hypertension is first diagnosed during pregnancy, the task of determining the specific cause is greater because PIH also must be considered. Frequently, the normal decrease in peripheral vascular resistance causes the BP to drop 30–40% during the first and second trimesters of pregnancy (14, p 810). When the BP then rises to its usual prepregnant level in the third trimester, it must be

distinguished from PIH. Because women with chronic hypertension from renal disease may have proteinuria and the normal edema of pregnancy, the diagnosis may not be clear until it can be made retrospectively several weeks after delivery. Another confounding factor is that preeclampsia may be superimposed on chronic hypertension. Indeed, chronic hypertension predisposes to preeclampsia.

Maternal and Fetal Outcome

The effects of chronic hypertension on the fetus range from minimal to death. The critical factor seems to be the adequacy of placental blood flow. With severe hypertension, often the placenta is quite small. Hyperplastic arteriosclerotic changes in the myometrial segment of the radial arteries cause impeded blood flow to the intervillous space. Frequently, the result is IUGR, which tends to correlate with the severity of the hypertension. With IUGR the perinatal mortality increases eightfold (12, p 861).

The incidence of preterm delivery also is increased in women with chronic hypertension. These babies tend to have accelerated lung maturity, possibly because of chronic stress, so the risk of respiratory distress syndrome is somewhat less than would be anticipated by gestational age alone.

Babies of chronic hypertensive patients have added risks because of conditions associated with hypertension, such as abruptio placentae and superimposed preeclampsia. The risk of perinatal death is five times greater with superimposed preeclampsia than with chronic hypertension alone (12, p 861). Compromised placental blood flow may cause fetal hypoxia during labor and delivery.

Maternal outcome varies depending upon the severity of chronic hypertension and any associated complications. Usually, the mother fares quite well, but occasionally complications are so severe as to cause death. There is a general risk of cardiovascular accident with very high BPs. Abruptio placentae is more common in hypertensive patients and may result in shock or DIC (see chapters 8 and 31). With superimposed preeclampsia there is increased risk of cardiovascular accident, cerebral edema, convulsions, DIC, and renal or liver failure. The course of chronic hypertension in pregnancy is not predictive of the long-term course of the disease.

Medical Management

The management of chronic hypertension should begin prior to conception, if possible. The workup to determine the specific cause is done ideally when the patient is nonpregnant. She can be counseled to make life-style changes as necessary (e.g., lose weight, begin regular exercise program, begin a healthy diet, and cease smoking) and taught how to monitor her own BP.

Prenatal care should begin as soon as possible in the pregnancy. Careful surveillance during pregnancy may require prenatal visits every 1–2 weeks. At the first prenatal visit the usual history, physical examination, and laboratory tests should be performed. In addition, BUN, serum creatinine, creatinine clearance, urine culture, and serum electrolytes should be taken. A chest x-ray and EKG can be done if needed (12, p 865). The patient should receive individualized diet counseling, and she should be encouraged to salt foods to taste unless there is a significant problem with water retention. If there is significant proteinuria, she may need to increase her protein intake above that normally recommended for pregnant women.

The cornerstone of management for the chronic hypertensive patient is bed rest. She should be encouraged to rest at least twice daily for an hour each time. Even a working patient should be encouraged to rest midday and as soon as she gets home from work. It may be necessary for her to curtail working partially or altogether during the pregnancy in order to rest. Rest should be in the left lateral position in order to enhance uteroplacental and renal blood flow. It will result in an increased GFR and mild diuresis (12, p 866).

Drug therapy during pregnancy is somewhat controversial. If the patient already is on antihypertensive drugs, some physicians prefer to leave her on them to avoid the risk of having the BP go out of control. Often, however, diuretics will be stopped gradually. A rebound in plasma volume expansion (and thus a sudden weight gain) may occur after diuretics are discontinued (7).

The only antihypertensive drug shown to be safe and effective during pregnancy is methyldopa. It is unclear whether methyldopa improves perinatal outcome, but it does prevent maternal complications. Other antihypertensive drugs may be safe to use, but they have not been studied sufficiently to verify their safety. Propranolol may cause IUGR, but since hypertension itself causes IUGR, the effect of propranolol is not clear. Oral hydralazine suppresses the release of renin but cannot be used long term. Labetalol is both an α and β-adrenergic blocker. So far, no major adverse effects are known during pregnancy, but it is still under investigation (12, p 868). When hypertension first is diagnosed during pregnancy, methyldopa is the drug of choice because its effects in pregnancy are known. The goal of drug therapy is to lower BP sufficiently to prevent maternal cardiovascular complications, but not so much as to interfere with uteroplacental blood flow (19, p 21).

Successful attempts at lowering BP in hypertensive pregnant women have been made using relaxation techniques with or without biofeedback (20). Because there are no known ill effects from relaxation, it has the potential to contribute to management of chronic hypertensive patients.

During the course of pregnancy, the hypertensive patient must be monitored carefully. Home BP monitoring is relatively easy for the patient to learn and can greatly increase the number of BP readings available for evaluation. Monitoring the BP at home eliminates the anxiety that may adversely affect office BP readings. Because BP can be taken several times a week at home, the patient may be the first to notice a significant change. For consistency, BP readings, both at home and in the office, should be taken with the patient in the same position, preferably left lateral.

Because chronic hypertension predisposes the patient to preeclampsia, and superimposed preeclampsia has a profound adverse effect on both maternal and fetal outcome, careful evaluation of the signs and symptoms of preeclampsia is a major component of each prenatal visit. After about 20 weeks' gestation, the SPT (rollover-test) may be done at each prenatal visit. Normally, a woman with chronic hypertension will maintain a BP that is normal for her when she rolls to her back. Such a test is negative and indicates that she probably will not get superimposed preeclampsia. A BP elevation of >20 mm Hg diastolic when the woman is turned to her back indicates that she is at risk for preeclampsia.

Laboratory tests that should be performed during the pregnancy include BUN, creatinine, and creatinine clearance at least every 2 months; a sonogram early in the pregnancy to establish gestational age, a second one at 20–26 weeks, and a third one at approximately 32 weeks if IUGR or oligohydramnios is suspected (12, p 863); a check for proteinuria at each prenatal visit; and perhaps serial checks of electrolytes, uric acid, serum iron, and antithrombin III concentration to detect subtle indications of preeclampsia.

Intensive fetal surveillance should begin at approximately 28–32 weeks' gestation. NSTs should be done biweekly or weekly until 36 weeks and weekly thereafter. A contraction stress test should be done if the NST is not reactive. A biophysical profile may be done weekly to evaluate fetal status. Fetal movement counts may be done by the patient beginning at 32–34 weeks or earlier if there is evidence of IUGR, oligohydramnios, or other fetal problems. Some physicians also may use human placental lactogen levels or estrogen/creatinine ratio to further evaluate fetal well-being (12, pp 863–864).

If there is evidence of superimposed preeclampsia, such as a rise in BP or the appearance or significant increase of proteinuria, the patient should be hospitalized at once. She should be treated as a severe preeclamptic, with the goals of preventing convulsions and controlling the BP. She is placed on bed rest, and $MgSO_4$ is given by either the intramuscular or intravenous route. Hydralazine is given as necessary to control the BP. The patient is worked up to evaluate any end-organ involvement, including the following: intake and output; BUN; creatinine; urine protein spot checks; urine specific gravity; 24-hour urine for protein, creatinine, and creatinine clearance; and serum electrolytes, liver enzymes, and clotting studies. External electronic fetal monitoring is done to evaluate fetal status. Delivery should be accomplished as soon as the patient is stable. Vaginal delivery is preferred, but cesarean section may be required if the cervix is unfavorable and speedy delivery is needed, or for obstetric indications.

When there is no superimposed preeclampsia, delivery may be required prior to term if there is IUGR and a mature L:S ratio; fetal distress; worsening maternal condition; or a maternal BP that cannot be maintained below 180/110 (19, p 22). If the fetus is immature, glucocorticoids may be given to try to enhance fetal lung maturity. It is not known whether glucocorticoids will aid fetal lung maturity, but they might, and they will not adversely affect the BP.

When there are no maternal complications and the fetus is doing well, the pregnancy may be allowed to continue until term but not beyond. At term, the patient should be induced if she does not go into labor spontaneously. Cesarean section is reserved for obstetric indications.

Conduction anesthesia should not be used during the labor and delivery of a chronic hypertensive patient since it sometimes causes a further reduction in uteroplacental blood flow. Electronic fetal monitoring should be used to evaluate fetal status. A pediatric resuscitation team should be present at delivery.

NURSING MANAGEMENT

Nursing care specific for a patient with
chronic hypertension:

☐ If possible, prior to conception, teach health-promoting behaviors:
   — Change eating patterns as necessary (e.g., eliminate excess dietary sodium);
   — Establish a regular exercise program;
   — Complete medical workup on cause of hypertension;
   — Maintain blood pressure control by taking medications regularly;
   — Monitor blood pressure at home;
   — Begin prenatal care as soon as pregnancy is confirmed.

☐ Teach relaxation techniques to promote lowering of blood pressure.
☐ Provide individualized dietary counseling regarding nutritional needs of pregnancy and any special needs she may have (e.g., increased need for protein).
☐ Teach the importance of rest periods at least twice daily.
☐ Teach changes in medication regime during pregnancy including rationale for changes.
☐ Teach patient how to keep a record of fetal movement according to accepted protocol for the institution (see Chapter 6).

NURSING MANAGEMENT

☐ Teach signs/symptoms of complications and how to report them (e.g., increasing blood pressue at home, headaches, visual disturbances, generalized edema).

☐ Teach the patient the importance and rationale for tests of maternal fetal status (e.g., creatinine clearance, sonograms, NSTs).

☐ During labor:
— Monitor fetus by continuous electronic monitoring;
— Monitor for signs/symptoms of preeclampsia;
— Be prepared for emergency cesarean section;
— Alert pediatrician to attend delivery; be prepared for neonatal resuscitation.

☐ After delivery, continue to monitor blood pressure; encourage patient to continue postpartum care for management of hypertension.

Nursing diagnoses most frequently associated with *chronic hypertension*:

☐ Knowledge deficit regarding etiology, disease process, treatment and expected outcome

☐ Knowledge deficit regarding medication regimen

☐ Altered fetal cardiac and cerebral tissue perfusion

☐ Altered maternal tissue perfusion

☐ Anxiety/fear

REFERENCES

1. Zuspan FP: Hypertension and renal disease in pregnancy. *Clin Obstet Gynecol* 27:797–799, 1984.
2. Harrison EE Jr: Why do pregnant women die? *Dallas Med J* (Sept–Oct):242, 1982.
3. Freidman EA, Neff RK: Pregnancy outcome as related to hypertension, edema, and proteinuria. In Lindeheimer MD, Katz AI, Zuspan FP (eds): *Hypertension in Pregnancy*. New York, John Wiley and Sons, 1976, p 13.
4. O'Shaughnessy R, Zuspan FP: Managing acute pregnancy hypertension. *Contemp OB/GYN* 18:85–98, 1981.
5. Worley RJ: Pathophysiology of pregnancy-induced hypertension. *Clin Obstet Gynecol* 27:821–835, 1984.
6. Willis SE, Sharp ES: Hypertension in pregnancy: prenatal detection and management. *Am J Nurs* 32:798–808, 1982.
7. Sibai BM, Anderson GD: Clues from blood volume changes in hypertensive pregnancies. *Contemp OB/GYN* 21:241–250, 1983.
8. Pritchard JA, MacDonald PC, Gant NF: *Williams Obstetrics*, ed 17. Norwalk, CT, Appleton-Century-Crofts, 1985, p 541.
9. Zuspan FP, Zuspan KJ: Strategies for controlling eclampsia. *Contemp OB/GYN* 18:135–142, 1981.
10. Hughes EC (ed): *Obstetric-Gynecologic Terminology*. Philadelphia, Davis, 1972.
11. Willis SE: Hypertension in pregnancy: pathophysiology. *Am J Nurs* 82:792–797, 1982.
12. Zuspan FP: Chronic hypertension in pregnancy. *Clinical Obstet Gynecol* 27:854–873, 1984.
13. DeVoe SJ, O'Shaughnessy R: Clinical manifestations and diagnosis of pregnancy-induced hypertension. *Clin Obstet Gynecol* 27:836–853, 1984.
14. Chesley LC: History and epidemiology of preeclampsia-eclampsia. *Clin Obstet Gynecol* 27:801–820, 1984.
15. Kelley M, Mongiello R: Hypertension in pregnancy: labor, delivery, and postpartum. *Am J Nurs* 82:813–822, 1982.
16. Oney T, Kaulhausen H: The value of the mean arterial blood pressure in the second trimester (MAP-2 value) as a predictor of pregnancy-induced hypertension and preeclampsia: a preliminary report. *Clin Exp Hypertension in Preg* 132:211–216, 1983.
17. Koontz WL, Cefalo RC: Do's and don't's of treating preeclampsia and eclampsia with MgSO₄. *Contemp OB/GYN* 22:163–167, 1983.
18. Chez RA Zuspan FP: Guide to MgSO₄ therapy for PIH. *Contemp OB/GYN* 22:65–66, 1983.
19. Berkowitz RL: Managing hypertension. *Contemp OB/GYN* 21:20–24, 1983.
20. ————: Relaxation techniques relieve hypertension in pregnancy. News from the literature. *Contemp OB/GYN* 23:233, 1984.

Chapter 14
Deviations of the
Neuromuscular System
Mary C. Fallon, R.N., M.S.N.

INTRODUCTION

The neuromuscular system undergoes several changes during pregnancy. Many of the discomforts commonly encountered in pregnancy can be attributed to these changes. (These changes and their relief measures are listed in Table 14.1.)

Neuromuscular Discomforts

As pregnancy progresses and the uterus grows heavier, greater stress is placed on the pregnant woman's back muscles and the round ligament that supports the uterus. This accentuates the dorsal and lumbar curves, causing progressive lordosis, and contributes to lower backache. The stress placed on the round ligament may contribute to pain experienced as a "stitch in the side" (1).

Many women experience lightheadedness and dizziness during pregnancy; there are several possible causes of this. The increased release of progesterone that occurs in pregnancy results in an increased distensibility of the blood vessels, including those of the lower extremities and the splanchnic and pelvic areas (2). Pooling of the blood occurs in those areas, particularly after prolonged sitting or standing. This pooling is enhanced further by the pressure exerted on the pelvic veins and inferior vena cava by the ever-enlarging uterus, impinging on blood return to the heart. Rapid alterations in position can result in faintness or lightheadedness. The pregnant woman also can experience a sense of dizziness as a consequence of alterations in her respiratory system (see Chapter 16). Dizziness and lightheadedness also can result from hypoglycemia. The expanding plasma volume can cause a dilutional anemia, resulting in less oxygen being carried to the brain and further contributing to dizziness.

Pregnant women frequently experience leg cramps, largely attributable to the large portions of milk and milk products that pregnant women are encouraged to include in their diet. These products contain a high level of calcium, but they also contain a higher level of phosphorus. It is believed that the disproportionate decrease of diffusable serum calcium and/or the disproportionate increase of serum phosphorus contributes to the leg cramps commonly experienced (2). In addition, as the uterus grows, it impinges on the inferior vena cava. This indirectly diminishes the return of oxygenated blood to the lower extremities and also potentially compresses nerves in the lower leg.

Numbness and tingling of the fingers occur in about 5% of pregnancies (2). It is believed to be due to the drooping of the shoulders during pregnancy (2) or to edema in the wrist and hands (1), either of which compresses the median nerve. The weight of the pregnant woman's enlarging breasts also may contribute to the phenomenon.

Many pregnant women experience headaches during their pregnancies. Causes for headaches can include the stress and fatigue associated with pregnancy or intermittent bouts of hypoglycemia as the woman compensates for the accelerated metabolic rate associated with pregnancy.

Estriol (E_3) production, which is increased one thousand-fold in pregnancy, stimulates many physiologic changes. One of these is the retention of sodium and water, contributing to tissue edema (3). Tissue edema in the nasal turbinates (resembling that of histamine reaction), the expanded circulat-

Table 14.1.

COMMON NEUROMUSCULAR DISCOMFORTS OF PREGNANCY[a]

DISCOMFORT	RELIEF MEASURES
1. Backache	1. Explain cause of discomfort to patient. 2. Advise local heat. 3. Advise back rub. 4. Advise exercises to strengthen back muscles, including pelvic rock. 5. Teach patient to use proper lifting techniques. 6. Instruct the patient to wear low heeled shoes or shoes with heels lower than toes (e.g., Earth Shoes) and to walk barefoot when possible. 7. Teach the patient to avoid overexertion and fatigue and to rest frequently in side-lying position. 8. Encourage the patient to perform total body relaxation exercises learned in childbirth classes. 9. Encourage good posture. 10. Encourage use of a maternity girdle for women with very lax abdominal muscles.
2. Dizziness, light-headedness	1. Explain cause of discomfort. 2. Encourage patient to rise slowly from sitting or lying position, to sleep in side-lying position, and to have support nearby when arising. 3. Encourage the patient to force fluids in order to prevent hypovolemia. 4. Advise the patient to eat smaller, more frequent meals to prevent hypoglycemia. 5. Assess the patient's hemoglobin; consider iron supplementation and diet counseling if the patient is anemic. 6. Assess factors in patient's life that may be stressful or distressing and make appropriate referrals as indicated. 7. Assess if the patient is hyperventilating to compensate for feeling of breathlessness; advise her of physiologic explanation for this and encourage her to attempt to moderate her breathing. 8. Teach the patient to keep feet elevated when possible and to avoid crossing legs or use of restrictive hose in order to prevent venous pooling. 9. If the patient should become acutely dizzy, teach her to lie down at once.
3. Tingling, numbness of fingers	1. Explain cause of discomfort. 2. Encourage good upper body posture (shoulders straight, head up). 3. Discourage sleeping on affected area. 4. Suggest maintaining the arm at the level of the waist when walking or sitting and flexing fingers to enhance circulation. 5. Encourage use of supportive, well-fitting bra. 6. Remind patient to be careful when handling hot, sharp, or breakable items.

4. Headache	1. Explain possible mechanisms responsible for headache.
	2. Carefully assess characteristics of headache (e.g., where experienced, for how long, nature of pain, triggering event, previous comfort measures attempted and their success/failure, associated symptoms).
	3. After learning nature of headache, recommend relief measures consistent with type of headache:
	  a. Tension or muscle strain—advise rest in quiet, dark room and use of relaxation exercises; explore measures to diminish triggering events (or refer to appropriate resources); consider use of guided imagery tapes.
	  b. Sinusitis: encourage use of humidity in the home (e.g., pan of water on radiator) and warm steamy showers; discourage use of over-the-counter decongestants; consider saline nose drops.
	  c. Eyestrain: encourage wear of prescription glasses if patient has them; refer to ophthamologist or optometrist if patient wears contact lenses since their fit may be altered due to changes in the cornea's contour.
	  d. Vascular headaches: encourage bed rest on left side to enhance circulation.
	4. If ordered, encourage the patient to take acetaminophen, 325–650 mg p.o. every 6 hours.

5. Leg cramps	1. Explain reason for cramps and reassure patient they occur commonly in pregnancy. 2. Evaluate patient's diet; if indicated, decrease amount of phosphorus in diet—antacids will bind the phosphorus; limit milk products to four servings daily; give calcium supplementation in the form of 1 g calcium carbonate chewable tablets three times daily. 3. Teach patient to dorsiflex foot when cramps occur. 4. Advise local heat for sore muscles.

Table 14.1.
(Continued)

	5. Encourage patient to avoid "toe pointing" stretch of the legs.
	6. Urge daily exercise to encourage circulation, alternated with rest periods (with legs elevated).
	7. Encourage "lead with heel walking."
6. Round ligament pain	1. Explain cause of discomfort to patient and reassure her this is a normal discomfort of pregnancy.
	2. Teach patient to bend toward the side that is painful.
	3. Suggest use of warm bath or heating pad after attack.
	4. Avoid sudden jerking or twisting movements that may strain round ligament.

[a]Adapted from Neeson J, Stockdale C: *The Practitioner's Handbook of Ambulatory Ob/Gyn*, New York, John Wiley and Sons, 1981, pp 3–7, and Buckley K, Kulb N: *Handbook of Maternal Newborn Nursing*, New York, John Wiley and Sons, 1983, pp 163–181.

ing blood volume, and increased heart rate also contribute frequently to headaches.

Headache in pregnancy must be evaluated carefully to rule out the underlying cause before attributing it to the normal physiologic changes associated with pregnancy. Table 14.2 details one system of classifying headaches, clearly outlining the multiple medical or organic etiologies associated with this symptom. The workup of headache should include a careful history of the nature, location, and successful relief measures associated with the headache; a thorough physical examination, including blood pressure, funduscopic and nasal examination, evaluation of the cranial nerves, examination of the urine for protein, and inspection for edema, particularly of the face; and possibly a referral for an ophthalmologic or dental examination. Abnormalities in any of these areas require further referral and evaluation and are beyond the scope of this discussion.

Diagnostic Procedures

Because of potential maternal and fetal risk from neuromuscular diagnostic procedures, the risk/benefit ratio must carefully be determined. Electroencephalography (EEG), echoencephalography, electromyography (EMG), and standard tests of the eye, ear, and nose can be performed safely (4). Lumbar puncture is considered safe to perform except when brain tumor is suspected, because it may cause a shift of intracranial structures, with herniation or coning through the tentorium (5). Caution and judgment must be exercised in the use of x-ray studies of the nervous system because of potential harm to the fetus. The probability of inducing malformations is greatest during the period of organogenesis, which begins 1–2 weeks after conception and extends through the tenth week postconception (4). However, it has been suggested that, with good equipment and careful technique, in fewer than 1 in 1000 radiographic examinations will the fetus be exposed to one or more rads (4).

Doses of less than five rads even during organogenesis would be unlikely to cause a measurable increase in maldevelopments in human populations (4). Consequently, x-rays of the head, cervical spine, and extremities can be performed safely with shielding of the abdomen; x-rays of the lumbar spine and pelvis should be done only upon urgent indications (4). Computerized axial tomography (CAT scan) of the head can be done as required. Cerebral angiograms require that the abdomen be shielded (4). Thoracic and lumbar myelography should be avoided because of the difficulty in adequately shielding the abdomen; however, cervical myelography may be performed safely with careful shielding (4). While pregnancy does not provide an absolute contraindication to neuroradiologic diagnostic studies, these studies should be ordered only when the benefit outweighs the risk.

MIGRAINE

Definition

Migraine headaches can be of special concern during pregnancy. It is estimated that 23–29% of the women in the United States experience migraines (6). The research group on migraine and headache of the World Federation of Neurology defined migraine as a:

familial disorder characterized by recurrent attacks of headache widely variable in intensity, frequency, and duration. Attacks are commonly unilateral and are usually associated with anorexia and nausea and vomiting. In some cases they are preceded by or associated with neurological and mood disturbances. All the above characteristics are not necessarily present in each attack or in each patient (7).

There are five types of migraines: classic, common, ophthalmoplegic, hemiplegic, and cluster. Diagnosis of the type of migraine is accomplished by review of the presenting signs and symptoms (Table 14.2).

Etiology

The etiology of migraine headaches is believed to be the abnormal dilatation and distention of the cranial arteries owing to the effect of vasoactive substances in the cerebral blood supply (e.g., catecholamines, histamine and serotonin, peptide kinins, and prostaglandins) (6). These substances interact with the cerebral vasculature, causing the equivalent of local sterile inflammations, which increase the vascular permeability and increase the sensitivity to pain (6). The inflammation stimulates the release of serotonin, which causes vasoconstriction (the aura phase of migraine). With the ensuing depletion of serotonin, the signs and symptoms of migraine develop (6). Serotonin, which is synthesized from dietary tryptophan, is present in high quantities in the chromaffin tissue of the intestine and in platelets. It has vasoconstrictor or vasodilator capacities, dependent on the specific vascular bed, its resting tone, and the dose of serotonin (8). Generally, it constricts arterioles and dilates capillaries (9), increasing their permeability.

Foods and factors that are believed to precipitate the release of the vasoactive substances include coffee, tea, cola, chocolate, cheese, fasting, alcohol, light, stress, sleep deprivation, fever, and decreased estrogen levels (6). Migraines appear to be genetically related since 60–80% of affected women report a positive family history.

Diagnosis

The diagnosis of migraine should begin with a careful history, with particular attention to previous history of migraines (type, severity, distribution, associated symptoms, relief measures and their success) (7) and a family history of migraines.

Other underlying disease(s) should be ruled out via the performance of electromyography; nerve conduction studies; EEG; evoked potential studies, including visual, auditory, and somatosensory; and CAT scan (10). In addition, a lumbar puncture and blood studies (complete blood count, prothrombin, platelet count) should be performed to rule out subarachnoid hemorrhage and thromboembolic stroke. An echocardiogram and real-time ultrasonogram should be performed to rule out thromboembolism of the heart or carotid artery (11).

Table 14.2.
HEADACHE CLASSIFICATION

---

1. Vascular—Due to tendency to vascular dilation and distention of one or more extracranial and probably intracranial branches of the external carotid artery with edema of the adjacent tissues.
    A. Migraine
       1. Classic—Preceded by 5–30 minute prodrome on side of head opposite the side that aches; results in pulsating and throbbing pain that lasts 1–6 hours; prodrome often includes nausea and vomiting sometimes diarrhea. Also, may see stars or flashes; pain tends to be localized.
       2. Common—No preceding prodrome; can last several days; pain is localized.
       3. Ophthalmoplegic—Associated with nausea; caused by abnormality of pupil or weakness of one or more eye muscles.
       4. Hemiplegic—Associated with nausea, vomiting, and headache; recurrent weakness of one arm or one arm and one leg occurs.
       5. Cluster—Occurs in clusters over a few days, weeks, or months, followed by remission; tend to begin suddenly, last a few minutes to 2 hours.
    B. Toxic vascular—Commonly produced by fever; vasodilation intensifies as fever rises; can be associated with pneumonia, tonsilitis, septicemia, etc.
    C. Hypertensive—Associated with sudden and extreme elevations of blood pressure in pregnancy-induced hypertension, or essential hypertension; is more or less continuous, generalized, pounding, difficult to relieve with simple analgesics; may be associated with blurred or double vision, proteinuria, facial edema, papilledema; can progress to hypertensive encephalopathy, with progression from severe headaches, nausea, and vomiting to convulsions, confusion, and ultimately coma.
II. Muscle contraction—Related to chronic muscular contraction occurring about the head, neck, face, scalp, and upper back; characterized by long, sustained contraction that causes the muscle to become tender, leading to restriction of motion and further contraction; produces dull, band-like, persistent pain that may last for days or months; is associated with cervical osteoarthritis, chronic myositis, affective disorders, and conversion reactions.
III. Traction—Evoked by organic disease of the skull or its contents, including the brain, meninges, arteries, veins, and paranasal sinuses; mass lesions of the brain including tumors, hematomas, abscesses, or brain edema, often result in nonspecific headache; subarachnoid and intracerebral hemorrhage and cortical venous thrombosis results in particularly intense headache.
IV. Inflammatory—Evoked by disease of special sense organs and the teeth, as well as allergic headache and major cranial neuralgia.

Maternal and Fetal Outcome

Women who have histories of migraine often experience relief in the first trimester, although there are some women who experience exacerbation or even first-time migraines during pregnancy (12, 13). There has been some speculation that women who experience migraines are more likely to develop preeclampsia; however, this has not been proven definitively. The association of fetal outcome and migraine has not been explored. Ergotamine tartrate, used to treat migraine headaches, has been associated with fetal wastage and growth retardation in animal studies (10).

Medical Management

The medical management of migraine in nonpregnant patients revolves around administration of one of the following medications: propranolol, a tricyclic antidepressant, phenytoin, methysergide, low dose ergotamines (6), clonidine (10), and fiorinal. These may be supplemented by antiemetics, mild sedatives, and codeine (6). Researchers have also recommended biofeedback, breathing 100% oxygen, attempting to increase the pCO_2 by use of a rebreathing bag, rest in a quiet dark room, yoga, transcendental meditation, hypnotherapy, and acupuncture (7, pp 61–67, 357–361).

In pregnancy ergotamine tartrate is contraindicated because of the animal studies revealing fetal wastage and because some of its derivatives can stimulate uterine contractions (14, p 89). Tricyclic antidepressants have been associated with neonatal withdrawal and should be avoided except for psychiatric indications (14, p 222). Propanolol in long-term therapy has been associated with fetal growth retardation, neonatal hypoglycemia, and bradycardia during the first day of life (14, p 185). Intermittent use to relieve migraine may be safe, but this has not been substantially documented (14, p 185). Methysergide's value is in the *prophylactic* treatment of migraine; as an ergot derivative it is contraindicated during pregnancy (14, p 140). Clonidine has been insubstantially evaluated to identify it as safe for use in pregnancy. Fiorinal contains butalbital (a barbiturate), aspirin, and caffeine and should not be used unless symptoms are severe.

NURSING MANAGEMENT

Nursing care specific for a patient with *migraine headaches:*

☐ Carefully evaluate all patients' complaints of headache; assist with diagnostic tests to determine cause.

☐ Teach patient to avoid stimuli (e.g., food, activities, stress) that trigger migraines.

☐ Teach patient to experiment with alternative therapies to prevent/treat migraines (e.g., yoga, biofeedback, hypnotherapy, guided imagery tapes, relaxation exercises).

☐ Teach comfort measures to use during an acute attack:

— Rest in a dark, quiet room or on the left side;

— Use an ice pack over the affected area; and

— Use medication as ordered.

☐ Encourage patient to maintain adequate nutritional intake, taking antiemetics as ordered, if necessary.

☐ Monitor for signs/symptoms of preeclampsia.

Nursing diagnoses most frequently associated with *migraine headaches:*

☐ Pain.

☐ Knowledge deficit regarding etiology, disease process, treatment, and expected outcome.

☐ Knowledge deficit regarding medication regimen.

☐ Altered nutrition: less than body requirements.

EPILEPSY

Definition

Epilepsy is defined as:

paroxysmal disorders of the nervous system that result in the loss of consciousness or other types of seizures in which convulsive movements or other motor activity, sensory phenomena, or behavioral abnormalities may occur (9, p 507).

The seizures are the result of "paroxysmal excessive neuronal discharges in different parts of the brain" (9, p 507), with the degree of involvement and triggering stimulus related to the type of epilepsy.

Etiology

Epilepsy can be categorized by its etiology and by the types of seizures the patient then experiences. "Idiopathic" or primary epilepsy, which comprises approximately 75% of the epilepsy that affects adults, is that epilepsy in which no definite etiology for the seizures has been determined. The etiology of "symptomatic" or secondary epilepsy is believed to be organic factors, including central nervous system infections, toxic agents or poisons, convulsive agents, parasitic infections, brain defects, metabolic imbalances, expanding brain lesions, cerebral hypoxia, anaphylaxis, degenerative brain disease, and hyperpyrexia (9, p 509).

Signs and Symptoms

Seizures may be convulsive or nonconvulsive, and they may be localized or generalized. The signs and symptoms of the seizures are determined by the type of seizure (see Table 14.3).

Diagnosis

The diagnosis of epilepsy is made with the assistance of a detailed history from the patient and/or the patient's family or friends, physical examination, and appropriate laboratory studies, including CAT scan, EEG, EEG telemetry (alone or in conjunction with video monitoring), serum chemistries (including electrolytes), fasting and postprandial glucoses, and complete blood count.

Maternal and Fetal Outcome

Young adults who suffer unexplained first seizures have a 50–60% chance of recurrence (10, p 362). The course of the pregnant patient's epilepsy throughout pregnancy is difficult to anticipate. In one study it was observed that in 45% of pregnancies the frequency of seizures increased, in 5% the frequency declined, and in 50% the frequency was unchanged (15). If the frequency of seizures increased, this happened more frequently in the first trimester, with a return to pregestational frequency after delivery (12, pp 325–329). Some prediction of the seizure rate during pregnancy can be based on the prepregnancy seizure rate: of those women experiencing more than one seizure a month, more than 60% will have an increased seizure incidence during pregnancy; only 25% of those patients with rare attacks (i.e., less than one every 9 months) can be expected to experience an increased number of seizures (10). Epileptic seizures occur rarely during labor (16).

The mechanism causing an increased number of seizures during pregnancy is uncertain. It has been attributed to the increased water retention and plasma volume that occur in pregnancy (17), to maternal hyperventilation and concurrent pH compensations (18), and to alterations in the concentration and/or absorption of the anticonvulsant medication(s) (12, pp 325–327, 18, 19).

Epileptics have a higher rate of pregnancy complications than nonepileptics, with an increased incidence of hyperemesis, vaginal bleeding, toxemia, and complications of delivery, including failure to progress in labor and failed induction (10, p 362).

In addition to the physical complications associated with maternal epilepsy, there are many psychosocial complications. All patients experiencing seizures have some damage to their self-image. Pregnant patients, with their dramatic and rapid body changes, frequently are particularly vulnerable to alterations in their self-image. Pregnant patients with a history of seizures especially will be anxious during their pregnancies. They may deny their seizures; elect to alter or terminate their medication regimens; fail to keep their prenatal appointments; or experience general anger, frustration, shame, or embarassment.

For any patient the unanticipated experience of a first seizure is very frightening. The pregnant patient will have the additional fear of the seizure's implications for her unborn child.

Infants born to epileptic mothers have less than a 2% chance of developing idiopathic epilepsy (17). Of more concern is the increased incidence of prematurity, intrauterine growth retardation, congenital malformations (10), and altered growth and performance (12, pp 325–327). The malformations, which include cleft lip and palate, congenital heart disease (17), unusual facies, distal phalangeal hypoplasia (20), and microcephaly (21), are believed to be associated with the anticonvulsant medication ingested by the mother. A "fetal hydantoin syndrome" has been described, which includes a variable pattern of craniofacial anomalies (low, broad nasal bridge; epicanthal folds; short, upturned nose; hypertelorism; ptosis; strabismus; prominent, low-set, malformed ears; wide mouth with prominent lips; variations in size and shape of head, including widening of the fontanelles and prominent ridging of the sutures) and limb defects (hypoplasia of distal phalanges and nails, finger-like thumbs, variations in palmar creases and hand markings). In addition, intrauterine growth retardation, which may result in permanent short stature and mild to moderate mental retardation may occur (4).

Table 14.3.

CLASSIFICATION OF SEIZURES[a]

I.	Focal Jacksonian seizures—	Seizure begins with convulsive twitching in one part of body and then involuntary movements spread to other areas.
II.	Sensory focal seizures—	Patient may experience transient abnormal sensations (e.g., numbness, tingling) in specific body areas; seizure may spread to entire body, resulting in loss of consciousness and possibly grand mal seizure.
III.	Grand mal seizure—	Typical sequence of signs and symptoms includes: a. Prodromal phase—vague change in emotional reactivity or affective responses; may last minutes or hours. b. Aura—often occurs at onset of seizure, is a brief sensory experience directly related to point of origin of seizure; (e.g., feeling of weakness, dizziness, strange sensation in arm or leg, numbness, or unpleasant odor); usually, aura precedes seizure by only a few seconds. c. Epileptic cry—sound caused by thoracic and abdominal spasm that expels air through narrowed spastic glottis. d. Tonic convulsions—usually last a few seconds; muscles are held in rigid tonic contractions; respirations may be suspended, face becomes cyanotic, eyes are opened widely with pupils dilated and fixed, jaws are fixed and hands clenched. e. Clonic convulsion—respirations become jerky and stertorous, jerky movements occur, saliva may be blown from mouth (creating froth at lips), urinary or fecal incontinence may occur, lips and inside of cheeks may be bitten. f. Postclonic phase—convulsion gradually subsides, excessive motor activity ceases, respirations become more normal, patient slowly returns to consciousness. g. Postictal state—general fatigue, confusion, headache, possibly specific residual neurologic symptoms (hemiparesis or monoparesis) that may last few minutes to several hours; patient may sleep for several hours, awakening with a headache, depression, nausea, sore muscles, and possibly complete amnesia for the seizure episode except some memories of prodromal phase or aura; seizures may vary in intensity and frequency from many times daily to once or twice yearly.
IV.	Petit mal seizures—	Usually affect children age 3–10; rare onset after age 20; patient experiences brief lapse or loss of consciousness and stops any activity and stares blankly; may blink rapidly, deviate eyes and head, or make minor movements of lips and hands; occasionally may stagger few steps, droop head, or lose bladder control; after completion of attack patient is immediately alert and pursues previous activities; seizures may last from 15–90 seconds; patients may have a few attacks daily or every few days; some patients may have hundreds every day.
V.	Myoclonic seizures—	Patient experiences sudden involuntary contractions of single muscle or small groups of muscles of trunk and extremities; may occur in petit mal or grand mal seizures.
VI.	Akinetic seizures—	Patient experiences sudden loss of muscle tone in all muscles of body; can cause patient to fall to the ground; may be accompanied by lapse of consciousness, but typically patient is on feet again so quickly that there is no awareness of the loss of consciousness; may be associated with petit mal or grand mal seizure.
VII.	Psychomotor attacks—	Characterized by brief lapse of consciousness during which patient does not fall or lose consciousness; last longer than petit mal seizures (30 seconds to 2 minutes); has a larger range of muscular movements than petit mal and a deeper and longer clouding of consciousness, including amnesia during attack; automatic activity occurs that may include asocial or inappropriate behavior.
VIII.	Status epilepticus—	Successively recurring grand mal seizures between which patient does not regain consciousness; if not terminated death will ensue; may be precipitated by sudden withdrawal of anticonvulsant medication.

[a]Adapted from Luckmann J, Sorensen K: *Medical Surgical Nursing: A Psychophysiologic Approach.* WB Saunders, 1974, pp 508–509.

Studies of the association between anticonvulsants and fetal malformations have shown a greater incidence of malformations in infants born to epileptics on anticonvulsants than in those not on anticonvulsants (22, 12, pp 325–327). However, because the various studies are inconsistent as to their methodology and reporting mechanisms (e.g., anticonvulsant plasma levels, type of seizures, frequency of seizures pre-pregnancy and during pregnancy, and multidrug therapy), it is difficult to draw absolute conclusions on this issue. The literature suggests the anticonvulsant with the highest association of malformations is phenytoin (12, 23), but phenobarbital, valproic acid (10), primidone (14), and trimethadione (12, 14) have also been associated with fetal malformations. Phenytoin and phenobarbital are heavily implicated, particularly when given concurrently.

Phenytoin and phenobarbital have been implicated in neonatal hemorrhage (10, 12, 24, 25). Many infants whose mothers received phenytoin or drugs metabolized to barbiturates have been shown to have a coagulation defect similar to that of vitamin K deficiency (12). Such bleeding usually occurs in the first 24 hours after birth (12). Occasionally, it involves somewhat unusual sites, including the pleural or abdominal cavities (12) in addition to the intraperitoneal and intracranial cavities (25). Some hemorrhages actually have occurred to the fetus while in utero.

The final potential difficulty for the infant born to a mother on antiepileptic drugs is withdrawal from the drugs themselves. A number of investigators have observed signs and symptoms of withdrawal in those infants whose mothers were treated with phenobarbital (26, 27). An additional group of investigators observed signs and symptoms of withdrawal in infants whose mothers had received mephobarbital (24, 26) (see Chapter 19).

Medical Management

For all patients the medical management of secondary epilepsy is directed at eradicating the underlying cause, while in primary epilepsy management is directed at achieving a seizure-free state, primarily with the use of anticonvulsant medications. Medical management of the pregnant patient's epilepsy is directed at maintaining her in a seizure-free state using anticonvulsants in as low a dose as possible. Anticonvulsant requirements have been shown to increase during pregnancy and decline after delivery (12, pp 325–327). Possible explanations for this phenomenon include the following:

1. The nausea and vomiting of the first trimester preclude the achieval of therapeutic levels.
2. The increasing weight and extracellular fluid volume dilute existing levels.
3. The increased metabolic rate of the maternal liver more rapidly metabolizes the anticonvulsant.
4. Additional metabolism of the anticonvulsant is provided by the fetus.
5. Folate supplements (which are particularly necessary for the patient on barbiturates and

drugs of the hydantoin group because of their interference with the absorption of folic acid) are administered to the extent that *they* then interfere with the absorption of phenytoin (12, pp 325–327).
6. The alterations in the pregnant woman's gastrointestinal tract (increased gastric and intestinal emptying time and increased pH and buffering capacity) all serve to affect the absorption rate of the oral anticonvulsants (28).
7. The general increase in the pregnant woman's metabolic rate (28).

Some authors encourage at least monthly monitoring of the anticonvulsant plasma levels throughout the pregnancy and puerperium (12, pp 325–327, 17). However, this then raises the issue of what to do with the data so gained. These authors argue for attempting to use the laboratory data as a guide to achieve therapeutic levels, while others are adamant that evaluation of the patient's clinical presentation (i.e., frequency and severity of seizures) should be the prevailing determinant (18). The most rational approach appears to be that of determining the prepregnancy plasma level that has maintained the patient in a seizure-free state, with subsequent monthly determinations of plasma level and then dosage adjustments to maintain the patient's level consistent with that already demonstrated to be therapeutic.

Folic acid should be administered to meet the increased requirements pregnancy imposes, but the anticonvulsant plasma levels and folic acid plasma levels should *both* be monitored to assure that neither drug is interfering with the other's absorption.

The infant should be assessed carefully for signs and symptoms of hemorrhage or withdrawal. One author (17) suggests administering 5 mg vitamin K intramuscularly to the mother each week for the last month of pregnancy. Another author encourages checking the prothrombin time of the cord blood at delivery. If it is less than 10% or if there is any evidence of bleeding during the neonatal period, this doctor recommends administration to the infant of vitamin K intravenously and transfusion of fresh frozen plasma or concentrates of factors II, VII, IX, and X (12).

NURSING MANAGEMENT

Nursing care specific for a patient with *epilepsy:*

☐ Assist with diagnosis of epilepsy and categorization of type by assisting with history, physical examination, and laboratory tests.

☐ Teach the patient the importance of taking prescribed medication as ordered to prevent seizures.

☐ Assist with monitoring anticonvulsant levels throughout pregnancy.

NURSING MANAGEMENT

- ☐ Monitor the patient for conditions associated with epilepsy (e.g., hyperemesis gravidarum, preeclampsia, anxiety, intrauterine growth retardation).
- ☐ Teach the patient signs/symptoms of preterm labor and how to report them.
- ☐ Encourage the patient to consume a diet high in folic acid and to take folic acid supplements as ordered; monitor folic acid levels as required.
- ☐ Administer vitamin K to the mother as ordered.
- ☐ Administer medications as required during a seizure:
  - — Valium, 10 mg intravenously over 2 minutes, then 2 mg/minute until seizure stops.
  - — Fifty percent dextrose and loading dose of a long-acting anticonvulsant as ordered.
- ☐ Prepare for general anesthesia if seizure is not controlled with intravenous medication.
- ☐ Prepare for use of a cooling blanket and curare if hyperthermia and rhabdomyolysis are present; protect the patient's safety (e.g., EKG monitor with alarms on, mechanical ventilation with ventilator alarms on, etc).
- ☐ Request the pediatrician to attend the birth; observe the baby for bleeding, congenital anomalies, or withdrawal from the anticonvulsant.
- ☐ Administer a double dose of vitamin K to the neonate as ordered.

Nursing diagnoses most frequently associated with *epilepsy*:
- ☐ Grieving related to potential/actual loss of infant or birth of an imperfect child.
- ☐ Ineffective family coping: compromised.
- ☐ Ineffective individual coping.
- ☐ Potential altered parenting.
- ☐ Disturbance in body image, self-esteem.
- ☐ Knowledge deficit regarding etiology, disease process, treatment, and expected outcome.
- ☐ Knowledge deficit regarding medication regimen.
- ☐ Anxiety/fear.
- ☐ Potential for trauma related to seizures.

MYASTHENIA GRAVIS

Definition

Myasthenia gravis is a disease causing weakness and easy fatigability of the striated muscles and is believed to be an autoimmune disease (29). Myasthenia occurs slightly more often among women than men, with the onset of symptoms usually between ages 20 and 40.

Etiology

The muscular weakness is attributed by many researchers to the presence of a circulating serum gamma globulin antiacetylcholine receptor immunoglobulin G (antiAChRIgG), which blocks acetylcholine receptors at the myoneural junction, thus inhibiting the contractile capability of skeletal muscle (29). In addition, the postsynaptic membrane has been noted to have loss or modification of the normally fine infolding clefts, so the distance for the acetylcholine to travel is increased (30). Other researchers have suggested that the reticulendothelial system, specifically the thymus, may react to end-plate protein as if it were a foreign protein when there is a disorder of the thymus (31).

Signs and Symptoms

Myasthenia gravis is characterized by weakness of the skeletal muscles, intensified by exercise and partially relieved by rest, and usually becomes more intense as the day progresses. All skeletal muscles or one group or a single muscle may be affected. The extraocular muscles are affected at some time in almost all myasthenics, and ptosis is the most common initial symptom. Myasthenia's course varies from patient to patient, generally with series of remissions and exacerbations. Occasionally, there is a rapid progression of involvement leading to death (due to respiratory failure, aspiration, or sepsis) or a gradual progression to a steady state of weakness (9, pp 504–505). The weakness affects the voluntary muscles, presenting difficulties in walking, climbing, swallowing, chewing, talking, breathing (due to weakness of the accessory muscles), coughing, holding the head up, brushing the teeth, and so on.

Exacerbations can present in the form of myasthenic crisis, nonreactive crisis, or cholinergic crisis. Because the treatment for each type of crisis is different (and if inappropriate may exacerbate the crisis), it is important to distinguish the nature of the crisis and to institute treatment promptly and appropriately. (See Table 14.4 for signs and symp-

Table 14.4.
DISTINCTION OF MYASTHENIC, CHOLINERGIC, AND NONREACTIVE CRISES: SIGNS AND
SYMPTOMS AND TREATMENT[a]

MYASTHENIC CRISIS	CHOLINERGIC CRISIS	NONREACTIVE CRISIS

Acute intensification of symptoms:
  Generalized muscular weakness
  Dyspnea
  Ptosis, diplopia
  Anxiety, restlessness
  Apathy
  Convulsions
Symptoms less intense with administration of more anticholinesterase medication or trial dose of edrophonium chloride
Treatment is increased anticholinesterase dose and supportive therapy as appropriate
	Overdose of anticholinesterases produces the following symptoms:
	  Increased salivation and secretions
	  Anorexia
	  Nausea
	  Abdominal cramps
	  Diarrhea
	  Diaphoresis
	  Anxiety
	  Convulsions
	  Pupillary constriction
	  Blurred vision
	  Pulmonary edema
	  Irritability
	  Headache
	  Confusion
	  Generalized muscular weakness
	Treatment consists of withholding all anticholinesterase medications, providing other supportive care, and possibly hospitalization with mechanical ventilation and parenteral nutrition
		Symptoms are the same as in myasthenic crisis, but there is no reduction in severity with administration of more anticholinesterase medications or edrophonium chloride
		Treatment is supportive therapy and possibly hospitalization with mechanical ventilation and parenteral nutrition

[a]Adapted from Szobar: *Crises in Myasthenia Gravis.* Hafner, 1970, p 50.

toms of the crises.) Myasthenic crises occur when the patient develops an acute intensification of symptoms and requires marked increases of anticholinesterase drugs. Cholinergic crises occur when the patient has received an overdose of anticholinesterase medications. Nonreactive crises are those that occur when the patient has experienced an intensification of symptoms that do not respond to anticholinesterase medications.

Diagnosis

The diagnosis of myasthenia gravis is made by administering edrophonium chloride intravenously after an initial assessment of skeletal muscle strength. Muscle strength is then reassessed 1 minute after the administration of the edrophonium; a transient increase in muscle strength following the edrophonium is considered confirmation of the diagnosis. For those patients known or suspected to be pregnant, edrophonium should not be administered intravenously since uterine irritability may result. Intramuscular neostigmine bromide may be used instead (31). Other diagnostic tests include electrical stimulation, which demonstrates fatigability of the muscle; electromyography; infrared pupillography; infrared nystagmography; electronystagmography; and immunological studies to test the presence of antiAChRIgG (30). In addition,

the use of motor point biopsy currently is being evaluated (30).

Maternal and Fetal Outcome

The course of myasthenia gravis in pregnancy is unpredictable; remission, exacerbation, and no change all have been observed. In a 30-year review of 292 pregnancies, exacerbation in the antepartum period occurred in 45% of the pregnancies, with postpartum exacerbation occurring in 30% of the pregnancies (29).

Maternal outcome is very dependent on the scrupulous attention to and management of the disease. Plauche reports nine maternal deaths among 202 myasthenics reviewed from 1938–1968; one because of cholinergic overdose crisis, four from nonreactive crisis, three from exacerbations of the myasthenia, and one from an unknown cause. Throughout the pregnancy and puerperium, careful management of anticholinesterase drug dosage, prevention and treatment of sepsis, education of the patient, and availability of intensive care facilities improve the possibilities for good maternal outcome.

It should be noted that these patients are particularly prone to respiratory infections because of their impaired ability to clear secretions. With advanced myasthenia they may also be nutritionally

Table 14.5.

ANTICHOLINESTERASE MEDICATIONS

MEDICATION	DOSE	DURATION	COMMENTS
		Maternal	
Neostigmine	15 mg every 2–3 hours p.o.	2–3 hours	Dose is titrated to muscle strength; serial recordings of hand strength may be performed.
Pyridostigmine	60 mg every 3–4 hours p.o.	3–4 hours	Medication is available in time-span capsules, has fewer gastrointestinal side effects

Intrapartally, parenteral route is preferrable for both medications, using the following formula:

0.5 mg neostigmine i.v. = 1.5 mg neostigmine i.m. = 15 mg neostigmine p.o. = 60 mg pyridostigmine p.o. 1/30th of oral dose may be given to augment strength in labor (given parenterally)

MEDICATION	DOSE	DURATION	COMMENTS
		Neonatal	
Neostigmine	0.1 mg i.m. or s.c. every 2–3 hours 1.0 mg p.o. every 2–3 hours	2–3 hours	Onset of symptoms may be delayed until 48/96 hours of age; condition lasts about 3 weeks, though may require medication up until 5 weeks.
Pyridostigmine	0.15 mg i.m. or s.c. every 2–3 hours 4.0 mg p.o. every 2–3 hours	Oral medication should precede feeding by 30 minutes, parenteral by 10–20 minutes.	Dosage should be reduced gradually over time, while also increasing the intervals between doses. Parenteral route may have the value of decreased likelihood of regurgitation, especially early in the disease. If diarrhea develops, decrease the dose; as in adults, pyridostigmine has fewer gastrointestinal side effects.

impaired, making them even less prepared to fight infection.

Antepartally, the myasthenic is at risk for exacerbation because of the ever increasing energy and nutritional demands of the pregnancy. Intrapartally, the myasthenic patient can anticipate difficulty in pushing. The puerperium has been identified as a particularly high risk time for the mother (29). It is speculated that this is because the hard physical work of labor, lack of rest and sleep, and general exhaustion may precipitate exacerbation of the myasthenia (30).

Fetal outcome does not appear linked to myasthenia. A spontaneous abortion rate of 4.7% has been observed, which is within normal limits. Neonatal outcome, however, is a separate issue. Transient neonatal myasthenia can occur because of the transplacental passage of the antiacetylcholine receptor antibodies from the mother to her infant (29). Its appearance may be delayed for up to 48 hours, possibly because of the concurrent transplacental passage of the maternal anticholinesterase drugs (29). Researchers have identified antiAChRIgG in infants of myasthenics, with high titers found up until day 12 of life and dropping to minimal levels by day 21 (32). Transient neonatal myasthenia definitely was observed in 17.7% of the infants. The severity of neonatal myasthenia does

not necessarily correlate to the severity and duration of the mother's illness (33). It is not possible to draw any definite conclusions regarding an association between myasthenia and prematurity. Congenital myasthenia occurs very rarely and is not associated with maternal myasthenia (33).

Medical Management

Recommendations for women contemplating pregnancy center primarily on attainment of optimum condition prior to conception, with weaning of corticosteroid therapy and preconceptual consideration of thymectomy and plasmapheresis (30).

Medical management of myasthenia during pregnancy centers around appropriate medication administration, rapid and aggressive intervention in the case of infection, and intensive supportive therapies (including respirator, intravenous therapy, tube feedings, etc.) when myasthenic crises occur.

Thymectomy and plasmapheresis are medical modalities also used in treating myasthenia. Thymectomy serves to remove the vestigial thymus, which may be producing the antibodies to the acetylcholine receptors, and plasmapheresis may serve to remove some of the anitAChRIgG in the circulatory system. (See Table 14.5 for a discussion of anticholinesterase medications.) However, thymectomy during pregnancy should be avoided except in the case of thymoma or intractable myasthenic crisis. Plasmapheresis can be conducted if done cautiously with careful attention to volume status (30).

Intrapartally, medical management includes shortening of the second stage by use of forceps and episiotomy, careful observation for signs of crisis, and parenteral administration of anticholinesterase medications (31). The use of narcotics and sedatives may precipitate respiratory arrest. Therefore, extreme caution must be exercised, including the administration of a small test dose before giving a "normal" dose. In addition, general anesthesia should be avoided, if possible, because many general anesthetics require liver and plasma cholines-terases to be metabolized. Also, the myasthenic patient is at very high risk for postoperative pneumonia. If general anesthesia must be used, nitrous oxide/oxygen, cyclopropane, or thiopental sodium/nitrous oxide/oxygen may be selected (31). No anticholinesterase medications should be administered if the patient is unconscious. Magnesium sulfate has been shown to diminish the depolarizing action of acetylcholine, and aminoglycosides have been shown to have the potential to block the neuromuscular junction, so both should be avoided as much as possible (29).

If it becomes necessary to induce labor, this should be done when hospital facilities are at peak efficiency.

NURSING MANAGEMENT

Nursing management specific for a patient with *myasthenia gravis*:

☐ Teach the patient the importance of taking medication at scheduled intervals; advise her that drug regimen may be altered during pregnancy.

☐ Teach the patient to notify the physician immediately if signs of myasthenic or cholinergic crisis occur.

☐ Schedule clinic appointments and tests close to the same time to conserve the patient's energy; make appointments late enough in the morning to allow the patient to compensate for weakness; encourage family/friends to assist her in transportation.

☐ Encourage the patient to eat small, frequent meals; a soft or liquid high protein diet may be easier to manage.

☐ Advise the patient that cooler environments and cold liquids or ice cream will sometimes combat signs of weakness.

☐ Administer anticholinesterase drugs to the hospitalized patient at the correct time.

☐ Time induction of labor when patient is strongest and hospital facilities are at their peak efficiency.

☐ Anticipate fatigue during labor; assess and document muscle strength carefully and regularly using predetermined parameters (e.g., grip, ptosis, swallowing, etc.). Administer additional anticholinesterase medication as required.

☐ Administer sedatives, narcotics, and tranquilizers cautiously and in small doses; ensure that an airway and ambu bag are available at the patient's bedside.

☐ Anticipate forceps delivery.

☐ Request the pediatrician to attend the delivery.

☐ Observe for neonatal myasthenia gravis.

☐ Assist the mother to rest as much as needed in the postpartum period:
  — Schedule activities to allow rest periods;
  — Limit visitors as required; and
  — Encourage and support the patient's mothering efforts, but acknowledge her limits and provide infant care if necessary.

☐ Assist the patient/family to make appropriate plans for care of mother and baby; make appropriate referrals.

Nursing diagnoses most frequently associated with *myasthenia gravis*:

☐ Anticipatory grieving related to actual/perceived threat to self.

☐ Ineffective family coping: compromised.

☐ Self-care deficit: feeding, bathing/hygiene, dressing, grooming, toileting.

☐ Disturbance in body image, self-esteem.

☐ Knowledge deficit regarding etiology, disease process, treatment, and expected outcome.

☐ Knowledge deficit regarding medication regimen.

☐ Potential for infection.

☐ Impaired gas exchange.

☐ Altered nutrition: less than body requirements.

☐ Potential altered parenting.

ABNORMALITIES OF THE SPINAL COLUMN— PARAPLEGIA AND QUADRIPLEGIA

Definition

Paraplegia is paralysis of both legs and the lower portion of the body, and quadriplegia is paralysis affecting all four extremities.

Etiology

Quadriplegia and paraplegia occur as a result of damage to the spinal cord from injury, disease, or surgery; birth trauma can result in paraplegia or quadriplegia, and certain congenital defects (e.g., myelomeningocele) also can contribute, depending upon the level of the lesion (9). The spinal cord injury causes "complete destruction of the nerve cells, disruption of the reflex arc, and flaccid paralysis of the muscles supplied from the destroyed segments of the cord" (34).

Signs and Symptoms

Signs and symptoms of paraplegia and quadriplegia center primarily around the inability to move an extremity or extremities and the loss of sensation in the affected area. (34).

Diagnosis

Diagnosis of spinal cord injury is made by physical and neurological examination, x-rays of the spine, lumbar puncture, and myelogram (34). It is extremely important to diagnose the nature and level of the spinal cord injury accurately to determine if treatment is possible.

Maternal and Fetal Outcome

Spinal cord lesions very rarely prevent conception (35). Maternal outcome, as measured by the ability to tolerate the antepartum period and to survive childbirth, largely is dependent of the level of the spinal cord injury. Of significant concern for those patients with high spinal cord injury (at or above T6) is the development of autonomic hyperreflexia (35, 36). Certain stimuli (including visceral distention, uterine contractions, stimulation of pain receptors, and stimulation of the skin) have the ability to trigger a "mass reflex response." Afferent impulses ascend the spinal cord and result in an autonomic response that originates from the lateral horn cells. Vasoconstriction and hypertension result, with the vagus nerve stimulating bradycardia as a compensatory mechanism. However, because of the spinal cord lesion, those impulses that would normally produce further compensation in the form of vasodilation and decreased blood pressure are blocked (35, 36). Signs and symptoms of hyperreflexia include bradycardia, flushing above the level of the lesion, diaphoresis, tingling, nasal stuffiness, pilomotor erection, headache, and severe hypertension (e.g., 250/150), potentially resulting in cerebrovascular accident, brain damage, and death (35, 36).

Quadriplegics and paraplegics have a very high incidence of urinary tract infections and pressure sores. While not at greater risk for anemia than other pregnant women, they are made more vulnerable to sepsis and tissue breakdown as a consequence of their immobility. Their immobility also increases the risk for respiratory tract infections and thrombophlebitis (35).

Fetal outcome generally can be anticipated to be good. The primary exceptions are the unanticipated home delivery or preterm delivery because of the patient's inability to perceive uterine contractions. Poor outcome also may occur if the mother sustains the injury resulting in spinal cord damage with accompanying anoxia during the pregnancy. Quadriplegics and paraplegics also are at risk for dysfunctional labor, potentially harming the fetus unless the progress of labor is monitored carefully. (35).

Medical Management

Medical management of paraplegia and quadriplegia is directed to optimizing function—providing treatment if possible, rehabilitation if not. At the same time, attention is directed to preventing and treating complications: urinary tract infections, renal calculi, pressure sores, anemia, respiratory tract infections, preterm labor, unanticipated home delivery, dystocia, supine hypotensive syndrome, orthostatic hypotension, and autonomic hyperreflexia. Some authorities discuss use of prophylactic antibiotics in pregnancy to prevent urinary tract infections (e.g., methenamine mandelate, 1 g orally, four times daily, in conjunction with an acidifying agent—e.g., ascorbic acid, 500 mg orally, four times daily) (35, 36). Any signs of infection in any system are followed with cultures and aggressive treatment appropriate to pregnancy.

Treatment of anemia is slightly controversial because of the constipating effects of oral iron supplements. Careful determination of the need for iron supplementation should precede any therapy. In the event supplementation is required, a parenteral route may be considered. The hematocrit should be monitored routinely. Several authorities even recommend blood transfusions (12, 37).

To prevent or decrease the likelihood of preterm or unanticipated term delivery, the condition of the cervix is evaluated at each antepartum visit after the 28th week, and some centers elect to hospitalize the patient beginning at 32 weeks' gestation to observe her for signs and symptoms of labor (12, 37).

Autonomic hyperreflexia must be differentiated from preeclampsia, and it is then treated primarily by eliminating the triggering stimuli (e.g., distended bladder, treatment/prevention of urinary tract infection or fecal impaction). In the intrapartum period a Foley catheter may be used even for the patient with bladder training, and it is virtually mandatory for the patient with a high lesion. Any insertion of rectal or urethral catheters or performance of pelvic examinations should be preceded by use of a topical anesthetic to avoid autonomic hyperreflexia (35, 36). Other measures include administration of ganglionic blocking agents, antihypertensives, and, particularly during the intrapartum period, close monitoring of blood pressure and pulse, with immediate access to surgical intervention should it be necessary.

Dystocia because of the inability of the patient to bear down may necessitate the use of forceps (12) or possibly cesarean section. After episiotomy, one author recommends repairing with nonabsorbable or delayed absorbable suture material because of poor absorption in patients with spinal injuries (38).

Because the potential for supine hypotensive syndrome is increased in patients with spinal cord injury, the patient should never be positioned on her back. When the patient assumes an upright position, she should proceed slowly and should be observed for signs of orthostatic hypotension.

NURSING MANAGEMENT

Nursing care specific for a patient with
paraplegia or quadriplegia:

☐ Evaluate the patient's ability to carry out activities of daily living; reinforce teaching, as needed; encourage frequent position changes, teaching the patient to avoid supine position.

☐ Observe for signs/symptoms of orthostatic hypotension when assisting patient to an upright position (e.g., nausea, perspiration, pallor dizziness).

☐ Teach the patient measures to prevent/recognize complications associated with paraplegia/quadriplegia:

— Coughing/deep breathing to prevent pooling of secretions in the respiratory tract.

— Use of support hose and periodic rest in the left lateral position with legs elevated to prevent thrombophlebitis; teach signs/symptoms of thrombophlebitis and how to report them.

— Consuming a diet high in fiber and fluids and adhering to previously established elimination patterns to prevent constipation.

— Self-palpation for contractions several times daily beginning at 28 weeks' gestation to prevent unrecognized labor.

☐ Assist the patient to develop a reliable communication system with medical providers/family in case she experiences signs of labor or complications.

☐ Encourage the patient to consume a diet high in protein, calories, and vitamins to prevent hypoproteinemia, and high in iron to prevent the need for iron supplementation.

☐ Assist the patient/family to make realistic plans for care of the baby; make appropriate referrals.

☐ Teach the patient the need for weekly pelvic examinations to detect signs/symptoms of labor beginning at 28 weeks and the possibility of hospital admission at 32 weeks to prevent unattended delivery.

☐ During labor, ensure that bowel and bladder remain empty. Use enema or urinary catheter as needed, ensuring that procedures are done with topical anesthesia.

☐ Monitor contraction status carefully to determine progression in labor. Limit the number of vaginal examinations, performing them under local anesthesia.

☐ Prepare for forceps delivery.

☐ If autonomic hyperreflexia occurs:

— Alleviate triggering stimulus immediately;

— Monitor vital signs frequently;

— Administer antihypertensives as ordered; and

— Prepare for cesarean section if needed.

Nursing diagnoses most frequently associated
with paraplegia or quadriplegia:

☐ Self-care deficit: feeding, bathing/hygiene, dressing, grooming, toileting.

NURSING MANAGEMENT

☐ Impaired skin integrity.
☐ Ineffective family coping: compromised.
☐ Disturbance in body image, self-esteem.
☐ Anticipatory grieving related to actual/perceived threat to self.

☐ Potential for infection.
☐ Altered patterns of urinary elimination.
☐ Altered sexuality patterns.
☐ Knowledge deficit regarding etiology, disease process, treatment, and expected outcome.

KYPHOSIS AND SCOLIOSIS

Definition

Kyphosis is the abnormally increased convexity in the curvature of the thoracic spine. Scoliosis is the lateral deviation in the normally straight vertical line of the spine (9, pp 1154, 1239). Kyphoscoliosis is the combination of both. Kyphoscoliosis occurs in about 1% of the population and in pregnancy has a reported incidence of 1:1400 to 1:12,000 (39).

Etiology

Causes of scoliosis include rickets, neuromuscular disorders, and vertebral disorders, but in 90% of cases it is idiopathic (9, p 1239). Girls are affected by idiopathic scoliosis 10 times more frequently than boys (9, p 1239). Kyphosis may be congenital or caused by disease—including tuberculosis, syphilis, and malignancy—or a compression fracture (40).

Signs and Symptoms

Scoliosis is characterized by poor posture: forward head and shoulders, dorsal kyphosis, winged scapulae, depressed chest, narrowed costal angle, lumbar lordosis, and sagging abdomen, possibly associated with disturbances in other weight-bearing areas (40). With increased lateral curves, other typical findings include difference in height of shoulders, one breast higher than the other, posterior bulging of the rib cage, difference in the distance between the hanging arms and the body, and the prominence of one hip (40). Some individuals experience functional symptoms, such as fatigue in the lumbar area, particularly after long periods of sitting or standing. Kyphosis is characterized by the exaggerated curvature of the thoracic spine, sometimes referred to as "hunchback" or "humpback." Kyphoscoliosis is characterized by a lateral curvature of the spine accompanied by an anteroposterior hump.

Diagnosis

Diagnosis begins with careful and detailed history taking, including questions regarding childhood diseases or injuries to determine if the deformity is congenital or the consequence of an illness or injury. Next, a physical examination based on observation of the patient standing and walking is performed. Complete spinal x-rays and a CAT scan are obtained to provide a three-dimensional sense of the deformity.

Maternal and Fetal Outcome

Because scoliosis or scoliosis associated with kyphosis has more implications for pregnancy than does kyphosis alone, the rest of this discussion centers on kyphoscoliosis and pregnancy. Maternal and fetal outcomes are dependent on the degree and location of the curvature (39). The deformities occurring higher on the vertebral column are associated with a higher incidence of complications because of compromise of cardiorespiratory function. Those curvatures located lower on the vertebral column are associated with more obstetric complications, including malpresentation and dystocia (39). The high curvatures result in "distortion and fixation of the thoracic cage with compression of the thoracic viscera resulting in diminished lung volume, ranging from large areas of segmental or lobar collapse" (39) and cause the lungs to be more vulnerable to infection. As the third trimester progresses and through the duration of the intrapartum period, the patient with a high level curvature increasingly is at risk for cardiorespiratory compromise because of the ever-enlarging uterus and nondistensible thorax. The curvatures occurring lower on the vertebral column may lead to increasing abdominal discomfort as the uterus grows because of the reduced height of the abdominal cavity. Backache and sensations of breathlessness would be expected to be increased in those pregnant patients with kyphoscoliosis; however, one study documented this in only 20% of the patients reviewed (41). The spinal deformity can cause abnormal fetal lie or malpresentation. Fetal outcome is dependent on appropriate and timely maternal care and intervention (e.g., administration of antibiotics for respiratory infections, initiation of oxygen therapy, etc.) and surgical intervention in the case of malpresentation and dystocia. There is a high incidence of low birth weight (less than 2500 g) associated with infants born to mothers with kyphoscoliosis (42).

Medical Management

Medical management during pregnancy is not directed at attempting to correct the spinal defect. If indicated by family history, genetic counseling may be advised. Baseline information about the patient is obtained, including cardiopulmonary function tests, arterial blood gas measurements, careful determination of the level and degree of the deformity, and x-ray pelvimetry (39). Particularly

careful monitoring of the patient's cardiorespiratory status should occur in the third trimester.

During labor, if a cesarean section is not anticipated immediately, the patient should remain in an upright position with supplemental oxygen on hand. Frequent vital signs, including central venous pressure, arterial blood gases, cardiac monitoring, and fetal heart monitoring should be obtained. Labor progress should be monitored carefully. The patient with a malpresentation almost certainly will require a cesarean section. General anesthesia with endotracheal intubation may be indicated to assure ventilatory assistance intra- and postoperatively. Depending on the level of the curvature, a classical cesarean section may be necessary because of the inaccessibility of the lower uterine segment (39).

NURSING MANAGEMENT

Nursing care specific for a patient with kyphosis/scoliosis:

☐ Refer the patient for genetic counseling if appropriate.

☐ Monitor the patient's cardiopulmonary status, especially in the third trimester and during labor.

☐ Encourage a diet high in iron, protein, and vitamin C to optimize the oxygen-carrying capacity of the blood.

☐ Teach proper body mechanics; encourage frequent rest periods.

☐ Anticipate intensive maternal monitoring during labor (e.g., electrocardiogram, central venous pressure, and arterial blood gas monitoring).

☐ Encourage the mother to labor in an upright position.

☐ Be prepared for cesarean section, as required.

Nursing diagnoses most frequently associated with kyphosis/scoliosis:

☐ Impaired gas exchange.

☐ Potential for infection.

☐ Spiritual distress.

☐ Disturbance in body image, self-esteem.

☐ Self-care deficit: feeding, bathing/hygiene, dressing, grooming, toileting.

☐ Anticipatory grieving related to actual/perceived threat to self.

REFERENCES

1. Buckley KA: Common discomforts of pregnancy. In Buckley KA, Kulb NW (eds): *Handbook of Maternal-Newborn Nursing*. New York, John Wiley and Sons, 1983, p 178.
2. Niswander K: Prenatal care. In Benson R (ed): *Current Obstetric and Gynecologic Diagnosis and Treatment*. Los Altos, CA, Lange, 1978, pp 591–592.
3. Neeson J, Stockdale C: *The Practitioner's Handbook of Ambulatory Ob/Gyn*. New York, John Wiley and Sons, 1981, p 4.
4. Dalessio D: Neurologic diseases. In Burrow GN, Ferris TF (eds): *Medical Complications During Pregnancy*. Philadelphia, Saunders, 1982, pp 435–436.
5. Taylor J, Ballenger S: *Neurological Dysfunctions and Nursing Interventions*. New York, McGraw-Hill, 1980, p 367.

6. Ambielli M: Drug stop migraine headache: current therapy. *Neurosurg Nurs* 14(4):203–205, 1982.
7. Wilkinson M: Recognition and management of migraine. *Practitioner* 227(1377):357–361, 1983.
8. Goodman L, Gilman A (eds). *The Pharmacological Basis of Therapeutics*, ed. 5, New York, Macmillan, 1975, p 622.
9. Luckmann J, Sorensen K: *Medical Surgical Nursing: A Psychophysiologic Approach*. Philadelphia, WB Saunders, 1974, p 804.
10. Bentley W: Neurological disorders. In Abrams R, Wexler P (eds): *Medical Care of the Pregnant Patient*. Boston, Little, Brown & Co, 1983, pp 357–372.
11. Migraine and mothers to be. *Emergency Med* 15(1):63–66, 1983.

12. Aminoff M: Neurological disorders and pregnancy. *Am J Obstet Gynecol* 132(5):328–329, 1978.
13. Migraine in pregnancy. *Briefs* 42(2):26–27, 1978.
14. Berkowitz RL, Coustan DR, Mochizuki TK (eds): *Handbook for Prescribing Medications During Pregnancy*. Boston, Little Brown & Co, 1981.
15. Knight AH, Rhind EG: Epilepsy and pregnancy: a study of 153 pregnancies in 59 patients. *Epilepsia* 16:99, 1975.
16. Willson JR, Carrington E: *Obstetrics and Gynecology*. St. Louis, Mosby, 1979, pp 220–241.
17. Rovinsy J: Diseases complicating pregnancy. In Romney S, Gray M, Little AB, Merrill J, Quilligan E, Slander R (eds): *Gynecologic and Obstetric Health Care of Women*. New York, McGraw-Hill, 1981, Chapter 31.
18. Hill R: The advisability of increasing antiepileptic drug dosage during pregnancy. In Janz D, Dam M, Richeus A, Bossi L, Helge H, Schmidt D (eds): *Epilepsy, Pregnancy, and the Child*. New York, Raven Press, 1982, p 163.
19. Hawkins DF: Human teratogenesis and related problems. In *Drugs in Pregnancy*. New York, Churchill-Livingstone, 1983, p 81.
20. Hanson J, Myrinthapoulos N, Harvey M, Smith D: Risks to offspring of women treated with hydantoin. *J Pediatr* 89(4):662–668, 1976.
21. Rating D, Jager E: Postnatal development of children of epileptic parents. In Selbeck GG, Doose H (eds): *Epilepsy: Problems of Marriage, Pregnancy, and Genetic Counselling*. New York, Thieme Stratton, 1981, pp 36–42.
22. Annegers J, Elvebank L, Hasuser W, Kurland L: Do anticonvulsants have a teratogenic effect? *Arch Neurol* 31(5):364–373, 1974.
23. Benson R: *Current Obstetric and Gynecologic Diagnosis and Treatments*. Los Altos, CA, Lange, 1978.
24. Hill R, Verniand W, Horning M, McCully N, Margan N: Infants exposed in utero to antiepileptic drugs. *Am J Dis Child* 127(5):645–653.
25. Speidel BP, Meadow S: Maternal epilepsy and abnormalities of the fetus and newborn. *Lancet* ii:839–843, 1972.
26. Rementeria J (ed): *Drug Abuse in Pregnancy and Neonatal Effects*. St. Louis, Mosby, 1977.
27. Rovei V, Sanjuan M, Sekeni F, Bossi L, Battino D, Caccermo M, Canger R, Como M, deGiambattist M,
    Marini T, Pardi G, Pifarotti G, Porro M: Plasma levels and clinical effects of antiepileptic drugs in newborns of chronically treated epileptic mothers. In Selbeck GG, Doose H (eds): *Epilepsy: Problems of Marriage, Pregnancy, and Genetic Counseling*. New York, Thieme Stratton, 1981, p 20–24.
28. Dam M, Dam H: Epilepsy, pregnancy, and delivery. In Selbeck GG, Doose H (eds): *Epilepsy: Problems of Marriage, Pregnancy and Genetic Counseling*. New York, Thieme Stratton, 1981, p 1–14.
29. Plauche W: Myasthenia gravis in pregnancy: an update. *Am J Obstet Gynecol* 135:691–697, 1979.
30. Lisak R, Barachi R: *Myasthenia Gravis*. Philadelphia, WB Saunders, 1982.
31. McNall P, Jafarma M: Management of myasthenia gravis in the obstetrical patient. *Am J Obstet Gynecol* 92(4):518–525, 1965.
32. Nakao, K, Nishitoni H, Suzuki M: Anti-acetylcholine receptor IgG in neonatal myasthenia gravis. *N Engl J Med* 297:169, 1977.
33. Namba T, Brown S, Grob D: Neonatal myasthenia gravis: report of two cases and review of the literature. *Pediatrics* 45(3):488–502, 1970.
34. Bromley I: *Tetraplegia and Paraplegia Guide for Physiotherapists*. New York, Churchill-Livingston, 1981.
35. Johnston B: Pregnancy and childbirth in women with spinal cord injuries: a review of the literature. *Maternal Child Nurs J* 11(1):41–45, 1982.
36. Nath M, Vivian J, Cherny W: Autonomic hyperreflexia in pregnancy and labor: a case report. *Am J Obstet Gynecol* 134(4):390–392, 1979.
37. Rossier AB, Ruffieux M, Ziegler WH: Pregnancy and labor in high traumatic spinal cord lesions. *Paraplegia* 7:210-215, 1969.
38. Tsoutsoplides G: Pregnancy in paraplegia: a case report. *Int J Gynecol Obstet* 20:79–83, 1982.
39. Kreitzer M, Gregory M: Maternal mortality in pregnancies complicated by kyphoscoliosis. *J Med Soc NJ* 78:36–38, 1981.
40. Hauser E: *Curvature of the Spine*. Springfield, IL, Charles C Thomas, 1962.
41. Siegler D, Zorab P: Pregnancy in thoracic scoliosis. *Br J Dis Chest* 75:367–370, 1981.
42. Kopenhager T: A review of 50 pregnant patients with kyphoscoliosis. *Br J Obstet Gynecol* 84(8):585–587, 1977.

Chapter 15
Psychiatric Disorders
Nancy DeVore, C.N.M., M.S.

INTRODUCTION

As discussed in Chapter 2, there are many stresses of the maternity period that demand psychosocial adaptations. When the underlying personality structure is weak, the potential for psychopathology is great. This chapter examines several psychiatric disorders associated with the maternity cycle—namely, pseudocyesis, hyperemesis gravidarum, depression, child abuse, mental retardation, neurotic reactions, and psychotic disorders.

PSEUDOCYESIS

Definition

Pseudocyesis is a condition in which the woman firmly believes she is pregnant and develops objective pregnancy symptoms in the absence of a pregnancy. It must be differentiated from hallucinatory pregnancy, which is caused by a psychosis, a simulated pregnancy in which the woman pretends to be pregnant, and a pseudopregnancy caused by endocrine changes secondary to a tumor or other structural defect (1). The incidence has been stated as 1:250 (2) to 1:160 true pregnancies (3).

Etiology

Study of the etiology of pseudocyesis has taken two tracks—psychological disorder versus a neuroendocrine disorder. With the former, the most common factors include an intense desire for pregnancy (women who have problems with infertility, have lost previous pregnancies, or are approaching menopause and strongly desire a child) or a great fear of pregnancy (women who have had illicit intercourse). Other stimuli may include a de-

sire for parity with other women (especially in cultures that determine a woman's social standing by her childbearing status) and a wish to improve disturbed family relationships (to save a faltering marriage or to acquire a substitute love object).

Psychodynamically, pseudocyesis is felt to be a defense against depression. The adult fear of losing the ability to bear a child can bring to awareness earlier fears of the loss of love, of body integrity, of sexual identity, or of self-esteem (4). Thus, the disorder may provide a defense against real or imagined feelings of separation, emptiness, or loss.

Although there is conflicting evidence about serum levels of gonadotropins and prolactin (most likely there is a high prolactin level with low or normal follicle-stimulating hormone [FSH] and low or elevated luteinizing hormone [LH]) and about the presence of a corpus luteum, it has been postulated that depression, via the cerebral cortex and limbic systems, can produce neuroendocrine changes (4). Depression, by causing a decreased availability of biogenic amines at the neuronal receptor sites in the hypothalamus, may lead to a suppression of FSH and LH releasing factors and of prolactin inhibitory factor. The anterior pituitary may then respond by decreasing FSH and LH secretion, which prevents ovulation and causes amenorrhea, and by increasing prolactin, which promotes lactation and may support the persistence of a corpus luteum.

In contrast to most defenses against depression, pseudocyesis has an intrinsic time limitation (usually 9 months). Once the defense breaks down, the underlying depression emerges—perhaps augmented by adverse social reaction and by conditions that normally contribute to the baby blues. Therefore, although the maternal outcome may include continuing symptomatology (indicating an enormous stress and a tremendous capacity for denial), more commonly it will involve a decreased self-image and depression with the potential for suicide.

Signs and Symptoms

A wide variety of symptoms is present with this illness. Menstrual disturbances—amenorrhea or oligomenorrhea—are the most common and usually first symptoms. These symptoms often may be attributed to the variations that occur in a young woman just establishing cycles, in an older woman approaching menopause, or in those at any age afflicted by severe stress. If some bleeding does occur, it may be misinterpreted as a sign of a threatened abortion or of placenta previa.

Although pseudocyesis is accompanied by abdominal enlargement, the shape of the abdomen may suggest an extrauterine gestation, and the umbilicus generally remains inverted (noneffaced). The change may be due to fat accumulation, gaseous distention, urinary or fecal retention, or age-related body changes. Breast swelling, tenderness, increased pigmentation, and secretion of a mucoid discharge may be secondary to fat deposits, hormonal changes, and continual manipulation.

Women with pseudocyesis often describe "fetal movements," which may be caused by increased peristalsis, violent contraction of the abdominal muscles, and imagination. The "fetal heart rate" when auscultated usually is a fast maternal pulse. If the movements or a heart rate are absent, the woman may fear the baby is dead.

Bimanual examination may reveal uterine or cervical changes not typical of any stage of pregnancy. The uterus rarely is more than 6 weeks in size but is often hard to delineate because of the abdominal distention. Nausea, constipation, and food cravings may be reported, but these are not specific for pregnancy. Labor pains, when described, may be due to gas or retained feces or urine, or they may have a psychological basis.

Diagnosis

The diagnosis of pseudocyesis becomes one of exclusion. False diagnoses usually are the result of failure to do a good examination—poor palpation, failure to perform the usual tests since the patient is so convincing, or refusal of the patient to be examined. Such mistakes are not so uncommon. In a study as recent as 1951, 9 of 27 women were told they were pregnant by 16 of 40 examining physicians (2).

To avoid such errors, the practitioner must proceed with a systematic examination of the patient. A careful history—medical, menstrual, sexual, contraceptive, obstetrical, and psychosocial—is needed to appreciate any significant factors impinging on this "pregnancy." This information must be correlated with the findings on abdominal examination (percussion for fundal height, Leopold's maneuvers, auscultation of fetal heart versus maternal pulse) and on pelvic examination (Chadwick's sign, uterine size and softening). When in doubt, laboratory tests should be employed, including pregnancy tests, ultrasonography, or x-ray. The pregnancy test may be either blood or urine, but its sensitivity and specificity must be known. Although a flat plate of the pelvis may provide a quick answer about pseudocyesis, the fear of radiation side effects has led to its replacement in the majority of centers by ultrasonography. Through these techniques it has been possible to rule out pregnancy, thus saving women from surgery for supposed ectopic pregnancy, placenta previa, or prolonged labor. Although x-ray and ultrasonography also have allowed detection of such confounding variables as tumors (abdominal or pelvic), ascites, urinary or fecal retention, or gaseous distention, an abdominal CAT scan may be required to rule out conclusively organic pathology (5).

Medical Management

Medical management of pseudocyesis currently involves establishing rapport, gently telling the diagnosis, and offering psychotherapy for support and insight. In some women hormonal therapy may be added to restore menses since for them its absence may be synonymous with pregnancy. Understanding the particular stresses leading to each woman's illness is essential.

The treatment of the future may involve more pharmocological interventions if one believes that depression is the core of the problem. Perhaps the use of levodopa (a catecholamine precursor) or monoamine oxidase (MAO) inhibitors (which increase the availability of catecholamines at neuronal receptor sites), combined with psychotherapy to alleviate the stresses precipitating the depression, may be the cure of the future.

HYPEREMESIS GRAVIDARUM

Since the medical aspects of hyperemesis gravidarum have been discussed at length in Chapter 11, only the psychological aspects of this disorder are mentioned here.

Etiology

Hyperemesis has been found to have a strong association with an hysterical or immature personality of the woman and with a disturbance of family relationships. Chertok (6), in a study of 100 women including 68 with nausea and vomiting, found a significantly positive relationship between vomiting and the woman's ambivalent attitude toward the fetus; a positive relationship between vomiting and her negative experience with quickening; and a negative correlation between vomiting and her husband's positive contribution to the marital partnership. This agrees with the more recent work of Wolkind and Zajicele (7), which indicated that these women have social stresses, including lack of support from parents and spouse. Often, however, the mother or husband and the patient are reunited by the illness as the support person physically tries to aid.

Medical Management

Medical management requires not only physical but also psychological care. Hospitalization may be required not only to improve the patient's nutritional status but to decrease environmental stress, provide relief from usual responsibilities, and display a profound interest by family and professionals. Psychological care must be directed toward treating the underlying personality problems and alleviating symptoms. Hypnotherapy, either individual or group, by way of trance induction and suggestions of comfort in the gastrointestinal tract, and behavior modification, with positive reinforcement for retaining food and gaining weight, have been two therapies employed. Psychotherapy, both supportive and more intensive, has aided through the establishment of a positive relationship, frequent reassuring conversations, and encouragement of the expression of thoughts and feelings. Stress areas frequently explored include mixed feelings about the pregnancy, the anticipated child, and the significant person, whether the father of the child or the woman's own parents. In addition, work is needed with the families who may be frightened, frustrated, and angry.

POSTPARTUM DEPRESSION

Definition

The illness known as postpartum depression can be defined as a depressive disorder occurring in proximity to activities related to childbirth.

Signs and Symptoms

The symptomatology does not define a specific entity but rather a continuum of the problem, including the following.

The *postpartum blues* (variously termed the baby blues, maternity blues, three-day blues, or milk blues) (8, 9) is a mild depressive reaction occurring 3 to 10 days following delivery in 50–80% of all postpartum women. Symptomatology includes tearfulness, anxiety, depression, restlessness, irritability, feelings of loneliness, decreased self-esteem, estrangement, increased vulnerability or hypersensitivity to possible rejection, and fears of an incapacity to control or master a new event. It is self-limiting, with spontaneous recovery without psychiatric intervention.

A *postpartum neurotic depression* (10) is thought to occur in 11–20% of puerperal women. Symptomatology includes fearfulness, feelings of inadequacy, an inability to cope, greater distress in the evening, guilt with self-reproach, labile mood, anxiety, hypochondriasis, irritability, undue fatigue and exhaustion, anorexia, insomnia, and decreased libido. The infant may reflect maternal difficulties by not eating or sleeping or by crying for long intervals.

A *postpartum psychotic depression* has a peak incidence in the first 4–6 weeks postpartum and is estimated to occur in 0.1% (11) to 2.9% (12) of puerperal women. The exact number is unknown since the American Psychiatric Association's diagnostic manual does not record puerperal reactions as a separate category—feeling that they are not distinct clinical conditions with a separate symptomatology, psychopathology, or prognosis. The disorder is marked by a sudden onset of physical and mental lethargy, retardation of thought and action, sadness, self-accusations, hopelessness, and thoughts of suicide or infanticide. Often there is clouding of consciousness (with disorientation, derealization, and delirium), and, when the illness is bipolar, there may be manic features. The woman may have hallucinations and delusions, most frequently of guilt involving the child, spouse, or self. Frequently, vegetative signs of anorexia, constipation, decreased libido, and early morning awakening are found. Rejection of the infant is a classic sign.

Etiology

The etiology of postpartum depression is poorly understood. A number of physiological theories have been advanced: high free plasma tryptophan levels (13), low tyramine levels (14), low norepinephrine levels (15), thyroid deficiency (16), and folate deficiency (17). In no instance have such correlations been confirmed by replicated controlled studies. Likewise, no association has been found between postpartum depression and circulating levels of estrogen, progesterone, prolactin, FSH, or LH.

The psychological postulates of the etiology include a disturbed ego identity of the woman and disturbed family dynamics. In one study with projective tests (18), the ill mothers perceived their children as a drain on their emotional resources, were symbiotically tied to a maternal figure, and were unable to develop a self-identity. When there is this symbiotic relationship with the husband or mother, the addition of a baby may threaten the equilibrium of the dyad and lead to overt or covert aggression against the woman by the dominant partner, precipitating a psychotic reaction (19).

Diagnosis

The diagnosis of a postpartum depression is based on the symptomatology plus an adequate history. A careful interview will elucidate not only stresses of the present maternity experience or life situation but, frequently, in the case of a psychotic depression, a family history of a psychotic reaction or the occurrence of a previous psychotic episode—puerperal or nonpuerperal.

. The differential diagnosis includes a schizophrenic reaction or an organic brain syndrome. In the former the affect is often flat, and delusions frequently are bizarre or paranoid, such as the baby was never born; was born by supernatural means; or is dead, ill, or malformed. Clues to an organic brain syndrome diagnosis include a negative family and past medical history for a psychotic reaction, sudden onset, fluctuating symptoms, disorientation to time and place (but not to person), deficit in short-term memory, decreased attention span with confused or concrete thinking, and worsening of the condition at night (20). The depressive affect is absent.

Maternal and Fetal Outcome

With a neurotic depression, the maternal outcome includes disturbance of activities of daily living and disruption of relationships with family and friends. Unfortunately, such sequelae merely serve to confirm the woman's poor self-image and further aggravate her support system, reinforcing her depression. The infant often responds by crying at long intervals and evidencing sleeping and feeding problems. This increased tension and the infant's failure to thrive may be further proof to the woman of her inability to mother well. With a psychotic depression, the maternal and infant outcomes may be more severe. Suicide or infanticide are the ultimate end points against which the woman and baby must be protected.

Medical Management

Medical management of a neurotic depressive reaction may include the use of antidepressants, short-term supportive therapy aimed at symptomatic relief through ventilation and ego support, and insight therapy to deal with unresolved conflicts and correct feelings of vulnerability, inadequacy, and low self-esteem. Psychotic depressions may require medication such as antidepressants, phenothiazines, or lithium. In recalcitrant cases of depression, somatic treatment such as electroconvulsive therapy may be needed. If institutionalization is required, ideally it would include the woman and her family or the woman and her infant. In these cases the staff could serve as role models in parenting. Supportive therapy is a useful adjunct to all other treatment.

OTHER PSYCHIATRIC DISORDERS

Other psychiatric disorders that may be seen in the high risk maternity setting include child abuse, mental retardation, other neurotic disorders (e.g., phobic reactions, anxiety reactions, and obsessive-compulsive reactions), and other psychotic disorders (e.g., schizophrenic reactions or paranoid reactions). The effects on the maternity experience and the implications for care providers will be discussed briefly for each category.

Child abuse consists of active acts of aggression, such as verbal assaults, physical batterings, and sexual abuse, as well as passive acts of neglect. It often occurs with abuse-prone parents (i.e., those who were abused themselves as children) or with a "special child" (one born prematurely or with another physical problem that required early separation from the mother, mental retardation, brain damage, psychosis, colic, or an identifiable quality of a hated person or situation). When a newborn requires special care, steps should be taken to minimize mother-infant separation and isolation. Maternity care givers must be alert to indications of abnormal maternal-infant attachment and make preventive referrals, as appropriate, for psychiatric counseling, Parents Anonymous, or other crisis intervention resources.

Problems of the mentally retarded woman related to the maternity experience may include failure to understand the importance of prenatal care or treatment, an increased chance of producing mentally retarded offspring, and the increased potential for parenting difficulties, including child abuse (21, 22). Implications for care therefore would include giving simple explanations and directions concerning prenatal care—demonstrating requests; providing kind, firm support; and giving behavioral reinforcement. To detect genetic disorders in the offspring, amniocentesis or chorionic villi biopsy may be offered (with the option of abortion for positive results), and adequate pediatric evaluation and follow-up for early diagnosis and treatment must be provided. Since many of the mentally retarded have been exposed to disruptive family settings, social service referrals for parenting supports or substitutes are essential. Homemaker services, surrogate or foster parents, and day care programs are a few of the interventions that may be beneficial.

The effects of other neurotic disorders on the maternity experience may include interference with following a treatment plan (e.g., a phobia for elevators may preclude visiting the genetic counselor whose office is on the 11th floor), interference with labor progress (e.g., a severely obsessive woman may persist with ineffective pushing efforts for fear of expelling some feces), and parenting difficulties. In the latter case symptomatology may interfere with activities of daily living and, therefore, of caring for oneself and a baby. The infant may reflect the parent's anxiety in eating, sleeping, and crying disorders, or the mother may be overwhelmed by the incessant demands of an infant when she feels she has no reserves for herself.

Implications for care include modification of obstetrical treatment plans to increase the rate of compliance. Such changes might include arranging for the genetic counselor to meet the woman in a ground floor office or encouraging the woman to push in labor while seated on the toilet. Treatment of symptomatology may necessitate referral of the patient for supportive or insight therapy plus the use of analgesia and anesthesia in labor to permit needed relaxation. Since medications should be discouraged in pregnancy whenever possible, the practitioner should substitute a firm supportive relationship for the usual antianxiety drugs. Parenting problems should be handled through social service referrals to determine family and friend support as well as to utilize community agencies, such as homemaker services.

Symptomatology of other psychotic disorders may affect the maternity experience by interfering with following an obstetrical treatment plan (e.g., fear that a B-scan will destroy the baby's brain) or interfering with labor progress (e.g., fear that her body will be torn in half). Parenting difficulties may occur since these women often have been subjected to poor care themselves. Their symptomatology may interfere with activities of daily living and therefore of caring for themselves and the baby, may cause rejection of the infant, and may include hallucinations that suggest infanticide.

Although the use of medication generally is discouraged in pregnancy, antipsychotic medications may be required to manage a psychosis. Neither phenothiazines (23) nor lithium (24) are absolutely contraindicated. In addition, however, the practitioner should try to form a kind, supportive relationship that will help the patient face the demands of the maternity experience. Social service referrals should be used for evaluation of family and friend support systems and for utilization of community agencies—homemaker services and surrogate or foster parents—that may avert or aid with parenting problems.

NURSING MANAGEMENT

Nursing care specific for a patient with psychiatric disorders:
- [ ] Ensure safety of mother/fetus/neonate.
- [ ] Encourage the patient to discuss fears/concerns regarding pregnancy, parenting, marriage, sex, plans for future child spacing.
- [ ] Encourage preparation for labor and delivery and parenthood; refer to preparation for childbirth classes.
- [ ] Provide referrals, as appropriate, for psychiatric counseling/therapy/peer support.
- [ ] Include family/significant others in plan of care, as appropriate.
- [ ] Contact patient after hospital discharge, as indicated, to assess adjustment to parenting.
- [ ] If rehospitalization is required, ensure that mother and baby can be cared for as a unit to minimize family disruption.
- [ ] Refer mother to visiting nurse for ongoing evaluation of parenting skills.

Nursing diagnoses most frequently associated with psychiatric disorders:
- [ ] Ineffective individual coping.

NURSING MANAGEMENT

☐ Ineffective family coping: compromised.

☐ Potential altered parenting.

☐ Self-care deficit: feeding, bathing/hygiene, dressing, grooming, toileting.

☐ Disturbance in body image, self-esteem.

☐ Anxiety/fear.

☐ Knowledge deficit regarding etiology, disease process, treatment, and expected outcome.

☐ Knowledge deficit regarding medication regimen.

☐ Knowledge deficit regarding pregnancy, process of labor and delivery, concerns of the postpartum period, parenting.

REFERENCES

1. Murray JL, Abraham GE: Pseudocyesis: a review. *Obstet Gynecol* 51:627–631, 1978.

2. Fried PH, Rakoff AE, Schopbach RR: Pseudocyesis: a psychosomatic study in gynecology. *JAMA* 145:1329–1335, 1951.

3. Lapido OA: Pseudocyesis in infertile patients. *Int J Gynaecol Obstet* 16:427–429, 1979.

4. Brown E, Barglow P: Pseudocyesis: a paradigm for psychophysiological interactions. *Arch Gen Psychiatry* 24:221–229, 1971.

5. Rosenberg HK, Coleman BG, Croop J, Granowetter L, Evans AE: Pseudocyesis in an adolescent patient. *Clin Pediatr* 22:708–712, 1983.

6. Chertok L: The psychopathology of vomiting in pregnancy. In Howells J (ed): *Modern Perspectives in Psycho-Obstetrics*. New York, Brunner/Mazel, 1971, pp 268–281.

7. Wolkind S, Zajicek E: Psychosocial correlates of nausea and vomiting in pregnancy. *J Psychosom Res* 22:1–5, 1978.

8. Vandenbergh RL: Postpartum depression. *Clin Obstet Gynecol* 23:1105–1111, 1980.

9. Hazle NR: Postpartum blues, assessment and intervention. *J Nurse-Midwifery* 27:21–25, 1982.

10. Pitt B: Atypical depression following childbirth. *Br J Psychiatry* 114:1325–1335, 1968.

11. McGowan M: Postpartum disturbance . . . a review of the literature in terms of stress response. *J Nurse-Midwifery* 22:27–34, 1977.

12. Tod EDM: Puerperal depression: a prospective epidemiological study. *Lancet* ii:1264–1266, 1964.

13. Stein G, Milton F, Bebbington P: Relationship between mood disturbance and free and total plasma tryptophan in postpartum women. *Br Med J* 2:457, 1976.

14. Sandler M, Carter SB, Reveley MA, Glover V, Rein G: Further light on the tyramine test in depression. *Can J Neurol Sci* 7:265–266, 1980.

15. Treadway CR, Kane FJ Jr, Jarrahi-Zadeh A, Lipton MA: A psychoendocrine study of pregnancy and puerperium *Am J Psychiatry* 125:1380–1386, 1969.

16. Hampton J: *Postpartum Psychiatric Problems*. St. Louis, Mosby, 1962.

17. Thornton WE: Folate deficiency in puerperal psychosis. *Am J Obstet Gynecol* 129:222–223, 1977.

18. Markham S: A comparative evaluation of psychotic and nonpsychotic reactions to childbirth. *Am J Orthopsychiatry* 31:565–578, 1961.

19. Ketal RM, Brandwin MA: Childbirth-related psychosis and familial symbiotic conflict. *Am J Psychiatry* 136:190–193, 1979.

20. Dubovsky SL: Psychiatric approach to high risk obstetrics. In Abrams RS, Wexler P (eds): *Medical Care of the Pregnant Patient*. Boston, Little, Brown & Co, 1983, pp 373–384.

21. Gillberg C, Geijer-Karlsson M: Children born to mentally retarded women: a 1-21 year followup study of 41 cases. *Psychol Med* 13:891–894, 1983.

22. Craft A, Craft M: Sexuality and mental handicap: a review. *Br J Psychiatry* 139:494–505, 1981.

23. Burgess HA: Schizophrenia in pregnancy. *Issues in Health Care of Women* 2:61–69, 1980.

24. Burgess HA: When a patient on lithium is pregnant. *Am J Nurs* 79:1989–1990, 1979.

Chapter 16
Pulmonary Disorders
Kathleen Buckley, C.N.M., M.S.N.

INTRODUCTION

Physiologic changes occurring in the respiratory system during pregnancy are the results not only of the increase in abdominal width and height but also of alterations of the hormonal composition during pregnancy. Total lung volume is progressively but slightly reduced over the course of pregnancy because of the enlarging uterus encroaching on the diaphragm. However, owing to the smooth muscle relaxation mediated by progesterone, airway resistance is decreased (as much as 50%); the chest is broadened because of musculocartilaginous relaxation, and therefore tidal volume increases up to 40%. Progesterone also is thought to cause the medullary centers to have a heightened sensitivity to pCO_2, which, in turn, increases the respiratory rate.

The greater tidal volume combined with the slight increase in respiratory rate (one to two respirations/minute) cause an increase in the minute volume from 6.5 liters/minute to 10 liters/minute (1, p 362). Changes in respiratory function during pregnancy are listed in Table 16.1.

Although controversy exists, it is thought that the increased alveolar ventilation produces a fall in the arterial pCO_2, which may in turn produce a slight arterial alkalosis (pH 7.40–7.44) (2, p 410).

Finally, as many as 70% of pregnant women complain of breathlessness during the first and second trimester. This well-documented normal phenomenon is thought to be due to the newness of the sensation of increased tidal and minute volume or an increased awareness of them. Since the symptoms can occur very early in pregnancy (9 weeks' gestation), it is not related to the

Table 16.1.

CHANGES IN RESPIRATORY FUNCTION VOLUMES DURING PREGNANCY[a]

FUNCTION	NOT PREGNANT	PREGNANT	CHANGE (%)
Respiratory rate	15	16	—
Tidal volume (ml)	487	678	+39[b]
Minute ventilation (ml)	7270	10,340	+42[b]
Minute O_2 uptake	201	266	+32[b]
Vital capacity (ml)	3260	3310	+ 1
Maximum breathing capacity (% of predicted)	102	97	− 5
Inspiratory capacity (ml)	2625	2745	+ 5
Residual volume (ml)	965	770	−20[b]

[a]Reprinted with permission from Cugell et al., *Am Rev Tuberc* 67:568, 1953.
[b]Highly significant differences.

mechanical obstruction of the growing uterus (2, p 410).

PHYSICAL ASSESSMENT

Physical assessment of the thorax and lungs requires skill and repeated practice. The reader is referred to a physical assessment text for discussion of the techniques of pulmonary evaluation. They are extremely useful in diagnosis of asthma, bronchitis, and pneumonia, which are discussed in this chapter. Prompt recognition of compromised maternal pulmonary status is crucial in preventing fetal hypoxia from decreased oxygen flow through the

Table 16.2.
PHYSICAL ASSESSMENT SIGNS IN SELECTED PULMONARY DISORDERS[a]

CONDITION	DESCRIPTION	PERCUSSION NOTE	BREATH SOUNDS	ADVENTITIOUS SOUNDS
Atelectasis	A collapsed or atelectatic lung is dull to percussion. Bronchial obstruction (not always present) prevents transmission of breath and voice sounds. The trachea may shift to the same side.	Dull	Decreased vesicular or absent	None
Lobar pneumonia	A consolidated lung is dull to percussion but as long as the large airways are clear, fremitus, breath, and voice sounds are transmitted as if they came directly from the larynx and trachea.	Dull	Bronchial	Rales
Bronchitis	In bronchitis the lungs themselves are normal. Signs are limited to breath sounds and adventitious sounds.	Resonant	Normal or prolonged expiration	Wheezes, rhonchi, or rales may be present
Asthma	A hyperinflated lung of obstructive lung disease is hyperresonant, but the enlarged alveoli muffle the voice and breath sounds.	Hyperresonant	Decreased vesicular, often with prolonged expiration	None or wheezes, rhonchi, or rales

[a]Adapted from Bates B: *A Guide to Physical Examination*. Philadelphia, JB Lippincott, 1974.

placenta. Findings of assessment of these conditions are noted in Table 16.2.

In addition, because functional capacity of the lung is measured mathematically using a spirometer, the nurse should be familiar with lung volumes and capacities (Table 16.3).

ASTHMA

Definition

Asthma (also called bronchial asthma) is a type of chronic obstructive pulmonary disease caused by spasmodic constriction of the main bronchi. It is marked by attacks of dyspnea with wheezing. Attacks may be chronic or acute. Severity differs widely from occasional wheezing and slight dyspnea to severe attacks that may cause suffocation. *Status asthmaticus* is an acute attack that lasts for days or even weeks. This is a medical emergency and has been known to be fatal (3, p 104).

Asthma is classified according to the causative factors. Thus, it is said to be extrinsic or allergic, intrinsic or nonallergic, and mixed (3, p 104).

Etiology

Extrinsic asthma is due to an allergy. Pollen, dust, smoke, animal hair, or even car exhaust are some of the allergic foci.

Extrinsic asthma is thought to be an inherited trait characterized by a heightened reaction of the immune system. Patients with this type of asthma typically have a family medical history of allergies and a past history of allergic disorders. Most cases in children and young adults are extrinsic.

Intrinsic or nonallergic asthma results from a hypersensitivity to certain bacteria. Usually, it develops secondary to chronic or recurrent infections of the bronchi, sinuses, tonsils, or adenoids.

Mixed asthma is due to a combination of allergic and bacterial hypersensitivity.

Secondary factors such as exercise, emotional stress, changes in humidity and temperature, or exposure to noxious fumes (e.g., smog) may trigger all three types of asthma.

Asthma is a common respiratory disorder occurring in about 3% of the general population. In pregnancy it is the most common form of obstructive lung disease. The incidence is thought to be from 0.4–1.3% (2, p 413).

Signs and Symptoms

The classical signs and symptoms are dyspnea, cough, and wheezing. However, cough may be the *only* symptom, and pulmonary evaluation should be performed for patients presenting with that complaint.

Table 16.3.
DEFINITIONS OF LUNG VOLUMES AND LUNG CAPACITIES[a]

	Definitions of lung volumes
Tidal volume (TV)	Volume of gas inspired and expired with a normal breath
Inspiratory reserve volume (IRV)	Maximal volume that can be inspired from the end of a normal inspiration
Expiratory reserve volume (ERV)	Maximal volume that can be exhaled by forced expiration after a normal expiration
Residual volume (RV)	Volume of gas left in lung after maximal expiration
Minute volume (MV)	Volume inspired and expired in 1 minute of normal breathing
	Definitions of lung capacities
Vital capacity (VC)	Maximal amount of air that can be expired after a maximal inspiration (TV + IRV + ERV)
Forced vital capacity (FVC)	Maximal amount of air that can be expelled with a maximal effort after a maximal inspiration
Maximal midexpiratory flow (MMEF)	Average rate of flow during middle half of forced vital capacity
Forced expiratory volume in 1 second (FEV$_a$)	Amount of air expelled in the first second of the forced vital capacity maneuver
FEV/VC ratio	Amount of air forcefully expelled in 1 second compared to total amount forcefully expelled
Maximal voluntary ventilation (MVV), also termed maximal breathing capacity (MBC)	Amount of air exchanged per minute with maximal rate and depth of respiration
Inspiratory capacity (IC)	Maximal amount of air that can be inspired after a normal expiration (TV + IRV)
Functional residual capacity (FRC)	Amount of air left in lungs after a normal expiration (ERV + RV)
Total lung capacity (TLC)	Total amount of air in lungs after maximal inspiration (TV + IRV + ERV + RV)

[a]Reprinted with permission from Phipps W, et al.: *Medical Surgical Nursing.* St. Louis, Mosby, 1979, p 936.

During an attack, the patient typically will assume a sitting position, leaning forward in order to use all the respiratory muscles. In mild to moderate attacks, the skin usually is pale and moist with perspiration. In severe attacks, as hypoxia increases, cyanosis of the nail beds and lips is seen.

Other physical findings include increased anteroposterior chest diameter and lowered diaphragm—both evidence of pulmonary hyperinflation. Ominous signs include:

1. Heart rate greater than 120 beats/minute;
2. Respiratory rate greater than 30/minute;
3. Peak expiratory flow of less than 120 liters/minute;
4. A pulse that becomes weaker during inspiration (pulsus paradoxus); and
5. Use of accessory respiratory muscles (4, p 9).

It should be noted that wheezing may decrease as the patient's condition worsens because of such severe reduction of the airway diameter, causing insufficient airflow to generate a wheeze. (2, p 413).

Diagnosis

Diagnosis is based on history, physical examination revealing the above signs and symptoms, and laboratory findings.

Historical data include family history of allergies and current complaints of wheezing and breathlessness, often triggered by exposure to specific allergies, infection, or emotional factors.

Laboratory data include evaluation of pulmonary function tests, arterial blood gases, sputum cultures, serum electrolytes, and chest x-ray.

Generally, pulmonary functions are depressed. A serious finding is a forced expiratory volume of less than 20% of the predicted value. The following blood gases signal impending respiratory failure (1, p 132):

1. pO$_2$ $\leq$ 70 mm Hg and pCO$_2$ $\geq$ 35 mm Hg; or
2. pCO$_2$ $\geq$ 40 mg Hg and pH > 7.3.

Sputum should be cultured to identify infection. Predominant organisms in such pulmonary infection are the pneumococcus bacterium and the hemophilus bacterium. Sputum also should be evaluated for presence of eosinophils or leukocytes.

The latter indicates infection, while the former suggests allergic reaction (1, p 365).

Serum electrolytes should be evaluated on an ongoing basis to determine any alterations in pulmonary status.

A differential diagnosis for asthma includes large airway obstruction, pulmonary edema, pulmonary embolism, bronchiolitis, and anaphylaxis (1, p 131). A chest x-ray will distinguish asthma from more severe forms of chronic obstructive pulmonary disease or other pulmonary disorders.

Maternal and Fetal Outcome

Pregnancy does not consistently affect the maternal asthmatic status for better or for worse. A clinical guideline in obstetrics has been the "rule of thirds." One third of patients improve, one third stay the same, and one third deteriorate. Some clinicians feel that patients with severe asthma tend to deteriorate, while patients with mild to moderate disease remain the same or improve (2, p 414). Asthma probably is more related to the patient's exposure to allergens and presence of respiratory infection (which are both dependent on the season) than to pregnancy itself. However, it has been noted that asthma may increase in severity in late pregnancy and the postpartum period. Moreover, asthmatic patients seem to respond to each subsequent pregnancy with a consistent pattern of disease (1, p 132).

Fetal status may be compromised with as much as a twofold increase in perinatal mortality due to low birth weight and hypoxia at birth. Fetal outcome correlates with the severity of maternal disease. The more hypoxic the mother, the more compromised the fetus becomes (2, p 414).

Medical Management

The aim of management is to provide a wheeze-free, oxygenated respiratory system. Bronchodilators, corticosteroids, and antibiotics are used in combination in order to improve oxygenation, to remove excessive secretions, and to prevent infection. Antihistamines generally are not used because they tend to harden bronchial plugs (See Table 16.4).

Table 16.4.
DRUGS USED TO TREAT ASTHMA AND RELATED PULMONARY DISEASES DURING PREGNANCY

A. Bronchodilators (xanthine derivatives)
   Indication: Symptomatic relief of asthma, bronchial spasms.
   Action: These drugs relax bronchial smooth muscle and inhibit the release of histamine and slow release substance A (SRS-A) from most cells. They are also mild diuretics and cardiac stimulants.
   Maternal side effects: Gastrointestinal upset, nausea, nervousness, frequency, diarrhea, insomnia, tachycardia, palpitations. Toxic levels may cause cardiac arrhythmias and seizures.
   Nursing implications: Use with care in clients with hypertension, hypoxemia, glaucoma, hyperthyroidism, and diabetes; monitor for central nervous system symptoms; give with food to decrease gastrointestinal upset; prohibit smoking.
   Drug of choice during pregnancy: Theophylline (Theo-Dur).
   Other drugs used: Aminophylline (Aminodur), oxytriphylline (Choledyl).
   Breastfeeding: Theophylline (and other xanthine derivatives) is excreted in breast milk (less than 1% of maternal dose). One infant became irritable after a rapidly absorbed dose. Therefore, *less* rapidly absorbed doses are advised.

B. Expectorants
   Indication: Facilitate productive cough.
   Action: These drugs facilitate removal of thick mucus from the lungs and act as a soothing demulcent by stimulating secretion of a lubricant. (May be no more effective at liquefying secretions than a high fluid intake and humidification.)
   Maternal side effects: Nausea/vomiting, gastrointestinal irritation, drowsiness.
   Nursing implications: Instruct client not to use these preparations for longer than 1 week without seeing physician and to use additional measures (high fluid intake and humidity) to help cough; do not follow administration with water.
   Drug of choice during pregnancy: Guaifenesin (Robitussin)
   Other Drugs Used: Ammonium chloride. Potassium iodide (SSKI) contraindicated because of possibility of maternal/fetal cardiac arrhythmias and fetal thyroid depression.
   Breastfeeding: No data available for guaifenesin, ammonium chloride, or potassium iodide.

C. Antitussives
   Indication: To treat dry, nonproductive coughs that interfere with sleep or other activities.
   Action: These drugs suppress the cough reflex. Nonnarcotics act peripherally within the tracheobronchial tree.
   Maternal side effects: In very *high* doses, may produce central nervous system depression.
   Nursing implications: Observe carefully if hepatic (excretory) function is impaired for overdose.
   Drug of choice during pregnancy: Unknown.

Table 16.4.
(Continued)

Drugs used: Dextromethorphan (Romilar), benzonatate (Tessalon), levopropoxyphene napsylate (Novrad).
Breastfeeding: No data available.
Note: Use of the narcotic antitussive (hydrocodone bitartrate, e.g., codeine) is prohibited because of possible fetal anomalies associated with first trimester use and fetal addiction and withdrawal associated with third trimester use.

D. Mucolytics
Indication: To liquefy thick secretions and minimize bronchiolar obstruction.
Action: These drugs act by disrupting the molecular structure of mucous secretions. They liquefy secretions throughout the tracheobronchial tree.
Maternal side effects: Nausea/vomiting, rhinorrhea, hypersensitivity reaction, bronchial spasms.
Nursing implications: Watch asthmatic clients closely: ensure that client either expectorates secretions or is suctioned in order to avoid aspiration; monitor client for nausea and vomiting.
Drug of choice during pregnancy: Unknown.
Drugs used: Acetylcysteine (Mucomyst), pancreatic dornase (Dornavac), multiple preparations (refer to *Physician's Desk Reference*).
Breastfeeding: No data available.

E. Autonomic Drugs
Indications: These drugs produce bronchodilation.
Action: These drugs stimulate the release of stored epinephrine and directly stimulate adrenergic receptors.
Maternal side effects: Hypertension, cardiac arrhythmias, electrolyte imbalance, palpitations, insomnia, tremor, anxiety.
Nursing implications: Monitor vital signs and mental status carefully.
Drug of choice during pregnancy: Unknown.
Drugs used: Ephedrine, terbutaline.
Breastfeeding: Unknown.

F. Corticosteroids
Indication: These drugs decrease the inflammatory process.
Action: These drugs inhibit the production and release of inflammatory mediators.
Maternal side effects: Fluid and electrolyte (especially sodium) imbalance, hyperglycemia, peptic ulcer, psychosis, Cushing's syndrome.
Nursing implications: Assess mental status, observe for signs or symptoms of electrolyte imbalance, glucose overload, and gastrointestinal bleeding. Consider greater susceptibility to Cushing's syndrome.
Drug of choice during pregnancy: Solu Cortef (i.v.), 100 mg every 8 hours. Used in asthmatic attack. Dose tapered rapidly.
Drugs used: See above.
Breastfeeding: Unknown. Drug is used during lactation upon indication.

NURSING MANGEMENT

Nursing care specific for patients with asthma:

☐ Encourage the patient to take prescribed medication for asthma, as ordered, and discuss the benefits and risks of medications during pregnancy.

☐ Teach patient to avoid triggering stimuli (e.g., known allergies, exposure to respiratory infections, stress).

☐ During an acute attack:
— Stay with the patient;
— Maintain bed rest in a quiet environment; place patient in Fowler's position;
— Administer oxygen and medications as ordered (e.g., epinephrine, aminophylline, expectorant, steroids, antibiotics); and
— Monitor maternal vital signs and fetal heart rate; prepare for chest x-ray as re-

quired, ensuring that abdomen is shielded; assist with blood gas testing; auscultate lungs at least hourly.

Nursing diagnoses most frequently associated with asthma:

☐ Anxiety/fear.

☐ Grieving related to potential/actual loss of infant or birth of an imperfect child.

☐ Anticipatory grieving related to actual/perceived threat to self.

☐ Knowledge deficit regarding etiology, disease process, treatment, and outcome.

☐ Knowledge deficit regarding medication regimen.

☐ Potential for infection.

☐ Impaired gas exchange.

ACUTE BRONCHITIS

Definition

Bronchitis is characterized by hypertrophy of mucous glands and inflammation of any of the larger bronchi conveying air to the lungs (right or left principal bronchus) and within the lungs (lobar and segmental bronchi). It may be either acute or chronic and frequently involves the trachea (tracheobronchitis) (3, p 167).

Etiology

Multiple causes of acute bronchitis have been identified. Viral causes include adeno, rhino, or parainfluenza. Acute bronchitis may be bacterial because of organisms such as *Haemophilus influenzae*. Other causes may be physical or chemical irritants such as pollen, dust, auto fumes, smog, or tobacco smoke. Smokers are 20% more likely to develop bronchitis than nonsmokers. Patients with a history of chronic or multiple respiratory infection are at risk to develop bronchitis. It is thought by some that heredity may be a predisposing factor. Debilitated, malnourished, or chronically ill women are susceptible to bronchitis with pneumonia as a secondary infection (4, p 18).

Signs and Symptoms

Symptoms of acute bronchitis usually begin with early symptoms of upper respiratory infection or the common cold. This progresses to fever; dry, irritating cough; and chest pain. As the inflammation of the bronchi increases, the cough becomes more productive of purulent sputum. A moderate fever may be noted. Auscultation of the lungs may reveal rales, ronchi, and wheezes (5, p 356).

Diagnosis

Diagnosis is based on history, physical examination, and sputum collection for culture, sensitivity, and cytology.

Maternal and Fetal Outcome

Maternal and fetal outcome are not compromised.

Medical Management

Medical management is conservative. Treatment consists of rest, hydration, and prescription of a broad spectrum antibiotic such as ampicillin, amoxicillin, or erythromycin. Treatment should also include use of a steam inhalor to liquify secretions, rather than iodine-containing expectorants because of their effect on the fetus (4, p 18, 6).

NURSING MANAGEMENT

Nursing care specific for patients with *bronchitis*:

- [ ] Teach patient to avoid exposure to upper respiratory tract infections.
- [ ] Encourage patient to stop smoking.
- [ ] Teach patient to report signs/symptoms of upper respiratory infection promptly.
- [ ] Teach patient to maintain adequate fluid intake (at least eight glasses of fluid daily) to liquefy secretions.
- [ ] Encourage patient to consume a diet rich in protein and vitamin C to promote healing.

- [ ] Teach the patient the importance of taking prescribed medications on time in order to maintain therapeutic blood levels.

Nursing diagnoses most frequently associated with *bronchitis*:

- [ ] Knowledge deficit regarding etiology, disease process, treatment, and outcome.
- [ ] Knowledge deficit regarding medication regimen.
- [ ] Potential for infection.
- [ ] Impaired gas exchange.

PNEUMONIA

Definition

Pneumonia is an acute inflammation of the respiratory bronchioles and aveolar sac—the parenchyma of the lung. Despite recent advances in antibiotic therapy, pneumonia still occurs in 1% of the United States population annually and ranks among the ten leading causes of death (5, p 353).

Pneumonia is classified as either lobar or bronchial. Lobar pneumonia affects a segment or an entire lobe. Both lungs may become affected, called "double pneumonia." Consolidation may be so severe as to block any air from entering the alveoli.

Bronchial pneumonia is more prevalent than lobar pneumonia, but usually runs a far more benign course. The area affected is smaller—usually limited to around the bronchi (5, p 353).

Etiology

Five basic classifications of etiology include bacterial, viral, fungal, aspiration, and hypostatic. The most common etiology of pneumonia in otherwise healthy women of childbearing age is *Streptococcus pneumonia*. Other bacteria are staphylococci and Gram-negative enteric bacteria. Patients with suppressed immune systems may acquire nosocomial pneumonia from *Pseudomonas aeruginosa*. Viral pneumonia may begin as influenza and may lead to a secondary bacterial pneumonia. Fungal pneumonia is a rare condition that mimics the same necrosis and casseation as tuberculosis. It is caused by inhalation of certain spores present in the soil (3, p 889).

Aspiration pneumonia occurs in anesthetized patients or those with a depressed gag or swallowing reflex. Pregnant women particularly are prone to aspiration during anesthesia due to the following factors:

1. Elevated gastric pressure because of mechanical compression of abdominal contents by the gravid uterus; and
2. Relaxation of smooth musculature of the gastroesophageal sphincter due to progestational effects (or due to effects of progesterone).

Hypostatic pneumonia results from shallow breathing, which causes accumulations of fluid in the lungs. Postoperative, hospitalized, and/or bedridden patients frequently fall victim to this type of pneumonia (3, p 889).

Signs and Symptoms

Symptoms of lobar pneumonia strike suddenly and are dramatic in their intensity. These include chills and fevers of 40.0–41.4°C (104–106°F), sharp chest pain, and cough productive of blood–tinged or brown sputum. Pulse and respirations have been known to increase to twice their normal rate.

Bronchial pneumonia is accompanied by milder symptoms, with a more gradual appearance.

Bronchial pneumonia is rarely fatal. However, relapses are more common.

Diagnosis

Diagnosis is based on history, physical examination, and chest x-ray. Laboratory testing should include complete blood count with differential, sputum gram stain, and blood culture and sensitivity. Gram stain in bacterial pneumonia usually reveals many polymorphonuclear leukocytes and gram-positive, lancet-shaped diplococci. Since many causative organisms are fragile and hard to grow outside the body, sputum cultures may be falsely negative and diagnosis may be based on presumptive criteria. Auscultation of the lungs in lobar pneumonia may reveal rales, wheezing, friction rub (due to pleurisy), and large areas of dull or diminished breath sounds (2, p 424).

Maternal and Fetal Outcome

Given an acute infectious process in a normally breathing pregnant patient, a healthy outcome may be expected for mother and baby.

However, with severe pulmonary disease and/or with predisposing chronic disease, maternal and fetal outcome may be jeopardized severely. For example, bronchial pneumonia has proved fatal to some patients with severe cardiac disease.

Medical Management

Medical management depends on the etiology and the severity of the pneumonia. Bedrest is essential in assisting the body to fight infection as well as to decrease the respiratory effort. Dehydration from fever and increased respiratory rate is a prime concern, and oral fluids should be forced and, if necessary, supplemented through intravenous infusion. Monitoring of vital signs also should include evaluation of mental status, which may become impaired from hypoxia and/or fever. Use of antibiotics is based on results of sputum culture and sensitivity. Antipyretics may be necessary in severe cases, as well as tepid sponging (5, p 354); analgesics may be necessary to encourage deep breathing.

Fetal status should be assessed carefully using nonstress testing and biophysical profile.

NURSING MANAGEMENT

Nursing care specific for patients with pneumonia:

☐ Encourage all pregnant women to report promptly signs and symptoms of upper respiratory tract infection.

☐ Screen all pregnant women for signs and symptoms of pneumonia (e.g., auscultate lungs; note temperature, respirations, skin color).

NURSING MANAGEMENT

- Stress the importance of smoking cessation in maintaining healthy lungs.

Nursing care specific for bedridden and postoperative pregnant patients with *pneumonia:*

- Teach patients preventive measures (e.g., turn, cough, and deep breathe at least every 2 hours).
- Observe sputum for color, amount, and consistency at least every 4 hours.
- During coughing spells, assist patient to an upright position and splint the chest with pillows.
- Change damp linen immediately to avoid chilling and fatigue.
- Maintain planned rest periods.
- Provide mouth care, as needed.
- Encourage adequate fluid intake, at least 3,000 cc of fluid daily.
- Encourage a diet high in protein and vitamin C to promote healing; small, frequent, soft or liquid diets may be required.

COCCIDIOIDOMYCOSIS

Etiology

This is a form of fungal pneumonia that may be dormant or become active and disseminate like tuberculosis. Although occurrence has been rare, with increasing incidence of AIDS, it is likely that more cases will be seen. Dormant, benign forms, are one hundred times more likely to disseminate in pregnant than nonpregnant patients. Left untreated, pregnant patients with the disseminated form have virtually a 100% mortality rate in comparison to a 50% rate in nonpregnant patients. Thus, pregnancy not only increases the incidence of occurrence of the lethal form but decreases chances for survival. Coccidioidomycosis primarily is a disease of the immune-suppressed patient (2, p 424).

Signs and Symptoms

Signs and symptoms are those of a severe lobar pneumonia.

Diagnosis

Diagnosis is based on sputum culture.

- Institute isolation precautions according to hospital policy and causative organism.
- Teach and encourage the patient to perform deep breathing exercises for at least six weeks after the hospital discharge.

Nursing diagnoses most frequently associated with *pneumonia:*

- Grieving related to potential/actual loss of infant or birth of an imperfect child.
- Anticipatory grieving related to actual/perceived threat to self.
- Disturbance in body image, self-esteem.
- Ineffective family coping: compromised.
- Knowledge deficit regarding etiology, disease process, treatment, and outcome.
- Knowledge deficit regarding medication regimen.
- Self care deficit—feeding, bathing/hygiene, dressing, grooming, toileting.
- Altered nutrition: less than body requirements.
- Potential for infection.

Maternal and Fetal Outcome

Maternal and fetal outcome are compromised. However, in the dormant form a good maternal and fetal outcome may be expected in the majority of cases. In the disseminated phase, maternal and fetal life are at stake.

Medical Management

Medical management is the same as that for other pneumonias. Use of amphotericin B has been reported to save some patients. Teratogenic effects of this medication on the fetus are not known (2, p 424).

TUBERCULOSIS

Definition

Tuberculosis is an infectious, inflammatory disease which commonly affects the lungs, although it may occur in any part of the body. Tuberculosis may be either primary or secondary. The primary disease is usually asymptomatic and results in the formation of specific antigen/antibody complexes. These, in turn, attack the site of infection and bring about progressive necrosis, fibrosis, and caseation of lung tissue—which processes render the disease inactive. However, if the formation of sufficient concentration of antigen/antibody complexes does not take place (e.g., due to debilitated health status or suppressed immunity), primary tuberculosis may progress to full blown disease. Secondary tuberculosis occurs as a result of endogenous or exogenous *reinfection*. This is the most common type of tuberculosis in the United States. Secondary tuberculosis is most likely to be endogenous, resulting from reactivation in patients with decreased resistance (e.g., the debilitated, chronically ill, and/or emotionally stressed) (5, p 360).

Although tuberculosis primarily affects the lungs, it may involve any organ. Other reported sites include (3, p 1145):

1. Bone, particularly the spine (Pott's disease);
2. Skin (lupus vulgaris);
3. Kidney and/or bladder;
4. Reproductive organs; and
5. Central nervous system (meningeal tuberculosis).

Etiology

Tuberculosis is caused by the tubercule bacillus (*Mycobacterium tuberculosis*). The most common mode of transmission in the United States is through inhalation of infected droplet nuclei from a person with active tuberculosis. In other parts of the world, consumption of milk and dairy products from infected cattle is a more common cause (5, p 360).

It is possible to destroy the tubercule bacillus. Autoclaving, boiling for 5 minutes, contact with phenol or other coal tar preparations, and/or exposure to sunlight (ultraviolet radiation) all have been proven to be effective agents (5, p 360).

Signs and Symptoms

Early signs can include loss of energy, listlessness, poor appetite, loss of weight, low grade fever, and/or vague chest pains. Other symptoms are development of laryngeal ulcers and/or inflammation and intestinal infection. Both of these are probably caused by swallowing infected sputum.

Unfortunately, the classic symptoms of chronic cough, night sweats, and hemoptysis occur quite late in the disease process—usually at least 1 year from onset of the disease.

Chest pain and dyspnea caused by pleurisy are the most common presenting symptoms (3, p 1145).

Diagnosis

A careful history is necessary to identify risks for tuberculosis. The following are significant risk factors (2, p 419):

1. Previous history of tuberculosis;
2. Known tubercular conversion;
3. Pleurisy;
4. Contact with known tuberculosis victim;
5. Presence of chronic disease (i.e., liver disease, diabetes mellitus, AIDS);
6. Severe psychological stress;
7. Malnutrition;
8. Crowded, unsanitary housing;
9. Recent travel in a country where tuberculosis is prevalent; and
10. Illegal United States immigration status.

Tuberculosis can be strongly suspected in patients who present with the following signs and symptoms (2, p 419):

1. Complaint of hemoptysis, night sweats, and productive cough.
2. Positive tine or purified protein derivative (PPD) after a known negative test.
3. Localized chest pain.
4. Chest x-ray indicating pleural effusion and/or areas of cavitation.

Positive diagnosis is based on positive sputum cultures for acid-fast bacteria. At least three cultures should be obtained to confirm a diagnosis. Ideally, cultures should be obtained in the morning. This provides time for pooling of secretions during the night, assuring a more representative sputum sample for culture. Since the tubercle bacillus is fragile and relatively slow growing (over 2 weeks), bronchoscopy and lung biopsy also may be used to confirm diagnosis (2, p 419).

Maternal and Fetal Outcome

The prognosis for the pregnant patient with tuberculosis is excellent, provided that she follows her medical regimen. However, side effects of the treatment regimen may be problematic (see Table 16.5).

Fetal outcome usually is good. No increased incidence of abortion or prematurity has been documented (2, p 419).

Teratogenic effects of certain antitubercular medications have been documented. However, use of chemotherapeutic agents have to be weighed against risks of untreated maternal disease. A recent study of fetal outcome is encouraging since

Table 16.5.
DRUGS USED IN TREATMENT OF TUBERCULOSIS[a]

DRUGS	DOSAGE DAILY	DOSAGE TWICE WEEKLY	MOST COMMON SIDE EFFECTS	TESTS FOR SIDE EFFECTS	REMARKS
Isoniazid	5–10 mg/kg up to 300 mg p.o. or i.m.	15 mg/kg p.o. or i.m.	Peripheral neuritis, hepatitis, hypersensitivity	SGOT/SGPT (not as a routine)	Bactericidal; pyridoxine 10 mg as prophylaxis for neuritis; 50–100 mg as treatment
Ethambutol	15–25 mg/kg p.o.	50 mg/kg p.o.	Optic neuritis (reversible with discontinuation of drug; very rare at 15 mg/kg), skin rash	Red-green color discrimination and visual acuity	Use with caution with renal disease or when eye testing is not feasible
Rifampin	10–20 mg/kg up to 600 mg p.o.	Not recommended	Hepatitis, febrile reaction purpura (rare)	SGOT/SGPT (not as a routine)	Bactericidal; orange-urine color; negates effect of birth control pills
Streptomycin	15–20 mg/kg up to 1 g i.m.	25–30 mg/kg	Eighth cranial nerve damage, nephrotoxicity	Vestibular function, audiograms; BUN and creatinine	Use with caution in older patients or those with renal disease

[a]Adapted from Phipps W, et al.: *Medical Surgical Nursing*. St. Louis, Mosby, 1979.

94% of births were normal, and only 3% of infants exposed to antitubercular medications in utero could be classified as having birth defects.

If the mother has active disease, the newborn has a great chance (>50%) of becoming infected with tuberculosis, unless treatment is begun (7).

Medical Management

Principles of management for the pregnant patient with active tuberculosis are the same as for the nonpregnant patient. This involves a chemotherapeutic regimen of a combination of two of the following drugs: isoniazid, ethambutol, rifampin, or streptomycin (see Table 16.5) (8, 9).

Most tuberculous patients can be managed at home with the help and supervision of public health nursing services. Attention should be placed on rest, good nutrition, and methods to prevent spread of disease as well as compliance with medication regimen.

Hospitalization is required only if complications occur. Possible complications include pulmonary hemorrhage, emphysema, and tubercular pneumonia. Hospitalization also may be advisable at the beginning of chemotherapy in order to ensure build-up of therapeutic blood levels of medication and to observe for possible side effects of medications (3, p 1145).

The pregnant patient with a history of adequate treatment including negative sputum cultures and stable chest x-ray should be observed carefully during the antenatal period. It is possible that the stress of pregnancy itself may be cause for endogenous reactivation of the disease.

The pregnant patient with a positive PPD (>10 mm wheal 72 hours after injection) but with negative sputum cultures and negative chest x-ray should not be treated routinely during pregnancy. Treatment usually is begun only in the postpartum period because of an increased risk of hepatitis associated with isoniazid use during pregnancy and the risk of fetal malformation (2, p 423).

The newborn of the active tuberculous patient also should be treated. Recommended therapy involves a one-time dose or vaccination of bacilli Calmette Guerin (BCG) vaccine. Alternatively, isoniazid (10–20 mg/kg/day) for 1 year may be prescribed. Obviously, the long-term isoniazid treatment is preferable, but the partial immunity conferred by BCG in one dose may be indicated if compliance is a problem or if long-term follow-up of the newborn is not possible (10).

Whether or not the newborn must be separated from the mother depends on the presence of active infection in the mother. The mother is considered inactive only if she is receiving treatment, her sputum cultures are negative, and her chest x-ray stable. Active disease—treated or untreated—should be cause for separation of the mother and infant until the mother meets the inactive criteria and the baby has a positive PPD from BCG vaccination or until isoniazid treatment is begun. Finally, breastfeeding is contraindicated if the mother has active tuberculosis because the disease is transmitted through breast milk (10).

Significance of Tubercular Testing

The commonly used Mantoux test consists of an intradermal injection of purified protein derivative (PPD) of the tuberculin bacilli. A positive reaction to the test is an indurated wheal of ≥10 millimeters in diameter occurring 48–72 hours after injection.

The test confirms the fact that sometime in the patient's life she has been exposed to the bacillus and developed antigen/antibody complexes against the disease. Further studies (e.g., sputum cultures and chest x-ray) need to be evaluated before the diagnosis of active tuberculosis is determined (3, p 1145).

It should be noted that patients who are vaccinated with BCG will continue to have a positive PPD. This results from the fact that the vaccine contains strains of bovine tuberculosis. Patients who were born in Europe and, indeed, in most countries other than the United States can be anticipated to have had BCG vaccine.

Finally, the tine test is a tuberculin test involving a multipuncture disposable device used to scratch the skin surface. However, it is less accurate than the PPD and false-positive results have been reported. Thus, while a positive reaction is the same as the PPD, it should be reevaluated with a PPD before a chest x-ray is warranted (3, p 1145).

False-negative results of either the PPD or the tine test should be considered in patients who are being immunosuppressed therapeutically (renal transplant) or those who have diseases that suppress the immunological system (Hodgkin's disease, AIDS).

NURSING MANAGEMENT

Nursing care specific for patients with *tuberculosis:*

☐ Screen all prenatal patients for tuberculosis (e.g., with PPD).

☐ For patient requiring chest x-ray, ensure that abdomen is shielded; delay screening x-rays until after 20 weeks of gestation, if possible.

☐ For patients with diagnosed tuberculosis in the hospital:

— Institute isolation if appropriate or if the patient has copious secretions; wear face mask when in close contact with patient;

— Limit number of visitors to provide rest and to control spread of disease;

— Encourage family to be screened for tuberculosis;

— Provide home follow-up through the visiting nurse service;

— Report contacts to Bureau of Infectious Disease for follow-up and treatment;

— Initiate isolation of infant if appropriate; and

— Prohibit breastfeeding if mother has active tuberculosis.

Nursing diagnoses most frequently associated with *tuberculosis:*

☐ Grieving related to potential/actual loss of infant or birth of an imperfect child.

☐ Disturbance in body image, self-esteem.

☐ Ineffective family coping: compromised.

☐ Knowledge deficit regarding etiology, disease process, treatment, and outcome.

☐ Knowledge deficit regarding medication regimen.

☐ Pain.

☐ Altered nutrition: less than body requirements.

☐ Impaired gas exchange.

AMNIOTIC FLUID EMBOLISM

Definition

In this catastrophic accident amniotic fluid and fetal skin cells, lanugo, hair, meconium, fat, or bile enter the maternal circulatory system, causing a blockage (embolism) in the pulmonary vasculature. Animal studies have documented the fact that amniotic fluid by itself is harmless in the maternal system. It is the combination of fluids with fetal debris that results in this unique disorder (1, p 419).

Although the incidence is rare (<0.05%) in pregnancy, its high mortality rate makes it responsible for as much as 15% of overall maternal mortality rates.

Etiology

The exact point of entry of the embolism as well as the etiology are unknown.

Theories regarding the point of entry include endocervical veins, known to be lacerated even in normal pregnancy; placental site; and uterine veins. Proposed rationales for the profound, life-threatening picture of this disorder include (11):

1. Mechanical occlusion of the pulmonary vasculature by fetal debris.
2. Anaphylactic reaction to fetal debris as foreign matter.
3. Secondarily, coagulopathy associated with uterine atony (postpartum hemorrhage usually is associated with this disorder).

Factors associated with the occurrence of amniotic fluid embolism have been identified. These are tumultuous labor, use of oxytocin induction/augmentation during labor, meconium staining, advanced maternal age, intrauterine fetal demise, and/or immediate postpartum hemorrhage (11).

Signs and Symptoms

The sudden onset of restlessness, hypotension, tachycardia, cyanosis, loss of consciousness, shock, seizures and/or cardiac arrest—especially coupled with positive identification of risk factors—compose the clinical picture of the disorder. Pulmonary edema and bronchospasm frequently are apparent.

Diagnosis

Laboratory findings confirming the diagnosis show right heart strain on electrocardiogram, low pO_2, and low fibrinogen. Chest x-ray reveals diffuse pulmonary infiltrates. However, presumptive diagnosis usually is based on the presence of the clinical signs and symptoms.

Maternal and Fetal Outcome

Maternal outcome is severely jeopardized. An 80% maternal mortality rate is reported. Twenty-five percent of these deaths occur within the first hour of onset of signs and symptoms (1, pp 419–420).

Because the infant has been delivered or the fetus is readily deliverable by cesarean section, infant outcome usually is not compromised.

Medical Management

Because the etiology of the embolism is poorly understood, medical management is controversial. Generally, management revolves around treatment of circulatory and respiratory collapse. Queenan and Hobbins (1, p 420) suggest the following regime:

1. Position the patient in a high Fowler's position.
2. Sedate the patient with 5–15 mg of morphine to relieve anxiety.
3. Intubate and ventilate the patient.
4. Infuse aminophylline, 250–500 mg in 50 ml of D_5W (5% dextrose in water) over a 20-minute period to relieve bronchospasm.
5. Digitalize the patient with 0.5 mg of digoxin intravenously, followed by 0.125 mg every 2 hours for 6 days to increase and strengthen cardiac contractility.
6. Give the patient hydrocortisone (1 g intravenously) to decrease pulmonary edema and follow with 250 mg every 4 hours.
7. Use bimanual uterine compression to control uterine atony and hemorrhage.
8. Combat disseminated intravascular coagulopathy by use of fibrinogen or fresh frozen plasma.

NURSING MANAGEMENT

Nursing care specific for patients with
amniotic fluid embolism:
☐ Be aware of factors associated with amniotic fluid embolism (e.g., oxytocin induction/augmentation, tumultuous labor, postpartum hemorrhage); monitor the patient closely during the intrapartum and immediate postpartum period for signs/symptoms of pulmonary embolism.
☐ If amniotic fluid embolism occurs:

— Stay with the patient, provide emotional support to her and her family;
— Offer patient the benefit of the clergy, if appropriate;
— Place the patient in Fowler's position;
— Administer oxygen, medication, and blood products, as ordered;
— Prepare for emergency cesarean section if undelivered;
— Prepare for transfer to intensive care unit, if appropriate; and

NURSING MANAGEMENT

— If the mother dies help the family through the grieving process.

Nursing diagnoses most frequently associated with *amniotic fluid embolism*:

☐ Anticipatory grieving related to actual/perceived threat to self.

☐ Knowledge deficit regarding etiology, disease process, treatment, and outcome.

☐ Impaired gas exchange.

☐ Fluid volume deficit.

☐ Altered maternal tissue perfusion.

REFERENCES

1. Queenan, J, Hobbins J: *Protocols for High Risk Pregnancy*. Oradell, NJ, Medical Economic Books, 1982.
2. Weinberger S, Weiss S: Pulmonary diseases. In Burrow G, Ferris T (eds): *Medical Complications in Pregnancy*. Philadelphia, WB Saunders, 1982.
3. Miller B, Keone C: *Encyclopedia and Dictionary of Medicine, Nursing and Allied Health*. Philadelphia, WB Saunders, 1983.
4. de Swiet M (Ed): *Medical Disorders of Pregnancy*. Boston, Blackwell Scientific Publications, 1984.
5. Mahoney E, Flynn J: *The Handbook of Medical-Surgical Nursing*. New York, John Wiley and Sons, 1983.
6. Schoenbaum S, Weinstein L: Respiratory infection in pregnancy. *Clin Obstet Gynecol* 22, 293–300, 1979.
7. Snider D: Pregnancy and tuberculosis. *Chest*, 863 (Suppl 3): 105–135, 1984.
8. American Thoracic Society: Treatment of mycobacterial disease. *Am Rev Resp Dis* 115: 185–187.
9. Sahn S: Tuberculosis in association with pregnancy. *Am Jour Obstet Gynecol* 140:492, 498, 1981.
10. Cloherty J, Stark A: *Manual of Neonatal Care*. Boston, Little, Brown and Co, 1984.
11. Letsky E: Blood volume, haematinics and anaemia. In de Swiet M (ed). *Medical Disorders of Pregnancy*. Boston, Blackwell Scientific Publications, 1984.

Chapter 17
Renal System Disorders
Kathleen Buckley, C.N.M., M.S.N.

INTRODUCTION

Pregnancy is associated with significant renal anatomic and physiologic changes. The renal system handles increased maternal fluid load and metabolic products, as well as fetal waste products.

Anatomic Changes

The main anatomic changes during pregnancy are dilation of the renal calyces and ureters. These changes begin in the first trimester and usually persist through the postpartum period. The dilation is thought to be the result of the hormone progesterone and is more pronounced on the right side due to the mechanical pressure of the dextrorotated pregnant uterus. The ureters are not only dilated, but become elongated, twisted, and laterally displaced. These changes result in a condition termed "physiologic hydroureters" of pregnancy in which the ureteral lumens are increased in diameter with a concurrent hypotonicity and hypomotility. This, in turn, causes a reservoir or backlog of fluids that are present in the ureters and that move more slowly to the kidney producing a delay in renal excretion. The kidney increases approximately 1.5 cm in size—probably because of the increased renal blood flow and renal macular change with some degree of hypertrophy, not an increase in the actual number of renal cells.

The bladder lies adjacent to the uterus. Its capacity is decreased early in pregnancy when the uterus is also a pelvic organ and again late in pregnancy when the fetal presenting part displaces it anteriorly and superiorly. Conversely, the tone of the bladder is decreased and during the second and early third trimester and the early postpartum period, the capacity may double in volume (i.e., to more than 1 liter). Due to progesterone, the vesicoureteral valve may become incompetent, allowing reflux from the bladder up into the ureters. Toward term, the bladder becomes edematous and easily traumatized. These changes increase the risk of injury during delivery and infection in the postpartum period (1).

Physiologic Changes

Renal blood flow increases dramatically during pregnancy with second trimester values up 60–80%, followed by a significant decrease in the third trimester. Increased renal blood flow, in turn, leads to an increased glomerular filtration rate and a concurrent decreased plasma level of creatinine and uric acid.

However, some selective renal tubular reabsorption rates are not increased and, as a result, nutrients such as amino acids and glucose are normally excreted in the urine of the pregnant woman. It is thought that this high nutritive content of urine during pregnancy may contribute to increased incidence of urinary tract infection. It should be noted that glycosuria during pregnancy is not necessarily indicative of endocrine malfunction (e.g., diabetes mellitus) but is more likely to be a byproduct of normal renal function.

The largest renal adjustment during pregnancy involves the handling of sodium. The amount of sodium filtered through the kidneys increases from the nonpregnant levels of 20,000 mEq/day to as much as 30,000 mEq per day. At the same time, selective tubular reabsorption not only equals the amount of sodium lost, but adds 2–6 mEq/day for maternal/fetal stores. While the etiology of the changes is unknown, these changes are thought to be mediated by increased levels of aldosterone, corticosterone, cortisol, estrogen, and/or prolactin. In any case, while the handling of sodium changes significantly during pregnancy, the alterations tend to cancel themselves out and a pregnant woman handles sodium as well as if not better than a nonpregnant woman (1, p 260).

Finally, water and sodium levels are markedly affected by maternal posture and diurnal activity. There is decreased excretion during the day when the woman is up and about resulting in dependent edema. At night, a left side lying position will increase water and sodium excretion by enhancing renal blood flow; and is the cause of the so-called physiologic nocturia during pregnancy.

ASYMPTOMATIC BACTERIURIA

Definition

Asymptomatic bacteriuria (ASB) is defined as the presence of actively multiplying bacteria within the urinary tract without urinary tract symptoms.

Etiology

The most frequent causative organism is *Escherichia coli* (80%) with *Klebsiella proteus* and *Enterobacter* accounting for the rest of cases. ASB is caused clinically by only one bacterial species; if more are recovered, the specimen should be considered contaminated and another obtained.

Incidence varies from 2–12%, depending on the population studied. Parity, race, and socioeconomic status influence incidence. For example, poor, black multiparas have the highest rates of ASB, whereas white, middle/upper-class primiparous women have the lowest rates. ASB is also markedly increased in pregnant women with sickle cell trait. Anemia also predisposes toward urinary tract infection.

Diagnosis

Diagnosis of ASB is based on obtaining two consecutive clean catch urines yielding a colony count of 10^5 of one type of the microorganisms mentioned above.

Maternal/Fetal Outcome

Between 20% and 40% of women with ASB progress to symptomatic infection of the urinary tract during pregnancy, including pyelonephritis. In addition, ASB may persist into the postpartum period and, untreated, may result in serious renal disease. ASB may also be indicative of undiagnosed chronic renal infection, obstructive lesions, and/or congenital anomalies of the urinary tract (2).

The fetus may be at increased risk of intrauterine growth retardation (IUGR) and preterm labor, although research at this time is still inconclusive. Clinically, there does seem to be an association between bladder infection and uterine irritability in general. IUGR may be more likely when ASB is a sign of undiagnosed chronic renal disease.

Medical Management

All pregnant woman should be screened for bacteriuria at the first prenatal visit. In addition, women with sickle cell trait and disease, history of recurrent urinary tract infection, or chronic renal disease, should be screened more often, at least once each trimester.

A 10-day course of either Macrodantin (100 mg/day) or sulfisoxazole (1 four times a day) will be effective in eradicating the common causative agents of ASB. In addition, because of client acceptability, a single dose regimen for treatment has been developed and also proven effective.

Treatment should always be followed by a test of cure 10 days after medication is complete. Because all women who are diagnosed with ASB are at risk for recurrence, monthly urine cultures should be obtained for the rest of the pregnancy. Reinfection with the same organism is indicative of underlying, chronic renal infection and usually occurs within 2–3 weeks of treatment. Subsequent infection with a different organism is usually localized to the bladder only and occurs 3 weeks or more after treatment.

URINARY TRACT INFECTION—CYSTITIS

Definition

Acute or chronic infection of the urinary tract that involves only the bladder and is symptomatic is termed cystitis.

Etiology

The most common causative organism, as with ASB, is *Escherichia coli*. Poor hygiene practice, trauma, or contamination of the urinary meatus during sexual intercourse increase the risk of infection.

Signs and Symptoms

Cystitis is characterized by localized symptomatology—dysuria, urgency, frequency, suprapubic tenderness, bladder spasm, and dyspareunia. Systemic signs are usually absent, although occasionally a low grade fever is present.

Diagnosis

Diagnosis is based on history and positive urine microanalysis and culture. A urine microanalysis will reveal increased bacteria and white blood cells (5 or more per high powered field). Occasionally, gross hematuria is present. Urine cultures will contain a bacterial count of 100,000/ml.

Cystitis may be concurrently present with vaginitis (especially *Trichomonas* or *Chlamydia*

trachamatis), but must be differentiated from secondary urethritis caused by vaginal pathogens (2, p 890).

Maternal/Fetal Outcome

Maternal prognosis is good as long as the infection is localized in the bladder and does not ascend to the kidney.

As with ASB, any bladder irritation can be associated with onset of labor (see Chapter 28).

Medical Management

Medical management is similar to management of ASB.

NURSING MANAGEMENT

Nursing management specific for patients with *urinary tract infection—cystitis*:

Prevention

- [ ] Teach all women methods to prevent urinary tract infection:
  - Increasing fluid intake to 8 glasses/day;
  - Washing hands before as well as after urinating/defecating,
  - Cleaning perineal region carefully from front to back;
  - Emptying bladder before and after sexual intercourse;
  - Avoiding perfumed soaps, feminine hygiene sprays, and bubble bath solutions;
  - Showering with antibacterial soap; and
  - Emptying the bladder at least every 2–4 hours while awake.
- [ ] Ensure that all pregnant women know how to collect a clean catch urine sample and are screened for bacteriuria at first prenatal visit, and that those with positive results are promptly contacted to return for treatment.
- [ ] Ensure that at-risk pregnant women (e.g., older, poor, minority women, and those with anemia or sickle cell trait or chronic renal disease) are screened on a more frequent basis.
- [ ] Follow up to ensure that all anemic pregnant women are prescribed iron and/or folic acid supplementation.
- [ ] Teach the patient the signs and symptoms of urinary tract infection and to report them promptly.

- [ ] Screen every pregnant patient for signs and symptoms of urinary tract infection at each visit and observe the routine urine specimen for color, odor, and viscosity.
- [ ] Encourage the laboring woman to void every 2 hours.
- [ ] Avoid routine catherization during labor, delivery, and postpartum period.

Treatment

- [ ] Review general health measures for any infection (e.g., rest, forced fluids, increased intake of vitamin C).
- [ ] Teach the patient to avoid bladder irritants (coffee, tea, cola, pepper).
- [ ] Teach the patient to take at least 6 oz of cranberry juice at bedtime to acidify the urine.
- [ ] Teach the patient the signs and symptoms of preterm labor and where to report them.
- [ ] Ensure that a test of cure is performed 2 weeks after a full course of treatment for ASB and/or cystitis. For that test *only*, the patient should be instructed to decrease fluid intake for at least 8 hours so that a concentrated urine specimen can be obtained.
- [ ] Continue to reculture pregnant women with ASB or cystitis on a monthly basis until delivery.

Nursing diagnoses most frequently associated with *urinary tract infection—cystitis*:

- [ ] Knowledge deficit regarding etiology, disease process, treatment, and expected outcome.
- [ ] Pain.
- [ ] Altered patterns of urinary elimination.
- [ ] Knowledge deficit regarding medication regimen.

URINARY TRACT INFECTION—ACUTE PYELONEPHRITIS

Definition

Pyelonephritis is an acute infection of the ureters, renal pelvis, and kidneys; it occurs in approximately 2% of all pregnancies. Acute pyelonephritis is considered one of the major medical complications of pregnancy (3).

Etiology

The infection is most commonly caused by *Escherichia coli*, which ascends to the kidney from the lower urinary tract or may extend to the kidney from the bladder through the blood vessels or lymphatics. The ascending route is most common.

Signs and Symptoms

Unlike ASB, which is asymptomatic, or cystitis, which has localized symptoms, acute pyelonephritis is a systemic disease. Symptoms are abrupt in onset and include (3, p 581):

1. Spiking temperature fluctuation from 34° C to as high as 42° C.
2. Nausea, vomiting.
3. Shaking, chills.
4. Severe malaise.
5. Unilateral (typically right-sided) or bilateral flank pain.
6. Abdominal tenderness, distention, rigidity.
7. Costovertebral angle tenderness (CVAT).

In addition, the localized symptoms of a cystitis may be present.

Diagnosis

The presence of these serious signs and symptoms are indicative of the condition. Urinary microanalysis will contain white blood cells almost always in clumps, *E. coli* and other numerous bacteria. Blood cultures may also demonstrate *E. coli*. However, differential diagnosis must include acute bowel disease (appendicitis, diverticulitis, regional ileitis), pelvic inflammatory disease, and ectopic pregnancy or placental abruption.

Maternal/Fetal Outcome

Acute pyelonephritis is a serious condition which jeopardizes both maternal and fetal well-being. Approximately 10% of women develop bacteremia and, of those, 3% will proceed into shock because of release of endotoxins from the infected kidney(s) into the bloodstream. Renal function may be impaired as evidenced by decreased creatinine clearance rates. Pyelonephritis is also associated with development of other life-threatening conditions such as thrombocytopenia, pneumonia, and volume overload congestive heart failure.

Medical Management

All pregnant women who develop acute pyelonephritis should be hospitalized. Because of severe nausea and vomiting, many patients will be dehydrated and require immediate treatment with intravenous fluid. In addition, because of the overwhelming systemic nature of the condition, antibiotics should be administered parenterally. Vital signs and urinary output should be frequently recorded in order to detect bacteremic shock. Hypotension, hypothermia, tachycardia, or decreased urinary output are all ominous signs.

The antibiotic of choice is Ampicillin—1–2 g every 6 hours intravenously. The addition of an amnioglycoside (gentamicin, tobramycin, or amikacin) in doses of 3–5 mg/kg/day in three divided doses is indicated in 48–72 hours if the urine culture is still positive or if clinical sepsis is present.

Preterm labor may ensue and accounts for reported increased incidence of low birth weight associated with pyelonephritis. Abatement of symptoms is not indicative of cure and antibiotic therapy should be continued for at least 10 days. Repeat cultures should be done 2 weeks after the course of treatment and monthly until delivery.

ACUTE RENAL FAILURE

Definition

Acute renal failure (ARF) is sudden cessation of renal function and is associated with a wide range of clinical conditions (4).

Etiology

Causes of ARF are usually classified into three groups: prerenal conditions, direct renal damage, and postrenal obstruction. A hemolytic uremic syndrome in the postpartum period has been described.

Prerenal conditions are caused by interference with renal perfusion. Examples of conditions that cause decreased renal perfusion include vomiting, diarrhea, hemorrhage, burns, and renal artery occlusion. Renal damage refers to parenchymal

Table 17.1.
COMMON CAUSES OF ACUTE RENAL FAILURE
IN PREGNANCY

Hyperemesis gravidarum
Antepartumpostpartum hemorrhage
Disseminated intravascular coagulation
Septic shock
Hepatic renal failure syndrome
Transfusion reaction
Nephrotoxins (x-ray contrast media, aminoglycosides,
    penicillins, diphenylhydantoin, phenylbutazone)

Table 17.2.
LABORATORY TEST FINDINGS
CHARACTERISTIC OF ARF

VALUE	FINDING
Blood urea nitrogen	Increased
Creatinine	Increased
Potassium	Increased
Sodium	Decreased
Magnesium	Increased
Phosphate	Increased
Calcium	Decreased
pH	Acidic
Hematocrit	Decreased

changes caused by disease or nephrotoxic substances. Acute tubular necrosis (ATN) accounts for 90% of cases of acute oliguria. Other causes include trauma, vasculitis atherosclerosis, and tumor invasion. Postrenal conditions refer to obstruction occuring anywhere in the urinary tract from the urinary meatus to the renal tubules. Common causes of obstruction include calculi, invading tumors, and surgical accidents (5).

Postpartum hemolytic uremic syndrome has no known cause and occurs usually within a month or less of a normal uncomplicated delivery.

The most common causes of ARF during pregnancy are hemorrhage caused by abruptio placentae, eclampsia, and disseminated intravascular coagulation caused by prolonged fetal death in utero. Other causes are listed in Table 17.1. ARF is an unusual complication of pregnancy occurring in one to 2000–5000 pregnancies.

Signs and Symptoms

Oliguria is usually present. Laboratory studies reveal evidence that the kidney has stopped functioning (see Table 17.2). The patient will appear acutely ill and the following medical complications may be present:

1. Confusion, lethargy, and seizures;
2. Hypertension, congestive failure;
3. Vomiting, gastrointestinal bleeding;
4. Respiratory or urinary tract infection, operative site infection.

Postpartum hemolytic uremic syndrome usually begins with nausea, vomiting, diarrhea or flu-like symptoms. This is followed by onset of anemia, intravascular coagulation, and severe hypertension.

Maternal/Fetal Outcome

While ARF is a relatively rare occurrence during pregnancy, the mortality can be as high as 60%, depending on causative factors. Direct damage to kidney cells has the poorest prognosis. In addition, a concurrent infection in the presence of ARF is associated with a 70% mortality rate.

The fetus, too, is at grave risk. ARF is associated with a high incidence of abortion, stillbirth, and preterm delivery. With hemodialysis, however, successful outcome has been achieved.

Medical Management

The following preventive practices can help ensure that ARF does not occur (4, p 290):

1. Prompt blood/fluid replacement;
2. Careful evaluation of kidney function in all preeclamptic patients;
3. Avoidance of nephrotoxic drugs in patients with oliguria;
4. Monitoring renal function if a nephrotoxic drug must be used;
5. Careful monitoring of intake/output and other signs of sepsis in patients with septic abortion, puerperal infection, chorioamnionitis, and pyelonephritis.

When ARF is present, management is based on causative classification. For example, prerenal hypovolemia can be corrected by replacing fluids. Postrenal obstruction can be surgically repaired. Direct damage to the kidney can be mediated with hemodialysis. Hemolytic uremic syndrome treatment includes antihypertensive mediation, supportive care, anticoagulation therapy, and dialysis if renal failure is present. In severe cases, some clinicians advocate nephrectomy.

Nutritional requirements include a diet low in protein (40 g), and sodium high in carbohydrates (100 g) and supplemented with essential and nonessential amino acids.

In some cases, parenteral hyperalimentation may be necessary to reverse negative nitrogen balance.

Because infection associated with ARF is the major cause of death (70%), careful evaluation of the patient's condition should be ongoing.

Usual signs of infection may be absent (e.g., fever, tachycardia), and many antibiotics are nephrotoxic. Thus, prophylactic antibiotics are generally not suggested. However, if the patient's condition continues to deteriorate with ongoing medical treatment, infection should be suspected and treatment begun against Gram-negative bacteria and *Staphylococcus aureus*.

NURSING MANAGEMENT

Nursing management for patients with *Acute Renal Failure (ARF)*:

☐ Be aware of conditions that cause ARF in pregnancy (e.g., antepartum or postpartum hemorrhage, DIC associated with fetal death in utero, preeclampsia, septic shock, hepatic failure syndrome, transfusion reaction).

☐ Be alert for ARF: maintain appropriate fluid replacement and meticulous intake and output records.

☐ Monitor vital signs including urine specific gravity.

☐ Monitor serum electrolyte levels (e.g., sodium, potassium, calcium, phosphate, magnesium).

☐ Assist with dialysis, as appropriate.

☐ Initiate seizure precautions, as appropriate.

☐ Take every measure to prevent secondary infection associated with ARF and encourage all other members of the health care team to do the same:

— Avoid skin breakdown by frequent position change, pressure mattress, etc.;

— Encourage coughing and deep breathing;

— Avoid unnecessary catheterization; and

— Use strict aseptic technique to dress wounds, start intravenous infusion, catheterize the bladder, and perform vaginal examination.

Nursing diagnoses most frequently associated with ARF:

☐ Anxiety/fear.

☐ Pain.

☐ Impaired tissue integrity.

☐ Altered fetal cardiac and cerebral tissue perfusion.

☐ Knowledge deficit regarding etiology, disease process, treatment, and expected outcome.

☐ Anticipatory grieving related to actual/perceived threat to self.

☐ Grieving related to potential/actual loss of infant or birth of an imperfect child.

CHRONIC RENAL DISEASE

As a general rule, women with chronic renal disease do not handle the increased renal demands of pregnancy as a healthy pregnant women would. Thus, more frequent visits will be necessary to observe for preeclampsia, prevent infection, assess renal function, avoid premature delivery, and make an early diagnosis of intrauterine growth retardation (6).

PREGNANCY AFTER RENAL TRANSPLANT

After renal transplant, as normal renal function returns, so does reproductive capability. Thus, since the first successful pregnancy in a renal transplant patient in 1963, thousands of women with renal transplants have had liveborn babies who have survived. However, increased incidence of preeclampsia, severe infection, or kidney rejection has been reported. A woman who is in general good health for 2 years after the transplant and has no evidence of graft rejection or proteinuria should not be discouraged from attempting pregnancy (7).

However, about half of the pregnancies will result in premature babies, and of these, respiratory distress is common. Because of maternal immunosuppressive therapy, mothers as well as newborns are at risk of infection. Long-term effects of maternal immunosuppressive therapy on the infants, such as increased incidence of cancer or adverse effects on their reproductive capability, are unknown.

REFERENCES

1. Davison J: The physiology of the renal tract in pregnancy. *Clin Obstet Gynecol* 28:257, 1985.
2. Harris R: Acute urinary tract infections. *Clin Obstet Gynecol* 27:877, 1984.
3. Pritchard J, et al: *Williams Obstetrics* (17th ed). Norwalk, CT: Appleton-Century-Crofts, p 580
4. Knuppel R: Acute renal failure in pregnancy. *Clin Obstet Gynecol* 28:288, 1985.
5. Doenges M, et al: *Nursing Care Plans*. Philadelphia, FA Davis, 1984, p 381.
6. Robertson E: Assessment and treatment of renal disease in pregnancy. *Clin Obstet Gynecol* 28:279-287, 1985.
7. Davison J: Pregnancy in renal transplant recipients—a clinical perspective. *Contrib-Nephrol* 37:170-178, 1984.

Chapter 18
Skin Disorders
Debra Brook Paparo, C.N.M., M.S.

INTRODUCTION

Dermatologic changes frequently accompany pregnancy. Cutaneous signs and symptoms that present during pregnancy may be related to normal pregnancy, to minor disorders, or they may be manifestations of systemic disease potentially dangerous to mother and/or infant. Pregnant women are susceptible to the same skin disorders as are nonpregnant women as well as skin disorders unique to pregnancy. This chapter focuses only on skin disorders associated with the childbearing process.

The integrity of the skin and mucous membranes is challenged by the systemic physiologic adaptations to pregnancy. The skin may respond to alterations in the endocrine, vascular, metabolic, and immunologic systems. Pregnancy-induced physiologic skin changes pose no threat to the well-being of the pregnancy. However, frequently they do become a focal point of concern for pregnant clients as they attempt to adjust to their rapidly changing body image.

Localized areas of hyperpigmentation commonly are encountered during pregnancy and are thought to be the result of increased melanocyte-stimulating hormone (MSH) mediated by elevated levels of estrogen and progesterone (1, 2, p 442).

PRURITUS GRAVIDARUM

Definition

Pruritus gravidarum (PG) is a recurring dermatologic disorder characterized by intractable itchiness that presents in the third trimester of pregnancy in genetically predisposed women. PG may occur with or without jaundice.

The reported incidence of PG varies from 0.02–2.4%. A higher incidence is reported in Scandinavia (3%) and in Chilean Indians (14%) and is thus reflective of the hereditary predisposition in these ethnic groups (3).

Etiology

PG is caused by a reversible and nonfatal intrahepatic cholestatic process. During pregnancy, the liver demonstrates a decreased capacity to excrete organic anions such as bile salts. This hepatic physiologic alteration is caused by complex synergistic biochemical actions mediated by the elevated levels of estrogens and progesterone. In the genetically predisposed pregnant client, these physiological phenomena manifest as PG. The specific basis for the symptom of itchiness is believed to be the detergent-like property of the bile salts that make lipid cell membranes soluble and stimulate the release of proteolytic enzymes that excite and aggravate free nerve endings. The pruritus is proportional to the concentration of bile acids in the skin, not in the serum (3, p 226).

Signs and Symptoms

The majority of cases of PG present in the third trimester with mild to severe itchiness of the abdomen, trunk, and/or extremities, especially noted at night. The pruritus becomes more generalized and more constant as the pregnancy progresses to term. Anorexia, nausea, and vomiting may occur. Primary skin lesions are absent; however, multiple secondary excoriations often result from scratching. In severe cases cholestatic jaundice manifests with icterus 2–4 weeks after the onset of pruritus. At this time urine color may darken, stools may turn clay colored, and the liver may become enlarged and tender (3, p 224) (see Chapter 12).

Diagnosis

Histopathological studies of the liver demonstrate normal parenchyma with bile pigments overflowing from the hepatocytes. Portal inflammation generally is absent. This cholestatic process is completely reversible; thus, permanent structural and/or functional damage does not occur (3, p 226).

PG is associated with elevated serum levels of direct bilirubin and alkaline phosphatase. Lactic dehydrogenase (LDH) and serum glutamic-oxaloacetic transaminase (SGOT) remain within normal limits. In the most severe cases, prothrombin times may be lengthened as a result of complete bile flow obstruction and malabsorption of vitamin K (3, p 224).

Differential diagnosis for PG must include other pruritic skin disorders. Scabies, pediculosis, drug reactions, atopic dermatitis, and neurodermatitis are frequent causes of itchiness in both pregnant and nonpregnant clients. When pruritus affects the female genitalia, trichomonal and monilial vaginitis must be considered.

The presence of jaundice demands careful scrutiny to distinguish benign PG from viral hepatitis and choledocholithiasis. Viral hepatitis is unlikely in the absence of markedly elevated transaminase levels. Choledocholithiasis is an unlikely diagnosis unless the client presents with an elevated white blood cell count, fever, and abdominal pain. When additional information is needed, ultrasound is a useful method for detecting stones. Also, liver biopsies may be performed safely during pregnancy (3, p 226).

Maternal and Fetal Outcome

The expected outcome for pregnant clients affected with PG is excellent. The pruritus usually subsides soon after delivery and completely resolves by 2 weeks postpartum. Jaundice may last up to 6 weeks postpartum, but it generally disappears along with the pruritus.

Controversy exists regarding fetal outcome. Usually, the fetus is not adversely affected by PG. However, a study of 56 clients with PG demonstrated an increased likelihood of premature delivery and intrauterine asphyxia. In this study poor fetal outcome was most often associated with frankly jaundiced mothers (4).

Medical Management

Medical management of mild cases of PG includes use of topical emollients and antipruritics. In more severe cases cholestyramine (Questran), a synthetic ion exchange resin, should be prescribed. Cholestyramine taken by mouth is nonabsorbable and therefore poses no threat to the fetus (3, p 226). This resin strongly binds bile acids in the gut, removing them from the enterohepatic circulation. Side effects from cholestyramine frequently include nausea, vomiting, bloating, abdominal pain, and/or constipation. When PG is severe, the clotting profile should be monitored. Vitamin K supplements should be given along with cholestyramine in cases of prolonged jaundice and when prothrombin times are lengthened. Antihistamines, including diphenhydramine hydrochloride (Benadryl), once thought to be helpful, are now believed to be of little use in the treatment of PG.

HERPES GESTATIONIS

Definition

Herpes gestationis (HG) is a rare and recurrent disorder associated with pregnancy and the puerperium. Unlike herpes types I and II, herpes gestationis is not a viral disease and is not infectious. The term "herpes" as defined by Galen was used to describe any skin disease characterized by the formation of small vesicles, often in clusters. It was in this context that the blistering disease specifically associated with pregnancy was given the name herpes gestationis (5). The incidence of HG frequently is reported as 1 in 4,000 pregnancies (2, p 444, 6); however, this statistic may be an overestimation. One recent study cites an incidence of only 1 in 60,000 pregnancies (7), and another demonstrates HG in only 2 out of 84,000 consecutive births (8). HG rarely affects primigravidas. Once occurring in multigravidas, it inevitably recurs, with varying intensities, in subsequent pregnancies.

Etiology

The etiology of HG remains unclear. Hormonal, autoimmune, and genetic processes have been identified as potential causative factors. In women who have had HG, exacerbations with menstruation, after administration of oral contraceptives, and in association with hydatidiform moles and choriocarcinoma have been documented and support the hypothesis that HG is triggered hormonally (3, pp 227–228, 5, p 610).

The basis for considering autoimmune factors as the stimulus for HG stems from concurrent presentation of HG with other autoimmune diseases such as Graves' disease, ulcerative colitis, alopecia totalis, and autoimmune thyrotoxicosis. One theory suggests a genetic predisposition for an immunologic abnormality that ultimately results in HG (5, p 610).

The clinically evident lesions of HG erupt in response to an inflammatory process. Whatever the stimulus, an IgG antibody is formed. This circulating antibody, designated the "HG factor," demonstrates a great propensity to localize in the basement membrane zone of the skin. The HG factor activates complement (C_3), which, in turn, activates an inflammatory process. Eosinophils found in the inflammatory exudate release lysosomal enzymes, which are believed to play a central role in mediating tissue necrosis. Ultimately, the epidermal basement membrane is destroyed, and cutaneous bullae (blisters) are formed (5, pp 608–609).

Signs and Symptoms

Herpes gestationis may present any time between 2 weeks' gestation and 1 week postpartum. Most often, onset occurs during the middle trimester. Once established, the clinical course of HG is one of alternating exacerbations and remissions. Exacerbations, sometimes severe, develop immediately postpartum in as many as 50–75% of cases (5, p 611).

Pruritus is a severe and constant symptom of HG and may antedate eruption of lesions by several days. Systemic symptoms of fever, malaise, nausea, and headaches also are commonly encountered.

Initially, lesions consist of urticarial papules. These hive-like eruptions undergo several metamorphoses into target lesions and asymmetric polymorphic vesicles; ultimately, in 4 weeks' time, they develop into large, tense bullae superimposed on an edematous erythematous base (6).

In the great majority of cases, lesions begin at the umbilicus and spread proximally to involve the remainder of the abdomen and the extremities. Eruptions have been noted on the palms and soles. Bullae tend to erupt in groups. Clustered together, they form rather grotesque multidimensional topographic patterns. The face and mucous membranes usually are spared.

Aging bullae become flaccid and eventually rupture. Their drying out process leaves denuded areas covered by hemorrhagic crusts. If secondary infection interferes with healing, lesions may become purulent and deeply ulcerated. Healing usually occurs without scarring, although hyperpig-

mented spots frequently do remain. In most cases HG gradually regresses over a period of weeks to several months.

Diagnosis

Skin biopsy is essential in confirming the diagnosis of HG. Direct immunofluorescence performed on lesional and perilesional skin provides the most useful information. The most diagnostic histological finding is the deposition of the third component of complement, C_3, in the basement membrane zone of the skin. IgG deposition also is a common finding. Ultrastructural studies show necrosis of basal cells, with blisters arising at the dermoepidermal junction (3, p 227).

Differential diagnosis for HG must include other blistering diseases. Contact dermatitis, herpes simplex, herpes zoster, and bullous impetigo differ histologically from HG in that their blisters are located intraepidermally. HG lesions are located in the subepidermis. Additionally, contact dermatitis affects only exposed areas, with lesions characterized by their sudden onset and short duration. Herpes virus may be confirmed via specific cultures or by demonstrating multinucleated giant cells in stained smears. The lesions of bullous impetigo contain very clear fluid with gram-positive cocci, and cultures of these lesion grow *Staphylococcus aureus* (5, pp 605–606).

Erythema multiforme, dermatitis herpetiformis, and bullous pemphigoid are rare, subepidermal, blistering diseases that must be included in the differential diagnosis for HG. Differentiation is made with histologic and immunologic data. Bullous pemphigoid and HG share many common immunopathologic factors. However, bullous pemphigoid most often affects patients between the ages of 60–80 and is thus an unlikely diagnosis in obstetric clients.

Maternal and Fetal Outcome

Herpes gestationis is not associated with increased maternal mortality. Duration of the disease process and its rate of infectious complications parallel the severity of each individual HG case. Clients treated with corticosteroid medications may expect the steroid-specific side effects such as cushingoid signs, serious gastrointestinal disorders, and psychological disturbances (9).

Transplacental transfer of the HG factor occurs infrequently; thus, clinical skin lesions in newborns are very rare. Most worrisome is the increased risk of prematurity (23% compared with 5% in the general population) and stillbirth (7.7% compared with 1.3%) (10). The advent of corticosteroids indirectly may be responsible for improving fetal morbidity and mortality. It is hypothesized that these medications safeguard fetal well-being by preventing serious systemic deterioration in the mother. Uncertainty prevails as to whether treated clients actually have an improved rate of uncomplicated deliveries.

Medical Management

The majority of patients affected with HG have severe cases that require systemic steroid therapy. Prednisone is the drug of choice, and the effective dosage usually is 20–40 mg taken by mouth in divided daily doses. For some clients doses as high as 120 mg/day have been required. Symptomatic relief usually is prompt and occurs within 48 hours. When the disease process is brought under control, attempts can be made to taper the steroid dosage. For the rare milder cases, antihistamines and topical steroid creams may be all that is necessary.

NURSING MANAGEMENT

Nursing care specific for a patient with *skin disorders*:

☐ Ensure that lesions are cared for properly to allow healing and to avoid infection.

☐ Help the patient cope with the discomforts of the condition.

☐ Encourage liberal use of sunscreens when exposed to the sun.

☐ Educate the patient regarding the following:

— Treatment (e.g., keep open lesions clean and dry; avoid constricting clothing; use mild soaps; avoid harsh detergents when washing clothes; avoid hot water, alcohol, scratching);

— medications (e.g., antihistamines, systemic/topical steroids as ordered; avoid self-treatment with over-the-counter preparations); and

— Signs/symptoms of infection (e.g., temperature; hot, reddened areas).

Nursing diagnosis most frequently associated with *skin disorders*:

☐ Impaired skin integrity.

☐ Knowledge deficit regarding etiology, disease process, treatment, and expected outcome.

☐ Knowledge deficit regarding medication regimen.

☐ Disturbance in body image, self-esteem.

☐ Ineffective individual coping.

REFERENCES

1. Black KE: Dermatologic complications. In Niswander KR (ed): *Manual of Obstetrics, Diagnosis and Therapy*, ed 2. Boston, Little, Brown and Co, 1983, p 155.
2. Ellis JW: Dermatologic disease. In Ellis JW, Beckman CR (eds): *A Clinical Manual of Obstetrics*. Norwalk, CT, Appleton-Century-Crofts, 1983.
3. Sasseville D, Wilkinson RD, Schnader JY: Dermatoses of pregnancy. *Int J Dermatol* 20:224, 1981.
4. Reid R, Ivey KJ, Rencoret RH, et al.: Fetal complications of pruritic cholestasis. *Br Med J* 1:870, 1976.
5. Lookingbill DP, Chez RA: Herpes gestationis. *Clin Obstet Gynecol* 26:606, 1983.
6. Holmes RC, Black MM: The specific dermatoses of pregnancy. *J Am Acad Dermatol* 8:405, 1983.
7. Kolodny RC: Herpes gestationis, a new assessment of incidence, diagnosis and fetal prognosis. *Am J Obstet Gynecol* 104:39–45, 1969.
8. Holmes RC, Black MM, Dann J, James DC, Bhogal B: A comparative study of toxic erythema of pregnancy and herpes gestationis. *Br J Dermatol* 106:499, 1982.
9. Rodman MJ, Smith DW: *Clinical Pharmacology in Nursing*. Philadelphia, JB Lippincott, 1974, p 231.
10. Hewlet TJ, Stingl G, Katz SI: Fetal and maternal risk factors in herpes gestationis. *Arch Dermatol* 114:552, 1978.

Chapter 19
Substance Abuse
Kathleen Buckley, C.N.M., M.S.N.

INTRODUCTION

It seems that there would be one commonly accepted definition of addiction. However, this is not the case. Addiction has been described as "feeling normal on drugs," "compulsive use of drugs," or "use of drugs as the central focus of life." The World Health Organization describes addiction as a mental and physical state resulting from an interaction between a living organism and a drug (1). Addiction is characterized by a compulsion to take drugs in order to experience positive euphoric effects or to avoid the discomforts of its absence. This state of dependency, then, presumes a physical and a psychological component. The psychological dependence is a drive toward pleasure or the relief of pain. It can be expected that the psychological component is much more powerful than the physiological dependence and less likely to be overcome. This explains the high relapse rate in any kind of drug rehabilitation program. Hunt et al. (2) underline these drug rehabilitation failures. In their study of rehabilitated heroin, nicotine, and alcohol addicts, less than 30% of the subjects still were abstaining after a 12-month period.

Two characteristics of drug addiction are tolerance and abstinence syndrome. Tolerance refers either to a decreased drug effect over a period of time or an increased need for larger doses of the drug. Abstinence syndrome refers to a group of physical symptoms that occur when the physically dependent individual refrains from drug use (2).

Chemical dependence in our society is subtle and all pervasive. It can be seen that not only heroin, barbiturates, amphetamines, and alcohol are addictive but also that nicotine and caffeine have been used to excess.

204

During pregnancy, it is probably safe to say that use of any substance to excess is not healthy for the mother and jeopardizes the fetus.

ETIOLOGIES OF DRUG ABUSE

Several theories have been proposed to explain the etiology of drug addiction. These attempt to correlate general characteristics of the addict (e.g., decreased assertiveness, impulsiveness, depression, need for immediate gratification) with an overall framework for treatment.

Psychodynamic psychotherapy views drug addiction as a need to experience the effects of drugs rather than the impulse to use them. That is, addiction occurs because it can produce euphoria and/or alleviate pain. Addiction represents an individual's regression to an infantile state of pleasure and omnipotence, associated with the functional oral state. Of course, as time and misuse of drugs progress, these positive feelings are more difficult to achieve and depression occurs. In an effort to regain these feelings of control, the addict will increase dosage and develop tolerance and physical dependence.

The "bad habit" theory proposes that addiction is a repetitious, harmful, semireflexive behavior, found only in *susceptible* individuals. Biobehavioral or genetic factors predispose the individual to addiction. An individual can be "susceptible" by his genetic inheritance, his psychosocial milieu, or some combination of the two. This theory attempts to explain why certain individuals experience more euphoria with drug use than others, resulting in a more powerful reinforcement to continue drug use. Relationship between agent-host-environment is postulated. Drugs produce powerful short-term euphoria in genetically susceptible individuals in specific psychocultural milieus.

The "self-medication" theory suggests that addiction is an attempt to alleviate psychic pain. Pain may be manifested in any number of ways—rage, loneliness, depression, or attempts to satisfy or control unacceptable wishes or fantasies. It is the people who have the very fewest resources and capacity for personality integration who will self-medicate with drugs as a type of healing. Narcissistic, borderline, or psychotic persons are typical drug abusers.

Finally, the "self-efficiency" or "locus of control" theory views drug abuse as a way for individuals who would otherwise feel powerless to control their environment. This theory postulates a relationship between external locus of control and affective experience of drug use.

From whatever theoretical base one views addiction, it is a complex problem. Also, drug-using behaviors may be influenced by a range of psychological profiles and societal reinforcements. For example, personal psychological characteristics are considered to be the key. On the other hand, something as abstract and unmeasurable as positive media presentation of alcohol or tobacco use may be the deciding factor in addiction. Certainly, the example of the family and the habits of peers are crucial in the teen and preteen years.

Looking at the problem from a different angle, the World Health Organization has identified the following motives for drug use (1, p 3):

1. To satisfy curiosity about the drug itself;
2. To achieve a sense of belonging;
3. To express independence or hostility;
4. To have new pleasurable experiences;
5. To break through to a new level of creativity;
6. To foster a sense of relaxation or to relieve tension; and
7. To escape from something.

NARCOTIC ADDICTION

Ninety-five percent of narcotic abusers use heroin and/or methadone (4, p 685). Other similar opiates abused are morphine, codeine, meperidine, and opium.

Heroin is sold illegally in "bags" of from 10–30 mg. Narcotic addiction develops in the majority of pregnant women and fetuses when the drugs are used regularly—usually by the intravenous route. Some women use narcotics irregularly. Although the latter use does not produce dependency, it predisposes the woman to serious overdose since the actual amount of heroin per bag may vary significantly. Heroin has a duration of 3–4 hours. Use may increase to 8 to 10 bags a day with a resulting cost of upwards of $200 per day.

Methadone can be given under medical supervision in a drug rehabilitation program. Doses range from 20–100 mg. Of course, this drug can also be obtained illegally.

After an initial intravenous injection of an opiate, a thrilling sensation originating in the abdomen occurs. This is called the "rush" and lasts for about 1 minute. Afterwards, the addict experiences a sense of well-being and euphoria. During the euphoric period, addicts either doze in a light sleep ("nod") or become very active ("drive") (3, p 41).

Chronic use produces tolerance; withdrawal will develop, and the euphoric period will become shorter. Withdrawal syndrome does not occur until 24–30 hours after the drug is taken. Thus, many pregnant addicts find it cheaper and easier to buy illegal methadone and to supplement its use with other drugs (i.e., tranquilizers or alcohol) to achieve heroin-like effects.

Withdrawal is the natural process that occurs when the opiate is withheld; it is abrupt and uncomfortable. Withdrawal commonly happens when the undetected addicted patient is admitted to the labor suite. If the addict's habit is of recent origin and low dosage, withdrawal will be mild and include yawning, sneezing, watering eyes, perspiring, and rhinorrhea. In those addicts with well-established, large dose habits, a much more severe pattern emerges—abdominal cramping, vomiting/diarrhea, muscle spasm, bone pain, and elevated blood pressure and pulse. Disturbances in acid-base balance occur because of severe nausea and vomiting, along with weight loss, dehydration, and ketosis. Cardiovascular collapse may follow (5, pp 296–297).

Even with severe symptomatology, the withdrawal process runs its course in 7–10 days. After that, a secondary rebound effect may occur at 6 weeks postwithdrawal and possibly last until the twenty-fourth week. Some of the above-mentioned parameters recur along with psychological disturbances—hypochondrias, tiredness, weakness, or depression (5, pp 296–297).

Physical signs and symptoms of narcotic abuse are associated with the following manifestations of low level of self-care that often are the first evidence of addiction for the health care team (4, p 687):

o   No prenatal care

Table 19.1.
GENERAL MEDICAL COMPLICATIONS ENCOUNTERED IN PREGNANT ADDICTS[a]

Anemia
Endocarditis
Cellulitis
Diabetis mellitus
Hepatitis B
Hypertension
Thrombophlebitis
Pneumonia
Tuberculosis
Starvation ketosis
Malnutrition
Poor dental hygiene
Urinary tract infections
  Cystitis
  Urethritis
  Pyelonephritis
Reproductive tract infections
  Gonorrhea
  Syphilis
  Herpes
  Condyloma acuminatum
  AIDS

[a]Adapted from Ostra J, et al.; *The Care of the Drug Dependent Women and Her Infant.* Michigan Department of Health, 1978, p 5.

o   Arriving at the hospital in transition or second stage of labor

o   History or presence of venereal disease

o   Tattoos or self-scarring over the arms to disguise needle marks

o   Fingertip burns (from diminished pain perception when smoking)

o   Cigarette burns in clothes

o   Jaundiced skin or sclera

o   Cellulitis or abscesses

o   Drowsiness (lethargy)

o   Pinpoint pupils

The literature shows that as many as 75% of pregnant addicts do not seek prenatal care (6). This, plus the low level of self-care (related to low self-esteem), produces many complications in pregnancy, labor, and birth for both the mother and the baby.

Needle-borne infections increase the risk of maternal mortality owing to increased incidence of hepatitis B and AIDS. Other serious medical complications are a result of the drug use itself, lifestyle, and nutritional deficiency (Table 19.1). Obstetric complications include abruptio placentae, abnormal presentations (e.g., breech), premature labor, premature rupture of membranes, amnionitis, chorioamnionitis, postpartum hemorrhage, postpartum uterine or urinary tract infection, and

Table 19.2.
MANIFESTATIONS OF NEONATAL NARCOTIC WITHDRAWAL[a]

CNS signs
  Hyperactivity
  Hyperirritability—incessant crying, high pitched cries
  Increased muscle tone
  Exaggerated reflexes
  Tremors
  Sneezing, hiccups, yawning
  Short, nonquiet sleep
  Fever
Respiratory signs
  Tachypnea
  Excess secretions
Gastrointestinal signs
  Disorganized, vigorous sucking
  Vomiting
  Drooling
  Sensitive gag
  Hyperphagia
  Diarrhea
  Abdominal cramps
Vasomotor signs
  Stuffy nose
  Flushing
  Sweating
  Sudden circumoral pallor
Cutaneous signs
  Excoriated buttocks
  Facial scratches
  Pressure point abrasions

[a]Reprinted with permission from Ostra J, et al.: *The Care of the Drug Dependent Woman and Her Infant.* Michigan Department of Health, 1978, p 30.

septic thrombophlebitis. Moreover, incidence of toxemia is increased significantly in narcotic addicts, probably partially effected by poor nutritional status (7).

The baby too is at risk. If the undiagnosed addict has a long labor, she and her unborn baby may experience signs of withdrawal that directly contribute to intrauterine demise. The addict's malnutrition not only affects her but also her unborn baby, increasing the incidence of intrauterine growth retardation (7). Nearly half of addicted babies are born prematurely and almost always weigh less than the average for any given gestational age. The infant, too, will undergo withdrawal. Heroin withdrawal usually occurs within the first 4 days after birth and can be treated successfully by sedation with paregoric, chlorpromazine, or diazepam and maintenance of hydration and nutrition (8). Signs and symptoms of neonatal withdrawal are listed in Table 19.2.

Methadone withdrawal takes longer to occur— up to 3 weeks after birth. It may not be as severe as heroin withdrawal, depending on the relative

Table 19.3.

AREAS OF SPECIAL CONCERN IN PHYSICAL EXAMINATION OF PREGNANT, NARCOTIC-DEPENDENT WOMEN[a]

SYSTEM	FINDINGS
Dermatological	Presence of infections, abscesses, thrombosed veins, herpes infections.
Dental	Status of dental hygiene. Existence of pyorrhea or abscessed cavities.
Otolaryngeal	Rhinitis, excoriation of nasal septum.
Respiratory	Presence of asthma, rales, signs of pulmonary disease.
Cardiovascular	Presence of increased pulmonary artery pressure or murmurs indicative of endocarditis or preexisting valvular disease.
Gastrointestinal	Hepatomegaly, scars from injuries, incisional or umbilical hernias.
Genitourinary	Presence of infections such as condyloma acuminatum, *Trichomonas vaginalis*, herpes vaginitis, gonorrheal ureteritis, salpingitis, tubal abscesses.
Musculoskeletal	Pitting edema, distortion of muscular landmarks because of subcutaneous abscesses.

[a]Reprinted with permission from Ostra J, et al.: *The Care of the Drug Dependent Woman and Her Infant.* Michigan Department of Health, 1978, p 7.

strength of maternal addiction (9, p 540). Maternal use of illegal methadone presents a special neonatal problem. The mother or her infant may not show withdrawal symptoms during her stay in the hospital. Thus, the first clue of neonatal addiction may be when the 2–3-week-old infant is hospitalized for severe dehydration due to nausea, vomiting, and poor feeding associated with withdrawal (10).

Other than withdrawal, other problems of the addicted newborn include:

1. Jaundice—etiology unknown;
2. Respiratory distress from prematurity or aspiration pneumonia;
3. Congenital abnormalities, especially genitourinary or cardiovascular; and
4. Infection (e.g., hepatitis B, syphilis, gonorrhea, herpes simplex, AIDS).

Finally, since the mother has such a low level of self-esteem/self-care, she may find it difficult or even impossible to mother her child adequately. Thus, the potential for child neglect or abuse is always present.

Medical Management

The pregnant narcotic addict requires a multifaceted team approach to achieve a successful outcome for both mother and baby. Management must include both supportive psychotherapeutic intervention, intensive medical management, primary nursing care, and social work support.

Evaluation of the patient is of paramount importance in discovering major medical problems. Special areas of concern in the physical assessment are listed in Table 19.3.

Other areas of management include (9, p 540):

Table 19.4.

QUEENAN/HOBBINS DETOXIFICATION REGIMEN[a]

1. Decrease dosage in small amounts *only* to prevent fetal withdrawal. Do *not* exceed the reduction by more than 2 mg every 10–14 days.
2. Aim for optimum intake of less than 20 mg of methadone/day.
3. Observe closely for increased fetal movements. (This signals fetal withdrawal).

[a]Adapted from Queenan J, Hobbins J: *Protocols for High Risk Pregnancy.* New Jersey, Medical Economic Books, 1982, p 6.

1. Nutrition—prevention of iron and protein deficits and maternal ketosis;
2. Prevention/treatment of infection;
3. Psychological support—team effort to support patient, prevent or ameliorate depression or low self-esteem, evaluate suicidal tendencies; and
4. Management of substance abuse—to promote careful, slow withdrawal or maintain consistent level of narcotics and to discover polydrug use.

These patients should be enrolled in a methadone maintenance program as soon as possible. Traditionally, it was thought that both the mother and the fetus would have a better chance for a healthy outcome if the mother was maintained on a consistent dose of methadone, even if that dose was high. However, Queenan and Hobbins (11) detail a detoxification regimen that they have found to be safe (Table 19.4) The goal of their detoxification program is to reduce the dose of methadone to less than 20 mg/day by the time of delivery. Data support the fact that fewer than half of babies born to

Table 19.5.
PHYSIOLOGICAL AND PSYCHOLOGICAL EFFECTS OF LOW TO MODERATE ORAL DOSES OF AMPHETAMINES[a]

PHYSIOLOGICAL EFFECTS	PSYCHOLOGICAL EFFECTS	
	POSITIVE	NEGATIVE
Increased blood pressure	Behavioral arousal	Increased irritability
Slowing of heart rate	Increased alertness	Increased restlessness
Heart palpitations	Increased wakefulness	Inability to sleep
Relaxation of bronchial muscle	Mood elevation	Blurred vision
Constriction of nasal mucous membranes	Mild euphoria	Mental confusion
Increased blood flow to musculoskeletal structures	Increased athletic performance	Hyperirritability
Decreased blood flow to internal organs	Decreased feeling of boredom	
Increased blood pressure	Decreased mental clouding	
Increased respiration rate	Clearer thinking	
Increased blood sugar	Increased sustained attention	
EEG signs of arousal	Increased activity level	

[a]Used with permission from Milby J: *Addictive Behavior and Its Treatment.* New York, Springer, 1981, p 51.

mothers taking low doses (less than 20 mg/day) experience withdrawal syndromes, while 90% of babies whose mothers took more have symptoms. The goal of either management is to prevent sudden maternal withdrawal—a major cause of fetal demise.

STIMULANTS

Amphetamines

Amphetamines produce addiction and tolerance, as well as withdrawal syndrome. Withdrawal consists of lethargy and profound depression.

Amphetamines—like all CNS stimulant—produce mood elevation, euphoria, decreased appetite, increased mental alertness, or decreased depression. Effects of low to moderate doses of amphetamines are listed in Table 19.5. In high doses these CNS stimulant produce anxiety, irritability, and, finally, psychosis.

With intravenous use of amphetamines, a "speed cycle" has been described. After the first injection, the addict experiences short-lived euphoria. Since intravenous amphetamine peaks in 10 minutes, the addict must continue to inject often to maintain the effect. During this period, she may not eat or drink because of the suppression of appetite by the drug. She frequently exhibits paranoid behavior (e.g., suspicion, violence) that may progress to full-blown psychosis. After the addict stops taking the drug, the reaction phase begins. The client may sleep for 24–48 hours or she may sleep as much as 18 hours per day for several weeks. Following this, profound depression occurs (3, pp 51–52).

Since amphetamines suppress appetite, during pregnancy it is especially important to prevent nutritional deficiency and ketosis. As with the heroin addict, needle-associated pathology such as hepatitis B, AIDS, cellulitis, and endocarditis must be evaluated. In a small number of patients, renal, cerebral, or pulmonary vasculitis may be severe. Maternal cardiac arrhythmias have been reported. These may be noted during labor and delivery, and they may be exacerbated during administration of obstetrical anesthesia (9, p 543).

The major fetal danger is from intrauterine growth retardation because of poor maternal nutrition. The fetus will become addicted to amphetamines, and withdrawal syndrome has been documented. Fetal abnormalities, such as congenital heart disease, urogenital defects, limb deformities, and cleft palate are associated with their use (12, p 108).

Cocaine

Cocaine either can be injected or inhaled. It is not known if cocaine produces tolerance. A physical withdrawal syndrome may not be as pronounced as psychologic dependence. This fact differentiates it from other addictive drugs, which leads to the conjecture that the drug must have powerful psychological addictive properties rather than physical ones (5, p 305). In order to reduce psychological withdrawal symptoms, cocaine routinely is used in conjunction with alcohol or barbiturates.

Cocaine is a short-acting drug, lasting only 30 minutes with inhalation and 10 minutes with injection. Thus, frequent use is necessary to maintain effect. The frequent injector of cocaine may complain of peculiar peripheral nervous system sensations, most commonly described as "bugs burrowing under the skin."

Because of its capacity to cause constriction of blood vessels, frequent inhalation can cause destruction of the nares and/or nasal septum. Concurrent health problems are associated with use of dirty needles and anaerobic infections from local ischemia. Poor nutrition is a major concern, along with starvation ketosis and dehydration (9, p 543).

The pregnant woman who uses crack places her life in jeopardy. Incidence of hypertension, stroke, and obstetric hemorrhage from placental abruption are all increased.

The newborn is at high medical and neurobehavoiral risk. A "snow baby" syndrome has been described and includes intrauterine growth retardation, malformations of the genitourinary trait, altered neonatal behavior patterns, and small head circumference. Newborns are also at risk for cerebral hemorrhage in utero, preterm delivery, increased incidence of SIDS, and perhaps, neural tube defects. Injection of cocaine has caused many cases of spontaneous abortion and placental abruption with subsequent fetal demise.

Because a mother who is involved with crack is mentally and physically consumed by the need for it, she may not be able to care for a child adequately, particularly one who may be jittery or unable to respond to maternal cues. Infants have been abandoned in the hospital of birth, or abused or neglected if they are taken home. Infant passive smoking of crack with subsequent seizures has been documented.

Caffeine

In our society coffee is the most popular beverage and is a very effective stimulant. The average American drinks three cups of coffee every day and buys about 16 pounds of coffee every year. The active ingredient in the coffee (as well as in tea, cola, and cocoa) is xanthine. It is important to note that xanthine belongs to the same anoleptic group as amphetamines, which produce very similar brain wave patterns and increased blood pressure and respirations—a "pick-me-up" feeling. In addition to caffeine, tea contains theophylline, and cocoa contains theobromine. These additional drugs are also cardiac stimulants and diuretics.

Caffeine does cause addiction. Both tolerance and a withdrawal syndrome are seen. Withdrawal consists of headache, lethargy, and depression (13, pp 100–101).

The American Psychiatric Association recently has described a psychoactive state of acute intoxication—"caffeinism." Symptoms include restlessness, nervousness, excitement, insomnia, flush, di-

Table 19.6.
COMMON SOURCES OF CAFFEINE[a]

SOURCE	AVERAGE AMOUNT
Instant coffee	66 mg/cup
Percolated coffee	74 mg/cup
Drip coffee	112 mg/cup
Decaffeinated coffee	3 mg/cup
Tea	30 mg/cup
Cola	50 mg/cup
Chocolate bar	25 mg
Cold tablet	23 mg
Allergy-relief tablet	16 mg
Headache-relief tablet	64 mg
"Stay-awake" tablet	150 mg

[a]Used with permission from Fried P: *Pregnancy and Life Style Habits*. New York, Beaufort Books, 1983, p 102.

uresis, and gastrointestinal complaints. These symptoms may range from very mild symptoms to full-blown psychosis. Doses of caffeine needed to induce symptoms may be surprisingly low (250 mg) in some individuals; however, the usual dosage needed is over 500 mg. With the typical dose of caffeine in a cup of coffee being ±100 mg, more people may experience these symptoms than is thought. Table 19.6 lists some common sources of caffeine.

Caffeine is in the bloodstream 5 minutes after ingestion, and it peaks within half an hour. It is broken down by the liver and excreted by the kidneys very quickly. After 12 hours 90% of caffeine consumed is cleared from the body. However, the body's ability to clear caffeine is altered during pregnancy. In the first trimester the time remains similar. In the second trimester, the clearance time is twice as long, and it increases to three times as long at term (14). The physiologic mechanism for this prolonged clearance time remains obscure. Many babies are born with caffeine in their bloodstream.

Fetal risks are nebulous. One study documented that with heavy caffeine intake (600 mg or more), there is an increased risk of spontaneous abortion, stillbirth, and premature birth (15). On the other hand, another recent study showed no association between coffee consumption and adverse outcomes during pregnancy (16).

However, because of the small amount of documentation of deleterious fetal effects and because of the delayed clearance time of caffeine during pregnancy, caffeine intake should be limited in pregnancy. Limitation during the first trimester is warranted in order to avoid possible teratogenic effects, while limitation in the third trimester (in light of decreased caffeine clearance) is necessary to avoid newborn withdrawal.

CANNABIS (MARIJUANA)

The active chemical in cannabis is one Δ^9-*trans* tetrahydrocannabinol (THC). The liver is responsible for the breakdown of THC, and it is excreted through the feces and urine. THC effects are felt within 5 minutes of inhalation, with peaks within 1 hour. However, the liver works at a very slow rate in the breakdown of THC. If one dose of THC is not cleared before another occurs, the chemical can accumulate in the liver, kidneys, lungs, and—important for the pregnant woman—the placenta. Traces of marijuana have been found as long as 8 days after use (3, p 57).

It seems clear that THC does *not* produce physical addiction in adults, nor is there any withdrawal syndrome. However, profound psychological addiction may be present. Smaller and smaller amounts of THC are needed to produce the same effect (reverse tolerance) (3, p 58).

Toxic effects of THC are psychological in nature and are similar to other hallucinogens (e.g., toxic psychosis). However, it is important to remember that toxic effects may not be from the THC itself but from other addictives, such as heroin, cocaine, or amphetamines.

Smoking large amounts of hashish (a concentrated form of marijuana) has produced severe respiratory syndromes (3, p 58).

Controversial studies with the chronic heavy user suggest the basis for a syndrome described as "amotivational." Symptoms include reduced activity level, lack of goals, slowed mental and physical responses, flattening of affect, mental confusion, and a slowed time sense. A postulated etiology of the syndrome is subtle brain changes associated with brain atrophy (17, 18).

Statistics suggest that as many as 10% of women 18–25 years old use marijuana (13, p 150). Despite widespread use, there are few data to document adverse effects of the drug on the pregnant woman or the fetus. However, the fact that the average adult marijuana user experiences altered neurological status is a compelling reason for ceasing drug use during pregnancy since the unborn fetus has none of the neural protective (blood/brain) barriers of the mother. Pregnant rhesus monkeys given an equivalent of 16 joints per day have experienced a pregnancy loss four times higher than controls (13, p 150).

In the human fetus and newborn, even less is known. In preliminary studies, newborns of heavy marijuana users were tested using the Brazelton Neonatal Assessment Scale. The babies of marijuana users had significantly decreased response to visual stimuli, a response postulated to be a withdrawal syndrome (19).

Congenital anomalies have not been documented (9, p 544).

TOBACCO

It was not until 1942 that tobacco was shown to be an addictive drug with tolerance and withdrawal symptoms. It took another 25 years before the increased risks of upper respiratory infection, bronchitis, emphysema, cancer of the lung, myocardial infarction, pregnancy wastage, and low birth weight were associated with tobacco use. Although any of these health problems is serious, tobacco still is one of the most commonly used drugs in the United States, and its use is on the rise in women and teenagers (9, p 544).

Tobacco is commonly smoked. It reaches the brain very quickly (5 seconds after the first puff). The most powerful and addicting drug in tobacco is nicotine. It is a potent vasoconstrictor and a carcinogen.

The second major component of cigarette smoke is carbon monoxide. This chemical reduces the oxygen-carrying capacity of the hemoglobin molecule by attaching itself to the oxygen's carrying sites. Since carbon monoxide has a much greater affinity for hemoglobin (200 times greater than oxygen), the amount of oxygen in the bloodstream is depleted rapidly. Furthermore, the oxygen that is left on the hemoglobin molecule is impaired from moving back into the body tissues. Therefore, carbon monoxide doubly depletes oxygen in the body by decreasing the amount available and by impairing transfer. It is interesting to note that carbon monoxide levels increase in low tar and low nicotine cigarettes (9, p 544).

Maternal hazards are thought to be due mainly to the effect of nicotine and carbon monoxide and include those listed above. Since more women are smoking and beginning the habit at a younger age, the incidence of lung cancer and myocardial infarction (previously thought to be male-dominated diseases) will rise in the female populations (9, p 544).

The fetus incurs severe risks. The overall frequency of spontaneous abortion in smoking mothers is increased 1.4 times, low birth weight 1.9 times, and perinatal mortality 1.2 times. Fetal risks increase with the number of cigarettes smoked. Babies born to mothers of smokers are significantly more irritable than babies born to non-

Table 19.7.
WHAT KIND OF A DRINKER ARE YOU? A QUESTIONNAIRE[a]

Define one drink as one bottle or can of regular beer, one glass (5 ounces) of wine, or one highball or shot of "hard" liquor (1.5 ounces of any distilled alcohol). Answer the following questions, remembering to consider all three kinds of drinks.

1. On average, how often during the past year did you have a drink?

   a. More than once a day.
   b. Approximately once a day.
   c. Three to five times a week.
   d. About one or twice a week.
   e. Less than once a week but more than once a month.
   f. Less than once a month but more than once a year.
   g. Once a year or less.

2. On average, how much do you usually drink at one sitting?

   a. More than six drinks.
   b. Five to six drinks.
   c. Three to four drinks.
   d. One or two drinks.
   e. Less than one drink.

3. How often during the past year did you have five or six drinks at one sitting?

   a. Nearly every time I drank.
   b. More than half the times I drank.
   c. Sometimes.
   d. Rarely.
   e. Never.

Your answers to these questions reveal both your usual drinking habits and any bursts of heavy drinking that you indulge in. Using your answers, put yourself in one of the following categories.

Abstaining/infrequent drinker: Includes nondrinkers to those who drink less than once a month and never drink more than three drinks in one sitting.

Light/intermediate drinker: Includes those who drink at least once a month but less than once a week and never more than five drinks at one sitting to those who drink once or twice a week and rarely more than three to four drinks at one sitting.

Moderate drinker: Includes those who consume an average of three drinks a week to one drink a day and rarely more than three or four drinks at one sitting or those who drink once or twice a month and often have five or six drinks in one sitting.

Heavy drinker: Includes those who have an average of at least two drinks a day or those who average a drink a day and sometimes have five or six in one sitting.

[a]Used with permission from Fried P: *Pregnancy and Life Style Habits.* New York, Beaufort Books, 1983, p 74–75.

smokers, and this may constitute a withdrawal syndrome (9, p 544).

Growth-retarded babies of smoking mothers continue to be behind in growth up to 11 years of age (20).

ALCOHOL

Today, alcohol is one of the most commonly used and/or abused drugs in much of the world, including the United States. More than 96% of American women have at least an occasional drink (13, p 72).

Alcohol abuse is difficult to quantify. A patient questionnaire that helps distinguish levels of alcohol use is given in Table 19.7.

A small but growing body of research postulates unique etiologies of alcohol abuse for women (Table 19.8). Although many of these data are conflicting and causal relationships are lacking, it is important to realize that alcoholism in women in the United States may be influenced by unique phenomena surrounding feminine role/status (Table 19.8).

Because of these unique stigmas associated with female alcoholism and other barriers to care,

Table 19.8.

POSTULATED ETIOLOGIES OF ALCOHOLISM IN WOMEN

Early childhood deprivation: The family background of women who abuse alcohol may contribute to its development. The typical family picture is a cold, distant mother and a warm, affectionate father. The father is perceived as weak and poorly organized. He is often alcoholic. Alcoholic women have been found to idealize their fathers and blame their mothers for all the problems at home. Fear, anger, and guilt arising from this dysfunctional family picture may create conflicts associated with sexuality, sense of feminine identification, and ambivalent feelings about drinking, and may predispose to alcohol abuse later.

Empty nest syndrome: There is an increased incidence of problem drinking women in the age group from 35–64. Female alcoholics usually can point to a specific life stress event that precipitated heavy drinking, such as death of a spouse or a child leaving home.

Sex role dysfunction: Sex role confusion and conflict may lead to alcoholism. A cold, distant mother may hinder the daughter's ability to develop a strong feminine identification. Drinking, then, may be a way to gain an artificial sense of femininity. On the other hand, the rise in alcoholism in women parallels the tremendous changes in modern mores, attitudes, and life-styles of women since the 1960s. The changes certainly are cause for confusion and conflict about sexual roles and norms.

Female physiology: Although studies are confusing, it does seem that physiologic events like premenstrual tension or menopause may be stressful and predispose toward abnormal coping behaviors—such as alcoholism. A higher incidence of infertility and gynecologic difficulties have been found. However, no causal relationship has been established.

Affective disorder: The major difference between male and female alcoholics may be a higher degree of psychiatric dysfunction specifically in the area of affective disorder. Depression, anxiety, and/or suicide are more common in the female alcoholic. This has led to the theory of "secondary" alcoholism in women. That is, alcohol abuse can be seen as a symptom of an underlying affective disorder.

women must overcome multiple barriers to reach treatment. In fact, alcoholic women are more likely than their male counterparts to receive *opposition* to treatment from their family, friends, and even physicians because of the "shame" of revealing to the community that a wife-mother-childbearer is an alcoholic.

Other barriers that cause women to under-utilize treatment services include:

o   Financial Concerns—Most women who do enter treatment programs are in serious financial difficulty and lack of insurance or other financial resources severely limits treatment options.

o   Knowledge/Attitude of Treatment Providers—Many providers are uncomfortable asking women about alcohol use (feeling that it intrudes their privacy) or do not know how to take an alcohol use history. Some providers say that they would be more comfortable asking a woman if she used heroin than if she drank to intoxication. Additionally, a long-standing misfounded belief concerning alcoholic women is that they are harder to treat and have a poorer prognosis than the male alcoholic. These negative outcome expectations

can and do negatively influence both therapists who provide treatment, and women who seek treatment.

o   Polydrug addiction—Women are more likely to abuse psychoactive drugs in combination because physicians prescribe tranquilizers, barbiturates, analgesics and amphetamines twice as often for women as men. In addition, the crack epidemic should also be viewed as an alcohol epidemic because these two drugs are *routinely* used in combination.

o   Codependency—Many alcoholic women have a spouse, lover, or family member who is also an alcoholic and these relationships reinforce the continued use of alcohol.

o   Battering/Incest—Physical and sexual abuse are frequently reported by alcoholic women who do seek treatment. The "conspiracy of silence" around such abuse prevents many others from ever approaching the treatment system.

Because of these special barriers, services in the targeted communities must provide child care and parenting counseling, support groups, therapy for battered women and incest victims, treatment for prescription drug addiction, job counseling as well as medical and nutrition counseling for pregnant women, and family therapy with a woman alcoholic's significant other (21–23).

Ethyl alcohol impairs nutritional status by specifically decreasing the amounts of folic acid and thiamine. It causes a general overall pattern of poor nutrition, inadequate weight gain, and increased incidence of hypoglycemia resulting in ketosis. Liver disease, bone marrow depression, and infectious complications also are associated with the use of alcohol.

Ethyl alcohol is addictive. Tolerance and withdrawal symptoms are seen. Withdrawal symptoms do not always correlate with the amount of alcohol consumed, perhaps mediated by nutritional or metabolic factors. Symptoms of withdrawal run a continuum of central nervous system (CNS) irritability, and a woman may experience none, one, or all of them. It is not possible to predict the severity of the withdrawal syndrome or the sequence of CNS manifestations.

Tremulousness, often accompanied by nausea, weakness, anxiety, and sweating, can occur as early as 2 or 3 hours after the last drink. Abdominal cramping and vomiting may ensue. Severity of tremors varies from mild to marked. The patient remains psychologically oriented, although she may begin to experience hallucinations ("seeing things"), especially when her eyes are closed. This tremulous state peaks within 24–48 hours. If they are going to occur, grand mal seizures ("rum fits") are most likely to occur within the first 24 hours after alcohol cessation (5, p 301).

If the syndrome continues after 48 hours, psychological orientation is impaired, and the woman becomes confused and agitated and experiences vivid hallucinations. A tirade of marked encephalopathy, severe hallucinations, and marked sympathetic overactivity characterizes delirium tremens ("DTs"). This is a life-threatening condition with a 15% mortality rate (5, p 301). However, all phases of alcohol withdrawal can be controlled successfully by use of sedation.

Alcohol withdrawal is a self-limiting process. If the patient survives through the first 5–7 days, she will recover.

Alcohol passes readily from the mother's bloodstream to the fetus until the concentration gradient is similar. The immature fetal liver is poorly equipped to handle the breakdown; thus, alcohol stays in fetal tissues much longer. Perhaps, as a result of this inability, a woman who drinks heavily (more than three drinks/day) has a three times higher risk of second trimester spontaneous abortion. The effects of abuse on the fetus were first

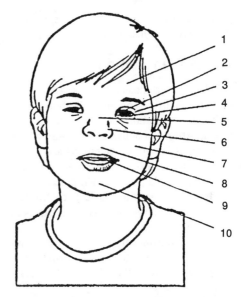

Figure 19.1. Facial features characteristic of the fetal alcohol syndrome. 1, Small head circumference. 2, Skin folds on nasal side of eyes. 3, Drooping eyelids. 4, Short eye openings. 5, Low nasal bridge. 6, Short nose. 7, Flat midface. 8, Indistinct ridges between nose and mouth. 9, Thin upper lip. 10, Small chin. Adapted from Fried P: *Pregnancy and Life Style Habits.* New York, Beaufort Books, 1983, p 63.

described by Jones (24) in terms of a fetal alcohol syndrome (FAS), comprising retardation of fetal and neonatal growth, CNS involvement, and specific facial abnormalities. Growth retardation may involve weight, length, and/or head circumference. One would postulate that the etiology may in part be due to poor maternal nutrition and anemia. FAS babies may be mistaken for failure to thrive babies since they continue to grow slowly after birth. A small but significant decrease in birthweight in babies whose mothers were infrequent drinkers and nonabusers has been documented (25).

CNS involvement may include mental retardation, developmental delay, or neurological coordination defects. Again, the severity of neurological damage is not always proportional to alcohol intake. The true effect may not be documented until the child reaches school age. It runs the gamut from hyperactivity, slow learning, and behavioral problems to significant intellectual deficits. It has been shown that these sequelae are not reversible over time. FAS children have a typical facies (Fig. 19.1). Also, FAS infants are more prone to cardiac or joint abnormalities and may have abnormal palmar creases.

It should be noted that the woman who drinks heavily *and* smokes may increase the risk of adverse physical and mental growth to the fetus. Some estimate a synergistic effect of as much as 400%.

Medical Management

Obtaining a complete data base about alcohol use is a crucial first step in identification of the actual abuser. Information about the amount of alcohol used, patterns of abuse, and concurrent use of other drugs is important. Questions about quality of life and psychosocial history are necessary in order to complete the identification process.

After identifying the problem, controlled detoxification in the hospital with careful fetal evaluation is recommended (26).

Maternal nutritional status should be monitored, with careful attention to identifying the presence of and correcting the following (9, p 541):

1. Megaloblastic anemia as a result of folic acid deficiency.
2. Alcoholic ketoacidosis as a result of heightened sensitivity to fasting hypoglycemia in pregnancy, and
3. Failure to gain weight as a result of overall poor nutritional status.

Liver enzymes must be evaluated to determine the extent of organ involvement. Seizure precautions should be observed, and sedation should be given if signs of tremulousness or irritability are observed.

Abstinence may be difficult to sustain. The patient surely may benefit from continued psychotherapeutic follow-up and referral to self-help groups such as Alcoholics Anonymous. It should be noted that the drug disulfiram (Antabuse), used in behavior modification treatment modalities to induce vomiting with any intake of ethyl alcohol, is contraindicated in pregnancy (12, p 128).

Fetal well-being should be assessed carefully through stress testing and biophysical profile. The amount of alcohol needed to produce any signs of fetal abnormalities has not been determined, nor can a "safe" level of use be established. Even as little as one drink a day has been associated with deleterious fetal effects. Women during childbearing years should be encouraged to refrain from alcohol use or to use it only in moderation. Women who drink regularly should stop before conception. Women who abuse alcohol should be counseled prior to pregnancy about adverse fetal effects and once pregnant should be encouraged to decrease alcohol intake as much as possible (5, p 298).

BARBITURATES

Barbiturates and hypnotic sedatives have similar CNS characteristics. They produce sedation or sleep. Common barbiturates and hypnotic sedatives are listed in Table 19.9.

Barbiturates can be injected as well as taken orally. Tolerance and abstinence syndrome are present. Signs of dosing are quite similar to those of alcohol.

Abstinence syndrome in the barbiturate addict can be more severe than opiate withdrawal. The syndrome includes all of the features of opiate withdrawal but also may be characterized by seizures. The psychiatric course of the withdrawal may be misleading. After 3 days the addict may seem to improve, but full-blown psychosis then may occur (5, p 298).

The barbiturate user is the one most prone to use other drugs such as opiates or hypnotic sedatives in combination. Alcohol and barbiturates are a frequent and deadly combination. As with other drugs in pregnancy, concern should be directed to monitoring maternal nutrition.

Whether or not barbiturates are teratogenic is controversial and unclear. One factor may be the "polydrug" or multidrug use pattern of barbiturate addicts, which may make it difficult to associate newborn outcomes with one specific drug (12, p 61).

The neonate will go through withdrawal symptoms similar to the opiates, but more seizures are seen.

Medical management of the barbiturate addict requires careful monitoring in hospitals to prevent seizures. Blood levels of barbiturates must be monitored daily. These should be titrated with doses of pentobarbital to prevent severe abstinence

Table 19.9.

COMMON BARBITURATES AND HYPNOTIC SEDATIVES[a]

TYPES AND SUBTYPES	GENERIC NAME	PRODUCT NAME
Barbiturates		
Long acting	Phenobarbital	Luminal
Intermediate	Amobarbital	Amytal
Short acting	Thiopental	Pentothal
Nonnarcotic hypnotics	Glutethimide	Doriden
	Methyprylon	Noludar
	Methaqualone	Quaalude
		Sapor
		Parest
		Somnafac

[a]Adapted from Milby J: *Addictive Behavior and Its Treatment.* New York, Springer, 1981, p 45.

syndrome. In labor the barbiturate addict may present with the same signs and symptoms as the narcotic addict. It is as important to recognize this addicted patient as it is to recognize the narcotic addict, since fetal risks are the same or greater and maternal risks include grand mal seizure and death (9, p 543).

SPECIAL NEEDS OF THE LABORING ADDICT

Labor is a most appropriate time to act as an advocate in behalf of the addicted mother and her infant. Probably there will be no other time when this mother will be more ready to reach out to another. The nurse—as a woman and a care giver—is a primary force in supporting the mother's attempts to cope with the stress of labor and delivery and to adjust to her new baby.

Lesser and Keane (27) in their classic study identified five needs of any laboring woman:

1. To be sustained by another human being.
2. To have relief from pain.
3. To be assured of a safe outcome for herself and for the baby.
4. To have attendants accept her personality toward and behavior during labor.
5. To receive bodily care.

Each of these needs is expressed differently by each woman during labor. These needs are *most* profoundly felt by the laboring addict. However, her behavior patterns many times prohibit care givers from meeting her needs.

To Be Sustained by Another Human Being

The laboring addict is convinced of her unworthiness to receive any support. She may never have had the support of another human being. Even under less stressful conditions, she feels depressed and has difficulty with interpersonal relationships. During labor, when the addict is experiencing discomfort, she can hardly adapt successfully to a strange hospital staffed by strangers who are often brusque and impersonal. Never having developed an ability to trust others, she will look on even the most sincere attempts to establish a therapeutic relationship with distrust. She will presume that doctors and nurses will reject her as unimportant or a menace. These attitudes promote negative feelings

and interaction with the members of the health care team. It is the obstetrical team that is in the best position to provide a sustaining, supportive presence. However, they *must* understand the addict's personality and behavior.

To Have Relief from Pain

The addict may experience labor pain more acutely than other women. She constantly has used a "pain reliever" to minimize any discomfort, so the birthing process now is perceived as exceptionally painful. She is most aware of not only uterine contractions but also other discomforts, such as an intravenous infusion.

When she tells the staff of her discomfort, she often is rebuked by staff who are accustomed to other laboring women who maintain a stoicism that the addict cannot. Health care providers may view the addict's complaints of pain with suspicion because they see them as illegitimate attempts to obtain narcotics. Even if the addict is given a narcotic pain reliever, she may not have relief because of cross-tolerance with the narcotic. This reinforces further the care giver's stereotypical response to the addict's plea for pain relief.

To Be Assured of a Safe Outcome Both for Herself and for Her Baby

Truly, there is no certainty of a safe outcome for mother or baby. This fact—certainly known to the laboring woman—increases anxiety for her and her guilt for the baby's fate and creates a "sense of impending death" during the birthing process.

To Have Attendants Accept Her Personal Attitude Toward and Behavior During Labor

Since the addict's behavior characteristically is dependent, needing constant gratification, and lacking in a sense of responsibility, it can be extremely difficult to accept her behavior. Even the most caring nurse needs encouragement and praise from other members of the health team.

To Receive Bodily Care

The addict herself has a very low level of self-care, which is associated with low levels of self-esteem. This is evidenced by the addict's poor nutritional state and poor general health. Thus, the laboring addict can hardly accept from others what she cannot give herself. Again, the addict's expectation may reinforce the care giver's behavior.

It is concluded, then, that the addict who is most in need of physical and psychological support during labor may not receive it. Her behavior and expectations create a progressive alienation from sources of support. This process can be conceptualized as follows:

Inability to trust others →
Inability to relate to obstretrical care givers →
Initial withdrawal of support by care givers →
Increased demand for pain medication as a way to cope with labor stress and pain →
Medication withheld →
Pain and anxiety increased →
Increased dependency and need for gratification →
Irresponsibility →
Further withdrawal by staff →
Increased maladaptive behavior →
Final withdrawal of physical as well as emotional support by staff

The obstetrical nurse is the care giver most consistently present. *She* is the one who must be willing to break this cycle. The following pattern of nursing support has been suggested during labor (4, p 687).

1. Continual consideration for the mother, remembering her founded and unfounded apprehensions;
2. Continual communication with the mother about her progress in labor and about the condition of the baby during labor, at delivery, and after birth;
3. Encouragement to the mother to hold the baby and to visit the nursery;
4. Encouragement to significant others to become involved in the laboring, birthing, and parenting process; and
5. Frequent communication with all health team members to provide continuity of care during

and after the hospitalization of mother and baby.

Furthermore, it would be helpful for care givers to create a "team" of support persons, since coping with the addict's behavior may be exhausting. The addict must have *consistent* support and information to establish a basis for a trusting relationship. She may need medication and within reasonable limits benefit from narcotic pain relief. Other drugs such as barbiturates or sedatives usually are avoided because their effects are not reversible in the infant. Significant others—family or friends—should not be allowed to bring street drugs surreptitiously to the laboring woman, but they should be encouraged to support the laboring patient.

The nurse must realize that labor is not the time to begin a program of behavior modification. She must allow and support the addict's need for dependency and instant gratification—within the bounds of reason and safety. The addict may not be able to be responsible for any of her care, she may present a more "out of control" picture than other women, and she should be encouraged and praised for even the smallest attempt to take charge of her labor and birthing experience.

The risk status of the mother and baby demands close supervision of parameters of maternal and fetal health.

Finally, the obstetric nurse should provide continuity of care and organize the efforts of the whole team (obstetrician, psychiatrist, social worker) to achieve the best possible outcome during the postpartum course of the addict. Moreover, the obstetrical nurse should take heart from the fact that caring labor support by a trusted supportive person can lay the psychological groundwork for sound bonding and family integration, as well as extinction of substance use.

NURSING MANAGEMENT

Nursing care specific for patients with *drug dependence*:

☐ Encourage all pregnant women to develop positive coping styles and to identify and maximize positive supportive relationships.

☐ Identify women at risk for drug dependency (e.g., family history of drug use, loss of child or spouse, absence of support systems, history of depression/suicide attempts, high stress levels).

☐ Maintain a nonjudgmental attitude when interviewing the patient for a history of substance abuse as well as the current status of abuse.

☐ Obtain a complete data base concerning type and route of drug use (e.g., illicit drugs, prescriptions, vitamins, over-the-counter drugs, caffeine, alcohol, and cigarettes).

NURSING MANAGEMENT

☐ Obtain a complete pattern of current substance abuse being aware of "binge" substance abuse.

☐ Schedule prenatal visits at least biweekly, but make appointments available whenever the patient comes to clinic, even if she is late or visits on the wrong day. Encourage her to "drop in" whenever she feels the need to.

☐ Observe for signs and symptoms of drug use (e.g., impaired neurologic state, track marks, cellulitis, destruction of nasal septum, etc.) and screen with urine toxicology, as appropriate.

☐ Ensure that women who are intravenous drug users (IVDUs) understand the risk of contracting AIDS and reinforce the need to refrain from sharing dirty needles.

☐ Offer HIV testing to all women who are IVDUs or who have IVDUs partners.

☐ Ensure that all pregnant drug users are screened for Hepatitis B, syphilis, chlamydia, and other sexually transmitted diseases, that results are prominently displayed in the medical record, that appropriate treatment regimens are completed, and that test of cure is documented.

☐ Coordinate the efforts of the health care team not only in providing comprehensive services to the patient; but also in giving *consistent* feedback regarding her health status and that of her baby.

☐ Praise any effort the patient makes to comply with treatment regimen.

☐ Work with social services to ensure that needed human services are coordinated on behalf of the patient, based on a comprehensive assessment of needs:

 — Mental health counseling;

 — Peer support groups (i.e., Narcotics Anonymous, Alcoholics Anonymous);

 — Medicaid;

 — Vocational training;

 — Day-care;

 — Income maintenance;

 — Job placement;

 — Housing;

 — Parenting support groups; and

 — Drug-free treatment modalities.

☐ Assist the patient/family to make realistic plans for care of the baby.

☐ Refer all pregnant women for prenatal public health nursing home assessment and continued postpartum evaluation of parenting skills and infant health assessment.

☐ During labor, monitor fetal status closely for deceleration of fetal heart rate and observe for meconium staining.

☐ Determine maternal drug intoxication at delivery if appropriate; have drug antagonist available.

☐ If mother tests positive, be aware that most states require that this be reported to appropriate authorities.

☐ Monitor neonatal respiratory and neurologic status closely after birth.

☐ If the patient is stable, encourage the family to be together immediately after birth, but observe closely.

☐ Postpartum—make a special effort to relive the labor/delivery with the mother, praising her for *any attempt* to assist the birthing process.

☐ If the infant requires intensive care, accompany the mother to the unit to meet the staff, discuss the baby's health as well as illnesses, encourage mother to touch and talk to the infant.

☐ Ensure that all drug-dependent patients leave the hospital with a method of birth control and know how to use it.

☐ Ensure that each patient has an early (1–2 week) newborn and postpartum check-up appointment, if at all possible on the same day in the same facility.

☐ Give every mother a number of both a drug and parenting hotline, as well as a number where she can reach designated hospital nursing staff (preferably someone chosen by the patient).

Nursing diagnoses most frequently associated with *substance abuse* (see Section V):

☐ Grieving related to potential/actual loss of infant or birth of an imperfect child.

☐ Disturbance in body image/self-esteem.

☐ Ineffective individual coping.

☐ Ineffective family coping: compromised.

☐ Potential altered parenting.

☐ Anxiety/fear.

☐ Knowledge deficit regarding etiology, disease process, treatment, and outcome.

☐ Knowledge deficit regarding pregnancy, process of labor and delivery, concerns of the postpartum period, parenting.

☐ Altered nutrition: less than body requirements.

REFERENCES

1. World Health Organization. Expert Committee on Drug Dependence. 20th Report, 1974, p 3.
2. Hunt, W, et al.: Relapse rates in Addiction Programs. *Clin Psychol* 27: 450–461, 1971.
3. Milby J: *Addictive Behavior and Its Treatment*. New York, Springer, 1981.
4. Finnegan L, MacNew B: Care of the addicted infant. *Am J Nurs* 74:685–693, 1974.
5. Goodman L, and Gillman A: *The Pharmacological Basis of Therapeutics*. New York, MacMillan, 1975.
6. Perlmutter J: Heroin addiction and pregnancy. *Obstet Gynecol Survey* 29:439–446, 1974.
7. de Swiet M (ed): *Medical Disorders in Pregnancy*. St. Louis, Blackwell Scientific, 1984, p 499.
8. Zelson C, et al.: Neonatal narcotic addiction," *N Engl J Med* 289:1216–1220, 1973.
9. Burrow G, Ferris T: *Medical Complications During Pregnancy*. Philadelphia, WB Saunders, 1982.
10. Zuspan F, et al.: Fetal stress from methadone withdrawal. *Am J Obstet Gynecol* pp. 43–45, 1975.
11. Queenan J, Hobbins J: *Protocols for High Risk Pregnancy*. Oradell, NJ, Medical Economic Press, 1982.
12. Finnegan L: Outcome of children born to women dependent upon narcotics. In *The Effect of Maternal Alcohol on the Newborn*, p 57.
13. Fried P: *Pregnancy and Life Style Habits*. New York, Beaufort, 1983.
14. Kirkinen P, et al.: The effect of caffeine on placental and fetal blood flow in human pregnancy. *Am J Obstet Gynecol* 147:939–942, 1983.
15. Weathersbee P, et al.: Caffeine and pregnancy: a retrospective study. *Postgrad Med* 62:64–69, 1977.
16. Lin S, et al.: No association between coffee consumption and adverse outcomes of pregnancy. *N Engl J Med* 306:141–145, 1982.
17. Maugh T: Marijuana: does it damage the brain. *Science* 185:775–776, 1974.
18. Chapra G: Man and marijuana. *Internat J Addictions* 4:215–247.
19. Fried P: Marijuana use by pregnant women: neurobehavorial effects in neonates. *Drug Alcohol Dependence* 6:415–424, 1980.
20. Abel E: Smoking during pregnancy: a review of effects on growth and development of offspring. *Hum Biol* 503–625, 1980.
21. Belfer M: Alcoholism in women. *Arch Gen Psychiatry* 25:540–544, 1971.
22. Tamerin J: The psychotherapy of alcoholic women. In Zimberg S, Wallace J, Blume S (eds): *Practical Approaches to Alcoholism Psychotherapy*. New York, Plenum Press, 1978.
23. Beckman L: Women alcoholics: a review of social and psychological studies. *J Stud Alcohol* 36:797–823, 1975.
24. Jones K, et al.: Patterns of malformation in offspring of chronic alcoholic mothers. *Lancet* i:1267–1271, 1971.
25. Kaminski M, et al.: Moderate alcohol use and pregnancy outcome. *Neurobehav Toxicol Teratol* 3:173–181, 1981.
26. Anderson C: Substance abuse in women. In Fogel C, Woods N (eds): *Health Care of Women*. St. Louis, Mosby, 1982, p 219.
27. Lesser M, Keane V: *Nurse-Patient Relationships in a Hospital Maternity Service*. St. Louis, Mosby, 1956, p 64.

Chapter 20
Trauma during Pregnancy
Debra Brook Paparo, C.N.M., M.S.

INTRODUCTION

Trauma complicates 6–7% of all pregnancies (1). Motor vehicle accidents account for the greatest number of injured pregnant women, and, in descending order of occurrence, falls, burns, and gunshot wounds follow as the next most frequent categories (2).

Maternal trauma is the leading cause of nonobstetric maternal deaths (3). Most trauma victims, however, do survive their accidents to seek medical treatment in an emergency room situation.

Emergency care for pregnant trauma victims is, as in nonpregnant patients, based on the ABCs (airway–breathing–circulation) of cardiopulmonary resuscitation and the acute stabilization of vital signs. However, normal physiologic adaptations to pregnancy produce unique baseline norms in laboratory and clinical data. Patterns of injury and systemic responses to trauma are altered as a result of the unique anatomy and physiology of pregnancy.

The maternal pulse rate normally increases by 15–20 beats/minute or approximately 15%. Blood pressure usually decreases by 5–15 mm Hg in the second trimester and then gradually returns to baseline during the third trimester. Maternal blood volume increases an average of 1000 ml or 45%. Cardiac output begins to increase early in the first trimester and peaks at about 40% above baseline by 28 weeks' gestation. The supine hypotensive syndrome, produced when the pregnant woman is supine and the gravid uterus compresses vena caval flow, may decrease cardiac output by as much as 30%. Central venous pressure (CVP) normally is elevated in pregnant women, but CVP increments will parallel those seen in nonpregnant individuals given equal volumes of fluid replacement (4).

The aforementioned normal physiologic cardiovascular changes make diagnosis of hypovolemic shock and evaluation of acute blood loss and fluid replacement formidable tasks. An increased heart rate and decreased blood pressure may reflect normal pregnant physiology or supine positioning; on the other hand, these fluctuations in heart rate and blood pressure may denote the cardinal signs of hemodynamic shock. The increased blood volume of pregnancy allows the gravid patient to tolerate a 1500 ml blood loss without an appreciable decrease in blood pressure. Severely hypovolemic pregnant patients have been reported to maintain a relatively stable blood pressure and pulse until nearly exsanguinated; in these cases, maternal decompensation is abrupt and severe, with blood pressure and heart rate suddenly becoming unobtainable (2, p 905).

Plasma volume increases disproportionately relative to red blood cell mass. Plasma volume increases 40–70 ml/kg while red blood cell (RBC) mass increases only 25–30 ml/kg. Differentiating the resultant physiologic anemia from an anemic state caused by acute blood loss is most difficult around 28 weeks' gestation when normal dilutional "anemia" reaches its lowest point.

The majority of clotting factors and plasma proteins normally are increased during pregnancy. Fibrinogen levels are elevated especially, with normal ranges changing from 80–180 mg/dl in nonpregnant clients to 350–450 mg/dl in pregnant women (5). Abruptio placentae, a relatively frequent complication of maternal trauma, can induce severe coagulopathies that deplete fibrinogen. Thus, practitioners must be aware that a normal nonpregnant fibrinogen value is an abnormal finding in a pregnant patient. The increase in clotting factors also produces a state of hypercoagulability,

219

which predisposes pregnant patients to the development of deep vein thrombosis.

The average leukocyte count during pregnancy varies from 10,000–18,000 μl. At term, white blood cell (WBC) levels may rise to 25,000 μl in response to minimal stress or labor. Erythrocyte sedimentation rate is elevated in uncomplicated pregnancies as a result of increased fibrinogen. Increased WBC count and increased sedimentation rate thus are less indicative of the presence of true infection.

The respiratory rate changes little during pregnancy, but the functional residual capacity normally decreases while the tidal volume normally increases. The result is a chronic state of respiratory alkalosis and a corresponding decrease in the blood's buffering capacity. $PaCO_2$ levels of 32 torr are considered within the normal range for pregnancy.

PaO_2 levels remain unchanged, but oxygen consumption normally is increased. The increase in oxygen consumption coupled with the decrease in functional residual capacity alters the pregnant woman's response to general anesthesia. Generally, pregnant clients undergo induction more rapidly and display a decreased tolerance threshold for general anesthetics (6).

After the first trimester, the uterus becomes increasingly vulnerable to injury as it grows to become an abdominal organ. The bladder also increasingly becomes predisposed to trauma as it rises passively from the pelvis into the abdomen, secondary to growth of the uterus. Injury to the genitourinary system may lead to massive and devastating intravascular blood loss because of the greatly enhanced blood supply directed toward the uterus, bladder, and kidneys during pregnancy. Furthermore, the hyperemic bladder of pregnancy is traumatized quite easily if compressed or otherwise injured.

When evaluating x-ray and sonographic studies of the urinary system, practitioners must consider that hydronephrosis and hydroureter are normally seen during pregnancy. Also, laboratory values considered normal in nonpregnant patients may indicate renal dysfunction in the injured pregnant client. An increase in renal plasma flow and glomerular filtration lead to physiologic decreases in serum blood urea nitrogen (BUN) and creatinine.

The gravid uterus displaces the bowel into the upper abdomen. Therefore, contrary to the nonpregnant state, the bowel is less likely to be traumatized in cases of lower abdominal injury, and it is more likely to be traumatized in cases of upper abdominal injury. Repositioning of the bowel also tends to make paracentesis more dangerous and less accurate (7).

Clinical evaluation of intraperitoneal hemorrhage is of little diagnostic value during pregnancy. Abdominal guarding and rebound tenderness, the hallmark clinical manifestations of an intraperitoneal bleed, normally are decreased during pregnancy because of distention of the anterior abdominal wall.

Progesterone stimulation causes decreased gastric motility and prolonged gastric emptying. Thus, an unconscious pregnant woman or a pregnant woman undergoing general anesthesia is at greater risk for serious aspiration complications.

ACUTE MANAGEMENT OF PREGNANT TRAUMA VICTIMS

All pregnant trauma victims should be evaluated by skilled perinatal personnel, even when injuries are believed to be superficial. Minor cuts, abrasions, and simple fractures are managed as in nonpregnant patients. Tetanus prophylaxis, either with toxoid or human tetanus immune globulin may be given as indicated (7). Those antibiotics not contraindicated during pregnancy may be prescribed as needed.

Assessment of the severely injured pregnant woman should progress systematically. The clinician rapidly assesses the patient's level of consciousness. Areas of maximum pain are evaluated, and a quick history is taken, including events surrounding the injury and existence of major medical disorders and allergies. If the patient is unconscious, the clinician should obtain information from an accompanying family member or friend.

Ventilatory function is assessed by noting color, respiratory rate, breath sounds, and chest wall movement. If respiration is compromised, an airway is established immediately in order to provide adequate ventilatory support. A bag and mask can be used initially. An oral airway and/or an endotracheal tube is employed as indicated according to patient response. Laryngoscopic evaluation may help rule out occlusion of the airway by foreign matter. If chest wounds are apparent, they must be sealed immediately to facilitate respiratory efforts. Maternal ventilation will provide fetal oxygenation.

The patient's circulatory status is evaluated by noting skin color, heart rate, and blood pressure. If possible, vital signs should be measured with the woman in the left lateral decubitus position. External cardiac massage is initiated as indicated.

Maternal blood pressure is supported with fluid replacement. When injuries are believed to be severe, two peripheral intravenous lines should be inserted using large bore catheters. Cross-matched whole blood is the fluid infusion of choice. However, a Ringer's lactate drip should be initiated immediately and then continued until blood for transfusion is available.

Aggressive management of volume replacement is essential in the pregnant trauma victim, because maternal blood pressure will be maintained at the expense of uteroplacental perfusion. A 30–35% reduction in maternal blood volume will produce no appreciable change in maternal blood pressure, yet it will cause a 10–20% decrease in uterine blood flow (8). Maternal hypoxia causes blood to be shunted away from the uterus and toward maternal vital organs.

Vasopressors are indicated when maternal blood pressure does not respond to volume replacement. Peripheral vasopressors will decrease uterine blood flow, but centrally acting drugs, such as ephedrine, may simultaneously increase maternal blood pressure and uteroplacental perfusion (9).

While starting the intravenous line, the clinician draws blood for laboratory evaluation, including blood type, Rh and cross-match, complete blood count (CBC), electrolytes, platelets, prothrombin time, partial thromboplastin time, fibrinogen and fibrinogen split products, liver function tests, amylase, creatinine, and BUN. Arterial blood gases are needed when respiration is compromised, chest injury is apparent or suspected, and when the patient is unconscious or is demonstrating an altered mental status. A Kleihauer-Betke stain to rule out fetomaternal hemorrhage is indicated when patients are severely injured. When stain results are positive, RhoGAM is indicated for nonsensitized Rh-negative patients.

Shock, absent bowel sounds, guarding, rebound tenderness, and dullness to percussion in the flanks are suggestive of intraabdominal hemorrhage or visceral rupture. Whenever internal injury is suspected, a CVP line is indicated for evaluation of intravascular volume status, and a Foley catheter is indicated to monitor urinary output and hematuria.

Inability to pass a Foley catheter signals the possibility of urethral injury. When a Foley catheter has been inserted, hematuria signals the life-threatening possibility of a ruptured bladder. Diagnostic suspicion of bladder injury should be corroborated by cystogram (2, p 909). Direct injury to the kidney is suspected when the bladder and urethra are proven intact but blood is found in the urine. Blunt injury to the back with bruising along the flank necessitates a diagnostic intravenous pyelogram (2, p 909).

A nasogastric tube is passed to rule out gastric bleeding and to assess the integrity of the esophagus and stomach.

Since interpretation of the clinical abdominal examination is so difficult during pregnancy, peritoneal lavage is used to evaluate the need for emergency laparotomy in any case where abdominal trauma is a possibility. Laparotomy is indicated when the lavage fluid returned meets any of the following criteria: erythrocyte count greater than 100,000; WBC count greater than 500/mm^3; gastric contents present; and amylase levels elevated, suggestive of small bowel injury. Laparotomy also is performed in the absence of a positive peritoneal lavage when free air is found under the diaphragm on an upright chest x-ray or when there is progressive abdominal distention accompanied by a falling hematocrit. Laparotomy is always appropriate when the abdominal wall is disrupted or perforated (2, p 907). When performing a laparotomy, the surgeon usually can work around the pregnant uterus. Laparotomy is not an indication for cesarean section; anticipatory management for vaginal delivery is appropriate even within a few hours of laparotomy (2, p 907).

A complete obstetric examination is indicated whenever a pregnant woman sustains a severe injury. The patient is examined for fetal size and fetal heart rate, as well as for signs and symptoms of placental abruption, uterine rupture, and contractions indicative of labor. A pelvic examination is needed to assess the Bishop's score (see Chapter 37) and to rule out vaginal bleeding, rupture of membranes, and hematoma formation. Evaluation of fetal well-being via a nonstress test, contraction stress test, and sonogram is an integral aspect of the data collection process when the fetus is considered viable. Ultrasound is helpful for confirming fetal size and maturity, fetal death, placental location, and uterine integrity. Appropriate perinatal management should be instituted as indicated, and aggressive intervention for a viable fetus in distress can be initiated as soon as the maternal condition is stabilized.

The clinician collects a complete history and performs a meticulous physical examination once maternal vital signs are stable. It must be emphasized that x-rays are not to be withheld because of the pregnancy. Omission of indicated x-rays may seriously compromise accurate diagnosis and optimal care of both mother and fetus.

PENETRATING TRAUMA TO ABDOMEN

Gunshot and stab wounds are, respectively, the number 1 and number 2 most frequent causes of penetrating trauma to the gravid abdomen (10).

As previously discussed, the pattern of injury sustained by pregnant women is altered by virtue of the enlarged uterus. Bullets and sharp penetrating objects are more apt to strike the uterus if it is a relatively large size. Stab wounds to the upper abdomen carry a high risk of severe visceral damage because of compartmentalization of abdominal organs into this area.

On the other hand, the uterus acts as a mechanical shield in cases of lower abdominal stab wounds. Interestingly, the gravid muscular uterus can protect other abdominal viscera by absorbing and dissipating projectile momentum from an invading bullet (10). In approximatey 80% of reported cases of penetrating abdominal trauma, the uterus alone is injured and other abdominal viscera are spared (10).

Signs and symptoms of acute intravascular blood loss frequently present in the patient who has sustained a penetrating abdominal injury. With respect to gunshot wounds, if bullets do not strike the uterus, multiple entry and exit wounds in the bowel can be anticipated because of crowding. Also, the erratic path of bullets may cause unexpected diaphragmatic and thoracic injury and, hence, mild to severe respiratory distress.

Maternal mortality from gunshot wounds is rare. In fact, a lower mortality in pregnant women, as compared with an expected 10% in nonpregnant individuals, has been documented (10). This low incidence of maternal mortality is attributable to the protective properties of the gravid uterus and the fact that the uterus, most commonly assaulted, is not a "vital" organ.

Maternal mortality from stab wounds is related directly to the incidence and severity of abdominal visceral injury. Visceral injury and mortality occur less often in stab wound victims than in gunshot victims. Stab wounds to the abdomen have an associated mortality of 1.4% in the nonpregnant individual; during pregnancy, the protective influence of the gravid uterus further decreases this incidence (9, p 35).

Injuries to the fetus, umbilical cord, and placenta have been documented as a result of both abdominal gunshot and stab wounds. Gunshot wounds are associated with a very high prevalence of fetal injury and perinatal mortality, 70% and 65% respectively (11). In this same study perinatal mortality was evenly distributed between direct fetal trauma and prematurity. In another study involving 14 case reports of stab wounds to the gravid uterus, 50% of the fetuses suffered injury (10).

Management of stab wounds to the gravid abdomen requires a great degree of individualization. Surgical exploration usually is not indicated when the peritoneal cavity is intact. Peritoneal integrity is evaluated by introducing contrast medium into the cleansed wound via a French catheter. Some surgeons choose conservative management when the peritoneum of the lower abdomen only has been damaged. In these cases peritoneal lavage, retrograde cystogram, and close monitoring of vital signs are relied upon to identify patients who require surgical exploration. Surgery is always indicated to assess upper abdominal stab wounds because of the increased likelihood of visceral damage and the decreased diagnostic reliability of peritoneal lavage. All pregnant patients with abdominal gunshot wounds require exploratory laparotomy to control bleeding, retrieve the bullet, and identify the nature and extent of injuries (10).

BLUNT TRAUMA TO ABDOMEN

Blunt trauma to the abdomen may result from car accidents, falls, and assaults with blunt weapons. Car accidents are the most frequent and significant cause of severe blunt trauma (12). Falls, on the other hand, rarely are associated with increased mortality or serious maternal or perinatal morbidity (13). The protuberant gravid uterus is the organ most commonly injured when pregnant women sustain blunt trauma to the abdomen (12).

Although relatively rare, uterine rupture has occurred following severe blunt abdominal trauma (12). Animal studies with primates have shown a tenfold increase in intrauterine pressure occurring immediately upon collision impact (14). This increased intrauterine pressure is believed responsible for uterine rupture. Hemorrhagic shock frequently develops if myometrial lacerations are significant or if injuries involve the uterine blood supply.

In a large prospective study, abruptio placentae reportedly occurred with a frequency of 5.9% after blunt abdominal trauma (15). Acute impact flattens the uterus against the abdominal wall and causes turbulent waves of amniotic fluid to develop. The uterine musculature responds by elongating and shortening along its vertical axis. The relatively nonelastic placenta is unable to compensate for these alterations in uterine shape and is thus torn from its implantation site, initiating the abruption process (15). Hypovolemic shock and coagulation disorders frequently accompany abruptio placentae.

Premature rupture of membranes also may occur following blunt abdominal trauma as a result of the aforementioned increase in intrauterine pressure and the accelerated pattern of intrauterine activity. Premature labor develops in approximately 10% of all cases. Pelvic fractures frequently are associated with blunt abdominal trauma and may be responsible for devastating intravascular blood loss (15, p 684). (Refer to "Fractures" section.)

The protective shock-absorbing quality of amniotic fluid usually safeguards the fetus from direct blunt trauma injury. However, some isolated cases of umbilical cord hematomas, intracranial injuries, and fractures of fetal extremities have been reported. Abortion is an infrequent complication of blunt trauma but a cause-effect relationship is difficult to prove. Cases of fetal demise reportedly have occurred secondary to uterine injury (15).

Medical management for the pregnant woman who has sustained blunt abdominal trauma should proceed as outlined in the section "Acute Management of Pregnant Trauma Victims."

CAR ACCIDENTS

In a large prospective study of pregnant patients involved in serious automobile accidents, researchers reported a 7.2% maternal mortality rate and a 13.5% injury rate among survivors. Head injury was the leading cause of maternal death, and intraabdominal injury fell a close second (16).

Maternal injuries from car accidents tend to be multiple. Internal injuries most often associated with maternal death include rupture of major blood vessels and rupture of the liver, spleen, and bowel. Placental separation occurs with relative frequency and is a much more common obstetric complication than uterine rupture. Multiple fractures of the ribs, extremities, and pelvis are also commonly found; extraperitoneal hemorrhage should be anticipated in cases of pelvic fracture (16).

In the prospective study referred to above, the reported fetal death rate was 15%. Maternal death was the leading cause of fetal death, and placental separation was the second most common cause of fetal demise.

Seat belts play an important role in reducing maternal and fetal morbidity and mortality. The three-point shoulder harness is superior to a lap belt because it provides an equal distribution of momentum force, which helps to prevent maternal head injury. Fetal survival rises from 50 to 92% when a shoulder harness is used instead of a standard lap belt restraint (16, p 633). Seat belts should never be fastened across the dome of the uterus; instead, they should be applied across the lap with an intervening soft pillow.

FRACTURES

Fractures are a common finding in pregnant trauma victims. The incidence of fractures, however, is not significantly different in pregnant as compared to nonpregnant individuals.

Pelvic fractures are of particular importance during pregnancy. The enormously increased vascularity of the retroperitoneum is quite vulnerable to injury and is disrupted easily by a pelvic fracture. Pelvic fractures during pregnancy have been reported as responsible for massive concealed retroperitoneal hemorrhage, rapid maternal decompensation, and hypovolemic shock. Furthermore, fractures of the pelvis often are associated with abruptio placentae and severe injury to the lower urinary tract, both of which may initiate significant blood loss. Skull fractures are the most common fetal injury resulting directly from pelvic fractures (9, p 36).

Pregnant patients who have sustained blunt abdominal trauma especially are at risk for pelvic fractures. Meticulous evaluation for signs and symptoms of acute blood loss thus is indicated in these women. When a definitive diagnosis of pelvic fracture has been confirmed via x-ray, patients must be assessed carefully for abruptio placentae, urinary tract injury, and retroperitoneal hemorrhage. Additionally, fractures of long bones may lead to unexpectedly large and significant blood loss (2, p 911).

Management of fractures during pregnancy is, for the most part, based on the same orthopedic principles that apply to nonpregnant clients. Whenever spinal column injury is suspected, immobilization from the time of initial stabilization is of paramount importance. Major fractures should be identified at the scene of the accident and immobilized with splints until x-rays can be taken and appropriate therapies instituted. Patients with compound fractures require anticipatory management for the potential problems of acute blood loss and sepsis.

Traction is not a favored treatment modality during pregnancy because of the pregnant woman's increased potential for thromboembolism when subjected to prolonged periods of immobilization. Furthermore, numerous logistical problems are associated with delivering a baby while the mother remains in traction. Thus, despite the inherent surgical risks, open reduction with fixation often is the treatment of choice when either traction or surgery is considered appropriate (3, p 434).

Casts may be applied during pregnancy; however, several situations require special consideration. Large casts that encroach on the abdomen or perineum are to be avoided whenever possible since they may interfere with the assessment and management of labor and delivery. Body casts and hip spica casts also should be avoided because they may restrict space needed for the growing uterus. Operative fixation in the aforementioned cases usually is preferable to application of an unyielding cast (2, p 911).

With respect to modes of delivery, a stable spinal fracture is not a contraindication for vaginal delivery, and a stable pelvic fracture rarely interferes with progression of spontaneous delivery. Cesarean section is indicated for unstable pelvic and spinal fractures; in these cases, vaginal delivery predisposes to further bony displacement and injury to adjacent viscera, blood vessels, and soft tissue (17).

BURNS

Approximately 4% of women of childbearing age who are badly burned are pregnant (18).

Burns can result from flames, hot surfaces, hot liquids, chemicals, radiation, electrical currents, or frostbite. Fire injuries cause two-thirds of all burns. Eighty-five percent of all burns occur at home (19).

A minor burn is a superficial or partial-thickness injury covering less than 10% of the total body surface. Partial-thickness burns, previously classified as first- or second-degree burns, are thermal injuries wherein epithelial cells remain to provide new epidermis for spontaneous healing (18, p 384).

A full-thickness burn, previously labeled third-degree, is characterized by destruction of the skin and, frequently, destruction of subcutaneous tissue, muscle, and bone. Regeneration of the skin is not possible in full-thickness burns, and skin grafts are needed to cover the injured area (18, p 384).

A major burn is defined as a partial- or full-thickness burn affecting more than 10% of the total body surface. Major burns are classified as moderate when 10–19% of the body is burned, severe when 20–39% of the body is burned, and critical when 40% or more of the body is burned (20). Burns also are classified as major when medical history reveals concurrent chronic or severe illness; the face, hands, or perineum have been burned; the burn resulted from an electrical current; or there has been an accompanying injury resulting, for example, in respiratory difficulty (18, p 384).

The face, neck, and extremities are the most common burn sites found in pregnant women. Burns of the abdomen and perineum are rare unless greater than 45% of the total body surface is involved (18, p 384).

Initially, a burn causes dilatation of capillaries and increased capillary permeability. As plasma seeps from blood vessels into surrounding tissue, edema accumulates and blisters form. With major burns, intravascular fluid loss may be so great as to place the pregnant burn patient at risk for severe hypovolemia, decreased uterine blood flow, hypotension, decreased renal perfusion, and renal shutdown.

The prognosis for the mother and fetus after a burn is contingent upon the extent of the injury. Maternal mortality is 3% when burns cover less than 40% of the body surface. Deaths in these cases are caused by complications such as fluid and electrolyte imbalances, respiratory distress, and sepsis. Approximately 25% of all women die when burns cover 50% of the body surface, and all women die if the burn is 80% or more. The gestational age at the time of thermal injury does not appear to be related to maternal prognosis (18, p 392).

When burns cover less than 40% of the mother's body, fetal mortality ranges from 17–27%. When burns extend over 50% of the total maternal body surface, the associated perinatal mortality is approximately 63%. Perinatal deaths result from both in utero deaths and complications arising from premature delivery. The following maternal burn complications are believed to predispose to fetal distress or spontaneous uterine activity: hypovolemia, hypoxia, acidosis, electrolyte imbalance, sepsis, and carbon monoxide poisoning (21).

Premature delivery or stillbirth most commonly occurs within the first 5 days following a burn. The risk of premature delivery increases with the extent of thermal injury (18, p 395). Severe burns and accompanying sepsis are associated with high levels of prostaglandins (22). Prostaglandins are believed to enhance spontaneous uterine activity, which may lead to abortion or premature labor.

Principles used to manage minor burns in nonpregnant individuals apply as well to the pregnant patient. Erythema usually subsides within 24 hours and hospitalization rarely is indicated. Wounds are cleansed twice daily with mild soap and tap water and are covered with sterile bandages. Bacitracin or a burn ointment may be applied topically, and mild oral analgesics may be prescribed as needed. A minor burn usually will heal within 2 weeks without significant risk to the fetus (21, p 130).

When pregnant patients sustain major burns, the first 48–72 hours are focused on assessing the severity of the injury, stabilizing vital signs, maintaining adequate oxygenation, replacing fluid volume, and initiating wound care.

Strict attention to volume replacement is essential. Infusion of enormous volumes of fluid may be required to compensate for the loss of fluid through the burn site. Fluid loss is greatest within the first 12 hours. Even if the burned area covers only 15% of the body's surface, fluid loss may be significant enough for the patient to become hypovolemic (21, p 132). Assessment of urinary output and CVP is the most reliable indicator of intravascular fluid status. Excess fluid in the interstitial space returns to the intravascular space after several days. Profound diuresis then will signal successful resuscitation (18, p 387).

Medical management from day 3 to approximately day 20 is focused on wound debridement, wound coverage with autographs, and prevention and treatment of any complications.

One of the most common and devastating complications from severe burns is infection. Infection at the burn site and bacteremia may lead to overwhelming systemic infection, maternal hypotension, septic shock, placental infection, and transfer of bacterial toxins to the fetus. Intravenous penicillin usually is begun initially, pending the clinical picture of sepsis and microbiology reports. Cultures of the wound, urine, blood, and sputum should be obtained on admission and at least weekly thereafter.

Since the mother's head and neck are common sites of extensive burn injury, immediate and delayed respiratory complications may occur. Injury to the respiratory tract may result from inhaled irritants, direct burn to the upper respiratory tract, carbon monoxide intoxication, and/or pulmonary edema.

Pregnant burn patients have extraordinary nutritional needs. Higher caloric demands normally required during pregnancy are increased further by burn trauma. In an attempt to repair burn wounds and maintain homeostasis, the body adapts a state of hypermetabolism. Goals for nutritional intervention include correcting caloric deficits and avoiding or correcting a negative nitrogen balance and ketoacidosis (18, p 390).

Providing adequate nutrition may require use of nasogastric feedings and/or hyperalimentation. Although daily requirements will vary, pregnant burn patients require a minimum of 2800 calories and 120 g protein (18, p 390).

Emotional support for the pregnant woman who is severely burned is a vital and integral aspect of patient care. Fear of death, guilt, disruption of life-style, pain, emotional dependence, altered body image, low self-esteem, and depression are some of the psychological sequelae experienced by patients who have been badly burned (18, p 392). Premature labor and fetal loss are sources of additional emotional stress.

Returning the severely burned pregnant patient to health is a long and arduous process. When healing has progressed to the point that only 20% of her total body surface is involved, the threat to life is reduced markedly, and efforts can be directed toward correcting functional and cosmetic deformities. Discharge planning should be initiated as soon as maternal survival is assured.

NURSING MANAGEMENT

Nursing care specific for a patient with a traumatic injury:

☐ Assess maternal/fetal status:
- Assess breathing pattern and circulatory status;
- Assess for chest injuries; evaluate breath sounds and chest wall movement to determine presence of pneumothorax;
- Monitor and record vital signs and fetal heart tones at frequent intervals (e.g., every 15–30 minutes);
- Assess patient's entire body for areas of visible hemorrhage;
- Perform obstetric examination as indicated (e.g., determine fetal size, presentation, position; assess signs/symptoms of uterine rupture, abruptio placentae, la-

NURSING MANAGEMENT

bor, hematoma formation; determine Bishop's score [see Chapter 37], status of membranes;
— Assess intravascular fluid status: monitor CVP and assess urinary output;
— Inspect and dipstick all urine to determine presence of hematuria; and
— Insert nasogastric tube (if appropriate) to decompress stomach and assess for gastric bleeding.
☐ Provide emergency care as indicated:
— Maintain patent airway;
— Initiate CPR;
— Seal sucking chest wounds; and
— Control blood loss:
  * Apply firm manual pressure over involved wound or artery and rotate tourniquets, as ordered;
  * Elevate involved extremity;
  * Remove gross foreign material from wound;
  * Apply pressure dressing; and
  * Apply tourniquet if hemorrhage is uncontrollable, placing it as low on the extremity as possible.
— Treat signs/symptoms of hypovolemic shock:
  * Insert two intravenous lines and
  * Administer intravenous fluids and blood as ordered.
☐ Position the patient on her left side whenever possible to maximize uteroplacental blood flow and to avoid maternal supine hypotensive syndrome.
☐ Anticipate the need for emergency medications (e.g., cardiogenic drugs, sodium bicarbonate, atropine); administer antimicrobials and tetanus prophylaxis as needed.
☐ Assist the burn victim to maintain adequate nutritional status; administer nasogastric feeding and hyperalimentation as needed; assess

for clinical signs of inadequate diet (e.g., slow healing, infection, worsening anemia, anorexia, muscle wasting, weight loss).
☐ Observe the patient for signs/symptoms of preterm labor; administer tocolytic medications as needed (see Chapter 28).
☐ Be prepared for emergency cesarean section (if fetus is of viable gestational age, alive but in distress, and maternal condition would permit surgery).
☐ Assess and manage pain.

Nursing care specific for patients with *burns*:
☐ Remove hot or burning clothing; assist with evaluation of thermal injury; determine causative agent and duration of exposure.
☐ Immerse small burn areas in cold water for 10 minutes; cover extensive thermal injuries with moist sheets, sterile if possible.
☐ Irrigate chemical burns with copious amount of running water.
☐ Anticipate the need for tracheostomy for the patient with deep facial, neck, or respiratory tract burns.

Nursing diagnoses most frequently associated with *trauma* (see Section V):
☐ Grieving related to potential/actual loss of infant or birth of an imperfect child.
☐ Anticipatory grieving related to actual/perceived threat to self.
☐ Pain.
☐ Disturbance in body image, self-esteem.
☐ Fluid volume deficit.
☐ Impaired tissue integrity.
☐ Altered maternal tissue perfusion.
☐ Altered fetal cardiac and cerebral tissue perfusion.
☐ Impaired skin integrity.
☐ Knowledge deficit regarding disease process, treatment, and expected outcome.
☐ Anxiety/fear.

REFERENCES

1. Baker DP: Trauma in the pregnant patient. *Surg Clin North Am* 62:275, 1982.
2. Crosby W: Traumatic injuries during pregnancy. *Clin Obstet Gynecol* 26:902, 1983.
3. Lavin JP, Polsky SS: Abdominal trauma during pregnancy. *Clin Perinatol* 10:423, 1983.
4. O'Driscoll K, McCarthy J: Abruptio placenta and central venous pressure. *J Obstet Gynaecol Br Commonw* 73:923, 1966.
5. Cruikshank D: Anatomic and physiologic alterations of pregnancy that modify the response to trauma. In Buchsbaum H (ed): *Trauma in Pregnancy*. Philadelphia, WB Saunders, 1979.
6. Gutsche B: Maternal physiologic alterations during pregnancy. In Schnider S, Levinson G (eds): *Anesthesia for Obstetrics*. Baltimore, Williams & Wilkins, 1979.
7. Buchsbaum H: Diagnosis and early management. In Buchsbaum H (ed): *Trauma in Pregnancy*. Philadelphia, WB Saunders, 1979.

8. Greiss FC: Uterine vascular response to hemorrhage during pregnancy with observations on therapy. *Obstet Gynecol* 27:549, 1966.

9. Patterson RM: Trauma in pregnancy. *Clin Obstet Gynecol* 27:34, 1984.

10. Buchsbaum H: Penetrating injury of the abdomen. In Buchsbaum H (ed): *Trauma in Pregnancy*. Philadelphia, WB Saunders, 1979.

11. Buchsbaum H: Diagnosis and management of abdominal gunshot wounds during pregnancy. *J Trauma* 14:425, 1975.

12. Crosby W: Automobile injuries and blunt abdominal trauma in pregnancy. In Buchsbaum H (ed): *Trauma in Pregnancy*. Philadelphia, WB Saunders, 1979.

13. Fort A, Harlen R: Pregnancy outcome for the non-catastrophic maternal trauma during pregnancy. *Obstet Gynecol* 25:912, 1970.

14. Crosby W, Snyder R, Snow C: Impact injuries in pregnancy. *Am J Obstet Gynecol* 101:100, 1968.

15. Crosby W: Trauma during pregnancy: maternal and fetal injury. *Obstet Gynecol Survey* 29:683, 1974.

16. Crosby W, Costile J: Safety of lap-belt restraint for pregnant victims of automobile collisions. *N Engl J Med* 284:632, 1971.

17. Buchsbaum H: Accidental injury complicating pregnation. *Am J Obstet Gynecol* 102:752, 1968.

18. Smith BK, Rayburn WF, Feller I: Burns and pregnancy. *Clin Perinatol* 10:383, 1983.

19. Feller I, Crane K: *Planning and Designing a Burn Care Facility*. Ann Arbor, National Institute for Burn Medicine, 1971.

20. Feller I, Archambeault C: *Nursing the Burned Patient*. Ann Arbor, National Institute for Burn Medicine, 1973.

21. Taylor J: Thermal burns. In Buchsbaum H (ed): *Trauma in Pregnancy*. Philadelphia, WB Saunders, 1979, pp 128–141.

22. Stage AM: Severe burns in the pregnant patient. *Obstet Gynecol* 42:259, 1973.

Chapter 21
Tumors
Nina Mimoni Daratsos, R.N.C., M.S.N.

INTRODUCTION

The consequences of a reproductive tumor for a pregnant woman are many. There may be a loss of the wanted pregnancy, loss of the woman's reproductive capabilities, and the potential for the loss of her life. Sometimes a decision must be made between prolonging the life of the mother with the risk of fetal demise or allowing the fetus time to grow and to develop while jeopardizing maternal survival.

HISTOLOGY OF NEOPLASTIC GROWTH

Normal tissues are composed of mature cells of uniform size and shape. Each cell contains a nucleus also of uniform size. Within the nucleus of each cell are the chromosomes containing DNA, the substance that controls RNA. RNA is found in both the nucleoli of the cell and the cytoplasm; it is the regulator of the growth and the function of the cell.

Malignant cells are those that have changed their basic structure and pattern into a bizarre pattern. The cells divide and grow but no longer resemble the parent cell. There are nuclei of varying sizes and in varying stages of mitosis. The mitotic divisions are rapid and disorderly.

Abnormal cells are classified according to their degree of variation from normal cells. A grade I tumor is most like the parent cell and the least malignant. A grade IV tumor is the least like the parent cell and the most malignant.

Malignant tumors are not encapsulated and can invade blood vessels or lymphatics. The tumors often break off and are carried by the blood and lymphatics to other parts of the body (1).

Benign tumors are composed of cells that resemble parent cells. Usually, they are encapsulated, localized, slow in growth, and harmful only because of pressure placed on surrounding tissue by the growth and diversion of blood supply from the normal tissue to the tumor. Although a benign tumor may not be life-threatening in the nonpregnant state, it can have a deleterious effect during pregnancy. The tumor can prevent placental implantation; cause hemorrhagic diseases, such as disseminated intravascular coagulation, in the mother; or cause mechanical obstruction, preventing vaginal delivery.

Tumors derive their names from the type of tissue involved. They may arise from one or all three of the embryonic tissue structures: mesoderm, ectoderm, and endoderm (see Table 21.1). Muscles, bones, fascia, and connective tissue form from the mesoderm. Skin cells and cells for hair follicles, sweat glands, and the nerves are formed from ectoderm. Lining membranes of the respiratory tract, gastrointestinal tract, and the genitourinary tract develop from the endoderm.

Benign tumors generally are of one tissue type. Malignant tumors are named by the type of tissue or tissues they arise from:

1. Carcinoma, from epithelial cells;
2. Sarcoma, from connective tissue cells; and
3. Teratoma, from all three embryonic layers.

The mode of treatment depends upon the type and the location of the tumor. Treatment may consist of surgery, radiation therapy, chemotherapy, or a combination of these.

Table 21.1.
TUMOR TYPES

EMBRYONIC TISSUE	CELL TYPE		BENIGN	MALIGNANT	GYNECOLOGIC TUMOR SITE
Mesoderm	Endothelial tissue			Endothelioma	
		Blood vessels	Hemangioma	Hemangiosarcoma	
		Lymph vessels	Lymphangioma	Lymphangiosarcoma	
		Lymph tissue		Lymphosarcoma	
	Connective tissue				
		Fibrous	Fibroma	Fibrosarcoma	Symphysis pubis
		Adipose	Lipoma	Liposarcoma	Breast
		Cartilage	Chondroma	Chondrosarcoma	
		Bone	Osteoma	Osteosarcoma	
		Blood		Leukemia	
	Muscle tissue		Myoma	Myosarcoma	Uterus, cervix
		Smooth muscle	Leiomyoma	Leiomyosarcoma	Uterus, cervix
Ectoderm	Epithelium		Papilloma	Carcinoma	
		Skin	Wart, verruca		Vagina
		Gland	Polyp	Basal cell	Vagina, cervix
			Adenoma	Adenocarcinoma	Breast, ovary, fallopian tubes
	Pigmented neoplasms		Nevus mole	Malignant melanoma	Metastases to placenta and fetus
	Nerve tissue		Neuroma	Neurogenic sarcoma	
		Nerve fibers		Neuroblastoma	Fetus
Mixed embryonal tissue				Teratoma	Ovary
				Dermoids	Ovary

BENIGN VULVAR TUMORS

During pregnancy, condyloma acuminatum is the most common tumor of the vulva. It is a sexually transmitted disease (refer to Chapter 22).

CARCINOMA OF THE VULVA

Definition

Vulvar carcinoma is a malignant cutaneous cancer of the external genitalia. The disease progresses from a dysplasia through intraepithelial neoplasia to invasive cancer. It is the fourth most common type of female genital cancer. The incidence is highest in women 50–60 years old. In pregnancy the occurrence of vulvar carcinoma is 1:8000. It is thought that pregnancy has no effect on the course of the disease.

Signs and Symptoms

Early symptoms may be complaints of vulvar pruritus, a sore, or a lump. Later symptoms may be persistent pruritus and pain.

Diagnosis

The tumor may be detected during a careful examination with a good light source. The actual diagnosis is made by a biopsy of the lesion. Staging is determined by size, location of the tumor, regional node involvement, and absence or presence of distant node involvement (2). During the childbearing years, vulvar carcinoma usually is limited to stage I or II. The difference between the two stages is the size of the tumor.

Maternal and Fetal Outcome

The 5-year survival rate with appropriate therapy is 90% for stage I disease. The rate drops to 64% for stage II disease. The risk to the fetus is due to anesthesia (see Chapter 38) and stress from surgery.

Medical Management

The standard form of therapy for stage I and II vulvar carcinomas is a radical vulvectomy with groin node dissection. The surgery is indicated regardless of the stage of pregnancy. Dissection includes a large segment of skin from the abdomen and the groin, the labia majora, labia minora, clitoris, mons veneris, and terminal portions of the urethra. The surgery may be done as a one- or two-step procedure (Fig. 21.1). Route of delivery will depend upon the level of healing from the vulvectomy. Ab-

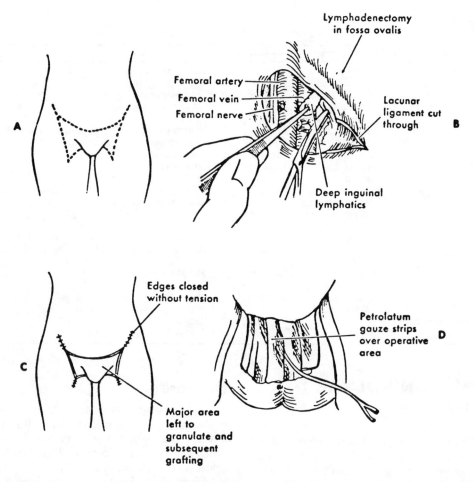

Figure 21.1. Radical vulvectomy. *A,* Outline of incisional lines for simple or radical operations for vulval cover. *B,* Dissection is completed, involving nerves, saphenous veins, and muscles, when dissection of distal half of femoral canal has been completed. *C,* Upper edges of abdominal incisions may be partially closed. *D,* With indwelling catheter in bladder, wound is dressed with layers of gauze and held in place with light pressure dressing. (From Gruendemann B, Huthmeeker M: *Alexander's Care of the Patient in Surgery,* ed 7. St. Louis, Mosby, 1983, p 316.)

dominal delivery therefore is not always indicated (3).

BENIGN VAGINAL TUMORS

Gartner's or Müllerian duct cysts are collections of fluid within an embryologic remnant that can extend down the vagina. The cysts can become large enough to cause mechanical obstruction of the birth canal. Simple drainage usually will relieve the dystocia they can create, allowing for a vaginal delivery. Surgical excision usually is postponed until after delivery and the puerperium (4).

BENIGN CERVICAL TUMORS

Cervical myomas are growths arising out of muscular tissue and are rare during pregnancy. If they do occur, the growth rate is rapid as a result of hormonal stimulation of pregnancy. The treatment is myomectomy. Treatment is postponed until after delivery because of the threat of abortion and/or hemorrhage. Delivery of the infant usually is by cesarean section because of mechanical obstruction and threat of hemorrhage from myoma.

Cervical polyps are the most common of the benign cervical tumors. Generally, they arise from the intracervical mucosa, are bright red in color, have a spongy texture, and are fragile; they are located usually at the external os. Polyps can cause slight bleeding, especially when provoked by muscular exertion, such as with defecation or coitus. This bleeding must be differentiated from other pathology, including spontaneous abortion, cervicitis, cervical carcinoma, abruptio placentae, or placenta previa. Polyps presenting at the external os tend to bleed early in pregnancy. The bleeding should disappear and not affect the course of pregnancy (3, p 371).

CERVICAL CARCINOMA

Definition

The epithelium of the cervix has two types of tissue. The portion of the cervix known as the external os is covered with stratified squamous epithelium. The internal os is lined with columnar epithelium. The point at which these tissues meet is the squamocolumnar junction. This point is the most common site of cancer cell growth.

The most common cervical carcinoma involves squamous epithelium. It accounts for 90% of all cervical cancer. Adenocarcinoma, the second type, accounts for less than 10%; it involves glandular epithelium.

The mean age of a woman with cervical cancer is 46 years. The incidence in pregnancy is 1:1240. There seems to be some correlation among parity, age, and cancer of the cervix. Women having sexual activity at an early age with an average parity of 4–4.5 develop the cancer at a younger age (5).

Etiology

Cervical carcinoma is found primarily in women of lower socioeconomic status. Intercourse at an early age with multiple partners and poor hygiene are believed to be predisposing factors. The disease has been associated with condylomata; it is more common in lower socioeconomic urban areas and rare in the Amish or Mennonites. Squamous cell carcinoma has never been reported in a virgin (2, p 3).

Signs and Symptoms

There are minimal signs and symptoms, and the cervix appears normal in over half the cases. Abnormal symptoms are indicative of cervical invasion; these include the following:

1. Postcoital bleeding
2. Abnormal discharge
3. Persistent bleeding
4. Profuse discharge

Pain in the presence of cancer of the cervix is a late symptom denoting very advanced disease.

Diagnosis

The Papanicolaou (Pap) smear is a diagnostic tool for screening cervical changes. A Pap smear should be a routine procedure at the initial prenatal visit for every pregnant woman. The Pap test is a cytological evaluation of cervical/vaginal cells. The classification, once done numerically, now is descriptive. There is more than one classification. Richart's classification (Table 21.2) is histological and provides a more accurate definition of the character of the cells than the original classification (Table 21.3). The Koss classification gives a description of the degree of dysplasia (see Table 21.4).

The histological classifications refer to changes in the tissues. Dysplasia refers to histologic changes that may be due to malignant or nonmalignant causes. Herpetic infections can cause benign dysplasia. Carcinoma in situ describes

Table 21.2.
RICHART'S CLASSIFICATION[a]

Findings inadequate for diagnosis
Findings essentially normal
Atypical cells present and suggestive of cytologic
    findings consistent with cervical intraepitheliai
    neoplasia (CIN)
        Grade I   Mild dysplasia
        Grade II   Moderate dysplasia
        Grade III   Severe dysplasia carcinoma in situ
Invasive squamous cell carcinoma
Endometrial carcinoma
Other

[a]From Baldwin KA, Goodwin K: The Papanicolaou smear. *J Nurse Midwifery* 30:327–332, 1985.

Table 21.3.
PAPANICOLAOU CYTOLOGICAL SMEAR CLASSIFICATION[a]

Class I	Normal
Class II	Normal with abnormal cells
Class III	Suspicious cells
Class IV	Sign of malignancy
Class V	Definitely malignant

[a]From Baldwin KA, Goodwin K: The Papanicolaou smear. *J Nurse Midwifery* 30:327–332, 1985.

Table 21.4.

KOSS CLASSIFICATION[a]

CIN grade I	Mild dysplasia, a borderline lesion
Grade II	Moderate dysplasia, 50% abnormal cells
Grade III	Severe dysplasia, carcinoma in situ of many types

[a]From Baldwin KA, Goodwin K: The Papanicolaou smear. *J Nurse Midwifery* 30:327–332, 1985.

Table 21.5.

RECOVERY RATES BY STAGE OF DISEASE[a]

STAGE		RECOVERY RATE
Stage 0	Carcinoma in situ	95–100%
Stage I	Carcinoma confined to cervix	70–80%
Stage IA	Microinvasion	
Stage IB	All other cases stage I	
Stage II	Carcinoma extends beyond cervix, has not reached pelvic wall, involves the upper two-thirds of vagina	
Stage IIA	No parametrial involvement	65–75%
Stage IIB	Parametrial involvement	50–65%
Stage III	Carcinoma has reached pelvic wall, involves lower one-third of vagina	20–30%
Stage IV	Carcinoma involves the bladder, rectum, or both or has extended past the limits described previously	5–10%

[a]From Brunner L, Suddarth D: *Textbook of Medical-Surgical Nursing*, ed 5. Philadelphia, JP Lippincott, 1984, p 348.

a cancer limited to the epithelial layer. Invasive carcinoma involves tissue beyond the epithelium.

While obtaining the cervical smear, the practitioner should inspect for fungating or ulcerating lesions. The presence of these lesions is indicative of a cancerous growth and may present prior to symptoms.

Colposcopy-directed biopsy has become the method of choice for the evaluation of abnormal cytology. During pregnancy it is considered a safer procedure than a cone biopsy (6). The epithelium and the underlying stroma within the cervical canal cannot be excised as they would be in the non-pregnant state. They are in too close proximity to the fetal membranes. While cone biopsy remains the most accurate method with which to diagnose and stage a cervical cancer, it has a significant complication rate when performed during pregnancy—as high as 20–30%. Maternal complications include blood loss requiring transfusion, cervical stenosis, cervical laceration during labor, phlebitis, pulmonary embolism, and chorioamnionitis. Fetal complications have been reported as spontaneous abortion, premature labor and delivery, premature rupture of the membranes, stillbirth, and infection. Generally, the risks do not outweigh the benefits during pregnancy. This diagnostic method usually is reserved for those cases in which a definitive diagnosis cannot be made by colposcopy (5, p 742). Fortunately, colposcopy performed by a skilled practitioner has a rate of accuracy approaching cone biopsy (5, p 742).

If colposcopy is not available, punch biopsies at the squamocolumnar junction may be obtained. The area is stained with Lugol's solution. Any area not picking up the stain is suspicious for malignancy, and a biopsy is obtained for further histologic examination. Bleeding from the site can be controlled by vaginal packing for several hours.

Maternal and Fetal Outcome

Pregnancy outcomes are dependent on the extent of disease, the chosen treatment, and the stage of disease. Carcinoma in situ without intervention does not impact negatively on the fetus. Therapy

involving radiation during the first trimester or early second will result in the death of the fetus. Exposure in the late second and third trimesters can cause microcephaly, bilateral hip deformity, and aplastic anemia. Pregnancies are interrupted prior to treatment to avoid these sequelae (7).

Women with mild disease have excellent recovery rates, while the rate is poor for severe disease (Table 21.5).

Medical Management

Once the tissue has been classified (Table 21.4), management can be planned. Generally, a normal colposcopy requires no further intervention except to repeat the Pap smear. If this smear is normal, then the next colposcopic examination is performed between 28–32 weeks' gestation. If the colposcopy is within normal limits at that time, the pregnancy is followed to term, with no treatment required. The woman must understand the importance for follow-up to monitor any changes in her cervical cytology. If a client hears a report of "normal," she may not be inclined to return for subsequent visits, unless she fully understands the potential for change.

The management of an abnormal colposcopic examination with an abnormal smear varies with the extent of the disease, stage of gestation, and the family's attitude toward the pregnancy.

Dysplasia and Carcinoma In Situ

Dysplasia and carcinoma in situ are managed conservatively during pregnancy. Pap smear and colposcopy are performed every 4–6 weeks until time of delivery to ascertain that the disease does not progress. There does not seem to be any significant change in the course of the disease based on the mode of delivery. After the puerperium, treatment of the disease can be accomplished through cryosurgery, electrocauterization, or laser therapy should the woman wish to retain childbearing capabilities. These women need to be followed closely and usually require cervical smears as frequently as every 3 months. After careful counseling and discussion, the woman who does not desire to have more children is advised to undergo a hysterectomy (5, p 740).

Microinvasive Carcinoma

Microinvasive carcinoma has no precise diagnostic criteria. The definition varies in different reports. The largest invasion to meet the criteria for microinvasion varies from 1–5 mm without vascular space involvement (5, p 738). A repeat colposcopy that demonstrates an increase in severity of a lesion, whatever its original size, requires a biopsy under colposcopic visualization.

Diagnosis in the first trimester requires a thorough discussion with the client, her significant other, and support staff if necessary. There is insufficient evidence to support a prolonged delay in undergoing surgery unless there is a strong desire on the part of the parents to maintain the pregnancy. Treatment consists of an extrafascial hysterectomy with the fetus in situ (5, p 744).

If the diagnosis is made in the late second or third trimester, the pregnancy usually is allowed to go to term without treatment. Delivery is either by cesarean hysterectomy or vaginal delivery with a postpartum hysterectomy (5, p 744).

If the woman chooses to maintain her childbearing capabilities, radiation therapy may be considered after termination of the pregnancy (5, p 738).

Frankly Invasive Carcinoma

Frankly invasive carcinoma needs immediate treatment. For stages IB and early IIA, a radical hysterectomy and pelvic lymphadenectomy with preservation of the ovaries has been shown to be an effective treatment (5, p 739). Up until 20 weeks' gestation, the hysterectomy is performed with the fetus in situ. From 20–26 weeks, a hysterotomy is performed prior to radical surgery in order to facilitate the dissection. After 26 weeks' gestation, the decision for surgery needs to be assessed taking into account the interest of the unborn child and the mother. The level of expert neonatal care may have an impact on the timing for interruption of the pregnancy. Any decision to delay therapy should involve the mother, the significant other, and other appropriate members of the health care team. It is not advisable to delay treatment for more than 6 weeks (5, p 739).

Radiation therapy is an alternate therapy for early stage disease and is the preferred treatment for late stages of frankly invasive carcinoma. The therapy varies among institutions, but most utilize a combination of external and intercavitary irradiation. For treatments prescribed during the first trimester, external therapy is the most common.

Spontaneous abortion usually occurs within a range of 27–50 days following treatment. During the second trimester, irradiation is less likely to cause spontaneous abortion. This is due to a decreased sensitivity of the fetus to radium (5, p 740).

If the fetus is less than 20 weeks' gestation and does not abort spontaneously, a hysterotomy should be performed. After 20 weeks' gestation, hysterotomy should be done prior to initiating radiation therapy. Pregnancies are not continued after radiation therapy because of the risks to the fetus. The effects on the fetus include mental retardation, microcephaly, bilateral congenital hip deformity, and aplastic anemia. For patients diagnosed in the third trimester, the therapy is postponed to 7 days postpartum. The decision regarding preterm cesarean section depends upon the level of neonatal care available and the family's decision to interrupt the pregnancy prematurely. Cesarean section is the preferred method of delivery as there is an increased risk of cervical lacerations with a vaginal delivery (4, p 493).

BENIGN TUMORS OF THE UTERUS: LEIOMYOMA

Definition

Leiomyomas (also called myomas) are benign tumors of the smooth muscle of the uterus. They are the most common tumors found during pregnancy. The incidence has been reported to be as high as 1% of pregnancies. Myomas are classified according to their location:

1. Submucous myomas are immediately beneath the endometrial or decidual surface.
2. Subserous myomas are on the outer peritoneal covering immediately beneath the serosa.
3. Intramural myomas are located within the muscular wall.

Table 21.6.

DIAGNOSTIC ULTRASOUND FINDINGS[a]

A mass larger than 3 cm in diameter is present.
The mass is spherical.
The myometrial contour is distorted by the mass.
The mass is of different acoustical structure than the myometrium.
A speckled pattern of internal echoes, increasing in density with an increase in ultrasound sensitivity, is present.
There is no enhancement of echoes behind the mass.

[a]From Muram D, Gillieson M, Walters JH: et al.: Myomas of the uterus in pregnancy: ultrasonographic follow up. *Am J Obstet Gynecol* 138:16–19, 1980.

4. Pedunculated myomas are submucous or subserous myomas connected by a stalk.

Etiology

It is assumed that estrogen stimulation is an important factor. During pregnancy, the myomas enlarge under the stimulation of hormones and the enhanced blood supply to the uterus (3, p 373).

Signs and Symptoms

Myomas usually are asymptomatic and first detected on a routine pelvic examination. Symptoms appear when a myoma undergoes a degenerative change during a pregnancy or there is torsion of a pedunculated subserous myoma. The symptoms include focal pain with tenderness on palpation and in some cases a low grade fever. The peritoneum overlying the infarcted myoma can become inflamed, and a peritoneal rub may develop. Differential diagnoses are appendicitis, placental abruption, ureteral stone, or pyelonephritis (4, p 689).

Diagnosis

Myomas may be discovered accidentally during ultrasound ordered for other reasons. This is not always an accurate method for diagnosis in the first trimester. The myoma may be misdiagnosed as a corpus luteum, cystic teratoma of the ovary, or other benign or malignant ovarian growths, or it may not be seen at all. In the third trimester the myoma may be masked by the fetus. Criteria to establish the diagnosis by ultrasound are listed in Table 21.6.

Maternal and Fetal Outcome

The prognosis for a pregnancy complicated by a uterine myoma depends on the location of the tumor rather than its size (8). Submucous myomas can have a deleterious effect on a pregnancy if they are of prominent size prior to conception. Implantation of the zygote rarely is successful. Even when it is, there often is difficulty with placental implantation, resulting in abortion.

Pedunculated myomas may undergo torsion and in some cases detachment from the uterus. Subserous (intramural) myomas may become parasitic, gaining their blood supply from the well-vascularized omentum.

It has been shown that myomas located near the placental implantation site generally adversely affect pregnancy outcome. Myomas may develop into a hemorrhagic infarction. The client may complain of focal pain with a low grade fever and tenderness upon palpation. There may be leukocytosis, which is indicative of inflammation of the peritoneum. There may be a release of thromboplastin into the maternal circulation, resulting in disseminated intravascular coagulation (see Chapter 8). In some cases enlargement may affect fetal development.

Medical Management

The overall treatment for uterine myomas during pregnancy is conservative. Surgical treatment is not indicated during pregnancy or at delivery. Intervention at that time has resulted in severe bleeding and bizarre histological changes (3, p 375) resembling sarcoma-type cells. Peduncular myomas are the only ones generally surgically ligated and then *after* the puerperium. Vaginal delivery is the preferred route unless the myoma obstructs the birth canal. Decisions on the mode of delivery should not be made until labor, since an obstructive myoma may grow upward during the pregnancy and thus allow a vaginal delivery. If a woman has had a myomectomy prior to the current pregnancy, cesarean section may be indicated. This depends upon the location of the myomas and the depth of penetration into the uterine wall. Labor is avoided in such cases if there is thought to be significant risk of uterine rupture.

Myomas developing into hemorrhagic infarctions are treated with bed rest, an analgesic agent for pain, and treatment of any resulting complications.

OVARIAN TUMORS

Definition

Ovarian tumors are difficult to classify because the organ is made up of four distinct cell types: epithelial, sex cord stroma cells, lipid cells, and germ cells. Each of these cells gives rise to a distinct or mixed tumor type.

Epithelial tumors are classified into three groups based on gross appearance and the fibrous stroma produced by the tumor. The three groups are benign epithelial, borderline epithelial, and invasive epithelial. Benign epithelial tumors are made up of three subgroups: cystadenoma, cystadenofibroma, and adenofibroma. Some of these tumors, such as cystadenoma, may be stratified, making it difficult to classify the tumor histologically. Invasive epithelial tumors are defined either as serous or mucinous cystadenocarcinomas. These are the most common type of epithelial ovarian malignancy (9).

Stromal tumors are made up of sex cord and stroma of either male or female origin. They exhibit sex steroid activity; those of female embryologic origin (granulosa cells or theca cells) produce estrogens; those of male embryologic origin (Sertoli cells or Leydig cells) produce androgens (9, p 789). Granulosa tumors have a low malignant potential.

Germ cell tumors generally are seen in the prepubescent period. There is a malignant change in primordial germ cells. The most common germ cell tumor is a dysgerminoma. It occurs 85% of the time in women under 30 years of age. Approximately 15% of these tumors occur during pregnancy or the puerperium. Endodermal sinus tumor is the second most common ovarian germ cell tumor. The immature teratoma is the third most common germ cell tumor. Primary choriocarcinomas of the ovary are rare and should be differentiated from mixed germ cell tumors. These tumors also can be confused with metastases from gestational trophoblastic disease (10).

Tumor-like conditions such as follicular cysts are, in reality, enlarged graafian follicles. They are located in the cortex of the ovary and contain fluid. A corpus luteum cyst occurs when there is a persistence of the corpus luteum follicle together with slow or irregular withdrawal of ovarian hormones, causing it to swell.

Etiology

Carcinoma of the ovary has been found in all trimesters of pregnancy. It is associated with tubal pregnancy and spontaneous abortions. The incidence of ovarian malignancy of all ovarian tumors complicating pregnancy is 2.2% to 5% (11). It is more common in blacks than whites and occurs in parous women less often than in nulliparous. Until the recent past, women using talc contaminated with asbestos were at increased risk for ovarian cancer. There has been recent research indicating that women with diets low in fiber and vitamin A may be at increased risk for ovarian cancer. Oral contraceptive use may have a protective effect from the disease.

Signs and Symptoms

In the early stages of the disease, generally there are no signs or symptoms. In about 50% of cases, the first suspicion of an ovarian tumor is during a routine pelvic examination. An accurate physical examination can be made only early in pregnancy, since the ovary will be elevated into the abdomen and obscured by the growing uterus. The most frequent symptoms include abdominal pressure on the gastrointestinal or urinary tracts. These symptoms may be considered part of the expected discomforts of pregnancy and not be considered abnormal. Virilization has been reported in stromal tumors.

Diagnosis

The actual diagnosis is by a histological classification that can be obtained only during a laparotomy.

Maternal and Fetal Outcome

The malignancy does not affect the fetus's growth and development. The risks to the fetus result from anesthesia and surgical trauma during the laparotomy (see Chapter 38). If the woman requires chemotherapy or radiation therapy, termination of the pregnancy is recommended, because no chemotherapeutic agent is considered safe for the developing fetus owing to teratogenic effects.

If a cystic teratoma or mucinous cystadenoma ruptures during spontaneous labor or during surgical removal, maternal death from granulomatous peritonitis may occur (4, p 691).

A tumor blocking the uterus may cause rupture of the uterus during labor. Virilization of mother and fetus have been reported in hormonally active stromal tumors.

Medical Management

The treatment is the same as in the non-pregnant state. In all cases a laparotomy is performed to classify the tumor histologically. The mass is removed intact, leaving the ovary unless a malignancy is present (see Fig. 21.2).

During the third trimester, a classical cesarean section is performed as soon as possible, with definitive surgery following. Timing of the surgery during the second trimester is dependent upon the feelings of the family about continuing the preg-

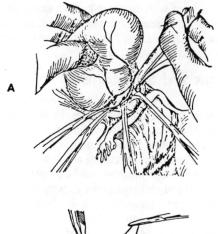

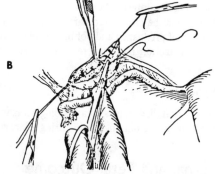

Figure 21.2. Resection of ovarian cyst. *A,* Incision made around ovary near junction of cyst wall and normal ovarian tissue. Knife handle is convenient instrument for shelling out cyst. *B,* Wound in ovary closed. (From Gruendemann B, Huthmeeker M: *Alexander's Care of the Patient in Surgery,* ed 7. St. Louis, Mosby, 1983, p 342.)

nancy, the level of expert neonatal care available, and maternal risk.

Following removal of a highly malignant tumor, chemotherapy may be used alone or in combination with radiation therapy (see Table 21.7 for agents used). Generally, radiation therapy has been less successful in tumors larger than 2 cm.

Dysgerminomas are removed by a unilateral oophorectomy if confined to one ovary.

Granulosa tumors confined to one ovary and histologically classified at stage IA are not an indication for terminating the pregnancy; it can continue to term with a vaginal delivery. If the tumor ruptures, treatment is delayed until 32 weeks' gestation; the infant then is delivered by cesarean section. The wound must heal and then abdominal radiation is given (11, p 849). For stages IB to IV during the first 28 weeks of the pregnancy, an abdominal hysterectomy, bilateral salpingo-oophorectomy, and excision of the metastatic disease is rec-

Table 21.7.
CHEMOTHERAPEUTIC AGENTS[a]

ALKYLATING AGENTS	SIDE EFFECTS
Cyclophosphamide (Cytoxan)	Immediate: nausea and vomiting; Delayed: bone marrow depression (lowering the bone marrow's production of blood cells), alopecia (hair loss), cystitis (inflammation of urinary bladder), late occurrence of acute leukemia (following long-term use).
L-phenylalanine mustard (melphalan, Alkeran)	Immediate: nausea. Delayed: bone marrow depression

[a]From *The Breast Cancer Digest.* U.S. Department of Health and Human Services (NIH publication No. 81–1691) National Cancer Institute, Bethesda, MD: 1980.

ommended. In the last trimester or late second trimester, the fetus is delivered by cesarean section and the definitive surgery follows.

CHORIOCARCINOMA

Definition

Choriocarcinoma is a malignant neoplasm of trophoblastic origin. It is a carcinoma of the chorionic epithelium but grows and metastasizes like a sarcoma (4, p 454).

Etiology

Choriocarcinoma follows some form of pregnancy: hydatidiform mole, ectopic pregnancy, abortion, or normal pregnancy (4, p 454). Approximately 40% of choriocarcinomas are preceded by a hydatidiform mole, 40% are preceded by a spontaneous abortion, and 20% are preceded by a normal pregnancy (2, p 16).

Signs and Symptoms

The most common sign is irregular bleeding after pregnancy. Other signs and symptoms are those in connection with the focus of the metastases. Metastatic foci include lungs, brain, vagina, vulva, liver, and cervix. Other symptoms include cough and hemoptysis and vaginal and vulvar tumors. The metastatic lesions can be identified grossly as purplish red, granular, and hemorrhagic (2, p 16). Women with a pregnancy complicated by

Table 21.8.

CHORIOCARCINOMA RISK CATEGORIES

	HCG TITERS	LOCATION OF METASTASES	APPARENT ONSET
Low risk	Urine excretion HCG <100,000 IU in 24 hours	Lung, vagina; no brain or liver	<4 months
High risk	Urine excretion HCG >100,000 IU	Tumor in association with term pregnancy or metastases including brain or liver	>4 months

Table 21.9.

CHORIOCARCINOMA LOW RISK THERAPY

AGENT	DOSAGE	COURSE
Methotrexate	0.4 mg/kg/day i.m.	1. 5 days or until toxicity appears 2. Resume when blood count is normal and no toxicity is present 3. Two subsequent courses after a normal HCG
Actinomycin D (used for individuals with hepatic or renal problems not caused by the cancer)	7–11 mg/kg/day	1. 5 days unless toxicity appears 2. Resume treatment when blood count is normal and no toxicity is present 3. Two subsequent courses after a normal HCG

a hydatidiform mole are watched closely for signs of choriocarcinoma (see Chapter 31).

Diagnosis

Suspected cases where chorionic gonadotropin levels remain persistently high in the absence of pregnancy are highly suspicious. The titers are evaluated together with chest x-rays, sonogram of the pelvic organs, liver chemistries (especially alkaline phosphatase and serum glutamic oxaloacetic tranaminase [SGOT]), renal function tests, liver scan, brain scan, EEG, and echogram. Elevated human chorionic gonadotropin (HCG) levels in cerebrospinal fluid indicate brain metastases. Biopsy of an accessible vaginal or vulvar metastasis with HCG assay will establish a diagnosis (2, p 16).

Maternal and Fetal Outcome

This is a curable disease in almost all cases. Mortality is related to delay in the diagnosis and treatment. The cause of death in the cases reported was found to be liver metastases or brain metastases.

Medical Management

The management is dependent upon the site of metastases and whether the client is high risk or low risk (Tables 21.8 and 21.9).

HCG titers are obtained each week until three consecutive normal titers have been obtained after completion of chemotherapy. HCG titers then are collected twice each month up to 6 months, then every month up to 1 year, and then every 2 months for another year (2, p 17).

If the HCG titer does not decrease significantly after two courses of either drug, therapy is discontinued, and the alternate chemotherapeutic agent is used in therapy as described above.

High Risk Therapy

Treatment is individualized. Chemotherapeutic agents are used in combination and depend upon the condition of the client. With brain metastases, radiation may be given in addition to multiple-agent chemotherapy.

CHORIOADENOMA DESTRUENS

Definition

Chorioadenoma destruens is a mole that invades the myometrium via molar villi. Hydatidiform mole is followed by chorioadenoma destruens in 15% of all cases (2, p 12).

Table 21.10.

FETAL EFFECTS OF CHORIOANGIOMA

SIZE OF TUMOR	CHANGE IN PLACENTAL PHYSIOLOGY	RESULT TO FETUS/MOTHER
Multiple small	Chronic fetal/maternal hemorrhage	Severe iron deficiency anemia in neonate
Large	A-V shunt in fetal circulation	Heart failure
		Consumptive coagulopathy, microangiopathic hemolytic anemia
Small	Asymptomatic	No effect

Etiology

The villous structure remains intact in the presence of myometrial invasion of the malignant trophoblast.

Diagnosis

This condition has a distinguishing feature of excessive trophoblastic overgrowth and extensive penetration of the trophoblastic elements, including whole villi, deep into the myometrium. At times, penetration can go to the depth of the peritoneum or vaginal vault. There are no metastases as with choriocarcinoma. The invasion differs from hydatidiform mole in that the villous structure always is preserved (2, p 13).

Medical Management

Treatment is with methotrexate. Remission can be brought about without hysterectomy once the treatment is instituted. Hysterectomy is necessary if there is uterine perforation by the tumor or massive intraabdominal hemorrhage.

CHORIOANGIOMA OF THE PLACENTA

Chorioangioma of the placenta is a tumor that histologically resembles the blood vessels and stroma of chorionic villi. The incidence is 1% (2, p 14).

Large tumors may be associated with hydramnios or antepartum hemorrhage. Small growths may be asymptomatic. See Table 21.10 for fetal effects of chorioangioma.

TUMORS OF THE BREAST

Introduction

The breasts, or mammary glands, are made up of many glandular lobes. These lobes are separated by connective tissue and adipose tissue. Each lobe is divided into lobules. Embedded in the lobules are secretory cells called acini. They are in close proximity to blood and lymph supply. Each acini drains into a lactiferous duct that ends in a nipple.

Externally, the breast is made up of epidermis, with the adipose and connective tissues beneath. The nipple is an erectile fibromuscular tissue. Encircling the nipple is the areola. This includes sebaceous glands—the tubercles of Montgomery. During pregnancy and lactation, the breast reaches complete morphologic maturity and functional activity. The breast has two compartments: the mesenchymal and the epithelial. The mesenchymal compartment consists of connective tissue, blood vessels, and lymphatics. The epithelial compartment consists of the breast fat and inter/intralobular fibrous stroma. Changes in the breast tissue during pregnancy and lactation make it difficult to evaluate the breast.

Pregnancy can have an adverse short-term effect and a beneficial long-term effect on subsequent breast cancer risk. A normal individual in the nonpregnant state is thought to be in a state of equilibrium between the production of actively growing malignant cells (of any type) and their subsequent destruction by the immune system. A malignant tumor appears when the equilibrium is upset. This can occur when an event prevents or reduces destruction of malignant cells or there is an increase in the number of malignant cells beyond the capacity of the immune system (12).

During pregnancy, there is an initial tendency for an increase in neoplastic growth. The immune system is depressed during the first 20 weeks of pregnancy, including a decrease in the number of T lymphocytes. In addition, there is hormonal stimulation on the growth of breast tissue. Thus, a latent breast carcinoma may be stimulated into active growth during this period (12, p 180).

Table 21.11.
RISK FACTORS ASSOCIATED WITH BREAST CARCINOMA

HIGHER RISK STATUS	LOWER RISK STATUS
Nulliparity	Multiparity
First parity after age 30	First parity before age 27
Natural menopause after age 50	Early artificial menopause
Family history	
Western cultures	Japanese women have lowest incidence
Constant psychological stress	

BREAST CARCINOMA

Definition

Cancer of the breast begins as a histologically atypical area located in breast tissue. The disease progresses to a carcinoma in situ of a duct or a lobule, then enters the minimally invasive state, and then finally enters the stage where lymph nodes and systemic circulation are invaded.

Etiology

The exact cause of breast cancer is unknown. However, some women have a higher predisposition to the disease than others (Table 21.11). Lactation, once thought to decrease the incidence of breast cancer, has not been proven statistically to do so.

Signs and Symptoms

The tumor may be palpated upon a self-examination or during an antepartum visit. During the palpation, a lump may be discovered that is nontender and fixed to the skin or underlying tissue. In the pregnant or lactating woman, a careful breast examination should be a routine part of the initial and postpartum visit. Palpation of a tumor may be difficult due to the normal enlargement of the breasts. The more obvious visible signs of breast cancer are dimpling of the skin, retraction, abnormal contour, increased venous prominence, and thickened skin with enlarged pores (peau d'orange). Suspicious signs of typical breast masses are shown in Table 21.12.

Diagnosis

Biopsy is indicated for all suspicious masses and can be performed under general or local anesthesia. If breast cancer is diagnosed during pregnancy or lacta-

tion, usually it is in the more advanced stages of the disease because of the difficulty in feeling a mass in the pregnant or lactating breast. This results in a delay of diagnosis. Approximately 75–85% of those women diagnosed during pregnancy have axillary node involvement (12, p 180).

Maternal and Fetal Outcome

Breast carcinoma during pregnancy or lactation has an outcome similar to that in nonpregnant women. That is, the prognosis is determined by the stage of the disease at the time of diagnosis. When surgery is necessary, the fetus is at risk because of the anesthesia and stress related to surgery. If the woman is undergoing radiation therapy or chemotherapy, a first trimester pregnancy will be aborted. Radiation therapy initiated in the second or third trimesters has no effect on the fetus (unless it cannot be shielded properly during the radiation therapy owing to the location of the metastatic disease).

Medical Management

Mastectomy is the preferred management (Fig. 21.3). The pregnancy does not have to be terminated, since it has not been proven to improve the prognosis for the mother. Oophorectomy has not had a positive effect on outcome either (12, p 181).

In those situations where the disease is extensive and the woman considered inoperable, radiation may be indicated. If treatment can be postponed until the second or third trimester, radiation therapy can be done safely with adequate shielding of the fetus. If there are metastases to an area where shielding is ineffective in protecting the fetus, then a decision is made about terminating pregnancy.

Chemotherapy is delayed until after delivery. If the diagnosis is made in the first trimester and there is axillary node involvement, the pregnancy is terminated so that adjuvant chemotherapy can be initiated. If the diagnosis is made during lactation, suppression of breast milk is done by means other than estrogen therapy.

Pregnancy subsequent to a mastectomy must be monitored carefully for recurrence of a cancerous growth.

GALACTOCELE

Definition

A galactocele is a cyst containing breast milk. It is occasionally formed when the glandular epithelium begins secreting late in the pregnancy. It

Table 21.12.

COMPARISON OF FINDINGS IN BREAST DISEASE[a]

	FIBROCYSTIC DISEASE	CARCINOMA	FIBROADENOMA
Median age	>30 years	>40 years	20 years
Pain or tenderness	Premenstrual, menstrual	None	None
Nipple discharge	Absent	Usually absent	Absent
Retraction	Absent	Present	Absent
Mobility	Mobile	Fixed	Mobile
Delineation	Discrete	Nondefined	Discrete
Consistency and number	Firm, multiple	Firm, usually single	Rubbery, usually single
Unilateral or bilateral	Bilateral	Usually unilateral	Unilateral

[a]Adapted from Neeson J, Stockdale C. *The Practitioners' Handbook of Ambulatory Ob/GYN*. New York: John Wiley & Sons, 1981, p 245.

may also develop by any process that obstructs the flow of milk. This can occur at the time of cessation of lactation. Milk remaining in the duct obstructs it and the acini.

It is important to carefully examine a galactocele as it may be secondary to a benign or malignant tumor. Diagnosis can be made by sonography (13). Aspiration of the galactocele may partially or completely decompress the mass. If the mass

should recur, an incisional biopsy is recommended to rule out carcinoma in the blocked gland or ductal system.

FIBROCYSTIC DISEASE

This is the most common breast lesion to occur in the childbearing age group. Generally, the

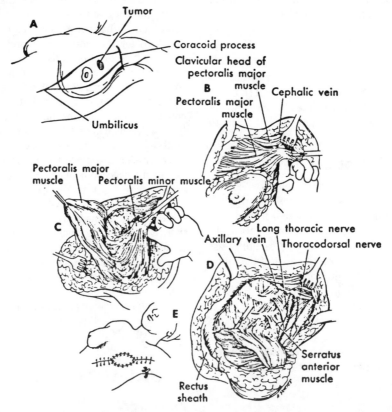

Figure 21.3. Radical mastectomy. *A*, Lines of incision. *B*, Resection of pectoralis major muscle at clavicular attachment. *C*, Resection of pectoralis minor muscle at coracoid attachment. *D*, Axillary contents are dissected free and resected. *E*, Incision is closed (skin graft may be necessary), and drain is placed. (From Gruendemann B, Huthmeeker M: *Alexander's Care of the Patient in Surgery*, ed 7. St. Louis, Mosby, 1983, p 173.)

Table 21.13.
ADENOMAS

TYPE	ORIGIN	TISSUE	CLINICAL CHARACTERISTICS (ALL TYPES)
Fibroadenoma	Lobular	Fibrous stroma epithelial	1. Discrete
Pure adenoma	Lobular	Epithelial	2. Freely mobile
Nipple adenoma	Tubular	Epithelial	3. Firm
			4. Approximately 3 cm diameter
			5. Round to lobulated
			6. Rubbery and firm
			7. No nipple or skin retraction

incidence increases until menopause when it abruptly diminishes. Breast cancer and fibrocystic disease occur most often in the same population. Differentiating between the two conditions often is difficult and requires a careful evaluation.

Definition

Fibrocystic disease usually is located in the upper outer quadrant. The following are characteristics of a fibrocystic lesion: it is firm, not fluctuant; aspirant is green, gray, or brown; and tenderness increases until menses and regresses during pregnancy. A malignant mass may not be painful and does not change in size or intensity with menstruation.

Breast carcinoma and fibrocystic disease can coexist. Therefore, a breast mass palpated in a pregnant woman with a history of fibocystic disease should not be dismissed but rather investigated further. Monthly breast examinations by a reliable patient or by the clinician will give early warning to changes in the fibrocystic breast. Mammography is not recommended in the early stages of pregnancy because of the risk to the fetus. It can be done in the second and third trimester with proper shielding of the fetus.

Aspiration of a breast mass with cytologic study is the most expeditious method for diagnosing a mass as malignant or benign. This can be accomplished under local anesthesia without significant risk to the mother or fetus.

Maternal and Fetal Outcome

There is no adverse effect on the fetus nor the mother.

Medical Management

Management includes careful monitoring of the tumors for changes. The client should be advised to restrict xanthine intake, which is thought to aggravate this disease (13, p 856).

ADENOMAS

Definition

Adenomas of the breast are neoplasms that rank as the third most frequent breast lesion in American women. There are three types of adenomas:

1. Fibroadenomas
2. Pure adenomas
3. Nipple adenomas

It is worth mentioning that lactating adenomas are a pure adenoma type. They are the only type of pure adenoma that arises during pregnancy and lactation (13, p 859). Table 21.13 gives a brief description of each type of adenoma.

In all cases diagnosis is made by biopsy. Ultrasonography can be used to determine if the mass is solid or cystic in cases where the fibroadenoma may be difficult to differentiate from a tense cystic lesion. Biopsy of the breast can be accomplished with limited risk as described before.

There is no need for medical intervention except careful follow-up and case management. Lactating adenomas that resolve spontaneously only to recur should be regarded as suspicious. They have been associated with carcinoma in situ (13, p 860).

MALIGNANT MELANOMA

Malignant melanoma is a tumor made up of melanocytes. During pregnancy a benign nevus may become malignant. The growth is rapid because most are sensitive to the changes in hormone levels during pregnancy, although at this time researchers have been unable to describe which type of melanomas are sensitive to these hormonal changes.

The prognosis for women diagnosed as having malignant melanoma during pregnancy is poor. Women diagnosed prior to pregnancy who are treated and then become pregnant may not have an increased risk. Rapid metastases are reported with these tumors. Sites may include the placenta and the fetus (14).

NURSING MANAGEMENT

Nursing care specific for a patient with a tumor:

☐ Participate in measures designed to minimize/prevent the complications of the following:
  — Disease process/condition and
  — Treatment (e.g., surgery, radiation, chemotherapy):
    * Radiation sickness: administer vitamin B, sedatives, antihistamines, and antiemetics as ordered.
    * Diarrhea from chemotherapy/radiation therapy: give the patient a low residue diet and replace fluid losses.
    * Skin rashes from radiation therapy: observe the patient for erythema, apply oil to radiation site when possible, avoid mechanical irritation to skin, and limit use of soaps and alcohol.
    * Bone marrow depression: observe for bleeding, protect from infection, and review the lab results and report them to the physician.
    * Wound infection: keep dressing clean, dry, and intact; monitor temperature at regular intervals; administer antipyretics and antibiotics as ordered, and monitor their effectiveness; encourage fluid intake.
    * Hemorrhage: monitor vital signs and evaluate lab data for changes; administer blood products as ordered; monitor stools, urine, and sputum for blood; observe wound site frequently for bleeding; note character and amount of blood from surgical drains.

☐ Assess for and manage discomfort (e.g., administer antiemetics and analgesics as necessary; teach relaxation techniques and visualization).

☐ Provide emotional support for the patient and family.

☐ Educate the patient regarding the following:
  — Diagnostic procedures;
  — Disease process (e.g., etiology, pathology, maternal/fetal prognosis);
  — Treatment (e.g., benefits and risks of surgery, chemotherapy, and radiation); and
  — Medications (e.g., compliance, comfort measures to relieve side effects).

Nursing diagnoses most frequently associated with tumors (see Section V):

☐ Anxiety/fear
☐ Anticipatory grieving related to actual/perceived threat to self
☐ Potential for infection
☐ Knowledge deficit regarding etiology, disease process treatment, and expected outcome
☐ Altered nutrition: less than body requirements
☐ Disturbance in body image, self-esteem
☐ Altered sexuality patterns
☐ Impaired skin integrity
☐ Impaired tissue integrity
☐ Grieving related to potential/actual loss of infant or birth of an imperfect child
☐ Spiritual distress
☐ Pain
☐ Knowledge deficit regarding medication regimen

REFERENCES

1. Brunner L, Suddarth D: *Textbook of Medical-Surgical Nursing*, ed 5. Philadelphia, JP Lippincott, 1984, p 302.
2. Downstate Medical Center, Division of Gynecologic Oncology: *Tumor Protocol*. Brooklyn, State University of New York, 1983.
3. Roberts JA: Management of gynecologic tumors during pregnancy. *Clin Perinatol* 10:369–378, 1983.
4. Pritchard JA, MacDonald P, Gant NF: *Williams Obstetrics*, ed 17. New York, Appleton-Century-Crofts, 1985, p 492.
5. Hacker N, Berek JS, Lagasse LD, Elsworth HC, Savage EW, Moore JG: Carcinoma of the cervix associated with pregnancy. *Obstet Gynecol* 59:735–745, 1982.
6. Ostergard DR, Nieberg RK: Evaluation of abnormal cervical cytology during pregnancy with colposcopy. *Am J Obstet Gynecol* 134: 756–758, 1979.

7. Lee RB, Neglia W, Park RC: Cervical carcinoma. *Obstet Gynecol* 58:584–589, 1981.
8. Muram D, Gillieson M, Walters JH: Myomoas of the uterus in pregnancy: ultrasonographic follow-up. *Am J Obstet Gynecol* 138:16–19, 1980.
9. Jolle C: Ovarian cancer: histogenic classification, histologic grading, diagnosis, staging, and epidemiology. *Clin Obstet Gynecol* 28:787–799, 1985.
10. Gershenson DM: Malignant germ-cell tumors of the ovary. *Clin Obstet Gynecol* 28:824–838, 1983.
11. McGowan L: Surgical diseases of the ovary in pregnancy. *Clin Obstet Gynecol* 26:843–852, 1983.
12. Hornstein E, Skornick Y, Razin R: The management of breast carcinoma in pregnancy and lactation. *J Surg Oncol* 21:179–182, 1982.
13. Canter J, Oliver GC, Zaloudek CJ: Surgical diseases of the breast during pregnancy. *Clin Obstet Gynecol* 26:853–864, 1983.
14. Sutherland CM, Wittlif J, Fuchs A, Mabie W: The effect of pregnancy on hormone levels and receptors of malignant melanoma. *J Surg Oncol* 22:191–192, 1983.

Chapter 22
Venereal Disease
Tina Duperret, C.N.M., M.S.

INTRODUCTION

Sexually transmitted diseases are epidemic in proportion, have no racial or socioeconomic barriers, tend to be asymptomatic, and always are inoculated in the patient by another person. These realizations should alert care givers of pregnant women to the need for increased screening and vigorous treatment of veneral disease. Moreover, care givers should be mindful that the emotional impact of the diagnosis can be devastating to the pregnant woman—divesting her of trust in her partner and inculcating guilt and fear for the safety of her unborn child.

GONORRHEA

Definition

Gonorrhea is a sexually transmitted infectious disease, most commonly affecting the endocervix, caused by the organism *Neisseria gonorrhoeae*. In prenatal patients the expected incidence of asymptomatic endocervical gonorrhea is 1–5% (1). Nongenital sites of infection may include the rectum and the oropharynx.

Etiology

Neisseria gonorrhoeae is a gram-negative, nonmotile, non-spore-forming diplococcus. Gonococci are difficult to destroy within the body but possess little resistance outside it. In moist, dark body areas, gonococci may live for 18–20 hours, thus explaining the possibility of transmission to the eyes and skin by direct inoculation. The skin-to-skin contact of sexual intimacy is the most common mode of transmission of the gonococcus. The

site of inoculation, although most commonly the columnar epithelium of the genitourinary tract, may include the rectum and oropharynx. Vaginal infection is not common because the cornified, stratified, squamous epithelial lining under the influence of estrogen is resistant to gonococcal infection.

Signs and Symptoms

Like other infectious diseases, the clinical presentation of gonococcal infection is the result of many factors, including the site of the infecting inoculum and the woman's condition and response at the time of exposure. The infection usually is superficial and localized to mucous membranes, and it is often asymptomatic—an acute inflammatory exudate may not be generated or may be insufficient for the woman to notice along with the increased secretions of normal pregnancy. A variety of coinfecting pathogens may also increase discharge and mask any alteration in secretions produced by the gonococci. These factors make it impossible to determine the incubation period of gonococcal infection in women, although it is estimated to be 1–6 days.

Women with symptoms of acute gonococcal infection are more likely to have an extension of the infection from the endocervix to the surrounding structures of the genitourinary tract or to have a primary infection at an extragenital site. After the first trimester, ascending infections do not occur because the uterine cavity is obliterated after the fusion of the chorion and decidua, and the cervical canal is sealed after the formation of the mucus plug.

Clinical manifestations vary according to the site involved. A woman with involvement of the urethra and urinary bladder may exhibit a red

244

edematous urinary meatus and purulent discharge from the Skene's glands and/or urinary meatus, and she may voice the complaint of pruritus, urgency, frequency, dysuria, and incontinence. Microscopic examination of the urine reveals pyuria and, occasionally, hematuria.

Two-thirds of women with rectal infections may be asymptomatic. The woman who is symptomatic may complain of mild perianal itching, burning on defecation, mucus in the stools, rectal pain, tenesmus, and a copious discharge with pus and blood in the stools.

Orogenital sexual activity is the source of gonococcal infection of the oropharynx. Although there are no characteristic features of gonococcal oropharyngeal infections, some women may exhibit symptoms of tonsillitis or pharyngitis.

Disseminated gonococcal infections are characterized by lesions on the hands and feet. These lesions may be observed as pustular, necrotic, or hemorrhagic, and they may be accompanied by symptoms of migratory polyarthralgia; polyarthritis; and tenosynovitis of the wrists, fingers, knees, or ankles.

When direct cultures of the rectum and pharynx are carried out on women with disseminated gonorrhea, the yield of disease seeded from the rectum is 20–50% and from the pharynx is 10%.

Other sites of extragenital infection reached by direct inoculation are the eyes, skin, and tongue. Gonococcal eye infection in adults is due to direct inoculation of the organism onto the conjunctiva. After an incubation period of 1–6 days, the early symptoms are the same as those of any conjunctivitis. However, if the infection goes untreated, a thick, creamy-white to yellow purulent discharge is produced. Also, corneal ulceration may occur, which ultimately may cause loss of visual acuity.

Primary cutaneous gonococcal infection is uncommon, because stratified and cornified squamous epithelium normally is resistant to invasion by the organism. When skin breaks are present, the gonococcus may invade and infect the fingers and hands as a result of self-infection or intimate contact with another infected person. The clinical manifestations visually are indistinguishable from other skin infections, and must be diagnosed by gram stain or culture. Localized infections of the perineal glands or the tongue may produce ulcerative lesions resembling those of syphilis and must be evaluated by gram stain and selective culture.

Diagnosis

Diagnosis is made after a careful history (including sexual history) and physical examination have been completed and after cultures of the endocervix and all other sites dictated by the history and physical examination have been taken. A culture on Thayer-Martin medium, which is a specially treated chocolate agar, usually establishes the diagnosis. An estimated 6–8% of gonococcal infections are missed with the initial culture. Urine culture and sensitivity are obtained to diagnose urinary tract involvement from *Neisseria gonorrhoeae*. A gram stain also may be used for those women with skin lesions.

Maternal and Fetal Outcome

With early recognition and treatment, the prognosis for mother and infant is good. Untreated gonococcal infection, however, increases the risks for both mother and baby. Studies imply a relationship between gonococcal infection and chorioamnionitis, resulting in an increased risk of prolonged rupture of the membranes, peripartum fever, premature delivery, and postpartum endometritis. There also is an increased risk of disseminated gonococcal infection (arthritis and dermatitis) in pregnancy.

Ophthalmia neonatorum, acquired while passing through the birth canal, is the most common infant consequence of maternal infection. Rarer neonatal consequences may be infantile sepsis, meningitis, or arthritis. There are no firm estimates of risk for these, nor are the predisposing circumstances known.

Medical Management

Since an estimated 75–90% of women are asymptomatic for gonorrheal infection, medical management is focused on screening all prenatal patients and treating those with documented infection. All prenatal patients should be screened for gonorrheal infection by a careful history (including sexual history), a physical examination, and a culture on selective medium from the endocervix and any other site determined by the history or physical examination. A complete urinalysis should be done on all patients and a clean-catch urine taken for culture and sensitivity on those women exhibiting urinary tract symptoms. A second culture, late in the third trimester, should be obtained from women at high risk of gonococcal infection. These women include those with multiple sexual partners, those having frequent infections prior to pregnancy, and those with partners who have a suspicious discharge. Since other sexually transmitted pathogens often coexist with gonorrhea, management should include a serological test for syphilis and a microscopic examination or culture for organisms such as *Trichomonas vaginalis* and *Candida albicans, Gardnerella vaginalis*, and *Chlamydia trachomatis*.

All cases of gonorrhea must be reported to the public health department, and the woman should be encouraged to inform her contact(s) and secure their treatment. She should refrain from intercourse until all cultures for both herself and her partner(s) are negative.

Drug regimens of choice for the infected prenatal patient are: Amoxicillin, 3.0 gm, or Ampicillin, 3.5 gm preceded by 1 gm of Probenecid (Benemid) to block excretion of the penicillin maintaining a high blood level. The treatment regimen is advantageous because it is a single dose regimen by mouth, which enhances acceptability and compliance. It is not effective if the woman has a pharyngeal or anorectal gonococcal infection or coexisting chlamydial infection. Women allergic to penicillin or probenecid should be treated with Spectinomycin (Trobacin), 2.0 gm i.m. Tetracycline is

contraindicated in pregnancy because of potential teratogenic effects. Erythromycin can be added to treat coexistent chlamydial infection. Follow-up cultures to test for cure should be obtained 4–7 days after completion of treatment. A rectal culture should be obtained at the same time.

Procaine Penicillin G (Bicillin) is effective and the preferred treatment for pharyngeal infection and is also effective for anorectal gonococcal infection. Spectinomycin is effective for pharyngeal but not anorectal gonococcal infection.

Gonococcal ophthalmia neonatorum is best prevented by prenatal diagnosis and treatment of the mother and her partner(s). Although the prevention of gonococcal ophthalmia neonatorum can be achieved by the use of silver nitrate eye drops, prophylaxis with erythromycin or tetracycline ointment is recommended for concurrent prevention of neonatal chlamydia.

If ascending intrauterine gonococcal infection is well established at birth (because of prolonged ruptured membranes), routine neonatal prophylaxis may not be enough. With established maternal infection, the infant should be treated with aqueous penicillin as soon after birth as the mother's infection is recognized, whether or not the infant has been diagnosed with the disease at the time.

NURSING MANAGEMENT

Nursing care specific for patients with gonorrhea:
- [ ] Screen all prenatal patients for gonorrhea.
- [ ] Administer treatment; encourage evaluation and treatment of sexual contact(s).
- [ ] Evaluate the patient for other sexually transmitted diseases.
- [ ] Teach comfort measures (e.g., Sitz baths, loose-fitting clothing, cotton underwear).
- [ ] Ensure that a test of cure is done after treatment.
- [ ] Teach prevention measures (e.g., abstain from sexual activity until patient and partner are treated).

- [ ] Administer prophylaxis for ophthalmia neonatorum, as appropriate.

Nursing diagnoses most frequently associated with gonorrhea (see Section V):
- [ ] Disturbance in body image/self-esteem.
- [ ] Ineffective individual coping.
- [ ] Ineffective family coping: compromised.
- [ ] Knowledge deficit regarding etiology, disease process, treatment, and outcome.
- [ ] Knowledge deficit regarding medication regimen.

SYPHILIS

Definition

Syphilis is a sexually transmitted infectious disease caused by the organism *Treponema pallidum*. Untreated, it is a chronic, progressive dis-

ease characterized by the stages of primary, secondary, latent, and late syphilis.

Each year 25,000 cases of primary/secondary syphilis are reported in the United States, with the highest incidence in the 15–39 year old age group. The incidence in pregnancy is low, but is increasing rapidly (1).

Etiology

Treponema pallidum (the pale spirochete) is an actively motile, slender, corkscrew-like organism. It is capable of living outside the body for 10–12 hours but is killed readily by heat and drying. It does not occur outside the body except on objects that have been contaminated by secretions containing the spirochetes. It can live in refrigerated whole blood or plasma for 24 hours.

Syphilis is contracted primarily through sexual contact. However, on rare occasions it is contracted by direct contact with lesions on the skin or mucous membranes.

Most fetal infections are transmitted transplacentally. Although rare, fetal infection can occur in the first trimester of pregnancy. Fetal infection occurs readily after the fourth month of gestation but is more common after the sixth month, when the placenta is established fully.

When the *Treponema pallidum* organism is introduced into the body, it begins to multiply at the site of the inoculation. Concurrently, many of the treponemes invade the lymphatic ducts, causing regional lymphadenopathy. The organism enters the bloodstream via the thoracic duct, disseminating rapidly to all organs of the body before the primary lesion appears. When the treponemes have multiplied in sufficient quantity to produce an inflammatory reaction, the characteristic primary lesion, known as a chancre, develops and ulcerates. The incubation period is inversely proportional to the size of the inoculum and ranges from 10–90 days, with an average incubation period of 21 days. Development of antibody and cellular immune response begins to be measurable about 3–6 weeks following inoculation.

Signs and Symptoms

The clinical manifestations of syphilis vary according to each stage. During the primary stage, one or more painless chancres develop on the genitals after an incubation period of about 21 days. Initially, these chancres appear as papules and then erode to form the characteristic painless, indurated, clear ulcers whose borders are sharply defined, raised, and smooth. These lesions contain spirochetes and are highly contagious. The regional lymph nodes become enlarged, firm, and minimally tender.

The most common genital sites for chancres in females are the labia, the fourchette, the cervix, the perineum, and the rectum. The most common nongenital site is the lips; other sites include the tongue, tonsils, face, breasts, and fingers. The primary lesion(s) usually disappear within 3–6 weeks.

Secondary syphilis is characterized by a generalized eruption of mucocutaneous lesions that can be highly variable in appearance: macular, papular, pustular, or nodular. The rash is generalized and well defined, with the characteristic copper hue and palmar distribution. Another manifestation of secondary syphilis is condyloma latum: a flat, moist, grayish-white papular growth that may involve the vulva, perineum, inner thighs, and buttocks.

All secondary lesions, especially those in moist areas such as skin folds and mucous membranes, contain abundant spirochetes and are highly contagious. Serologic tests are always positive during this stage. A flu-like syndrome may be present. Symptoms may include headache, rhinorrhea, myalgia, anorexia, sore throat, malaise, and a low grade fever. Generalized lymphadenopathy of a rubbery, firm character is present. Alopecia may occur, and nails may become pitted and brittle. Untreated, the secondary lesions heal in 4–12 weeks, and the patient becomes asymptomatic.

Latent syphilis is characterized by a reactive reagin and treponemal test without any clinical or historical findings. If serological tests were nonreactive within the previous year or if the patient gives a history of symptoms highly suggestive of primary or secondary syphilis within the past year, the diagnosis of early latent syphilis is given.

When the infection is less than 4 years' duration, the patient must be considered potentially contagious since the recurrence of infectious mucocutaneous lesions is possible. After 4 years the patient enters the late latent stage. Two-thirds of patients with untreated syphilis in the late latent stage remain asymptomatic until death. The remaining one-third of patients progress to late stage symptoms.

Late syphilis is the final, destructive, noninfectious stage of the disease. During the late benign stage, gummas (chronic, superficial, painless, asymmetric nodules or deep granulomatous lesions that are solitary and indurated) develop on the skin, bones, mucous membranes, upper respiratory tract, or stomach. They can develop between 1 and 10 years after the initial untreated infection.

Cardiovascular syphilis develops approximately 10 years after the initial infection in about 10% of patients with late untreated syphilis. Neurosyphilis develops approximately 5–35 years after the initial infection in about 8% of patients with late untreated syphilis. Symptomatology may include personality changes, weakness of the arms and legs, or paresis. These symptoms are suggestive of meningitis and widespread central nervous system damage.

Diagnosis

At the time of the initial prenatal visit, all pregnant women should have a nontreponemal test for syphilis, such as the RPR (rapid plasma reagin) or VDRL (Venereal Disease Research Laboratory) tests. These tests are economical and detect nonspecific antibodies within 1–2 weeks after the primary lesion appears or 4–5 weeks after the onset of the infection. Those women who have multiple sexual partners or a previous history of syphilis should be retested in the third trimester. Cord blood should be tested for syphilis antibody on all babies, especially when third trimester screening is not employed.

Seroreactive patients need an immediate evaluation. This should include a thorough history and physical examination, dark field examination of any lesions, a quantitative nontreponemal test, and a confirmatory treponemal test such as the FTA-ABS (fluorescent treponemal antibody-absorption test). The FTA-ABS is the most sensitive, reliable, and convenient serologic test for antitreponemal antibodies at the present time.

False-positive nontreponemal tests represent an estimated 20–40% of all positive nontreponemal tests. This fact emphasizes the importance of doing a specific treponemal test before establishing a diagnosis or, when a woman has been treated previously for syphilis, of observing for a fourfold increase in titer.

Pregnancy is one cause of a biologic false-positive nontreponemal test. Biologic false-positive tests are due to substances in the patient's serum that react like the reagin antibody and result in positive flocculation or complement fixation reactions. Biologic false-positive results occur in about 1% of all pregnancies.

Maternal and Fetal Outcome

Untreated syphilis in the mother is a chronic, destructive disease for both mother and baby. Most fetal infections are transmitted transplacentally. Fetal infection can occur readily after the fourth month, when the placenta is completely established. When fetal infection occurs, one-half of the babies are stillborn, premature, or suffer intrauterine growth retardation or neonatal death.

A good prognosis for both mother and baby can be expected if syphilis is treated early in pregnancy. The treatment of choice for patients not allergic to penicillin, regardless of the gestational age of the pregnancy, is penicillin in the dosage appropriate to the stage of syphillis.

Medical Management

For early syphilis (defined as primary, secondary, and latent syphilis of less than 1 year's duration), the treatment regimen is penicillin G benzathine (Bicillin), 2.4 million units (total) intramuscularly at a single session (1.2 million units in each buttock) (2).

For syphilis of more than 1 year's duration, the treatment is penicillin G benzathine (Bicillin), 2.4 million units intramuscularly once a week for 3 successive weeks (7.2 million units total) (2).

For those patients who have a documented allergy to penicillin and who are reliable and able to comply with the treatment regimen, oral outpatient treatment and follow-up can be planned. If compliance in taking medication and follow-up cannot be assured, hospitalization is indicated.

For early syphilis the oral treatment regimen consists of erythromycin, 500 mg every 6 hours for 15 days (2). For syphilis of longer than 1 year's duration, the treatment is erythromycin, 500 mg by mouth every 6 hours for 30 days, (2, p 51S). Infants born to mothers treated during pregnancy with erythromycin should be treated with penicillin.

It should be noted that once treponemal antibodies have developed, they tend to persist for life but do not confer immunity. Adquate treatment of primary syphilis should yield a nonreactive serologic test for syphilis in 6–12 months. Adequate treatment of secondary syphilis should yield a nonreactive serological test for syphilis in 12–18 months. Although a low positive titer may remain after the treatment of early latent syphilis, it usually converts to negative in 18–36 months. Quantitative measurement of nontreponemal antibodies therefore is important both in diagnosis and evaluation of treatment.

Pregnant women who have been treated for syphilis should have monthly quantitative nontreponemal serologic tests for the remainder of their pregnancies. Women who show a fourfold rise in titer should be considered reinfected and should be retreated.

All patients with early syphilis should be encouraged to return for repeat quantitative nontreponemal tests at 3, 6, and 12 months after treatment. Those women with latent syphilis (defined as infection of more than 1 year's duration) should have repeat quantitative nontreponemal serology tests for 24 months after treatment.

It is extremely important that those women treated with antibiotics other than penicillin have careful follow-up with nontreponemal serologic tests to ensure adequate treatment. The length of the treatment period depends on the stage of the disease when treatment is begun and on the results of an examination of the cerebrospinal fluid at the last follow-up visit (to rule out neurosyphilis).

All cases of syphilis must be reported to the public health department, and the woman should be encouraged to inform her contact(s) and secure his or their treatment.

NURSING MANAGEMENT

Nursing care specific for patients with
syphilis:
☐ Screen all prenatal patients for syphilis, ensure that a confirmatory treponemal test is used to establish the diagnosis since pregnancy can cause false-positive nontreponemal results.
☐ Evaluate the patient for other sexually transmitted diseases.
☐ Monitor treated patients with monthly quantitative nontreponemal serologic test to rule out reinfection.
☐ Evaluate for congenital syphilis by evaluating presence of syphilis antibody in cord fluid; evaluate presence of signs/symptoms after the first week (e.g., jaundice, anemia, snuffles, copper hue rash); administer treatment as required.

☐ Advise patient that nontreponemal antibody titers are likely to remain elevated for months to years, requiring serial titers or treponemal tests to detect reinfection.
Nursing diagnoses most frequently associated with *syphilis* (see Section V):
☐ Grieving related to potential/actual loss of infant or birth of an imperfect child.
☐ Disturbance in body image, self-esteem.
☐ Ineffective individual coping.
☐ Ineffective family coping: compromised.
☐ Knowledge deficit regarding etiology, disease process, treatment, and outcome.
☐ Knowledge deficit regarding medication regimen.
☐ Impaired skin integrity.

GENITAL HERPES

Definition

Genital herpes is a very contagious, sexually transmitted viral infection that occurs on or around the genitalia. It may be chronic and recurrent. To date, there is no known cure.

Genital herpes is not a reportable disease in the United States. It is estimated that five million Americans have genital herpes, with approximately three hundred thousand new cases each year. The incidence of primary or recurrent genital herpes infection during pregnancy is 1% (1). Of these, one in a thousand women will have documented infections at or near term. This number increases to 1 documented case per 250 women when tested with viral cultures, which give the fastest results.

Etiology

Genital herpes infection is caused by the herpes simplex virus (HSV). HSV type I (usually oral) and HSV type II (usually genital) are the two strains that may cause disease in humans. About 15% of all genital herpes infections are caused by HSV type I and 85% are caused by HSV type II.

Mucous membranes, such as those in the mouth or genital area, are very susceptible to herpes invasion. However, herpes infections can be transmitted when any part of a person's body directly touches active HSV. Although intact skin usually is resistant to the HSV, skin in which the integrity has been jeopardized through cuts, burns, or other infection may become infected. It is controversial and unknown whether people who are exposed become asymptomatic carriers of the disease even if they do not have overt symptoms.

Following the initial infection, the virus "hibernates" (i.e., remains latent or dormant) in the ganglia of the sensory nerve that serves the site of the lesions. During recurrence, the virus becomes reactivated and probably travels down the same nerve and multiplies on the skin at or near the site of the primary infection.

Infants of mothers with genital herpes almost always acquire the infection from the mother's infected birth canal, either as an ascending infection through ruptured membranes or during passage through the birth canal. In rare cases infants are infected in utero, acquiring the initial viremia transplacentally from the mother.

Signs and Symptoms

The incubation period begins with the initial exposure to the virus and lasts until symptoms appear 2–10 days later. The woman with a primary infection of the genitalia may experience burning and tingling, followed by eruption of fluid-filled vesicles that either resolve spontaneously or rupture to form shallow, painful ulcerations. The ulcerations then scab and heal. Regional tender lymphadenopathy also may be present. Other features of the primary mucocutaneous infection may include edema of the involved area; dysuria; and the constitutional symptoms of sore throat, fever, and malaise. The initial infection lasts from 14–28 days. It is believed that the infection is contagious until the scabs have fallen off and the lesions have healed completely. It should be noted that cervical and vaginal herpes infections often are asymptomatic, which increases the probability that the infection will go undetected.

The number of recurrences is very unpredictable. They are triggered in some women by infection, sexual intercourse, sunlight, or emotional stress. The most distressing part of recurrence for some women is the prodromal symptoms: pain running down the buttocks or knees and genital itching, burning, or tingling. The constitutional symptoms of recurrent infections usually are mild. Lesions usually are localized and heal more rapidly than the primary infection; lesions of recurrent infection generally last about 7–14 days.

Diagnosis

Diagnosis and/or typing can be done only when lesions are present. Diagnosis of genital herpes infection is based on the patient's history and physical examination. A Pap smear of the lesion(s) will accurately identify the virus by its characteristic multinucleated giant cells in approximately two-thirds of all cases. Serial blood antibody titers, which determine levels of antibody against herpes, are useful in establishing whether it is a primary or recurrent infection. They do not distinguish between type I and type II infection. The most definitive means of diagnosis is a viral culture of the lesion. Unfortunately, this technique is not available in all communities. It is difficult to distinguish, both clinically and by available laboratory tests, between primary and recurrent genital infection.

Genital reinfection (defined as exogenous genital infection in those with previous nongenital herpes) may further confuse diagnosis. Data on reinfections are limited. The clinical course resembles recurrent rather than primary infection and disease.

Maternal and Fetal Outcome

Studies suggest that herpes genital infection predisposes women to cervical cancer. Epidemiologically, both diseases have similar predisposing factors. Both occur in young, sexually active groups and generally in women who have frequent intercourse with multiple partners. More antibodies to herpes simplex have been found in cervical cancer cells, and women who develop cervical cancer have a history of herpes infection more often than controls.

Genital herpes, especially a primary infection, is potentially dangerous for an unborn child. During a primary infection, the amount and duration of virus production are considerable, creating an excellent opportunity for the virus to spread. Herpes simplex virus can cause severe disease in infected infants. If the mother is infected at 32 weeks' gestation or later, there is a 10–20% chance that the infant will be infected. The risk is greatest (40–50%) if the infant is exposed to active infection in the mother's birth canal during delivery. In rare cases infants may acquire the virus transplacentally during maternal viremia. Transplacental infection has a mortality rate of up to 50%.

Primary genital herpes infection in the mother may result in neonatal herpes, which is a rare but devastating disease. Fortunately, primary infections are rare at the time of delivery. The incidence is 0.03 to 0.5 per one thousand infants (3). Neonatal herpes either may be disseminated (with an 80% mortality rate and 11% of those surviving having serious sequelae), localized to the central nervous system (with a 30% mortality rate and 50% of those surviving having serious sequelae), or restricted to the skin and mucous membranes (with a negligible mortality rate but frequent serious sequelae. Serious sequelae include brain damage and blindness).

If the mother has a recurrent genital herpes infection, the risk of transmission to the infant may be less than 10%. Recurrent infection is much more common. Neonatal disease usually is localized in the central nervous system or is restricted to the skin or mucous membranes.

Medical Management

The primary goal of medical management of genital herpes in pregnancy is the prevention of neonatal infection. The incidence of neonatal infection can be greatly reduced by:

1. Identifying those women with genital herpes in pregnancy.
2. Screening all high risk patients for the presence of disease by observing for visible lesions and taking weekly cervical virus cultures or Pap smears for virus isolation from 34 weeks' gestation until delivery. (High risk women are defined as those women with clinically suspect or documented genital herpes and women with a history of herpetic lesions below the waist.)
3. Avoiding the use of fetal scalp electrodes in all patients with unidentified lesions.
4. Delivering the infants of women with active herpes lesions in labor by cesarean section (providing the membranes are intact or have ruptured within the past 3–6 hours).

Women excreting virus at or near term are advised to have a cesarean section, provided the fetal membranes are intact or have ruptured within the past 3–6 hours. For those with ruptured membranes of 12 hours or more, cesarean section seems to provide no benefit in preventing neonatal infection. Within 24 hours fetal infection usually is present. The so-called gray zone seems to be between 6 and 12 hours, during which time each case must be evaluated individually to determine the most favorable method of delivery.

When two viral cultures or cytological smears are negative for HSV (taken at least 7 days apart prior to the onset of labor) and no lesions are found during labor, vaginal delivery is indicated.

During pregnancy, the treatment of HSV is palliative. Treatment consists of the following:

1. Warm soaks with solutions such as boric acid or Epsom salts to keep the area clean and to promote healing by reducing edema;
2. Drying agents such as alcohol and local heat to hasten healing of lesions;
3. Rest; and
4. Analgesics, such as acetaminophen (Tylenol, Datril).

Since stress seems to be related to recurrence of lesions, implementation of stress-reducing techniques may be beneficial.

Women with herpes also should be educated in the importance of obtaining yearly Pap smears because of the potential increased risk of cervical cancer.

During labor, delivery, and the postpartum period, women with active or clinically suspect HSV should be isolated in a private room, with gown and glove precautions being taken for the disposal of contaminated articles. Peri-pads and bed linen should be double bagged.

Women with HSV may feed their infants under supervised conditions following strict aseptic isolation procedures (skin and wound isolation procedures). Breastfeeding is not contraindicated after breast and nipple lesions are ruled out and careful hygienic measures are implemented.

The same isolation procedures, with the addition of a mask or dressing to cover lesions, should be taken for the woman with HSV type I infection (oral). Breastfeeding is contraindicated if breast or nipple lesions are present.

A woman with inactive herpes at term requires no special precautions.

Continuous rooming-in may be a viable alternative for the mother who understands the risks to the infant and who has proven her ability to carry out appropriate protective measures. This can promote maternal infant attachment in an otherwise sterile environment.

The newborn with the potential for herpes virus infections because of active maternal disease should be isolated. Gown and glove precautions should be taken by personnel having contact with contaminated articles or lesions. Linen and clothing should be double bagged. The infant should be taken to the mother under supervision.

Once infants of mothers with HSV type I are in contact with their mothers, they also should be isolated since the clinical course of the disease is the same as HSV type II in infected newborns.

NURSING MANAGEMENT

Nursing care specific for patients with *genital herpes*:

☐ Screen all patients for genital herpes by history; ensure that diagnostic tests (preferably viral cultures) are performed on all suspicious lesions.

☐ Teach comfort measures for active lesions (e.g., warm soaks with boric acid or Epsom salts, drying agents, rest, acetaminophen).

☐ For the patient with documented or suspected genital herpes:

NURSING MANAGEMENT

— Perform weekly cervical viral cultures or Pap smears beginning at 34 weeks' gestation;

— Teach the patient the importance of reporting to the hospital promptly after membranes rupture;

— Advise the patient of the possibility of cesarean section if active lesions are present at the time of delivery to prevent neonatal infection.

☐ For the patient with active herpes lesions or suspicious lesions in labor:

— Institute strict isolation precautions (gowns, gloves, double-bagging of contaminated articles);

— Avoid use of fetal scalp electrode;

— Allow breastfeeding if no breast lesions are present, using strict aseptic isolation procedures.

☐ Teach the patient the importance of obtaining yearly Pap smears.

☐ Instruct the mother, or anyone with oral herpes, to avoid kissing or fondling the baby and to employ good handwashing technique.

☐ Refer the patient to the American Social Health Association for more detailed information. (It has a program run by the Herpes Resource Center which provides a quarterly news letter, a telephone hotline, and organizes local self-help groups. Address: P. O. Box 110, Palo Alto, California 94302.)

Nursing diagnoses most frequently associated with *herpes* (see Section V):

☐ Grieving related to potential/actual loss of infant or birth of an imperfect child.

☐ Disturbance in body image, self-esteem.

☐ Ineffective individual coping.

☐ Altered sexuality patterns.

☐ Knowledge deficit regarding etiology, disease process, treatment, and outcome.

☐ Pain.

☐ Impaired skin integrity.

CONDYLOMA ACUMINATUM

Definition

Condylomata acuminata are wart-like growths found most commonly where the stratified squamous epithelium is thin, moist, and warm. They are caused by a virus that is transmitted sexually.

Etiology

Condylomata acuminata are caused by one of five distinct human papilloma viruses. These are DNA viruses belonging to the herpes group. The wart virus invades the cell, assisted by the microscopic degree of trauma occurring during intercouse, enters the nucleus, and replicates and sheds viral particles that become the source of new lesions.

During pregnancy, the cervical glands hypertrophy, mucus secretion increases greatly, and the consistency of the mucus is altered by steroid hormone activity. This increased vaginal secretion seems to accelerate viral growth, causing the condylomata to proliferate.

Growth also is enhanced by poor perineal hygiene, tight-fitting clothes of synthetic material, and perspiration. Autoinoculation can spread the condylomata to adjacent areas. The incubation period is 1–2 months but may be as long as 9 months.

Because of its increasing incidence and potential for carcinogenic changes, condyloma acuminatum no longer should be considered a minor sexually transmitted disease.

Signs and Symptoms

The woman with condylomata acuminata may present the complaint of wart-like growths in the vulva, pubic, or anorectal area. These growths also can be found in the vagina and on the cervix. They are less commonly found in the mouth. The patient may complain of pain and a malodorous discharge and express the concern that the warts have spread or grown. A secondary vaginal infection often is present. Regional lymphadenopathy does not occur.

Diagnosis

Diagnosis is based upon clinical observation in conjunction with the woman's medical and sexual history. Condylomata appear as papillomas with a central core of connective tissue in a tree-like structure covered with epithelium. These warts may grow and coalesce into cauliflower-shaped lesions.

Since 20–25% of women with genital warts have a coexisting sexually transmitted disease, appropriate laboratory tests should be done (i.e., wet preparation, gonorrhea culture, chlamydia culture, serologic test for syphilis).

Cervical inspection should be done on all women with condylomata of the vulva since 10% will have cervical warts. A Pap smear of the cervix should be taken since there have been reports of metastatic changes in warts that give the appearance of cervical neoplasia. Since 50–75% of exposed sexual partners have or develop genital warts, contacts should be examined.

Maternal and Fetal Outcome

The physiologic changes of pregnancy can produce a dramatic stimulus to the hyperplasia of the condylomata. This effect is not only painful but also psychologically disconcerting for the woman because of the alteration in body image caused by the appearance of large condylomata.

Massive condylomata can interfere with delivery and necessitate a cesarean section or surgical excision. If delivery occurs while the condylomata are still present, care must be taken to avoid tearing or cutting into them because they may bleed excessively. Spontaneous regression following childbirth can occur because of the withdrawal of the hormonal stimulus that caused increased vaginal secretions.

Research is being done on the relationship between anogenital warts and cervical carcinoma. There is epidemiologic evidence linking laryngeal papillomas in newborns to the existence of condylomata acuminata in the mother.

Medical Management

The approach to the medical management of condylomata acuminata in pregnancy primarily is palliative. Treatment is difficult because of the persistent stimulation of the condylomata by the continuing copious vaginal secretions of pregnancy, often complicated by increased discharge produced by secondary infection. The increased vascularity that occurs with pregnancy may contraindicate surgical incision. Secondary vaginal infections should be treated to decrease the volume and alter the character of the discharge, thus containing the growth of the virus. Measures to decrease moisture and to promote comfort should be suggested.

The treatment of choice in nonpregnant patients for condyloma acuminatum is podophyllum resin (10–25%) in tincture of benzoin, but this is contraindicated in pregnancy owing to reports of fetal death and premature labor following its use.

During pregnancy, small warts are observed to see if they will regress spontaneously. Electrocoagulation may be useful especially when large lesions have developed during pregnancy. Thompson and Grace have developed a scissor dissection method that spares normal tissue and prevents the scarring and resultant pain caused by other methods of excision (4). Excision can be performed under caudal anesthesia. Women with genital warts should be followed after delivery with yearly Pap smears, and atypical or persistent warts should be biopsied. Sexual contacts should be examined and treated as needed.

NURSING MANAGEMENT

Nursing care specific for a patient with condylomata acuminata:

☐ Teach patients with condylomata acuminatum measures to promote comfort and perhaps inhibit growth (e.g., sitz baths, perineal hygiene, use of cotton panties, avoidance of tight-fitting, synthetic clothing).

☐ Evaluate the patient for other sexually transmitted diseases or vaginal infections.

☐ Advise evaluation of sexual partner(s).

☐ Ensure that a Pap smear is performed; advise the patient to get regular yearly Pap smears.

☐ Provide teaching appropriate to the size, location, and planned treatment for the condylomata, e.g.:

— Advise that condylomata often regress in size after delivery;

— Provide pre- and postoperative teaching if surgical excision or electrocoagulation is planned;

— Advise that cesarean section may be required if condylomata prohibit vaginal delivery;

— Advise that postpartum treatment may be required since there are more options and treatment may be more successful in a nonpregnant patient.

☐ During the postpartum period, be aware of possibility of hemorrage due to condylomata. Frequently, observe perineum for bleeding and apply ice packs as needed.

Nursing diagnoses most frequently associated with condylomata acuminata (see Section V):

☐ Disturbance in body image, self-esteem.

☐ Altered sexuality patterns.

NURSING MANAGEMENT

- ☐ Knowledge deficit regarding etiology, disease process, treatment, and outcome.
- ☐ Knowledge deficit regarding medication regimen.

- ☐ Pain.
- ☐ Impaired skin integrity.

REFERENCES

1. Alexander RE: Maternal and infant sexually transmitted diseases. *Urol Clin N Am* 11:132, 1984.
2. Sexually transmitted diseases: treatment guidelines. *MMWR* supplement 31(2S):50S, 1982.
3. Devore N, Jackson V, Piening S: Torch infections. *Am J Nurs* 1662, 1983.
4. Margolis S: Therapy for condyloma acuminatum: a review. *Rev Infect Dis* 4 (Suppl):S829, 1982.

Chapter 23
Viral Infections in Pregnancy
Tina Duperret, C.N.M., M.S.

INTRODUCTION

Physiologic changes in pregnancy tend to increase the severity of most viral infections. However, viral disease in pregnancy is a most serious concern not only because of the increased maternal morbidity but also because of the profound teratogenic potential to the fetus in the first trimester and because of the serious risk of neonatal infection after exposure in the third trimester.

This chapter discusses the following viral infections during pregnancy: toxoplasmosis, cytomegalovirus, rubella, and varicella. See Chapter 22 for a discussion of herpes simplex virus and condyloma acuminatum.

TOXOPLASMOSIS

Definition

Toxoplasmosis is a common infectious disease caused by the intracellular protozoan parasite *Toxoplasma gondii*. Although it occurs worldwide, it is most prominent in warm climates. The incidence in pregnancy is 1 to 10 per 1000 pregnancies (1).

Etiology

Humans can become infected with *Toxoplasma gondii* by eating infected meat that is raw or undercooked or through contact with the feces of infected cats. Blood transfusions also are a potential mode of transmission. During an acute infection of the mother, the fetus can become infected transplacentally.

In an acute infection the *Toxoplasma gondii* invades many types of cells and forms a cyst around itself. It is not able to survive freezing, thawing, drying, or exposure to digestive juices. Tissue cysts are found in infected animals and humans. Oocysts (microscopic egg-like structures) are a form of the parasite found only in cats.

Humans and other warm-blooded animals can become infected when they inadvertently eat the mature oocysts. The intestinal wall is penetrated and the organisms spread throughout the body via the bloodstream. They multiply within the cells, where the parasite is transformed into cysts by the body's immune defenses. Although they remain there throughout the life cycle of the host, they usually remain dormant unless the immune system becomes suppressed. Reactivated toxoplasmosis is dangerous and often fatal.

It should be noted that cats are infectious only around the time of the initial infection, when they shed oocysts.

Signs and Symptoms

Infection with *Toxoplasma gondii* in adults often is asymptomatic. When symptoms do occur, they usually appear 1–2 weeks after infection and subside within a few weeks to several months. The most common clinical manifestation in adults is swollen lymph nodes, the posterior cervical chain being the one most frequently involved. Other symptoms that may occur are fatigue, labile fever, rash, depression, malaise, headache, and sore throat.

Diagnosis

The differential diagnosis must include infectious mononucleosis, because of the similarity of symptoms. Diagnosis of toxoplasmosis is made by testing for toxoplasma antibodies. Serial blood samples drawn 3 weeks apart are compared. A sample should be taken during the active disease and compared to one taken after convalescence. Toxoplasmosis infection is confirmed if the second sample has a significantly higher antibody titer than the first sample. Specific interpretation of titers depends on which of the several available laboratory tests is used.

The serologic tests most commonly used in the United States are the Sabin-Feldman dye tests, the complement fixation test, and the indirect fluorescent antibody test. The diagnosis of acute toxoplasmosis is established by demonstrating rising serologic titers.

The Sabin-Feldman dye test is based on the observation that *Toxoplasma gondii* incubated with normal serum for 1 hour become swollen and deeply stained when alkaline methylene blue is added to the suspension. The parasites expand in serum containing antibody under the same conditions, appear thin and distorted, and are not stained when the dye is added.

In the complement fixation test the antibodies appear later than those demonstrable by dye tests. Therefore, active infection is indicated by a negative complement fixation test that becomes positive or by a fourfold rise in complement fixation titer in conjunction with a stable, high dye test titer.

Indirect fluorescent antibody test does not require living organisms. It is equal in specificity to the dye test, and it has been used successfully to establish the diagnosis of congenital and acquired infection. An indirect fluorescent antibody titer of 1:512 or greater correlates with active infection.

If a woman has antibodies against toxoplasmosis at any time prior to conception, she and her fetus will be protected since permanent immunity usually is conferred with the disease.

Maternal and Fetal Outcome

Although *Toxoplasma gondii* infection is common in adults, maternal effects are minimal because symptomatic disease is uncommon.

The incidence of congenital toxoplasmosis in the United States is 0.25 to 1.0 per 1000 live births (1, p 1662). When the primary infection takes place during pregnancy, transmission of the parasite to the fetus occurs in 40% of cases. The most severe disease occurs when the fetus is less than 24 weeks' gestation. When toxoplasmosis is present in early pregnancy, spontaneous abortion is a frequent result, perinatal mortality is increased, and the prognosis for those who survive is poor. Abortion, stillbirth, or severe congenital infection occurs in 10–15% of pregnancies complicated by toxoplasmosis. Twenty percent of offspring infected in the first trimester are affected severely.

Most infected neonates are asymptomatic at birth. Despite the lack of overt neurologic manifestations, abnormalities of cerebrospinal fluid (lymphocytosis and elevated protein) are detectable in asymptomatic infants. Less than 10% without overt disease escape without residual cerebral or ocular damage.

Approximately 10% of infected infants born with congenital toxoplasmosis manifest severe disease. Ocular involvement in the form of chorioretinitis is the only overt manifestation in half of these. If the infection is generalized at birth, cyanosis, pneumonia, hepatosplenomegaly, jaundice, and thrombocytopenic purpura are the presenting signs. The classic triad of chorioretinitis, hydrocephaly, and cerebral calcifications occurs in only a few cases.

Fifty to sixty percent of infants with overt toxoplasmosis have central nervous system involvement, which is manifested by convulsions, microcephaly, hydrocephaly, or brain calcifications. Ten to fifteen percent of those infants die, with most of the remainder sustaining permanent neurologic damage.

Medical Management

Medical management consists primarily of prevention through education of all women of childbearing age. They should be warned to avoid eating raw or undercooked meat and to avoid exposure to infected cats. All cats in the house should have texoplasmosis titers. If positive, the cat's feces should be cultured for oocysts. If the titer is negative, the cat should be prevented from roaming freely outdoors to prevent contact with contaminated meat or rodents. Women also should avoid contact with the cat's litter box during pregnancy.

Optimally, serologic testing should be done periodically during pregnancy in those women who have cats or eat raw meat. If this is not feasible, it is advisable to test maternal serum at the time of delivery. If the mother demonstrates a high titer, her infant should be monitored carefully for clinical and serologic evidence of disease.

The treatment of toxoplasmosis in pregnancy should be limited only to active forms of the disease or to those women with immunologic impairment. Women should understand that treatment of the acute stage of toxoplasmosis acquired during pregnancy can only decrease but not totally eliminate the risk of having a congenitally infected infant. Little or nothing can be done to reverse any damage already done.

The only effective treatment in the United States is a combination of pyrimethamine (Daraprim, an antimalarial drug) with sulfadiazine or triple sulfa drugs. The standard dosage for adults is pyrimethamine, 25 mg twice a day for 1 day, followed by 25 mg every day along with sulfadiazine in a total daily dosage of 2–6 g for 3–4 weeks. The combination of pyrimethamine and sulfonamides is synergistic against sporozoites, but has no effect on the dormant encysted forms of toxoplasmosis. Therapy should be combined with 6–10 mg of folinic acid (leucovorin) or 5–7 g of baker's yeast daily, to try to minimize the toxic hematologic effects of pyrimethamine (a folic acid antagonist). During treatment, biweekly laboratory testing should be done to monitor patients for thrombocytopenia, agranulocytosis, or megaloblastic anemia.

During the first trimester, treatment with pyrimethamine should be withheld since it has been teratogenic in mice during the period of organogenesis. If the emotional or physical well-being of the mother is not compromised, therapeutic abortion can be discussed. Sulfonamides should be discontinued 2–3 weeks prior to the expected date of confinement (EDC) to avoid hyperbilirubinemia in the neonate. Since sulfonamides are known to compete with bilirubin for albumin-binding sites, hyperbilirubinemia can become so severe as to cause kernicterus. An alternative approach to those requiring treatment in the last trimester of pregnancy is to postpone treatment and to treat the neonate after delivery.

Neonatal therapy is indicated for all neonates whose mothers were treated for acute toxoplasmosis during pregnancy, for all infants with symptomatic infection, and for all asymptomatic infants with positive cerebrospinal fluid.

NURSING MANAGEMENT

Nursing care specific for a patient with
toxoplasmosis:
- ☐ Teach all patients measures to prevent toxoplasmosis:
  - — Wash hands after working with soil or changing cat litter;
  - — Cook meat thoroughly, avoid eating raw meat, and freeze meat promptly;
  - — Keep flies away from food;
  - — Have cats tested for toxoplasmosis, prevent cats from roaming to prevent contact with infected meat, and avoid changing cat litter during pregnancy, if possible; and
  - — Provide written information to all women of childbearing age to reinforce instruction.
- ☐ Counsel patient regarding disease, including risk to fetus; support her in making an informed decision on therapeutic abortion versus drug therapy.

- ☐ Explain the drug regimen; monitor hematologic tests to detect side effects; teach the patient to report side effects (e.g., nausea/vomiting, bad taste, anorexia, gingivitis, headache, weakness, dizziness, skin rashes, jaundice, bruising, mental depression, convulsions).
- ☐ Report all cases of toxoplasmosis to local health department.

Nursing diagnoses most frequently associated with *toxoplasmosis* (see Section V):
- ☐ Grieving related to potential/actual loss of infant or birth of an imperfect child.
- ☐ Knowledge deficit regarding etiology, disease process, treatment, and outcome.
- ☐ Spiritual distress.
- ☐ Ineffective individual coping.
- ☐ Knowledge deficit regarding medication regimen.
- ☐ Anxiety/fear.

CYTOMEGALOVIRUS INFECTION

Definition

The cytomegaloviruses (CMVs), members of the herpes family, are among the oldest known viruses. CMV infection is caused by one of the strains of CMV. CMVs are DNA ether-sensitive viruses that are widely distributed in the human population.

The prenatal incidence is 10 to 70 per 1000 pregnancies (1, p 1662). The incidence at delivery rises to 30 to 140 per 1000 pregnancies (1, p 1662).

Etiology

Although the exact mechanism of transmission is unknown, CMV infection is thought to take place after contact with infected secretions. As with other herpes viruses, viral shedding can occur for months or years. Since CMV has been isolated in cervical secretions, saliva, urine, breast milk, semen, feces, and blood, many modes of transmission are possible. Epidemiological data show it occurs more frequently and at a younger age in lower socioeconomic areas, where crowded and poor sanitary conditions prevail. It is frequently a life-threatening superinfection in AIDS patients.

Signs and Symptoms

Acquired CMV infections usually are subclinical, documented only by a positive antibody titer. A mild mononucleosis-like syndrome has been seen in young adults and in recipients of blood transfusions. The viral infection reacts like herpes infections, becoming latent for months or years and thus complicating the question of immunity. Reactivation of the infection occurs in response to a variety of stimuli, as in herpes simplex infections. Immunity to the specific CMV strain is conferred on the host after the latent period. Although unusual, it is possible for a mother to give birth to a second infant infected by the same virus. Also, since CMVs exist in multiple strains, reinfection of a woman with a different strain also can result in a second infected infant.

In rare cases an individual will have a symptomatic primary CMV infection. Although the symptoms resemble mononucleosis (i.e., fever, lymphocytosis, many atypical lymphocytes, and abnormal liver function tests), the lymphadenitis, pharyngitis, and presence of heterophil antibody in mononucleosis are absent.

Diagnosis

Diagnosis of CMV infection in the mother is made by obtaining a negative heterophil antibody titer to rule out mononucleosis; by isolating the virus from the urine, saliva, cervix, liver, blood, or cerebrospinal fluid; and by demonstrating a fourfold or greater rise in complement fixation or immunofluorescent titers between the pre- and postconvalescent sera (i.e., serum obtained at onset of disease compared to serum obtained after recovery). It is important for accurate diagnosis that both sera be run under identical test conditions at the same time.

Maternal and Fetal Outcome

Intrauterine infection seems to occur either during the initial viremia of the mother or as an ascending infection from the virus-laden cervical secretions, especially in the latter part of pregnancy. The overall incidence of neonatal CMV infections is 0.5 to 1.0% (2). The effects on the fetus can be mild or severe. The mild form of the infection is much more frequent than the severe form. Hearing loss and learning disabilities are the most common manifestations. Severely affected neonates demonstrate intrauterine growth retardation (birth weight less than 2500 g), pneumonitis, hepatitis, and necrotizing meningoencephalitis. Severe neurologic degeneration, causing microcephaly, obstructive hydrocephalus, and periventricular calcifications (seen on x-ray) can be attributed to the necrotizing meningoencephalitis. Diffuse purpura caused by thrombocytopenia, anemia, jaundice, and hepatospenomegaly are temporary short-term effects of the disease. Profound mental retardation, deafness, seizures, spasticity, optic atrophy, and chorioretinitis are long-term effects of severe CMV infection.

Since most cases in adults are subclinical, maternal effects are minimal.

Medical Management

Currently there is no satisfactory means of preventing CMV infection or of treating congenital neonatal infection. Although a vaccine has been developed, it must be studied clinically before its effectiveness can be evaluated.

NURSING MANAGEMENT

Nursing care specific for a patient with cytomegalovirus:

- ☐ Teach all patients measures to prevent CMV:
  - — Avoid contact with persons with viral infections (especially known or suspected CMV infections) and
  - — Use good handwashing techniques.
- ☐ Screen patients with mononucleosis-like symptoms or with AIDS/ARC for presence of CMV.

- ☐ Teach the patient to avoid individuals with known CMV infection (e.g., AIDS patients).

Nursing diagnoses most frequently associated with cytomegalovirus (see Section V):

- ☐ Grieving related to potential/actual loss of infant or birth of an imperfect child.
- ☐ Knowledge deficit regarding etiology, disease process, treatment, and outcome.
- ☐ Anxiety/fear.

RUBELLA

Definition

Rubella (German measles or three-day measles) is an acute, mild, contagious disease caused by the rubella virus. It is distributed worldwide and is most prevalent in big cities during spring. In the United States it occurs most frequently in adolescents and young adults who have not been immunized. It is estimated that 5–15% of women of childbearing age are susceptible (1, p 1660).

Etiology

The rubella virus is a medium-sized RNA virus that is transmitted by direct contact with blood, urine, stools, or nasopharyngeal secretions. The incubation period is 10–21 days. The period of communicability lasts from approximately 10 days prior to the appearance of the rash to 5 days after. The virus is transmitted to the fetus transplacentally.

Signs and Symptoms

The clinical manifestations of rubella infection in the mother start when viral shedding occurs (approximately the fourth day following exposure). The most common sign is postauricular and occipital lymphadenopathy, which is followed by a low-grade fever 99.5–101.7°F (37.5–38.7°C), malaise, coryza, and conjunctival irritation. Ten to fourteen days after exposure, a maculopapular rash starts on the face and then spreads rapidly to the trunk and upper extremities. The rash usually disappears by the third day, distinguishing it from rubeola, which lasts approximately 10 days. In rare cases individuals exhibit more severe manifestations, such as high fever 104°F (40°C), thrombocytopenia, arthritis, arthralgia, and encephalitis. An equal number of individuals are asymptomatic during rubella infection.

Diagnosis

When the woman gives a positive history of exposure to a rubella infection and has obvious symptoms of disease, a presumptive diagnosis can be made by clinical examination. In those women with subtle clinical manifestations, the disease may go unnoticed. Diagnosis can be confirmed by obtaining a hemagglutination inhibition (HI) antibody titer immediately after exposure and then by repeating it in 2–3 weeks after exposure. Titers of less than 1:8 indicate the absence of previous rubella infection. A fourfold or greater rise in antibody titer 2–3 weeks after exposure indicates infection. The initial titer should be rerun at the same time that the second titer is determined to prevent error due to interassay variations.

Maternal and Fetal Outcome

Maternal effects of rubella infection are not more severe than those of nonpregnant women, nor are there more complications.

Rubella infection, although relatively benign for the mother, is devastating for the fetus. Sixteen to eighteen percent of pregnancies complicated by early rubella infection terminate in spontaneous abortion or stillbirth. Of those that survive, 61% have anomalies if infection occurs in the first 4 weeks of pregnancy, 26% in weeks 5–8, and 8% in weeks 9–12. Thirty percent of infants infected in the first 16 weeks will be deaf.

Maternal viremia and infection of the placenta are sources of transmission of the virus to the fetus. Although 50% of all rubella-infected pregnancies result in transmission of the virus to the fetus, the transmission rate reaches 100% when the infection occurs prior to the tenth week of gestation. Rubella virus acquired in utero persists throughout pregnancy and can be recovered from the infected infant for months after birth.

The rubella syndrome for years has been known to cause defects in the eyes, ears, and heart of infected fetuses. Malformations are caused by cell destruction or disturbed cell division. Intrauterine growth retardation has been attributed to inhibition of cell multiplication.

Ocular defects associated with congenital rubella, occurring in 50% of infected infants, are nuclear cataracts, which develop during the first year of life; retinopathy, which consists of disturbances in pigment homogeneity; glaucoma; microphthalmia; and myopia.

Auditory defects, occurring in 30–50% of infected infants, are the most difficult to diagnose at birth and may be unilateral or bilateral. Chronic postnatal otitis media is responsible for additional hearing loss in those children with atrophic and degenerative changes already present in the inner ear. In rubella infections occurring after the first trimester, hearing loss may be the only effect.

Patent ductus arteriosus and pulmonary artery stenosis are the two most common cardiovascular lesions in congenital rubella infection. Ventricular septal defect is the most common intracardiac lesion. Other cardiac defects that have been reported are pulmonary and aortic valvular stenosis.

Fifty percent of infants infected with rubella have decreased head circumference (i.e., head circumference below the third percentile) and central nervous system damage resulting in mental retardation. Poor childhood growth, poor language and motor development, and seizures are associated with encephalitis.

Disruption of the cartilagenous development of the distal femur and proximal tibia also may be seen. Recently, it has been demonstrated that early onset diabetes mellitus may be caused by congenital rubella infection (3).

Medical Management

There is no specific treatment for the rubella syndrome. All pregnant women should be screened for rubella antibody on their initial prenatal visit. Those women who are susceptible should be counseled to avoid contact with anyone with a rash, and they should be encouraged to be immunized during the postpartum period.

Women receiving vaccine postpartum should be instructed to avoid pregnancy for at least 3 months following vaccination because the rubella vaccine is a live attenuated virus that is known to cross the placenta. Maximum risks of fetal infection after maternal vaccination are 5–10%. However, some recent studies assess the risk to be only 2%.

Pregnant women exposed to the rubella virus early in pregnancy should have an antibody titer done within a few days after exposure. Ideally, the antibody titer should be obtained before the rash appears or within 5 days of its appearance. If the specimen shows the presence of antibody, the patient can be reassured that she is immune and not at risk.

If the woman is susceptible, a second blood specimen should be taken 2–3 weeks after exposure and retested along with the first specimen. The presence of antibody in the second specimen indicates disease, and the woman should be counseled as to the risk to the fetus according to the gestational age of the pregnancy. Her decision to continue or to terminate the pregnancy should be supported.

NURSING MANAGEMENT

Nursing care specific for a patient with *rubella*:

- [ ] Ensure that all pregnant women are tested for rubella and that each woman knows her rubella status.
- [ ] Be aware of your own rubella status and the need for vaccination as appropriate.
- [ ] Teach measures to prevent rubella to all women of childbearing age:
  - — Have a rubella antibody test prior to pregnancy and get vaccinated if susceptible; emphasize the importance of using a reliable method of birth control for at least 3 months after receiving the vaccination;
  - — Ensure that unprotected pregnant women receive rubella vaccination in the postpartum period to protect future pregnancies; after inoculation teach the patient to use a reliable method of birth control for at least 3 months; and
  - — Avoid contact with persons known or suspected to have rubella.

Nursing diagnoses most frequently associated with *rubella*:

- [ ] Grieving related to potential/actual loss of infant or birth of an imperfect child.
- [ ] Knowledge deficit regarding etiology, disease process, treatment, and outcome.
- [ ] Spiritual distress.
- [ ] Anxiety/fear.

VARICELLA

Definition

Varicella (chickenpox) and herpes zoster (shingles) represent two phases of activity of a single virus referred to as the varicella zoster (VZ) virus. It is an acute, highly contagious infection. Since it is a common disease of childhood, it is rare during pregnancy.

Etiology

Varicella and herpes zoster infections are transmitted primarily by direct contact with the VZ virus in secretions from the respiratory tract. It is less often acquired through contact with skin lesions and air transmission of the virus from room to room. Varicella has an incubation period of 14 days, with a range of 10–21 days. Diseases caused by the VZ virus are contagious from 1 day before the appearance of the rash until 2–6 days after, when the lesions have crusted over. The first time the body is invaded by the virus, the generalized infection, varicella, occurs. Viremia is a regular feature of the infection, but transmission to the fetus is unpredictable. Herpes zoster represents a localized infection, which may be either a reinvasion of an immune person or the activation of a latent virus.

Signs and Symptoms

Varicella is manifested by characteristic vesicular eruptions generalized in the skin and mucous membranes that develop in crops, are centripetally distributed, and are most prominent on the trunk. New vesicles continue to appear for 3–4 days, so the rash contains a combination of red papules, vesicles, and scabs in various stages.

The rash is accompanied by pruritus. Prior to the vesicular eruptions, the woman may notice a fever of 101–103°F (38.3–39.4°C), malaise, and anorexia.

Herpes zoster almost always is unilateral, and vesicular eruption is distributed along dermatomes, usually corresponding to peripheral nerve areas most commonly involved in varicella.

Diagnosis

Diagnosis is made by assessment of a patient's history and the presence of characteristic clinical signs. The virus can be isolated from vesicular fluid within the first 3–4 days of the rash. Serum contains antibodies as early as 7 days after onset. Complement fixation testing is satisfactory for demonstrating a rise in antibodies, thus confirming the diagnosis, but it is unreliable for diagnosing susceptibility since the antibody is not long lasting. Fluorescence antibody membrane antigen (FAMA) titer is a rapid and reliable way to determine immunity in the mother. Unfortunately, its availability at present is limited.

Maternal and Fetal Outcome

Varicella is more severe in adults than children because they have higher fevers, more severe rashes, and are more prone to complications, including potentially fatal pneumonia.

Although congenital defects from maternal infection with varicella prior to 16 weeks' gestation have been reported, they are extremely uncommon. There has been no increased incidence of spontaneous abortion, prematurity, or fetal demise in pregnancies complicated by maternal varicella.

Maternal infection 5–15 days prior to delivery seems to allow sufficient antibody production in the mother to mediate or prevent disease in the newborn. If disease in the newborn does occur, it is not fatal. Maternal infection 4 days or less before delivery leads to neonatal death in approximately 20% of cases.

Medical Management

Zoster immune globulin (ZIG) prevents varicella when given to susceptible infants within 24 hours of exposure. ZIG is a hyperimmune serum prepared from pooled blood of persons convalescing from herpes zoster and therefore is in short supply. It is available only for infants whose mothers develop varicella between 4 days before and 2 days after delivery and for immunosuppressed people who are at high risk for severe disease. The Centers for Disease Control in Atlanta, Georgia, can direct hospitals to the source of the available globulin.

Treatment of maternal varicella is symptomatic, with local antipruritics such as cool bicarbonate of soda baths, local application of calamine lotion, and systemic antipyretics, such as acetaminophen (Tylenol), to bring down the fever. Antibiotics are not warranted unless a superimposed bacterial infection develops. Women should be isolated until all vesicles and most of the scabs have disappeared, which is usually 7 days after the rash appears.

Women in labor with varicella should be isolated in a private room. Respiratory and skin precautions should be taken (gowns, gloves, masks, double-bagging procedure). Nurses who have not had varicella and those who are pregnant should not care for patients with varicella.

NURSING MANAGEMENT

Nursing care specific for a patient with varicella:
☐ Teach patients to avoid contact with persons known or suspected to have varicella.
☐ Educate the patient regarding care of lesions:
  — Avoid scratching, piercing, or squeezing;

  — Use good hygiene;
  — Maintain cool environmental temperature;
  — Use topical antipruritics (e.g., calamine lotion; cool bicarbonate of soda baths); and

NURSING MANAGEMENT

— Use acetaminophen for analgesia and to reduce fever.

☐ Institute appropriate isolation procedures when the patient is hospitalized:

   — Isolate the mother with varicella from her newborn until lesions are crusted over; and

   — Isolate infants with varicella.

Nursing diagnoses most frequently associated with *varicella* (see Section V):

☐ Grieving related to potential/actual loss of infant or birth of an imperfect child.

☐ Disturbance in body image, self-esteem.

☐ Knowledge deficit regarding etiology, disease process, treatment, and outcome.

☐ Impaired skin integrity.

REFERENCES

1. DeVore N, Jackson V, Piening S: Torch infections. *Am J Nurs* 83: 1662, 1983.
2. Monif G: *Infectious Diseases*. Tallahassee, FL, Rose Printing, 1982, p 142.
3. Simpson JL, Goebus MS, Martin AO, Sarto GG: *Genetics in Obstetrics and Gynecology*. New York, Grune and Stratton, 1982, p 229.

Chapter 24
Early Pregnancy Loss
Kathleen Buckley, C.N.M., M.S.N.

INTRODUCTION

Cessation of menstruation is one of the first signs of pregnancy. For some women it is a wanted occurrence; for others it is a tragedy. For those who elect to carry the pregnancy—whatever their feelings about it—the sudden recurrence of vaginal bleeding is a frightening event. The patient may fear her own death and begin to grieve the loss of her unborn child. She may question her feminine identity, or her partner may view the potential loss as a reason to end a "nonproductive" union.

This chapter discusses the potentially emotionally charged crises of spontaneous abortion and ectopic pregnancy.

ECTOPIC PREGNANCY

Definition

An ectopic pregnancy is one in which the fertilized ovum implants in a site other than the endometrial lining of the uterine cavity. Implantation can be intrauterine, occurring in the cervix, or extrauterine, occurring in the abdominal cavity, ovary, or fallopian tube (Fig. 24.1). However, 95% of all ectopic pregnancies occur in the fallopian tube. The most common implantation site in the tube is the fimbriated end (1).

Overall incidence varies with the population studied and has increased rapidly over the years as specific etiologic factors (e.g., salpingitis) have become more widespread. Current incidence ranges between 1 in 100 pregnancies and 1 in 200 pregnancies (2).

Etiology

Factors precipitating ectopic pregnancy can be conceptualized as any condition that prevents or delays the passage of the fertilized egg through the fallopian tube or into the uterus. Conditions include occlusion of the tube, impaired tubal ciliary action, impaired tubal contractility, and decreased sperm motility (1, pp 36–38).

Common etiologies include (1, pp 36–38, 3):

1. Adhesions because of endosalpingitis (35% of cases and incidence is rising).

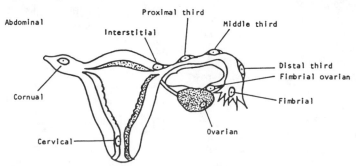

Figure 24.1. Sites of ectopic pregnancies. (From Buckley K, Kulb NW (eds). *Handbook of Maternal-Newborn Nursing.* New York, John Wiley & Sons, 1983, p 419.)

2. Use of an intrauterine contraceptive device (IUCD), which impedes intrauterine but not extrauterine implantation.
3. Distortion of the fallopian tube because of anatomical malformation, tumor, or structural damage after tuboplasty or other surgery that blocks the tube and prevents intrauterine implantation.
4. Use of a progesterone-only oral contraceptive because the hormone decreases tubal ciliary action.

Signs and Symptoms

The classic presentation of ectopic rupture follows a progressive pattern. The patient will have a history of 1 or 2 months of amenorrhea accompanied by other signs of early pregnancy. Onset of mild vaginal bleeding and sharp unilaterial abdominal pain mark the onset of rupture and hemorrhage, and the pain forces the patient to seek emergency medical attention. Abdominal pain becomes generalized and associated with shoulder pain as the hemorrhage becomes extensive, irritating the diaphragm. The patient complains of dizziness and may faint. Pelvic examination reveals marked vaginal vault tenderness and excruciating pain when the cervix is moved. A tender adnexal mass may be palpated. If culdocentesis is performed, blood is found in the cul-de-sac. Signs of shock become worse, and the patient deteriorates rapidly (3).

However, this clear picture of an obvious, life-threatening medical emergency occurs in only 15% of cases (4). Most often, signs and symptoms of ectopic rupture are vague or subacute. Some history of menstrual irregularity, crampy abdominal pain, and mild vaginal bleeding always are present. Thus, ectopic rupture must be considered when any woman of childbearing age complains of them, no matter how mild the complaints may seem. It must be noted that mild signs and symptoms do not indicate a small amount of bleeding—hemorrhage indeed may be massive.

Signs and symptoms are further related to site of implantation (4). Tubal pregnancy most often will present as has been described above. Cervical pregnancy is associated with painless bleeding very early in pregnancy and presence of a cervical mass. The rare ovarian pregnancy also shows the signs described above. In addition, an ovarian mass may be palpated.

In tubal, ovarian, and cervical ectopic pregnancy/rupture, signs and symptoms always occur in the first trimester of pregnancy. However, abdominal pregnancy has been carried to term. Thus, signs and symptoms of abdominal pregnancy *may* be completely different, including (1):

1. Exaggerated gastrointestinal disturbance as the pregnancy enlarges.
2. Transverse fetal lie.
3. Ease in palpating fetal small parts.
4. Loud fetal heart tones.

Diagnosis

Diagnosis is difficult because signs and symptoms are vague and overlap many other types of pathology. Differential diagnoses of ectopic rupture include salpingitis, appendicitis, rupture or torsion of an ovarian cyst, or pelvic abscess. One of the most difficult distinctions is between ectopic rupture and spontaneous abortion (see Table 24.1). In order to safeguard the life of the woman, every woman complaining of amenorrhea, vaginal bleeding, and abdominal pain should be considered a candidate for ectopic rupture until proven otherwise (5).

After 8 weeks' gestation, a clear sonogram revealing an intrauterine gestational sac and fetal movement rules out ectopic pregnancy except in the very rare case where an ectopic pregnancy coexists with an intrauterine pregnancy. Conversely, a positive pregnancy test and an empty uterine cavity confirm the diagnosis (if the patient is over 8 weeks' gestation). If the patient is less than 8 weeks' gestation or a clear sonogram cannot be obtained, other evaluative measures must be used (5).

If ectopic pregnancy is suspected, serum radioimmunoassay of beta-subunit human chorionic gonadotropin (HCG) should be the pregnancy test of choice because it is highly reliable. Urine tests are associated with a 50% false-negative rate in ectopic pregnancy because of the smaller, poorly developed implantation site's inability to produce normal amounts of HCG (Fig. 24.2) (5).

Culdocentesis may be done to evaluate presence of intraperitoneal bleeding, which then would imply ectopic rupture. If blood is obtained from the cul-de-sac and does not clot within 10 minutes, it is freelying in the intraperitioneal cavity, indicating hemorrhage. However, if the patient is unable to tolerate this procedure or the procedure is contraindicated because of a severely retroverted uterus, attempts should be abandoned. Considering the risk-benefit ratio, when there is doubt, surgery is the safest, surest diagnostic test.

Maternal and Fetal Outcome

Maternal health is greatly jeopardized. Uterine infection, septicemia, hemorrhage, shock, and disseminated intravascular coagulation are common. Ectopic rupture is one of the main causes of maternal mortality in the United States—occurring in 1

Table 24.1.
SYMPTOMS OF TUBAL PREGNANCY AND EARLY THREATENED ABORTION[a]

TUBAL PREGNANCY	EARLY THREATENED ABORTION
1. Scanty vaginal bleeding	1. Scanty vaginal bleeding
2. Enlargement on one side of the uterus, due to embryo in the tube	2. Possible enlargement on one side of the uterus, due to corpus luteum cyst of pregnancy
3. Sharp, cramp-like pain on the affected side	3. Pain, if present, less severe; located in the middle rather than to the side
4. The time between the last menstrual period and the onset of bleeding is apt to be shorter, usually 6–8 weeks	4. The time between the last menstrual period and the onset of bleeding is apt to be longer, usually 8–10 weeks
5. Anemia, if present, out of proportion to observable blood loss from internal bleeding	5. Anemia not usually present, except if there is profuse bleeding, and then it is in line with observable blood loss
6. Uterus not enlarged, cervix not softened	6. Uterus enlarged, cervix softened
7. Nausea, vomiting, faintness	7. No nausea, vomiting, faintness

[a]Reprinted with permission from Madaras L, Patterson J. *Woman Care.* New York: Avon Books, 1981, p 645. Copyright 1981 by Lynda Madaras and Jane Patterson. Used by arrangement with Avon Books.

out of 100 ectopic pregnancies (6). Besides the physical sequelae, the distress of pregnancy loss as well as the loss of reproductive capacity may be emotionally overwhelming.

In tubal, ovarian, and cervical pregnancies, the fetus has no chance of survival beyond the first trimester. In abdominal pregnancy perhaps 1 out of 10 may survive to viability.

Medical Management

Once the diagnosis of tubal pregnancy has been made, the pregnancy should be evacuated *immediately.* There is no reason to delay until the ectopic pregnancy ruptures and the patient's life is at stake. If the initial diagnosis is ectopic rupture, the necessity for surgery is absolute. The usual procedure is salpingectomy. However, in some tubal pregnancies the conceptus simply can be pushed manually from the implantation site out to the end of the tube. The choice of procedure depends on the condition of the affected tube, the normalcy of the opposite tube, the patient's desire for another pregnancy, and the clinical condition of the patient. Whether or not oophorectomy is needed depends on the damage to the ovaries during the tubal pregnancy and the resultant hemorrhage (5).

Cardiovascular stability should be maintained through use of plasma expanders and blood transfusions, if necessary. Careful evaluation of Rh status is essential and an Rh immunoglobulin injection is indicated in the Rh-negative patient.

Follow-up and counseling are essential. The unaffected tube's condition is assessed during surgery. The assessment should be discussed with the patient. Generally, she should know that her chances of conceiving are greatly reduced (only 50% of normal) and that her chances of another ectopic pregnancy are high (25–30%). If the woman decides to attempt another pregnancy, a preconceptual evaluation of uterine and tubal patency should be scheduled and the conceptual environment optimized by surgical intervention (e.g., lysis of adhesions) if necessary. The patient should know that menstrual irregularity, abnormal vaginal bleeding, and abdominal pain are highly suggestive of a recurrence of an ectopic pregnancy. The health care team must maintain the highest level of suspicion for these symptoms and evaluate them with the utmost urgency.

NURSING MANAGEMENT

Nursing care specific for *ectopic pregnancy*:
- [ ] Ensure that every woman of childbearing age who complains of amenorrhea, vaginal bleeding, and abdominal pain is screened for presence of ectopic pregnancy.
- [ ] If ectopic is diagnosed, provide emotional support to the patient, prepare for emergency surgery, and monitor the patient for shock.

- [ ] Postoperatively, ensure that:
  - — All Rh-negative patients receive RhoGAM;
  - — Any anemic patient is discharged with appropriate iron/folic acid therapy; and
  - — Every patient has a 2-week follow-up appointment before discharge.
- [ ] Postoperatively, teach the patient the following before hospital discharge:

NURSING MANAGEMENT

— Signs of postsurgery infection (e.g., abdominal pain, fever, excessive lochia, foul-smelling lochia) and where to report them;

— Signs of ectopic pregnancy (e.g., amenorrhea, vaginal bleeding, abdominal pain) and where to report them;

— Need for tests/procedures to be scheduled to evaluate future reproductive status; and

— Use of birth control until reproductive potential is determined.

☐ Be aware that the patient/significant others have a real need to grieve both the pregnancy loss and the potential reproductive capacity loss. Encourage them to verbalize their feelings.

Nursing diagnoses most frequently associated with *ectopic pregnancy* (see Section V):

☐ Grieving related to potential/actual loss of infant or birth of an imperfect child.

☐ Anticipatory grieving related to actual/perceived threat to self.

☐ Disturbance in body image, self-esteem.

☐ Knowledge deficit regarding etiology, disease process, treatment, and outcome.

☐ Fluid volume deficit.

☐ Altered maternal tissue perfusion.

☐ Pain.

☐ Anxiety/fear.

☐ Impaired tissue integrity.

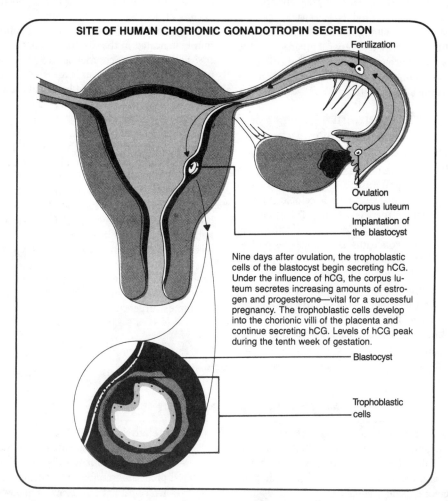

SITE OF HUMAN CHORIONIC GONADOTROPIN SECRETION

Fertilization

Ovulation

Corpus luteum

Implantation of the blastocyst

Nine days after ovulation, the trophoblastic cells of the blastocyst begin secreting hCG. Under the influence of hCG, the corpus luteum secretes increasing amounts of estrogen and progesterone—vital for a successful pregnancy. The trophoblastic cells develop into the chorionic villi of the placenta and continue secreting hCG. Levels of hCG peak during the tenth week of gestation.

Blastocyst

Trophoblastic cells

Figure 24.2. Normal site of human chorionic gonadotropin secretion. (From *Diagnostics.* Springhouse, PA, Nurse's Reference Library, p 192.)

SPONTANEOUS ABORTION

Definition

Spontaneous abortion is the unintentional termination of pregnancy before the fetus is viable. A nonviable fetus is defined as one expelled at or before 20 weeks' gestation and/or weighing 500 g or less. In general, about 20% of all pregnant women experience some signs and symptoms of spontaneous abortion, and about half of these (10%) progress to pregnancy loss.

However, as maternal age increases, clinical loss rates increase. Spontaneous abortion occurs in 15% of the 30–34 year old age group, 17% in the 35–39 year old age group, and 25% in the over 40 years old age group. Most recognized spontaneous abortions occur after 7–8 weeks' gestation (3, p 417, 5, p 22).

Main classifications of spontaneous abortion are as follows (5, p 26):

1. Threatened: pregnancy loss is possible, but the pregnancy may continue without further complications.
2. Inevitable: the pregnancy cannot be salvaged.
3. Incomplete: products of conception have been passed, but some—usually the placenta—remain.
4. Complete: all products of conception have been expelled.

Other classifications include the following:

1. Missed: retention of a dead fetus for more than 8 weeks.
2. Early: pregnancy loss before 12 weeks' gestation.
3. Late: pregnancy loss between 12 and 20 weeks' gestation.

Etiology

In many cases the etiology is unknown or multifactorial in nature. However, specific factors have been associated with pregnancy loss and can be classified according to maternal, fetal, and uterine categories. Almost all of the chronic, systemic diseases or infectious processes discussed in this book are associated with increased incidence of pregnancy loss, including endocrine disorders, blood group incompatibility, radiation, trauma, pyelonephritis, or bacterial or viral infection. Specific microorganisms that are well known to increase risk of spontaneous abortion

Table 24.2.

CHROMOSOMAL STATUS OF FIRST-TRIMESTER ABORTIONS[a]

COMPLEMENT		
46,XX or 46,XY		54.5%
Abnormal		45.5%
Autosomal trisomy		20.7%
No. 16	9.9%	
No. 22	2.8%	
No. 21	2.6%	
No. 15	2.4%	
Other	3.0%	
Triploidy		7.8%
Tetraploidy		2.6%
Monosomy X		8.6%
Sex chromosome polysomy (XXY, XXX, XYY)		0.6%
Structural abnormalities		1.5%

[a]Reprinted with permission from Simpson S. What management for repeated abortions? *Contemp. OB/GYN,* p 103, June, 1985.

include *Brucella, Toxoplasma gondii, Mycoplasma hominis, Chlamydia trachomatis,* and *Ureaplasma urealyticum. Ureaplasma urealyticum* is the most frequent cause, and chronic, undiagnosed infection may lead to repeated abortion.

Life-style habits such as smoking and drug abuse increase the risk of pregnancy loss. Smoking increases the risk of spontaneous abortion 1.4 times in the general population (see Chapter 19).

Abnormalities of the uterus, such as leiomyomas, bicornuate uterus, and incompetent cervix, increase the abortion rate. A pregnancy coexisting with an IUCD in situ will be expelled in approximately 50% of cases.

Abnormal fetal development, such as blighted ovum or severe chromosal anomalies incompatible with life, are diagnosed in many spontaneous abortions and probably constitute a natural species-protective mechanism (3, p 419).

In the first trimester more than 50% of spontaneous abortions are the result of chromosomal abnormalities. Table 24.2 details the most frequent chromosomal abnormalities found. When abortion becomes repeated or habitual, specific subsets of the above-mentioned factors are implicated (Table 24.3).

Signs and Symptoms

Signs and symptoms include varying degrees of severity of uterine cramping, vaginal bleeding, low back pain, and passage of the products of conception (2, p 106, 4, p 135). Table 24.4 lists these signs and symptoms according to type.

Table 24.3.
SIGNIFICANT CAUSES OF HABITUAL
ABORTION[a]

Endocrine disorders
  Diabetes
  Thyroid Disease
  Reproductive hormone deficit (e.g. luteal phase)
Infection
  Ureaplasma urealyticum
Autoimmune disorders
  Lupus erythematous
Uterine defects
  Submucous leiomyoma
  Adhesion
  Bicornate uterus
Incompetent cervix
Chromosomal abnormalities
  Numerous fetal abnormalities (i.e., aneuploidy)
    parental translocation or inversion

[a]Adapted from Simpson J. What management for repeated abortion? *Contemp. OB·GYN*, p 100, June, 1985.

Diagnosis

Diagnosis is based on history, physical examination, and laboratory findings. A history of previous second trimester fetal loss without contractions is usually considered diagnostic of incompetent cervix. Differential diagnoses of bleeding in pregnancy also includes malignancy, cervicitis, ectopic pregnancy, and hydatidiform mole.

A thorough history will elicit the presence and the severity of signs and symptoms of spontaneous abortion, as well as the progression of symptoms over time. It is important to carefully reevaluate the gestational age of the fetus and the growth to date. An abdominal examination that reveals a regressing uterine size and/or absence of fetal heart tones by doppler after 12 weeks is indicative of a missed abortion. Pelvic evaluation—including speculum and bimanual examination—will confirm the amount of bleeding, passage of tissue, dilation of the cervical os, and documentation of uterine size (5, p 22).

After 8 weeks' gestation, sonography (B scan or real time) can identify the gestational sac and confirm fetal motion—a sign that all is still within normal limits. It should be noted that presence of a gestational sac in the uterus rules out ectopic pregnancy except in those rare cases (1 out of 10,000) where an ectopic pregnancy coexists with an intrauterine pregnancy. Sonography before 8 weeks' gestation is very inaccurate, and failure to find a gestational sac or to document fetal movement are not prognostic indicators (7).

Serum radioimmunoassay of beta-subunit HCG is a highly sensitive diagnostic tool. Production of HCG rises rapidly in early pregnancy, peaks at 10 weeks' gestation, and then falls to 10% of first trimester levels for the rest of the pregnancy. Figure 24.3 details the rate of HCG production during pregnancy. HCG levels in early pregnancy should double every 2.2 days. Thus, serial HCG levels that do double are reliable indicators of a favorable prognosis (5, p 22).

Maternal and Fetal Outcome

Psychological as well as physical maternal complications may occur. It has been shown that spontaneous abortion results in as much grief reaction as the loss of a full-term pregnancy or neonatal death (see Chapter 3). A questionnaire has been developed to help elicit maternal grief reaction (see Table 24.5). It should be noted that repeated episodes of weeping (six or more times) has been associated with development of significant clinical depression. Inability to carry a pregnancy may carry with it guilt or disturbance in self esteem or feminine role performance.

Table 24.4.
SYMPTOMS OF ABORTION BY TYPE[a]

TYPE	BLEEDING	CONTRACTIONS	UTERINE SIZE	CERVICAL OS	EXPULSION	PROGNOSIS
Threatened	Slight	Slight	Compatible with dates	Closed		Variable with therapy
Inevitable	Moderate	Moderate	Compatible with dates	Dilated		Poor
Incomplete	Heavy	Strong	Compatible with dates	Open	Tissue	Poor
Complete	Diminished	Stop	Decreases to normal prepregnancy state	Open/closed	Fetus	Poor
Missed	Initially absent/ delayed, severe	None	Slowly decreases over months	Closed		Negative

[a]Reprinted with permission from Perez R. *Perinatal Nursing Practice*. St. Louis: C.V. Mosby Company, 1981, p 106.

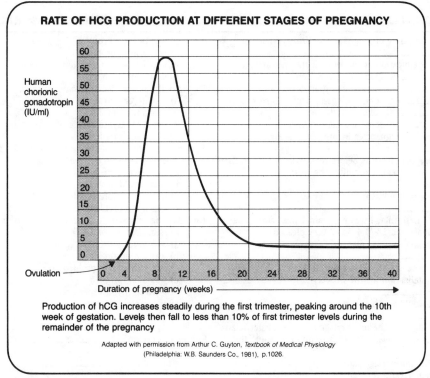

RATE OF HCG PRODUCTION AT DIFFERENT STAGES OF PREGNANCY

Human chorionic gonadotropin (IU/ml)

Ovulation

Duration of pregnancy (weeks)

Production of hCG increases steadily during the first trimester, peaking around the 10th week of gestation. Levels then fall to less than 10% of first trimester levels during the remainder of the pregnancy

Adapted with permission from Arthur C. Guyton, *Textbook of Medical Physiology* (Philadelphia: W.B. Saunders Co., 1981), p.1026.

Figure 24.3. Rate of HCG production at different stages of pregnancy. (From *Diagnostics.* Springhouse, PA, Nurse's Reference Library, p. 191.)

Maternal physical complications include hemorrhage and the possibility of superimposed disseminated intravascular coagulation, uterine infection, septicemia, or calcification of a missed abortion (uterine lithopedion). If the mother has had at least one live-born infant, her risk of repeat abortion is approximately 25–30%. However, the risk rises to 40% if the mother has had no live-born children (5, p 22).

About half of all pregnancies exhibiting signs and symptoms of threatened abortion progress to inevitable abortion, and the pregnancy is lost. However, the other half of the cases exhibiting signs of threatened abortion are salvaged and progress to term with no further complications (4, p 134).

Medical Management

Treatment of incompetent cervix is surgical and involves reinforcing the cervix with a "purse-string" suture. The suture can be removed at term when labor begins.

In all other cases of threatened abortion, management is palliative, including (1, p 32; 7, p 364):

1. Rest *in bed*.

2. Pelvic rest (no sexual intercourse, no douching, and no insertion of anything into the vagina).

3. Prompt reporting of any of the following: increased vaginal bleeding, passage of clots/tissue, gush of fluid, fever, uterine cramping, and back pain.

As long as the patient is symtomatic, weekly or biweekly office visits should be scheduled to document progressive uterine growth and evaluate worsening symptoms or the possibility of missed abortion. Serial complete blood counts should be done to evaluate hematologic status over time and to observe for evidence of infection. C-reactive protein also may be used to detect infection and is a more timely indicator of infection than a rising white blood cell count (5, p 24).

In all cases of fetal death or incomplete or inevitable abortion, the uterus should be evacuated immediately in order to prevent hemorrhage and infection. Controversy centers around whether the emptying of the uterine cavity should be allowed to occur naturally or should be assisted medically. Often, women who are thought to have a "complete" spontaneous

Table 24.5.

EVALUATION OF WOMEN'S PERCEPTIONS OF FIRST TRIMESTER SPONTANEOUS ABORTION[a]

1. Age at the time of pregnancy and miscarriage.
   _____

2. Level of education at the time of the miscarriage:
   _____ a) grade level completed
   _____ b) high school graduate
   _____ c) some college or professional school
   _____ d) college graduate
   _____ e) some graduate school

3. Number of pregnancies before the miscarriage.
   _____

4. Number of live births before miscarriage. _____

5. Number of pregnancies after the miscarriage.
   _____

6. Number of live births after the miscarriage.
   _____

7. When I first knew I was pregnant I was (circle one)
   disappointed 1 2 3 4 5 6 7 very pleased

8. The pregnancy was "planned." Yes _____
   No _____

9. Did you have a roommate during your
   hospitalization for the miscarriage? Yes _____
   No _____

10. If yes, would you have preferred to be alone?
    Yes _____ No _____

11. How long after the miscarriage did your obstetrician
    suggest you wait before becoming pregnant? (fill
    in) _____

12. After the miscarriage *sadness*
    a) was never a problem
    b) was a mild problem
    c) was a moderate problem
    d) was a big problem

13. After the miscarriage *sleeping*
    a) was never a problem
    b) was a mild problem
    c) was a moderate problem
    d) was a big problem

14. After the miscarriage *eating*
    a) was never a problem
    b) was a mild problem
    c) was a moderate problem
    d) was a big problem

15. After the miscarriage *preoccupation, thinking and
    dreaming about the baby*

    a) was never a problem
    b) was a mild problem
    c) was a moderate problem
    d) was a big problem

16. After the miscarriage *my own irritability*
    a) was never a problem
    b) was a mild problem
    c) was a moderate problem
    d) was a big problem

17. After the miscarriage *thinking I had done something
    to cause the miscarriage*
    a) was never a problem
    b) was a mild problem
    c) was a moderate problem
    d) was a big problem

18. After the miscarriage *anger (at self, husband,
    nurses, doctors, or God)*
    a) was never a problem
    b) was a mild problem
    c) was a moderate problem
    d) was a big problem

19. Please check if you experienced any of the following
    after your miscarriage.

	Yes	No	Comments
Episodes of crying	_____	_____	_____
Praying for baby	_____	_____	_____
Depression	_____	_____	_____
Couldn't believe what had happened	_____	_____	_____
Wanted to be left alone	_____	_____	_____

20. Compared with before the pregnancy, after the
    miscarriage my husband and I became
    closer 1 2 3 4 5 6 7 more distant

21. Additional comments or anecdotes around the time
    of your miscarriage that you might think useful in
    conveying your feelings would be appreciated.

[a]Adapted from Wall-Haas C. Women's perceptions of first trimester abortion. *JOGN,* 14: 22–28, 1985.

abortion continue to bleed or become febrile—both sequelae of retained fetal/placental tissue.

Many obstetric authorities support instrumental evacuation of all spontaneous abortions. Evacuation in early abortions can be done on an outpatient basis and requires only suction curettage (5, p 22).

Late terminations carry with them increased maternal risks of hemorrhage, and hospitalization is indicated. Dilation and sharp curettage will be used. However, curettage should be gentle in order to avoid denuding the endometrium, thus causing adhesions that destroy sites for future implantation.

Cervical and endometrial culture and sensitivity to detect infection should be done routinely for every case. Diagnosed infection must be treated vigorously in both partners. Doxycycline (250 mg four times a day for 10 days) is the treatment of choice for *Ureaplasma urealyticum*. In fact, many clinicians treat couples prophylactically after spontaneous abortion. Tissue from the evacuation is sent to pathology in order to assess presence of chorionic villi (indicating presence of fetal tissue) and to evaluate chromosomal composition. Hematologic studies to be done include:

1. Complete blood count to assess for anemia and infection.
2. Type and cross match to evaluate Rh status and to be prepared for transfusion in case of hemorrhage or low baseline hematocrit/hemoglobin.
3. Coagulation studies in missed abortions to detect disseminated intravascular coagulation (see Chapter 8).

All Rh-negative women who are unsensitized should receive an Rh immunoglobulin injection within 72 hours to prevent future hemolytic disease of the newborn (see Chapter 29).

The health care team must support the patient and her significant others in grieving the loss of the pregnancy. The patient's plans for future pregnancy should be discussed. If the patient desires another pregnancy, contraception for 4–6 months will allow the uterine lining to regenerate and will help ensure the optimal environment. Counseling regarding cessation of life-style habits (i.e., smoking or drug use) that predispose to spontaneous abortion is important. If any genetic defect in the abortus was diagnosed, the patient must be informed, referred for genetic screening, and made aware of the possibility (if any) of future recurrence.

Nutritional status should be evaluated carefully, including presence of anemia. The goal is to optimize maternal status before the next pregnancy. If the patient is anemic, iron therapy is begun immediately after the abortion.

The patient should return for evaluation 2 weeks after the abortion occurred. Until that appointment, the patient is instructed to maintain pelvic rest (i.e., refrain from vaginal intercourse, douching, tampons). At the follow-up appointment, if the uterus is normal size, firm, and nontender, the patient will be able to choose a contraceptive method. A barrier method is preferable since it will allow normal hormonal functioning. If the birth control pill is chosen, the patient must be instructed to discontinue it at least 3 months before she plans to conceive in order to ensure that the fetus is not affected by the exogenous hormones.

The patient should be instructed in the importance of early prenatal care and to return for a pregnancy test at the first sign or symptom of pregnancy.

NURSING MANAGEMENT

Nursing care specific for *threatened abortion*:
☐ When abortion is threatened, teach the importance of:
  — REST IN BED;
  — Pelvic rest;
  — Prompt reporting of increased vaginal bleeding, passage of clots/tissue, gush of fluid, fever, uterine cramping, and back pain; and
  — Collection of tissue/clots passed.
☐ Ensure that all women who abort spontaneously are tested for Rh type and that all Rh-negative unsensitized women receive an Rh immunoglobulin injection within 72 hours.
☐ Educate the patient who aborts spontaneously regarding:
  — The course of normal recovery and the importance of reporting any deviation (fever, excessive bleeding, foul-smelling lochia, or back/abdominal pain);
  — The need for contraception for 4–6 months before attempting another pregnancy in order to allow for full maternal recovery, including regeneration of an optimum uterine lining;
  — Potential outcomes of future pregnancies; and
  — The need for gynecologic follow-up examination in 2–3 weeks.
☐ Ensure that the products of conception are sent for genetic evaluation, if appropriate, and that the patient receives the results of it.
☐ Advise patients with repeated pregnancy loss to seek preconception evaluation to try to determine and treat the cause.

Nursing diagnoses most frequently associated with *spontaneous abortion* (see Section V):
☐ Anxiety/fear.
☐ Grieving related to actual/potential loss of infant or birth of an imperfect child.
☐ Disturbance in body image, self-esteem.
☐ Knowledge deficit regarding etiology, disease process, treatment, and outcome.
☐ Pain.
☐ Altered maternal tissue perfusion.

REFERENCES

1. Neeson J, Stockdale C: *The Practitioner's Handbook of Ob/Gyn.* New York, John Wiley and Sons, 1981, p 36.
2. Perez R: *Protocols for Perinatal Practice.* St. Louis, Mosby, 1981, p 107.
3. Buckley KA, Kulb NW: *Handbook of Maternal-Newborn Nursing.* New York, John Wiley and Sons, 1983, p 412.
4. Varney H. *Nurse-Midwifery* (2nd ed.) Boston: Blackwell Scientific Publications, 1987, p 133.
5. Friedman E: *Obstetric Decision Making.* St. Louis, Mosby, 1982.
6. Pritchard J, MacDonald PC, Gant NF: *Williams Obstetrics,* ed 17. Norwalk, CT, Appleton-Century-Crofts, 1985, p 431.
7. Nursing Reference Library: *Diagnostics.* Springhouse, PA, Springhouse, 1986, p 192.

Chapter 25
Congenital Anomalies
Margherita Modica Hawkins, R.N., M.S.

INTRODUCTION

Throughout recorded time—in literature, art, and historical writings—man has chronicled his fascination with the mysteries of congenital defects. Only in the past 15–20 years, as much has become known about the basis of human genetic disorders, has the subject been approached with any clarity. Intense study has led to discoveries, which, in turn, has led to the development of a new field—prenatal diagnosis. Advances such as karyotyping and gene mapping have greatly enhanced our capcity to understand and predict the occurrence of genetic abnormalities. Currently, the list of detectable metabolic, biochemical, and structural genetic abnormalities approaches 200.

Today, advances in medical science are front page news. As a result, the public has developed a sophisticated body of knowledge, often of esoteric and highly expensive treatments, and individuals have come to expect those treatments when they seek health care. Also, recent court decisions awarding huge sums to plaintiffs because of health care providers' failures to employ certain testing have increased demand for services. This creates a special problem for the field, since expansion requires complex equipment and highly trained personnel, all of which cannot be acquired rapidly.

There is another point to consider here. Americans are having fewer babies; instead, they expect a perfect outcome for the pregnancies/children they do have. To ensure that end, many families take full advantage of newer technologies. This approach has pitted them against other segments of society that abhor manipulation of the reproductive process. There is, then, an open controversy as to the advisability of employing prenatal diagnosis, continuing biological research, and applying genetic engineer-

ing techniques. Such issues are far beyond the pages in this chapter, but the nurse must keep them in mind when caring for patients.

PRENATAL DIAGNOSIS

Simply stated, prenatal diagnosis is the detection of selected abnormalities before birth based upon results of certain examinations of the mother and/or conceptus. The objectives of such a process are to provide the patients with information that will allow them to make better preparations and decisions about their pregnancies.

Genetic counseling is a process whereby an individual receives information about possible genetic risks in childbearing and the results of testing so as to make informed decisions. The counselor usually is a person who has had specialty training in this field.

Referral for genetic counseling can be made either by a health care provider who suspects that an individual might carry a greater than normal risk for a particular problem or by the individual.

Increasingly, individuals are seeking this service in preparation for marriage or pregnancy as a screening that might uncover problems before a union is formed.

Essentially, the counseling session occurs between the counselor and the individual(s) concerned. A family history is taken, drawing upon data gleaned from a variety of places: memory, birth certificate data, medical records, family chronicles such as a family tree in a family bible, and any other sources available; family members and friends may be brought in to complete the history. The probable risks of having an affected child are outlined, options for genetic testing are discussed, and the tests themselves are described.

If any testing is done, the counselor then may provide support as indicated during the procedures. Afterward, the counselor provides support during the anxiety-producing waiting period until results are known and then provides information once the results are received. Difficult decisions often are made during these times, and it is not unusual for the counselor to provide support long afterward. Bereavement counseling, in particular, falls into this support classification as individuals grieve the loss of the perfect child. In some instances patients may require more intensive support, in which case the counselor draws upon other members of the health team.

PROCEDURES

The following procedures are used to determine congenital anomalies (1–6) (see also Chapter 6.)

X-ray

Because of the development of other technologies that do not convey the risks of harm to the fetus from radiation, this method of visualization of the fetus is not often used. It is used, however, in cases where no other method is available or when the mother has another medical problem that can be diagnosed properly only by x-ray. Such an indication might be renal obstruction, requiring an intravenous pyelogram (IVP). The patient should be informed of the possible risks versus benefits; these risks vary according to gestational age of the pregnancy and may not be as deleterious as once thought.

Ultrasound

By far, this is the most widely used method to detect structual and some functional abnormalities in the fetus. Recent technological developments have resulted in high resolution real-time scanners that are capable of a high degree of diagnostic accuracy. While there has been concern as to its safety, no harm has been demonstrated, despite investigative studies that include longitudinal follow-up data spanning some 8 years or more. The national consensus report prepared by a panel of experts who reviewed all the findings concluded that this test is safe and should be used where indicated for improved patient management.

Amniocentesis

When performed properly under the guidance of ultrasonography, this procedure carries a 0.5–1.5% risk of spontaneous abortion, fetal death, trauma, perinatal morbidity, or infection (4).

Patients should be counseled about the potential risks. Decisions to proceed with testing are made after weighing the risks of having an affected child against the risk of this or any other invasive procedures.

Maternal Blood Sampling

Recent studies have shown that from 80–85% of open neural tube defects can be detected by elevated alpha-fetoprotein (AFP) levels in the maternal serum. Therefore, the FDA has approved the marketing of testing kits to be used by laboratories. This approval initially met with some controversy from organized medicine, which felt that the testing mechanism itself, with the high rate of 1.2% positive from which only one in three actually will have a defect, required that the testing center have a coordinated team of obstetrician, laboratory, medical geneticist, and ultrasonographer able to execute a complicated protocol in order to avoid undue anxiety and needless overtesting (5).

At the time of this writing it is safe to say that since the test is available, it is used frequently, at least in those populations at the highest risk of having an affected child. Some experts advocate using it as a routine screening test since a rather large percentage of these defects are de novo—that is, there is no family history to suggest an increased risk.

Fetoscopy

This highly invasive procedure has, in the past decade, come to be used in the detection of some 50 genetic abnormalities. The risks include abortion (6.7%), trauma to the mother or fetus, infection, leakage of fluid, and prematurity (8%) (6).

Because of its value in providing access to the fetus for blood sampling, examination, and skin and liver biopsy, it has become widely adopted. Its use, however, should be in the hands of skilled operators so as to minimize the risk. It is also believed that the procedure will become even more important in the application of fetal therapies, such as the administration of drugs or nutrients.

Chorionic Villi Sampling

Probably the most exciting breakthrough in this field has been the development of chorionic villi sampling (CVS) for first trimester prenatal diagnosis. For the obvious reasons that this testing provides earlier information, both because it can be done earlier and because the test results can be obtained within a couple of days rather than weeks, it is being hailed as a virtual replacement for amniocentesis. At this time, the procedure is not widely available. This is a highly invasive and delicate procedure that requires a skilled operator to minimize the risk of spontaneous abortion that goes with the test *and* this stage of gestation. Patients who opt for this testing must be fully aware of the risks and weigh that against the benefits of early information. As long as an adequate amount of material has been recovered from the products of conception, the results virtually are 100% accurate.

FORMS OF INHERITANCE

All defects that appear at or date from the time of birth are called congenital. That does not mean, though, that they are inherited in terms of being passed from parent to child. For example, a disorder that results from a teratogenic insult either to the gamete or conceptus, such as in x-radiation exposure, does not confer parental inheritance in the strictest sense. Another example would be one of de novo mutation, which is labeled as such when there is no parental explanation for the occurrence. This latter one is a problem since the triggers of this process are not known; conceivably, an undetected teratogen was at work or a yet-to-be-discovered gene was responsible.

Transmission of defects from parent to child usually occurs either through chromosomal abnormalities, such as trisomy, or in the passage of a single gene that causes the disorder, as in Tay-Sachs disease. In this section some of the more commonly seen disorders are outlined. In order to assist the reader, a glossary of terms is provided (see p 283).

CHROMOSOMAL ABNORMALITIES

This category of congenital defects accounts for a major portion of reproductive waste or inefficiency, such as in spontaneous abortion, stillbirth, neonatal death, and so on. By extrapolation of survey data, it has been suggested that 0.59% of all births have such a defect.

Classification of Chromosomal Changes

1. *Numerical.* Also called aneuploidy, this condition is evidenced by either fewer or greater than the required two in a pair. There can be none (nullisomy) of a pair, one (monosomy), or more (polysomy: trisomy, tetrasomy, etc.).

2. *Structural.* Aberrations can occur either in the number of genes in a chromosome (deletion, duplication) or to the location of genes in a chromosome (inversion, translocation).

3. *Mosaicism.* This disorder arises from an abnormal process in meiosis, producing an individual with a mixed genotype.

Relationship to Spontaneous Abortion

It was once thought that spontaneous abortion largely resulted from the body's rejection of an abnormal conceptus. Recent large-scale study has demonstrated that only 42.3% of abortions in recognized pregnancies showed abnormal karyotypes (7). Thus, it has been suggested that environmental factors, such as low socioeconomic status, play a large role in chromosomally normal abortions, particularly in younger women. It is interesting to note that the same study showed a higher proportion of trisomic abortions in patients under private care as opposed to those in public clinics. Also noted was a decreasing gestational age of the conceptus at time of abortion as the maternal age increased.

Relationship to Advanced Maternal Age

The higher incidence of spontaneous abortions in older women has been thought to result basically from natural selection and rejection of chromosomally abnormal conceptuses. However, this has not been supported in work on spontaneous abortuses wherein the same rejection patterns were found across all ages (8,9). Certainly, the incidence of chromosomal abnormalities rises dramatically after the age of 35, most specifically with the incidence of trisomies. The most common is trisomy 21, but the others, including trisomy 13, trisomy 18, and Klinefelter's syndrome (XXY), also occur more often in this group.

The exact reason why these abnormalities occur more often with advancing age is not clearly understood. It had been suggested that the ovum, which was formed in utero, is old and therefore subject to disintegration. However, that theory no longer stands against newer findings regarding continually generated sperm cells. Recent evidence has shown that 20% of trisomy 21 cases can be attributed to the paternal source. Whether the paternal source is a function of advanced age has not, however, been established, because unions of individuals customarily occur at comparable ages, thereby making it difficult to isolate the paternal age factors. More research is needed to determine what mechanisms cause the aging effect in female and male germ cells.

The search for an understanding of causes will continue. New lines of inquiry will widen in scope as more is learned about genetics. For example, in today's environmentally conscious society, many have come to believe that exposure to certain toxins has made man vulnerable to a host of carcinogens and chromosomally toxic agents. With that understanding in mind, could it be suggested that increasing exposure over one's lifetime could contribute to the inceasing risk of abnormalities associated with higher ages?

While the search for a cause continues, so does the pursuit of methods that can help couples face this increased risk by giving them knowledge and alternatives through prenatal diagnosis.

The Expression of Chromosomal Disorders

While in theory there is an infinite number of possible chromosomal aberrations, only a small number actually are seen. The majority are essentially incompatible with life and therefore expelled, largely before pregnancy is even suspected. Of the few remaining to delivery, some are extremely rare. Table 25.1 describes those most commonly seen, along with information the nurse might find helpful in working with this group (10–12).

AUTOSOMAL DOMINANT DISORDERS

This is a category of single gene inheritance wherein the characteristic, or condition, is expressed in every generation. An affected individual will pass that characteristic/condition on to about half of his or her offspring. An unaffected child will not transmit the trait. This form of inheritance appears with equal frequency in both sexes. New mutations of many dominant conditions can appear in a family, thereby establishing it within that line. Table 25.2 describes some conditions of clinical significance.

AUTOSOMAL RECESSIVE DISORDERS

In this form of single gene inheritance, a particular trait appears in the individual's genotype but is not expressed in the progeny unless there is mating with another individual who carries the trait. Each offspring of the pairing has about a 25% chance of getting the trait expressed, a 50% chance of carrying the trait, and a 25% chance of being free of it. This form of inheritance occurs equally in both sexes; parents of an affected child often are consanguineous. Table 25.3 describes some conditions of clinical significance (10–12).

X-LINKED RECESSIVE SYNDROMES

This is a more complex form of inheritance, where a trait is passed from an affected father through all his daughters, who pass it on to about half their sons. The nature of sex chromosomes actually dictates how this disorder appears. Each parent carries 22 autosomes plus a sex chromosome; the female gamete is always 22 + X, the male gamete 22 + X or Y. X chromosomes usually carry a lot of genetic information; the Y carries little, mainly maleness. When an X carries a particular trait, that trait can be suppressed if it is matched with another X that does not carry it. However, when the father contributes a Y chromosome, the trait is not counterbalanced, and the condition thereby is expressed. Table 25.4 describes some conditions of clinical significance (10–13).

OPEN NEURAL TUBE DEFECTS

A category of congenital malformations arises when the neural tube fails to close around the 25–28th day in embryonic development.

Upper end openings produce anencephaly; lower end openings cause spina bifida. The cause is considered to be multifactorial, arising from a combination of genetic predisposition toward slow closure and environmental factors. The incidence is 2 in 1000 live births in the United States; the rate is 10 times higher in the United Kingdom. In the United States 95% occur in the absence of a family history of the disorder; the recurrence risk for siblings of affected individuals is 2–3% (3, 14–16).

Table 25.1.
CHROMOSOMAL ABNORMALITIES

SYNDROME	INCIDENCE	PRENATAL DIAGNOSIS	EXPRESSION	OUTCOME
Trisomy 13 (Patau)	1:7000–20000 (advanced maternal age a factor)	Yes: amniocentesis, CVS	Severe CNS malformations, growth retardation, sloping forehead, ocular hypertelorism, cleft lip and palate, polydactyly, clenched fists, rocker-bottom feet, cardiac and urogenital defects	50% live-born infants die within the first month
Trisomy 18 (Edwards)	1:8000 (advanced maternal age a factor)	Yes: amniocentesis, CVS	Mental retardation, failure to thrive, prominent occiput, receding jaw, lowset/malformed ears, clenched fists, rocker-bottom feet, simian creases, arch patterns on fingers, hypoplastic nails, severe cardiac defects	95% abort spontaneously; live-born infant survival about 2 months
Trisomy 21 (Down)	Advances with maternal age: 1:1923 at age 20, 1:32 at age 45	Yes: amniocentesis, CVS	Variable: hypotonia, low set ears, epicanthic folds, low nasal bridge, protruding tongue, among other facial deformities: short, broad hands, simian crease; mental retardation; cardiac defects, leukemia	Depending upon expression, can have life span to 40 years
Turner (46,XO; also XXX, XXXX)	1:5000 live births	Yes: amniocentesis, CVS	Appear as females; sterile; short stature, abnormal jaws, webbed neck, shield-like chest; unexplained hypertension	Normal life span if hypertension does not intervene
Klinefelter (46,XXY; also XXYY, XXXY, XXXXY, XXXXXY)	1:500 individuals	Yes: amniocentesis, CVS	Appear as males, with tendency toward femaleness; sterile; underdeveloped testes and prostate, scanty body hair, enlarged breasts; mental retardation higher in those with higher numbers of sex chromosomes	Life span presumably normal
XYY	1:1000	Yes: amniocentesis, CVS	Normal males, somewhat taller	Recent research has found this group to be more prevalent in prison, but link to criminality not established.

Prenatal detection can be made by ultrasonography and screening for AFP levels. AFP is a protein substance synthesized by the yolk sac and, later, the fetal liver and gastrointestinal tract. Excreted in the fetal urine, it can be recovered from the amniotic fluid and, upon its diffusion, in the maternal serum. Diagnosis by AFP measurement is complicated. Usually, AFP levels are markedly higher in the presence of open neural tube defects. However, elevations also can occur in multiple gestations, inaccurate gestational dating, abdominal wall defects, and fetal demise, among others. In addition, some defects that are encapsulated by skin may not release elevated AFP amounts.

Because 95% of cases occur in the absence of family history, routine maternal serum screening has been advocated strongly (15). There is opposition to this, though, since the test currently available has a high proportion of false-positives, which therefore produce needless anxiety in families. Table 25.5 lists the full five-part screening program that should be followed in turn with a positive finding at each level.

As mentioned above, the United Kingdom has a high incidence of defects. Clinical research there has shown that dietary folic acid deficiencies before or during early pregnancy were linked to a higher incidence of this malformation. Trials of vitamin supplementation suggested that this incidence

Table 25.2.

AUTOSOMAL DOMINANT DISORDERS

DISORDER	CLINICAL FINDINGS/COMMENTS
Marfan syndrome	Elongated extremities, dislocation of the lens, cardiovascular anomalies, reduced subcutaneous tissue, muscle hypoplasia, inguinal hernia, and lung cysts. Life span is variable, with early death reported from cardiac disorder.
Cleft lip/palate	Usually, the cause is unknown or multifactorial. However, in some cases combination with "lip pits" or filiform fusion of eyelids conveys autosomal dominant transmission. Plastic surgery is treatment; life span not affected.
Heart-hand syndrome	The cardiac anomaly is usually atrial septal defect in two-thirds of cases, with others including patent ductus arteriosus, coarctation of aorta, ventricular septal defect, transposition of great vessels. Skeletal anomalies are of the upper limb, usually thumb hypoplasia, triphalangism or absence, and phocomilia. Life span and function depend upon severity of cardiac and bone anomalies.
Achondroplasia	Short limb dwarfism characterized by large head with bulging forehead, "scooped-out" nasal bridge, shallow thoracic cage. Motor development delayed, intelligence usually normal. Life span is normal in the absence of complications that stem from spinal cord compression.

could be lowered. Upon evaluation of the data, problems with the study design were identified, which hindered the applicability of findings to the United States population. However, since the United Kingdom diet is very low in fresh fruits and vegetables, it was felt that the research was valid for that population. A completely randomized study would be necessary in the United States before vitamin supplementation could become standard practice here (16).

TERATOGENESIS

A teratogen can be defined as an agent that causes the formation of abnormal structure in a developing embryo. The understanding of teratogenesis has broadened in the past two decades as much has been discovered regarding substances that cause disordered development. Although there is a growing body of knowledge, much is yet to be learned. Traditionally, investigators have used both epidemiological study and animal experimentation upon which to base conclusions about particular agents. In analyzing the former method, firm cause and effect relationships are elusive, resulting in conclusions based upon strong associations. In the latter, it must be kept in mind that results from experiments on one species may not be applicable to others. The most classic example of that is the case of thalidomide, where testing upon lower animals found no effect, but it was devastating to humans. There is considered opinion, however, that positive animal results can justify their use as predictors of human effects (17).

For the purposes of this review, the teratogenic agents are divided as follows: macroenvironmental (including occupational exposure), microenvironmental (mainly recreational drugs), and therapeutic. Since microenvironmental substances are covered in Chapter 19 and therapeutic agents under the various chapters that cover specific disorders, this section deals with the effects of macroenvironmental exposure.

Heavy Metals (17–21)

Mercury

Used in industry as an antifungal agent, this metal has the greatest potential for embryotoxicity and teratogenicity. Fetal exposure through accidental poisonings causes brain damage and neuromuscular defects. Mercury crosses the placenta easily by facilitated diffusion and binds tightly, with a four times greater concentration in the fetal brain. It also reaches the newborn in breast milk.

Lead

This metal is embryotoxic, fetotoxic, and teratogenic on the central nervous system. It has been associated with an increased rate of spontaneous abortions, low birth weight, brain damage, and an increase in premature rupture of membranes. Lead has been found to collect in the placenta, with higher concentrations on the maternal side. Men exposed occupationally have been found to have decreased fertility; women exposed at work are subject to sterility, spontaneous abortion, and fetal and neonatal loss.

Cadmium

Not well documented for teratogenicity and fetotoxicity, this agent has been found to be re-

Table 25.3.
AUTOSOMAL RECESSIVE DISORDERS

DISORDERS	PRENATAL DIAGNOSIS	MECHANISM	CLINICAL COURSE AND TREATMENT
Galactosemia	Yes: amniocentesis	Absence of galactose-1-phosphate uridyl transferase, resulting in inability to convert galactose into glucose	Symptoms develop upon milk feedings. Untreated, death is inevitible after a course of vomiting, jaundice and sepsis-like symptoms. With treatment, life span should be normal.
Tay-Sachs	Yes: amniocentesis	Absence of hexosaminidase A allows accumulation of fatty deposits in brain, causing gradual diminution of function	Appears around 6 months of age; by 18 months blindness, paralysis, lack of cognition. Treatment is merely palliative. Death usually is around 3–4 years.
Glycogen storage disease	Yes: amniocentesis	Inability to store glycogen	Grave course, including lethargy, coma, convulsions, sweating, poor feeding and weight gain, microcephaly, delayed motor development. Even with diet treatment, prognosis is not good.
Maple syrup urine disease	Yes: amniocentesis	Deficiency of branded-chain ketoacid decarboxylase with abnormally high concentrations of leucine and other amino acids in blood	Onset usually by end of first week with feeding difficulty, vomiting, shrill cry, and characteristic odor of urine. Neurologic signs leading to convulsions, coma, and death. Early, vigilant dietary treatment can save life.
Phenylketonuria	Yes: amniocentesis	Absence of liver enzyme causes accumulation of phenylalanine in brain	Undetected, mental retardation and seizures with a reduced life span. Early detection can allow for palliative dietary treatment and normal life span.
Cystic fibrosis	Yes: amniocentesis	Dysfunction of exocrine glands that produce abnormal secretions	Excessive sweat electrolytes, pancreatic insufficiency, chronic pulmonary disease, and cirrhosis of liver. With supportive treatment, may live into adulthood.
Sickle cell anemia	Yes: fetal blood by fetoscopy	Malformed sickle-shaped red blood cells become clogged flowing through blood vessels, thereby causing loss of circulation	Classic signs of anemia: paleness, fatigue, shortness of breath, low resistance to infection. Treatment is palliative; repeated severe crises can be fatal.
Thalassemias	Yes: fetal blood by fetoscopy	Class of diseases with disordered erythropoiesis and a major hemolytic component	Classic signs of anemia, varying in degrees, requiring exchange transfusions. This therapy can lead to cardiac or liver failure from overload of iron. Survival upwards of 20 years.

tained by the fetus in the liver and kidneys. It has been associated with craniofacial defects and is bound in breast milk. Industrial exposure has been linked to chromosomal breaks and other damages.

Nickel

Neonatal death and structural birth defects have been associated with this metal.

Pesticides (17–20, 22)

Dioxins

The main human exposure to these substances has been to its form as a contaminant of the defoliant "Agent Orange" when it was used in Vietnam. It is known as a powerful teratogen in animal models, but its effect upon humans has not been proven (23).

Table 25.4.
X-LINKED SYNDROMES

DISORDER	CLINICAL FINDINGS/COMMENTS
Hemophilia	Type A: Caused by the production of disordered factor VIII, which is essential to the clotting process, this disease is characterized by excessive bleeding into the tissues after even slight trauma. Bleeding into the joints is common, and crippling may occur in severest forms. Treatment is replacement therapy, which is usually successful in allowing relatively normal life.
	Type B: Resulting from decreased or disordered production of factor IX, this is often a milder disease with clinical manifestations similar to type A. Replacement therapy permits ability to live a long and active life.
Duchenne muscular dystrophy	This disease of progressive muscle weakness can be seen as early as the age of 3, but occurrence is more usual around 6 or 7. The child usually is confined to a wheelchair by age 10 or 11; death generally occurs around age 20 from pulmonary infection or cardiac failure. Intelligence is about 10% lower.
Glucose-6-phosphate dehydrogenase deficiency	This is a hemolyzing disorder of blacks and Mediterranean peoples brought on by a deficency that causes the destruction of red blood cells upon contact with certain agents such as oxidizing drugs. Treatment for this anemia is supportive blood transfusions. Survival usually goes into adulthood.
Fragile X syndrome	A disorder of varying expression, this syndrome is characterized by a moderate intellectual handicap; some have autistic traits or hyperactivity. Facial features include high forehead, big jaw, long ears. Life span is not affected.

Adverse effects have been suggested in the following studies:

1. Increased rate of spontaneous abortions in women in Oregon after the spraying of farms.
2. Two cases of myelomeningocele in New Zealand; dose was not known.
3. Increased incidence of cleft palate in Australia after sprayings.
4. Increased number of spontaneous abortions at Love Canal after illegal dumping.
5. Limb defects noted in the Midwest, but the causal relation was not established.

The difficulty with all these studies has been that they were not controlled; that is, those exposed were not matched against a comparable nonexposed population. Until that occurs, a definitive answer is not available. Such a study is very difficult to do amongst developed societies because we all have been exposed to low levels of many chemicals

Table 25.5.
MATERNAL SERUM SCREENING FOR AFP

Step 1.	Initial maternal blood screening at 15–20 weeks.
Step 2.	Repeat serum screen; ultrasonography.
Step 3.	Genetic amniocentesis for amniotic fluid AFP.
Step 4.	Measurement of amniotic fluid acetylcholinesterase; high resolution ultrasound.
Step 5.	Genetic counseling.

that in combination could skew results. There is, however, a chance that a good study might be conducted. A research group out of Binghamton, New York, has been awarded a grant to study the Vietnamese population itself. Spraying of "Agent Orange" was done only in the south. As it happens, people in the north have been found to be virtually free of any levels at all. Therefore, researchers have a perfect laboratory in that country to sort out the question, matching the relatively homogenous population that has been exposed to relatively few other chemicals at all. Both governments are cooperating on the study, and while it will take some years to be completed, it is a promising opportunity.

Organochlorine Pesticides (DDT, DDE)

The damaging effects of these substances have been well documented in avian species, but conclusions have not been made in humans. They have been found in human tissues, cord blood, and breast milk. Associations have been made with increased abortion, prematurity, low birth weight, and toxemia.

Food Additives/Contaminants (17–19, 22)

Polychlorinated Biphenyls (PCBs)

This is a substance used in industry as a heat exchanger, such as in transformers. Accidents that release it into the environment are serious because PCBs tends to accumulate and persist. Usually, PCBs reach humans by being passed through the marine food chain or milk supply. The human experience with this chemical, which crosses the placenta, includes stillbirth, intrauterine growth retardation, and "Yusho" syndrome, which is a collection of skin and nail disorders that appeared in Japan after an industrial accident. Neurologic and developmental deficits in breastfed infants have prompted the American Academy of Pediatrics to recommend that exposed mothers' milk be assayed. In the human body PCBs are stored in fat tissue; therefore, pregnant women are cautioned against weight loss for fear of mobilizing the chemical. They are also advised against the ingestion of sport fish to decrease exposure; commercial fish are acceptable since they are caught in presumed safe waters and are sampled for acceptable levels.

Polybrominated Biphenyls (PBBs)

A fire retardant, this substance accidentally was mixed in cattle feed and reached the food chain when slain carcasses were used as pig feed and fertilizer. While devastating to cattle, the effects in humans have been undocumented; high concentrations have been found in breast milk.

Air Pollutants

Carbon Monoxide

There is information on effects because of widespread exposure from industrial combustion, auto exhaust, and cigarettes. Human effects include increase in stillbirths, neurologic deficits, mental retardation, seizures, spasticity, and retarded psychomotor development. The federal Clean Air Act set maximum allowable limits for humans; however, pregnant women should be exposed to less because of their increased oxygen consumption.

Ozone

A constituent of the earth's upper atmosphere, this gas is hazardous to humans in high concentrations. Smog alerts usually are called at one-tenth the danger level. Higher altitude aircraft have clocked four times the allowable occupational exposure. Flight attendants have reported an increase in spontaneous abortions and defects, but the conclusive cause has not been confirmed.

Anesthetic Gases

Exposure through occupational contact has been the subject of a number of studies that have attempted to link them to increased abortions, birth defects, low birth weight, and infertility for the workers themselves and even extending to the mates of exposed workers. Recent exhaustive review of the studies' methodologies has questioned these findings (24).

Radiation

The devastation caused by radiation is relatively well known, leading to its classification as a known teratogen. Exposure at critical times in embryonic development was, until recently, considered to be absolutely harmful; however, a growing number of case reports of women with unrecognized pregnancy exposed during diagnostic procedures has altered thinking. This has led to recommendations that each case be considered on an individual basis, with predictions of teratogenic risk calculated by the dose and stage of gestation.

Concluding Remarks

The foregoing review is by no means exhaustive in its coverage of teratogens but is instead a compilation of illustrative common agents that will serve as a quick reference. The reader is encouraged to consult the references for more extensive coverage of less common substances.

Once again, it is worthwhile to mention that precise effects of agents upon humans are hard to evaluate. Part of the reason perhaps lies in the fact that the susceptibility to teratogenesis varies from one individual to another. While exposure during critical development carries a higher risk of teratogenesis, that risk does not necessarily lead to abnormality. It has been suggested that inherent genetic or polygenic factors may confer susceptibility to increased uptake and, therefore, effect of agents. In addition, much is yet to be learned about the effects of stress and nutrition on the occurrence of disease. Such factors could, then, explain why many individuals are unaffected by high exposure.

FETAL MEDICINE: PREVENTION AND TREATMENT

Advances such as prenatal diagnosis have led the way toward providing more information about the fetus than we have ever had, thereby allowing the development of new strategies in care. Increasingly, we are able to correct disorders before delivery. Along with these actions have come both enthusiastic approval and serious questions regarding risks and benefits. While it is not within the scope of this chapter to air the merits and drawbacks of

Table 25.6.
FETAL TREATMENTS

DISORDER	TREATMENT
Erythroblastosis fetalis	RhoGAM; transfusion
Lung immaturity	Corticosteroids
Paroxysmal atrial tachycardia	Digitalis
Hypothyroidism	T_4 intraamniotic
Neural tube defects	Vitamin therapy
Vitamin-responsive inborn errors of metabolism	Vitamin therapy
Adrenogenital syndrome	Dexamethasone
Hydronephrosis	Catheter shunt
Hydrocephalus	Catheter shunt

established. This is particularly so in the case of in utero shunts. When these procedures were introduced, they were hailed widely. An international registry, which has been keeping data on these procedures, has published a report wherein outcomes of 117 cases collected between 1982–1985 showed discouraging results. While the operations technically are feasible, the outcomes may not be worth the effort, although there might be some promise in urinary tract obstruction correction. It was advised that further work in this area be conducted in carefully controlled studies (27).

such interventions, it is worthwhile to keep them in mind.

Technically, fetal treatment is not new. In the broadest sense prenatal care with vitamin supplementation, maternal treatment for diseases that were also harmful to the fetus, and intrapartum management of fetal stress are fetal treatments that have been used for a long time. What is new, and the focus here, is the ability to diagnose and correct an increasing number of disorders (25, 26). Table 25.6 presents a list of these interventions.

As mentioned earlier, some of these treatments are controversial and their efficacy not well

CONCLUSION

The study of genetics has contributed to an expansion of knowledge about human reproduction, allowing the development of new treatment techniques that result in better perinatal outcome. With still more development upon the horizon, it may even be possible soon to see the day when genetic engineering techniques can be used to prevent or reverse genetic abnormalities. At the same time, ethical dilemmas related to implementation of anticipated advances need to be addressed.

NURSING MANAGEMENT

Nursing care specific for patients with *potential/actual congenitally abnormal fetus/neonate:*
- ☐ Screen all pregnant women for risk for congenital anomalies including assessment of teratogens in the workplace; refer for genetic counseling as appropriate.
- ☐ Provide continuing education and emotional support during prenatal testing, waiting for results of tests, and the decision whether to continue or terminate the pregnancy.
- ☐ If the family decides to terminate the pregnancy, provide emotional support and stay with the patient throughout the procedure.
- ☐ If the patient/family decides to continue the pregnancy:
  - — Provide anticipatory guidance about the diagnosis (e.g., degree of physical or mental handicap, anticipated medical costs);
  - — Assist them in identification of sources of support (family, friends, community organizations, organizations to help children with similar defects);

- — After birth, provide opportunity for bonding;
- — Demonstrate special care needs for the baby; assist parents to assume responsibility for meeting baby's needs;
- — Point out to parents normal/endearing characteristics of the baby; be a role model demonstrating that the baby is acceptable and pleasing; and
- — Observe for abnormal bonding/parent-child attachment.
- ☐ Provide anticipatory guidance about the possibility of recurrence of the anomaly in subsequent pregnancies.

Nursing diagnoses most frequently associated with *congenital anomalies* **(see Section V):**
- ☐ Grieving related to potential/actual loss of infant or birth of an imperfect child.
- ☐ Spiritual distress.
- ☐ Ineffective individual coping.
- ☐ Potential altered parenting.

GLOSSARY OF TERMS

Aneuploidy——Having an abnormal number of chromosomes, either fewer or more than the normal.

Autosome——Non-sex-determining chromosome.

Chromosome——One of 46 rod-shaped bodies contained in every human cell that carries hereditary factors; the mature ovum and sperm each carries only 23.

Congenital——Existing before or at birth; not necessarily due to genetic causation.

Deletion——Absence of a part of a chromosome.

Dizygous——Having developed from two fertilized ova at single birth.

Dominant——Quality of causing a trait to be expressed even though it was received by only one parent.

Duplication——A chromosome segment is repeated in a set of chromosomes.

Expression——Variable severity of a given genetic trait.

Gamete——Male or female reproductive cell; egg or sperm.

Gene——Single unit that transmits hereditary factors.

Genotype——Genetic makeup.

Homozygous——Having identical genetic composition.

Inversion——The arrangement of a chromosome structure has a portion reversed.

Karyotype——Standard arrangement of chromosomes.

Meiosis——Process of cell division that reduces chromosome pairs to half, as is carried in the sex chromosome.

Mitosis——Process of cell division into two identical daughter cells.

Mosaicism——Presence of cells containing different genetic composition within the same individual.

Multifactorial——Having resulted from more than one genetic and/or nongenetic factor.

Mutation——An alteration of the hereditary material.

Phenotype——Total traits that characterize members of a given group.

Penetrance——Percentage of individuals actually showing a genetic trait that is within its genetic composition.

Proband——Affected individual who brings a given family to study.

Recessive——Attribute of a trait that is not expressed unless it is received from both parents.

Sex-linked——Applied to genes located on the X chromosome.

Trait——Characteristic, quality, or property of an individual.

Translocation——Displacement of part or all of one chromosome onto another.

Trisomy——The appearance of three of a given chromosome rather than the normal two.

Zygote——The fertilized ovum.

REFERENCES

1. Gordon JE: Assessment of occupational and environmental exposures. In Bracken MB (ed): *Perinatal Epidemiology* New York, Oxford University Press, 1984, p 450.
2. Neilson JP: Indications for ultrasonography in obstetrics. *Birth* 13:16–19, 1986.
3. Chervenak FA, Isaacson G, Mahoney M: Advances in the diagnosis of fetal defects. *N Engl J Med* 315:305–307.
4. McNay J: Prenatal diagnosis. Amniocentesis. *Br J Hosp Med* 31:406–416, 1984.
5. Milunsky A: Results & benefits of a maternal serum alpha-fetoprotein screening program. *JAMA* 252:1438–1442, 1984.
6. Elias S: Fetoscopy in prenatal diagnosis. *Clin Perinatol* 10:357–367, 1984.
7. Warburton D, Kline J, Stein Z, Strobino B: Cytogenic abnormalities in spontaneous abortions of recognized conceptions. In Porter IH, Willey A (eds): *Perinatal Genetics: Diagnosis and Treatment*. New York, Academic Press, 1986, pp 133–148.
8. Ayme S, Lippman-Hand A: Maternal-age effect in aneuploidy: does altered embryonic selection play a role? *Am J Hum Genet* 34:558–565, 1982.
9. Hook EB: Down syndrome rates and relaxed selection at older maternal ages. *Am J Hum Genet* 35:1307–1313, 1983.
10. Bergsma D (ed): *Birth Defects Compendium*, ed 2. New York, Alan R. Liss, 1979.
11. Ayala FJ, Kiger JA: *Modern Genetics*. Menlo Park, Benjamin/Cummings, 1981.
12. Epstein CJ, Cox DR, Schonberg SA, Hogge WA: Recent developments in the prenatal diagnosis of genetic diseases and birth defects. *Annu Rev Genet* 17:49–77, 1983.
13. Turner G, Robinson H, Laing S, Purvis-Smith S: Preventive screening for the Fragile X syndrome. *N Engl J Med* 315:607–609, 1986.
14. Cramer A, Hirschhorn K: Prenatal diagnosis. *Birth Defects: Original Article Series* 21:9–35, 1985.
15. Macri JN, Weiss RR: Prenatal serum-fetoprotein screening for neural tube defects. *Obstet Gynecol* 59:633–639, 1982.
16. National center for Education to Maternal and Child Health: Open neural tube defects. *Genet Pract* 1:1–6, 1984.

17. Hemminki K, Vineis P: Extrapolation of the evidence on teratogenicity of chemicals between humans and experimental animals. *Terat Carcin Mutag* 5:251–318, 1985.

18. Kurzel RB, Cetrullo CL: Chemical teratogenesis and reproductive failure. *Obstet Gynecol Surv* 40:397–424, 1985.

19. Meurer SJ: The impact of environmental hazards on reproduction. *NAACOG Update Series* 1:1–8, 1984.

20. Monteleone-Neto R: Birth defects and environmental pollution. The cubatao example. *Prog Clin Biol Res* 163B:65–68, 1985.

21. Rogan WJ, Gladen BC: Study of human lactation for effects of environmental contaminants: the North Carolina breast milk and formula project and some other ideas. *Environ Health Perspect* 60:215–221, 1985.

22. Rogan WJ, Gladen BC, Wilcox AJ: Potential reproductive and postnatal morbidity from exposure to polychlorinated biphenyls: epidemiologic considerations. *Environ Health Perspect* 60:233–239, 1985.

23. Hatch M, Stein Z: Agent orange and risks to reproduction. *Terat Carcin Mut* 6:185–202, 1986.

24. Tannenbaum TN, Goldberg RJ: Exposure to anesthetic gases and reproductive outcome. *J Occup Med* 27:659–668, 1985.

25. Behrman RE: Fetal medicine. *Birth Defects: Original Article Series* 21:55–61, 1985.

26. Brent RL: Maternal nutrition and congenital malformations. *Birth Defects: Original Article Series* 21:1–8, 1985.

27. Manning FA, Harrison MR, Rodeck C: Catheter shunts for fetal hydronephrosis and hydrocephalus. *N Engl J Med* 315:336–340, 1986.

Chapter 26
Nutritional Abnormalities
Nancy W. Kulb, C.N.M., M.S.

INTRODUCTION

Many anatomic, physiologic, and biologic changes occur during pregnancy. These changes are required for fetal growth and development and to prepare the mother for labor, birth, and lactation. They significantly alter the nutrient needs of the pregnant woman.

Nutrient transport across the placenta to the fetus is by simple diffusion, facilitated diffusion, active transport, and pinocytosis. For example, fatty acids and fat-soluble vitamins cross by simple diffusion. Glucose, amino acids, B and C vitamins, calcium, sodium, and iron cross by active transport. Some nutrients are maintained in the fetal circulation because of differences in the concentration gradient or chemical alterations in the nutrients that prevent them from reentering the maternal circulation. When the basic nutrients are present, the fetus is able to synthesize its own proteins, carbohydrates, and fats (1).

Additional nutrients are needed to support the maternal adaptations to pregnancy. For example, maternal blood volume increases by about 50%, peaking near term. This extra blood volume provides for nutrient transport and removal of fetal metabolic waste. It requires additional fluid, protein, minerals, and vitamins for the additional plasma and blood cells. Breast and uterine tissues also grow during pregnancy, and fat stores are normally laid down in the early part of pregnancy to support fetal growth toward the end of pregnancy and during lactation.

All of these changes require additional nutrients during pregnancy. Approximately 30,000 additional calories are required to support pregnancy itself. It is estimated that 40,000 calories are needed if physical activity is maintained at a normal level because of the extra energy expended with the greater body weight in pregnancy (2). An average of 10 calories/day extra is needed in the first trimester, 85 in the second trimester, and 200 in the third trimester. Of course, the actual daily caloric requirement for an individual depends upon her basal metabolic rate, point in gestation, and physical activity. The total daily caloric need for the average woman during pregnancy is 2300 calories (3). The increase is *not* a large amount; if the woman has been maintaining a steady weight, 1½ glasses of whole milk each day will supply the additional calories. If the woman does not get the extra calories she needs from her diet, she will use the fat stores in her body to meet her energy requirements.

In addition to calories, 30 g protein per day in addition to normal requirements is recommended for a singleton pregnancy. An additional 25 mg is recommended for each additional fetus in a multiple gestation; 18 mg iron, an amount that is almost impossible to get without supplements in the normal American diet, is recommended. Increased amounts of other vitamins and minerals are needed (Table 26.1). Therefore, it is crucial that the food choices made by the pregnant woman are wise ones—foods that are rich in essential nutrients. Many practitioners routinely prescribe prenatal vitamins and iron for their patients to ensure adequate intake.

Weight gain during pregnancy consists of the weight of the products of conception (fetus, amniotic fluid, placenta) and of maternal growth (breasts, uterus, blood volume, and adipose tissue stores) (Table 26.2). Average weight gain can be summarized as follows (4):

First trimester: minimal gain
13–18 weeks: 0.36 kg/week (0.8 lbs)

285

Table 26.1.

RECOMMENDED DAILY DIETARY ALLOWANCES[a, b]

	AGE	WEIGHT		HEIGHT		PROTEIN	FAT-SOLUBLE VITAMINS			WATER-SOLUBLE VITAMINS		
							VITAMIN A	VITAMIN D	VITAMIN E	VITAMIN C	THIAMIN	RIBO-FLAVIN
	years	kg	pounds	cm	inches	g	μg RE[c]	μg[d]	mg α-TE[b]	mg	mg	mg
Females	11–14	46	101	157	62	46	800	10	8	50	1.1	1.3
	15–18	55	120	163	64	46	800	10	8	60	1.1	1.3
	19–22	55	120	163	64	44	800	7.5	8	60	1.1	1.3
	23–50	55	120	163	64	44	800	5	8	60	1.0	1.2
	51+	55	120	163	64	44	800	5	8	60	1.0	1.2
Pregnant						+30	+200	+5	+2	+20	+0.4	+0.3
Lactating						+20	+400	+5	+3	+40	+0.5	+0.5

	WATER-SOLUBLE VITAMINS				MINERALS					
	NIACIN	VITAMIN B6	FOLACIN	VITAMIN B12	CALCIUM	PHOSPHORUS	MAGNESIUM	IRON	ZINC	IODINE
	mg NE[f]	mg	μg	μg	mg	mg	mg	mg	mg	μg
Females	15	1.8	400	3.0	1,200	1,200	300	18	15	150
	14	2.0	400	3.0	1,200	1,200	300	18	15	150
	14	2.0	400	3.0	800	800	300	18	15	150
	13	2.0	400	3.0	800	800	300	18	15	150
	13	2.0	400	3.0	800	800	300	10	15	150
Pregnant	+2	+0.6	+400	+1.0	+400	+400	+150	[g]	+5	+25
Lactating	+5	+0.5	+100	+1.0	+400	+400	+150	[g]	+10	+50

[a]Reproduced from *Recommended Dietary Allowances*, ed 9. Washington, DC, National Academy Press, 1980.
[b]The allowances are intended to provide for individual variations among most healthy persons in the United States. Diets should be based on a variety of common foods in order to provide other nutrients for which human requirements have been less well defined. See text for detailed discussion of allowances and nutrients.
[c]Retinol equivalents, 1 retinol equivalent = 1 μg retinol or 6 μg β-carotene.
[d]As cholecalciferol, 10 μg cholecalciferol = 400 IU vitamin D.
[e]α-Tocopherol equivalents. 1 mg d-α-tocopherol = 1 α-TE.
[f]Niacin equivalent. 1 NE is equal to 1 mg of niacin or 60 mg of dietary tryptophan.
[g]The increased requirement during pregnancy cannot be met by the iron content of habitual American diets nor by the existing iron stores of many women. Therefore the use of 30 to 60 mg of supplemental iron is recommended. Iron needs during lactation are not substantially different from those of nonpregnant women, but continued supplementation of the mother for 2 to 3 months after parturition is advisable in order to replenish stores depleted by pregnancy.

18–28 weeks: 0.45 kg/week (1 lb)
28–40 weeks: 0.36 kg/week (0.8 lbs)

Average weight gain at term is approximately 27 pounds (3, p 172, 5). Any weight gain greater than 19 pounds normally is retained in the immediate postpartum period. It is lost slowly over a period of about 3 months. The weight loss may be dramatic if the woman is breastfeeding. Nursing mothers may burn as much as 700–800 calories/day from their body stores (3, p 172).

Scientific studies on nutrition in pregnancy are limited severely. Controlled studies in humans are impossible since it would be morally abhorrent to induce dietary deficiencies deliberately. Therefore, "controlled" studies must observe women at their various economic and nutritional levels. Any interventions must be in the direction of improving their situation. It has been possible to observe women with restricted diets at specific points in

Table 26.2.

AVERAGE COMPONENTS OF WEIGHT GAIN IN PREGNANCY (CUMULATIVE GAIN AT END OF EACH TRIMESTER)[a]

COMPONENT	FIRST	SECOND	THIRD
	kg	kg	kg
Fetal			
Fetus	Negligible	1.0	3.4
Placenta	Negligible	0.3	0.6
Amniotic fluid	Negligible	0.4	1.0
Fetal subtotal		1.7	5.0
Maternal			
Increased uterine size	0.3	0.8	1.0
Increased breast size	0.1	0.3	0.5
Increased blood volume	0.3	1.3	1.5
Increased extracellular fluid	0.0	0.0	1.5
Maternal subtotal	0.7	2.4	4.5
Total gain accounted for	0.7	4.1	9.5

[a]Reprinted from the American College of Obstetricians and Gynecologists, 1972.

Interviewer:_____

Patient's Name:_____   Date:_____

TIME	PLACE	FOOD EATEN	AMOUNT	SUMMARY
				Protein foods / Milk and Products / Grain Products / Vitamin C Products / Leafy Green / Other fruits & vegetables
INFLUENCES ON DIET:			SUMMARY: Svgs. eaten	
			Svgs. needed	4 4 3 1 2 1
			Difference	

Figure 26.1. An example of a 24-hour diet intake recall chart. (From California Department of Health: *Nutrition during Pregnancy and Lactation*. Sacramento, CA, California Department of Health, 1975.)

history, such as during the Dutch famine and the seige on Leningrad. Data collection is quite difficult under those circumstances. In these and other studies of human nutrition, it is also difficult to sort out the effects of other environmental factors (e.g., poor sanitation, stress, poor health care, poor economic status). Animal studies help to fill in some gaps in knowledge, but the applicability of the results to humans must always be questioned (6).

Nutritional status is difficult to assess in an individual. The three available methods of determining nutritional status are diet history, physical signs and symptoms, and laboratory measurements.

There are several types of dietary histories. Most common are the 24-hour recall, in which the patient reports types and amounts of foods consumed in the previous 24 hours, and the written diet history, in which the patient records her intake over a 3 to 7-day period. Figure 26.1 is a sample

form for recording a diet history. Both types of histories are subject to some inaccuracies (e.g., the 24-hour period covered by the recall may not be representative of the patient's usual diet; the patient may not be able—or motivated—to maintain an accurate record of her intake for several days; or she may alter her intake because of the difficulty in recording ingredients of dishes or sauces containing many different foods). In both types of histories, the patient may report what she believes the practitioner wants to hear rather than what she actually consumed.

Analysis of the diet history usually consists of categorizing foods by food groups and then comparing the number of servings in each group with the recommended number (Fig. 26.2). Recently, computer analysis of diet histories has become available and practical to use.

Physical assessment of nutritional status consists of assessment of weight for height, the weight

Interviewer: _____

Patient's Name: _____   Date: _____

Food Group	Servings Eaten (3 days)	Daily Serving Average	Servings Needed	Sug- gested Changes
Protein foods (animal & vegetable)			4	
Milk & milk products			4	
Grain products			3	
Vitamin C rich fruits & vegetables			1	
Leafy green vegetables			2	
Other fruits & vegetables			1	

Comments and Follow-up:

Figure 26.2. Diet history evaluation sheet. This type of form provides a quick, easy-to-read reference for the client's specific dietary deficiencies and excesses and can aid greatly in client diet counseling. (From California Department of Health: *Nutrition during Pregnancy and Lactation.* Sacramento, CA, California Department of Health, 1975.)

gain pattern during the pregnancy, assessment of fetal growth, and assessment of physical signs and symptoms of nutrient deficiencies (Table 26.3). Laboratory assessment of nutritional status during pregnancy usually is limited to hematology tests for iron and folic acid deficiency (see Chapter 8).

Nutrition intervention must be based on the assessment of the individual's nutritional and medical status. Eating behaviors are ingrained deeply and are difficult to change. To effect change, nutrition counseling must be consistent with the individual's financial status, cooking and food preparation facilities, cultural or ethnic background, religion, personal psychology, and personal food preferences. Often, the nutritional habits of individuals are influenced by the needs and preferences of other family members. Therefore, it may be helpful to include family members in nutrition counseling, especially if the patient is not responsible for buying and preparing food.

Because eating habits are difficult to change, it may be necessary to establish a long-term nutrition goal, with smaller, short-term objectives that are possible for the patient to meet. Sometimes it is helpful to establish a contract with the patient to help her maintain the motivation to change. With a contract the patient is given some reward (by herself or others) when she meets her goal(s). The patient should be praised for positive changes in eating patterns.

It is important to support nutrition counseling with food or financial assistance when necessary. Prenatal care providers should be aware of all available sources of assistance for their patients, including the Supplemental Food Program for Women,

Infants, and Children (WIC), Food Stamps, local food pantries, soup kitchens, and so on.

One particularly successful nutrition intervention program has been developed by Agnes Higgins at the Montreal Diet Dispensary in Montreal, Quebec, Canada. This method is based on accurate assessment of nutritional status by a detailed diet history, focusing on protein and calorie intake, and on weight assessment. Intake is compared to the protein and calorie requirements that are calculated for the individual woman. These requirements are based on her height, prepregnancy weight, stage of gestation, prior nutritional status, and high risk factors (i.e., poor obstetrical outcome, close pregnancy spacing, hyperemesis gravidarum, maternal stress, and failure to gain 10 pounds by 20 weeks' gestation) (Table 26.4). When dietary requirements and intake are compared, specific corrections to her current diet can be suggested. The woman is counseled, for example, to "eat what you have already been eating, but add. . ." the specific foods that are suggested. Frequent corrections include drinking a quart of milk a day, eating an egg and an orange each day, and eating liver once a week. It is emphasized that the woman must eat to provide the needs of the fetus since the fetus cannot yet eat for itself. Food supplements are given to those women who need them.

The results of the first 10 years of study of the Montreal Diet Dispensary method are excellent. The mean daily intake for all patients was increased by 529 calories and 33 g protein, although it varied greatly according to individual needs. The average birth weight was 3274 g, and that included women

Table 26.3.
SYMPTOMS OF NUTRIENT DEFICIENCY[a]

NUTRIENT	SYMPTOMS OF DEFICIENCY
Protein	Flaky dermatosis Hair easily plucked Mild wasting of fat and muscles Apathy Diarrhea Edema Mild anemia
Protein and calories	Hair easily plucked, sparse, dyspigmented Severe wasting of fat and muscles Impaired mental development Diarrhea Severe anemia Low body weight Flaky paint dermatosis, diffuse skin pigmentation
Vitamin A	Follicular hyperkeratosis, xerosis Eye abnormalities: night blindness, dryness of the conjunctiva, photophobia, swelling and redness of the lids, cloudy ulcerated cornea, blindness, Bitot's spots
Thiamine	Calf muscle tenderness Weakness, numbness, tingling of legs Loss of knee and/or ankle jerks Malaise Polyneuritis Loss of immediate memory Disorientation Ataxia Anorexia Nausea, vomiting Constipation Tachycardia, palpitations Edema of legs, trunk, face Hypertension Heart failure Dyspnea
Riboflavin	Cheilosis Angular fissures Seborrheic dermatitis Fatigue Neuropathy Photophobia Corneal inflammation, vascularization Soreness of mouth and tongue Glossitis Tongue: papillae hypertrophied, atrophied, or purple in color
Niacin	Dermatitis Mental apathy Depression, anxiety, disorientation, confusion Glossitis Anorexia Indigestion Weight loss Diarrhea Stomatitis Tongue: scarlet, raw, atrophy of papillae
Pyridoxine	Nausea In pregnancy, may be associated with toxemia, gestational diabetes, neurological symptoms, or mental retardation in the newborn
Vitamin B_{12}	Megaloblastic anemia Central nervous system abnormalities

NUTRIENT	SYMPTOMS OF DEFICIENCY
Folacin	Megaloblastic anemia In pregnancy, may be associated with toxemia and damage to the central nervous system of the fetus
Vitamin C	Dry, rough skin Petechiae, ecchymoses Inadequate wound healing Hemorrhages in muscles and joints Sunken chest Swollen, bleeding gums Anemia In pregnancy, may be a cause of spontaneous abortion and premature delivery
Vitamin D	Failure of calcification, skeletal abnormalities: head appears enlarged and flattened; bowed legs; knock-knees; knobbing at wrists; bowing of arms; rachitic rosary Decreased muscle tone Kyphosis Protuberant abdomen
Vitamin E	Deficiency in pregnancy has been associated with neonatal jaundice
Iron	Anemia Pallor of mucous membranes Koilonychia Atrophy of papillae of tongue
Iodine	Enlarged thyroid

^aAdapted from Ganella JG: *Nutrition for the Childbearing Year*. Wayzata, MN, Woodland Publishing Co., Inc., 1979; and Green ML, Harry J: *Nutrition in Contemporary Nursing Practice*. New York, John Wiley & Sons, Inc., 1981.

who entered the pregnancy underweight and/or undernourished and those who did not begin nutrition intervention until the last trimester of pregnancy. The incidence of low birth weight in their high risk population was 6.87%, less than the incidence for Canada (7.65%) or Quebec (9.02%). Their perinatal mortality rate was 14.32 compared to 24.99 for Canada and 26.01 for Quebec. (7).

Entire books are written on the subject of nutrition during pregnancy and lactation. This chapter deals only with selected specific nutrition problems: pica, obesity, low pregravid weight, and extremes of weight gain during pregnancy. The reader is referred to chapters on specific complications of pregnancy (e.g., diabetes mellitus, hyperemesis gravidarum) for nutritional management of those problems. Nutrition texts should be used for additional information on normal nutritional needs of pregnancy and techniques of nutritional assessment and intervention.

PICA

Definition

Pica is the ingestion of nonfood items. The word is derived from the Latin for magpie, "a bird who picks up a variety of things to satisfy its hunger or curiosity" (8). Among common types of pica are:

1. Geophagia—the ingestion of dirt or clay.
2. Amylophagia—the ingestion of starch.
3. Pagophagia—the ingestion of ice.
4. Trichophagia—the ingestion of hair.
5. Lithophagia—the ingestion of stones or gravel.

Other substances that have been reported to be eaten by pregnant women include refrigerator frost, charcoal, soap, ashes, soot, plaster, paint, Vicks Vaporub, coffee grounds, paraffin, dry Milk of Magnesia, baking powder, baking soda, air fresheners, mothballs, balls of dirt found in dried pinto beans, and "jarritos"—unfired clay jars made especially for eating.

Geophagia, amylophagia, and pagophagia are the most common forms of pica practiced during pregnancy. Clay may be eaten wet or may be baked. It may be eaten throughout the day or only after meals. White clay usually is preferred and may be valued so highly that it is mailed by rural people to their urban friends and relatives who cannot otherwise obtain it. Up to 5 ounces per day may be consumed.

Cornstarch usually is consumed in addition to foods but may occasionally replace a meal. Up to 2

Table 26.4.
THE HIGGIN'S INTERVENTION METHOD FOR NUTRITIONAL REHABILITATION DURING
PREGNANCY[a]

PROCEDURE FOR ESTIMATION OF CALORIC AND PROTEIN REQUIREMENTS

NORMAL REQUIREMENTS

The normal caloric and protein requirements for mothers 20 years of age or more are determined on the basis of ideal body weight, physical activity, and weeks of gestation, according to the recommendations in the Dietary Standard for Canada (1948) prepared by the Canadian Council on Nutrition. For mothers 19 years of age or less, use the Recommended Dietary Allowances (1958) prepared by the Food and Nutrition Board, National Research Council, United States. For all mothers add 500 calories and 25 g protein after 20 weeks of gestation as recommended in the Canadian Standard.

ADDITIONAL CORRECTIVE ALLOWANCES

Corrective caloric and protein allowances are given in addition to the normal requirements according to the degree of *underweight, undernutrition,* or for special high risk conditions that may be indicative of *nutritional stress.* A mother may have none or one or more of these conditions.

Underweight assessment and rehabilitation

Underweight. Underweight status is determined if the mother's pregravid weight is 5% or more under the weight recommended in the Table of Desirable Weights, prepared by the Metropolitan Life Insurance Company.

Underweight correction. Underweight correction should provide sufficient additional calories and protein to ensure that the mother gains during pregnancy the number of pounds she was underweight prior to conception; 20 g protein and 500 calories a day are added to the normal pregnancy requirements to permit a gain of 1 pound per week.

Undernutrition assessment and rehabilitation

Undernutrition. Undernutrition is determined if a protein deficit is found between actual dietary intake and requirement. The method used is a 24-hour recall diet history, cross-checked with a food list and family market order compared with the appropriate standard.

Undernutrition correction. Undernutrition correction is equal to the amount of protein deficit allowing 10 calories for each gram of protein added to the normal pregnancy requirements.

Nutritional stress assessment and rehabilitation

Nutritional stress. Nutritional stress is determined if any one of the following maternal conditions is present: pernicious vomiting, pregnancies spaced less than 1 year apart, previous poor obstetrical history, failure to gain 10 pounds by the 20th week of gestation, serious emotional problems.

Nutritional stress correction. Nutritional stress correction provides for the addition of 20 g protein and 200 calories for each stress condition added to normal pregnancy requirements to an upper limit of 40 g protein and 400 calories.

[a]From Higgins AC: Nutritional status and the outcome of pregnancy. *Can Diet Assoc J* 37:17-35, 1976.

---

pounds per day may be consumed. One brand may be preferred over others.

Pagophagia is defined as the consumption of at least one tray of ice per day for at least 2 months. Patients who practice pagophagia may also consume refrigerator frost.

The incidence of pica in pregnancy is somewhat difficult to determine since some women are ashamed of it and are therefore reluctant to admit it. Although it occurs in all geographical locations, races, creeds, cultures, ages, socioeconomic groups, and sexes, it is more prevalent in childhood and pregnancy. It is more common in the rural South, especially among blacks; in the Southwest among Spanish Americans; and in people of lower socioeconomic status. The practice may be preserved by immigrants from those areas, especially if their socioeconomic status remains low (9).

Studies that do look at the incidence of pica indicate that it is not a rare phenomenon. Bullough and Bullough, in Chicago in 1969, reported that 23.8% of the obstetric population admitted starch ingestion (10). O'Rourke et al., in Augusta, Georgia, reported that 55% of the obstetric population admitted eating clay or starch or both; most stated that they practiced pica only during pregnancy (11).

Etiology

Studies regarding the etiology and effects of pica are difficult or impossible to generalize because of the socioeconomic, cultural, geographic, and time differences of the groups being studied and because of the vast differences in the types of substances ingested. The etiology probably is multifactorial. It may be different for each substance and may be different in children and adults. Reported rationales for ingestion of nonfood items have included the following: substitute for food during times of famine, disease remedy, weight reduction, cosmetic purposes, condiments, or for religious ceremonies.

A strong and persistent relationship between pica during pregnancy and anemia has been demonstrated. It is not clear which is the cause and which is the effect. Several studies support low iron stores as the cause of pica, since after administration of iron, pica was eliminated, even before the anemia was corrected.

On the other hand, there is evidence to support the notion that pica causes anemia. Pica substances may replace iron-containing foods in the diet, resulting in iron deficiency. Certain pica substances may bind dietary iron or block its absorption. Magnesium oxide (found in antacids) is known to prevent iron absorption. Clay, because of its high cation exchange, may allow the formation of nonabsorbable iron compounds within the gastrointestinal system. Amylophagics were found to have a 50% decrease in iron absorption in one study (12). Another study, however, showed *no* alteration in iron absorption or utilization in either starch or clay eaters (13). Thus, the controversy over whether low iron stores cause pica or vice versa remains.

Another theory of the etiology of pica is that the pica substance compensates for some dietary deficiency. Clay often is high in calcium, magnesium, and potassium—nutrients that are often deficient in the diets of pregnant women. Some women actually relate their craving for dirt or clay to the need to supplement their diet with mineral sources. There is no scientific evidence, however, to support the theory that pica provides needed nutrients.

It may be that the basis for pica is psychological rather than physiological. It may be the result of the desire for special treatment during pregnancy. White clay, a "delicacy," may be a special gift from relatives or friends. Pica may satisfy the need for oral gratification that other people satisfy through smoking or chewing gum. Similarly, it may be practiced to relieve nervous tension.

In some cultures the desire for social approval may encourage a woman to practice pica. Traditions, passed on by older women, may include pica and certain food prohibitions during pregnancy and the postpartum period. The desire to be a part of the cultural community may be the reason for pica, as well as other health and nutrition practices.

Beliefs regarding the benefits of pica may be the reason some women practice it. Among reported beliefs are (14):

1. Cigarette ashes prevent preterm birth.
2. Dirt or clay is a cleansing agent for the organs.
3. Starch will cause the baby's skin to be lighter in color.
4. Starch will help the baby slide out at delivery.
5. Cravings result from the baby signalling the mother regarding its needs; if the cravings are not satisfied, the baby will be "marked."
6. Pica will ensure beautiful children.
7. Pica will relieve nausea and vomiting, dizziness, headaches, swelling, and a weak stomach.

Some women report that they like the taste, feel, and odor of clay and/or starch in the mouth. Dry pica substances may ameliorate the excessive salivation that often occurs during pregnancy, although it may actually cause ptyalism. Pica may suppress abdominal motility (due to hunger, worms, or uterine activity) by absorbing gastric juices, by quieting intestinal spasms, or by creating an environment unfavorable for the growth of disease-producing organisms. It may satisfy an appetite disorder that results from the alteration of taste and smell that is common during pregnancy.

Some women practice pica despite negative feelings and beliefs about it. They may disapprove of pica in general but feel that the unsatisfied craving is worse. Others believe pica is acceptable if not excessive—for example, too much starch could cause low blood pressure, obesity, or the baby to stick to the uterine wall, requiring a cesarean section. Others believe that pica could cause "hard delivery, kill the woman, cause constipation, dry up the blood, cause the child to 'lump up' and cause yellow jaundice, dropsy, tumors, or gas" (15).

Maternal and Fetal Outcome

The effects of pica on both mother and baby depend upon the substance ingested, the quantity, the duration of the practice, and the point in pregnancy when it is practiced.

Iron deficiency anemia commonly is associated with pica, although the cause-effect relationship is unclear (see above). Pica may replace nutritious foods in the diet or hinder absorption of nutrients, resulting in generally poor nutritional status. Excessive ingestion of starch or flour may result in excessive weight gain. Clay ingestion can cause impaction of the large bowel and result in perforation. Parasites (e.g., hookworm) may be ingested in dirt or clay. Toxic substances may be ingested inadvertently. The incidence of preeclampsia is doubled in pica practitioners, but whether one causes the other or both are the result of another cause is unknown (11). Other reported maternal complications of pica include hypokalemia, parotid enlargement (in starch eaters), hypertension, and dysfunctional labor.

Fetal effects of pica include an increased incidence of spontaneous abortions, stillbirths, and prematurity. Maternal anemia with poor oxygen transport may result in placental dysfunction and fetal anoxia. Congenital lead poisoning was reported in a baby whose mother had pica for wall plaster, and hemolytic anemia was reported after maternal ingestion of mothballs.

Medical Management

Medical management of pica begins with an awareness of the phenomenon and sensitivity to clues that it is being practiced. Although it is more common in certain groups (e.g., black women in or from the South), it is not restricted to any geographical, racial, cultural, or socioeconomic group. A nutrition history should be taken on all pregnant women early in the pregnancy. During this history, the patient must be made to feel that she can trust the practitioner and answer questions honestly without fear of punishment for "unacceptable" answers. It must be remembered that many women are ashamed of their pica and are reluctant to admit that they practice it. The woman should be asked whether she craves anything in particular. Questions regarding nonfood items can be intermingled with questions regarding foods.

During the initial general history and physical examination, and throughout the pregnancy, the practitioner should look for iron-deficiency anemia or a history of poor obstetrical outcome, both of which may suggest underlying pica.

Once pica is identified, additional information should be obtained, such as what substance(s) is (are) ingested, how much, for how long, and whether pica is practiced only during pregnancy. The patient's beliefs and motivations regarding pica should be explored. Since pica may have a deep-rooted psychological as well as physiological basis, change may not be easy.

Immediate attention should be placed on nutrition education, emphasizing positive nutrition habits and a well-balanced diet. The hazards of pica should be discussed but not to the extent that the patient will feel guilty or unable to discuss honestly her pica practice on future visits. Acceptable substitutes for the pica substance(s) should be explored. If needed, food assistance programs such as WIC should be made available to the patient. Social and psychological support services should be provided as needed. Counseling regarding pica and techniques for helping the patient eliminate it should be based on the patient's motivations and beliefs regarding pica. Specific techniques for dietary change may be used (e.g., a contract system, in which the patient receives some reward from herself or others if she meets an agreed upon dietary goal). Dietary goals should be reasonable and attainable; it may be that the patient will need to decrease pica gradually rather than eliminate it at once. The attainment of intermediate goals should be praised.

The patient with pica should be screened for anemia, and she should be given supplemental iron (usually oral, but parenteral if necessary) with explanations why it is important and specific instructions for taking oral iron. A multivitamin containing folic acid should be given. Hematologic status should be monitored throughout the pregnancy.

Until the pica has been eliminated, the patient should be cautioned about signs and symptoms of complications relating specifically to the substance she ingests (e.g., bowel impaction in dirt eaters). Specific tests may be required to screen for complications of pica (e.g., stool for ova and parasites in a patient with geophagia). Because of the increased incidence of preeclampsia, the patient should be monitored closely for signs and symptoms of its development.

NURSING MANAGEMENT

Nursing care specific for the patient with *pica*:
- [ ] Screen all pregnant women for the presence of pica.
- [ ] Explore reasons for pica; provide accurate information regarding pica.
- [ ] Teach importance of good nutritional habits; suggest nutritious alternatives for pica substances.
- [ ] Provide prenatal vitamin and iron supplements; teach the patient how to take them.
- [ ] Provide psychological evaluation and support, as needed; refer for psychiatric evaluation/treatment, as needed.

- [ ] Praise the patient for progress toward a nutritious diet.

Nursing diagnoses most frequentiy associated with *pica* (see Section V):
- [ ] Altered nutrition: less than body requirements.
- [ ] Knowledge deficit regarding etiology, disease process, treatment, and outcome.
- [ ] Ineffective individual coping.
- [ ] Disturbance to body image, self-esteem.
- [ ] Altered maternal tissue perfusion.

Table 26.5.
1983 METROPOLITAN HEIGHT AND WEIGHT TABLES

	MEN					WOMEN			
HEIGHT		SMALL	MEDIUM	LARGE	HEIGHT		SMALL	MEDIUM	LARGE
FEET	INCHES	FRAME	FRAME	FRAME	FEET	INCHES	FRAME	FRAME	FRAME
5	2	128-134	131-141	138-150	4	10	102-111	109-121	118-131
5	3	130-136	133-143	140-153	4	11	103-113	111-123	120-134
5	4	132-138	135-145	142-156	5	0	104-115	113-126	122-137
5	5	134-140	137-148	144-160	5	1	106-118	115-129	125-140
5	6	136-142	139-151	146-164	5	2	108-121	118-132	128-143
5	7	138-145	142-154	149-168	5	3	111-124	121-135	131-147
5	8	140-148	145-157	152-172	5	4	114-127	124-138	134-151
5	9	142-151	148-160	155-176	5	5	117-130	127-141	137-155
5	10	144-155	151-163	158-180	5	6	120-133	130-144	140-159
5	11	146-157	154-166	161-184	5	7	123-136	133-147	143-163
6	0	149-160	157-170	164-188	5	8	126-139	136-150	146-167
6	1	152-164	160-174	168-192	5	9	129-142	139-153	149-170
6	2	155-168	164-178	172-197	5	10	132-145	142-156	152-173
6	3	158-172	167-182	176-202	5	11	135-148	145-159	155-176
6	4	162-176	171-187	181-207	6	0	138-151	148-162	158-179

TO MAKE AN APPROXIMATION OF YOUR FRAME SIZE...

Extend your arm and bend the forearm upward at a 90 degree angle. Keep fingers straight and turn the inside of your wrist toward your body. If you have a caliper, use it to measure the space between the two prominent bones on *either side* of your elbow. Without a caliper, place thumb and index finger of your other hand on these two bones. Measure the space between your fingers against a ruler or tape measure. Compare it with these tables that list elbow measurements for *medium-framed* men and women. Measurements lower than those listed indicate you have a small frame. Higher measurements indicate a large frame.

Height in 1" heels	Elbow
Men	Breadth
5'2"–5'3"	2½"–2⅞"
5'4"–5'7"	2⅝"–2⅞"
5'8"–5'11"	2¾"–3"
6'0"–6'3"	2¾"–3⅛"
6'4"	2⅞"–3¼"
Women	
4'10"–4'11"	2¼"–2½"
5'0"–5'3"	2¼"–2½"
5'4"–5'7"	2⅜"–2⅝"
5'8"–5'11"	2⅜"–2⅝"
6'0"	2½"–2¾"

[a]Courtesy Statistical Bulletin, Metropolitan Life Insurance Co.
[b]Weight at ages 25–59 based on lowest mortality. Weight in pounds according to frame (in indoor clothing weighing 5 lb for men and 3 lb for women; shoes with 1" heels).

OBESITY

Definition

Obesity is the excessive accumulation of fat. Body fat is evaluated by skinfold thickness and body density determinations. Obesity is diagnosed when the triceps skinfold measurement is greater than the 85th percentile. Alternatively, body fat greater than 20% of body weight in males and greater than 30% in females is considered obesity. However, because of the difficulty in determining body fat percentages, or even skinfold thicknesses, obesity is often defined as weight greater than 20% above normal weight for height. Of course, it is possible to be overweight because of muscle, rather than fat, as many athletes are. And the problem of determining what is "normal" or "desirable" body weight has not been solved satisfactorily. Usually, a standard table based on average weight for height in a healthy population is used (Table 26.5). Studies of obesity in pregnancy use various definitions. Many use a weight of greater than 200 pounds (90 kg) or 250 pounds (114 kg) at any point in pregnancy as evidence of obesity.

Variations in the definition of obesity result in variations in the reported incidence. It is estimated that some 20% of Americans are overweight (16). The incidence of obesity in pregnancy has been reported as 5.6% by Calandra et al. (17) and as 6–10% by Kliegman et al. (4).

Etiology

Obesity results when caloric intake exceeds caloric expenditure. Controversy still exists as to whether it is primarily the result of nature (genetic heritage, altered physiology) or nurture (environment, learned dietary and exercise habits). Probably both contribute.

The population of the United States generally has an abundant food supply and a sedentary lifestyle. This contributes to overeating and low energy expenditure. As many adults age and their activity and basal metabolic rate (BMR) decrease, they maintain their same caloric intake, resulting in slow, steady weight gain.

Heredity is probably a factor contributing to obesity, but the evidence is conflicting. Eating and activity patterns are learned within families and may be more important in explaining why obesity tends to run in families; 42% of obese women were obese as children (18), and another 30% become obese in relation to gestation from poor eating habits, "eating for two," satisfying cravings, or compulsive eating.

Some reasons given to explain overeating are that it has an emotional basis, that it is learned (e.g., that sweets should be used to reward good behavior or to celebrate), or that there is an alteration in the appetite control center in the hypothalamus. Disturbances in the pituitary or thyroid gland also may affect appetite or utilization of foods.

Much research has gone into studying the development of fat cells in the body. Fat cells begin developing in the first trimester of fetal life and continue at a rapid rate through the first 6 months of life. The rate of fat cell production decreases during childhood and then accelerates again at puberty, with females developing more fat cells than males. By early adulthood the body has most of the fat cells it will ever have (about 30–40 billion on the average). Subsequent increases in body fat are due to increases in fat cell size rather than number (except in extreme obesity). Fat cells may shrink with weight reduction but do not disappear (16). There is speculation that people with a larger than normal number of fat cells tend to gain weight readily and retain it.

Research is conflicting and inconclusive about whether birth weight is related to subsequent obesity or whether fat babies become fat children, who become fat adults.

There is evidence that people prone to obesity do not necessarily consume more calories than their lean counterparts but that they expend calories at a slower rate. Obese patients have been found to have a decreased response to dietary- or cold-induced thermogenesis; therefore, they store energy that would have been dissipated in lean people. There may be an alteration in brown fat metabolism or in hypothalamic function, since the hypothalamus controls appetite and functions in

Table 26.6.
OBSTETRIC COMPLICATIONS ASSOCIATED WITH OBESITY[a]

COMPLICATION	INCIDENCE IN OBESE GRAVIDAS
Diabetes mellitus	10%
Hypertension	50%
Preeclampsia	41.7%
Pyelonephritis	10%
Breech presentation	8%
Operative delivery	35%

[a]From Tracy TA, and Miller GC: Obstetric problems of the massively obese. *Obstet Gynecol* 33:204, 1969.

thermoregulation and systemic catecholamine release (4).

Maternal and Fetal Outcome

Obesity in the general population is associated with diabetes mellitus, hypertension, cardiovascular disease, and a shortened life expectancy. The reports of incidence of complications in pregnancy vary because of variations in the definition of obesity and variations in the precision of diagnosis of complications. However, Tracy and Miller estimate that 62.5% develop some obstetric complication (19). Table 26.6 lists some of the common obstetric complications associated with obesity and the reported incidence. It should be noted that the incidence of diabetes mellitus is increased tenfold, preeclampsia sevenfold, and pyelonephritis fivefold over that in nonobese gravidas. Among other complications commonly reported in obese gravidas are multiple gestation, low weight gain, psychiatric disorders, aspiration under general anesthesia, postpartum hemorrhage, wound complications, thromboembolism, and puerperal infection.

Data regarding labor abnormalities and incidence of cesarean section are conflicting. Calandra et al. report an increased need for induction of labor in obese patients, primarily because of associated complications (e.g., diabetes mellitus, hypertension). They found the cesarean section rate to be slightly greater than in the general population, but the rate of forceps delivery was slightly less (17).

A British study reported that the incidence of prolonged labor was doubled in obese women (3). A 1950s study found no increased incidence of prolonged labor, but the cesarean section rate was increased about 40%, primarily as a result of cephalopelvic dysproportion (32). Gross et al. report no increase in labor dystocia, oxytocin augmentation, or primary cesarean section rate. Their increase in oxytocin induction of labor was due primarily to hypertension and diabetes; their increased overall cesarean section rate was due to repeat cesareans because of the higher parity of the obese population (20).

In spite of the high rates of serious maternal obstetric complications, reports of fetal outcome vary. Naeye (5) reports an increased perinatal mortality rate in the obese woman. He reports that obese women with low weight gains (less than 15 pounds) have twice the perinatal mortality rate of normal weight women with a low weight gain. Another study reports a stillbirth rate of 10.9% (3). Calandra et al., on the other hand, report no increase in perinatal mortality in spite of maternal complications and an increased incidence of low Apgar scores (less than 6 at 1 minute of life) (17). Gross agrees that there is no increased mortality (20), and Kliegman (4) and Eastman and Jackson (21) report that it actually is decreased.

It is suggested that the good perinatal outcome often reported for obese gravidas is primarily the result of higher birth weights. Kliegman reports that the incidence of prematurity is decreased, the incidence of intrauterine growth retardation (IUGR) is cut in half, and the incidence of large for gestational age infants is tripled (4). Gross et al. agree that the incidence of prematurity and IUGR are both halved and that macrosomia is increased 2½ times. The incidence of large for gestational age infants (31%) is not explained by the increased rate of diabetes mellitus (9–10%) in the obese population. Obesity and diabetes do not appear to have an additive effect on birth weight (21).

In spite of positive reports of fetal outcome with maternal obesity, there are risks, including an increased risk of asphyxia at birth and birth trauma. Reluctance to perform operative delivery because of the technical difficulties may contribute both to asphyxia and birth trauma. Shoulder dystocia is a risk because of the risk of fetal macrosomia.

A transient fasting asymptomatic hypoglycemia, not because of hyperinsulinism, has been reported in neonates, especially in the first 6 hours of life (4). The long-term outlook for large for gestational age babies in terms of risk for childhood and adult obesity is not yet clear (4, 22).

Medical Management

The optimum management of obesity in pregnancy is to prevent it by a program of weight reduction and fitness prior to pregnancy. Often, women retain weight after pregnancy, so if weight reduction and an exercise program are not implemented before pregnancy, the postpartum period is an ideal time to initiate them. The nutritional goal is to improve overall intake with a slow, progressive weight loss and then weight maintenance. An interdisciplinary approach often is beneficial: the physician must rule out endocrine abnormalities and evaluate the overall health of the patient; a psychologist and/or social worker can help assess and manage psychosocial aspects, such as body image and self-esteem; the nutritionist can assess dietary patterns and habits and assist in developing therapeutic alternatives. The nurse can coordinate efforts of the team, providing referrals, education, and support where necessary. Ultimately, the patient must assume responsibility for her dietary and exercise habits (23).

Weight gain requirements and dietary instructions for the obese woman during pregnancy are somewhat controversial. A study by Churchill et al. (24) indicated that ketonuria in pregnancy had a harmful effect on neurological development of the fetus; specifically, intelligence quotient (IQ) scores at 4 years of age were affected adversely. This study has been the basis for advising obese women not to lose weight during pregnancy and instead to gain enough weight to account for evident growth required by pregnancy (i.e., 15–16 pounds to account for fetus, placenta, amniotic fluid, and growth of maternal uterus, breasts, and blood volume). It is assumed that obese women do not need the additional fat stores that normally are laid down in early pregnancy to support fetal growth late in pregnancy and during lactation. Indeed, Naeye found that grossly overweight women had the best outcomes if they gained 15–16 pounds (5).

Recently, data supplied by Naeye and Chez suggest that ketonuria may not be a risk factor for poor neurological development and probably should not be a factor in determining the best dietary management of the obese gravida (25). The best dietary management of the obese woman obviously still is not clear, but most experts currently recommend a slow weight gain totaling 15–16 pounds.

The obese woman should be screened carefully in pregnancy for common complications, especially diabetes mellitus, hypertension, and preeclampsia. Each of these disorders should be managed as in the nonobese woman.

Induction of labor and/or operative delivery should be done as indicated. Reluctance, especially to perform cesarean section, while understandable because of greater operative risk, may result in increased maternal and perinatal morbidity and mortality. During labor, the risks of macrosomia, dysfunctional labor, shoulder dystocia, birth trauma, and birth asphyxia should be kept in mind. The pediatrician should be called to attend the delivery if any complications are anticipated.

When cesarean section is required, regional anesthesia is the method of choice since pulmonary insufficiency from increased pressure on the intercostal muscles and diaphragm may increase the risk of general anesthesia. Both midline vertical and Pfannenstiel's incisions are possible. The Pfannenstiel's incision has the following advantages and disadvantages for the obese gravida (4):

Advantages:
  o Decreased postoperative pain, allowing earlier ambulation and a decreased risk of atelectasis or embolism.
  o More secure closure.
  o Less adipose tissue to cut.
Disadvantages:
  o Warm, moist area predisposes to infection.
  o Delivery of a large baby may be difficult.
  o Retraction of the panniculus may compromise respiratory function.

A Smead-Jones closure with nonabsorbable suture may decrease the risk of dehiscence. Postoperatively, local skin care with antiseptic scrubs may be used to prevent wound infection. A course of prophylactic antibiotics may be given (4).

During the immediate postpartum period, early ambulation will help decrease the chance of pulmonary or thromboembolic complications. The lower extremities should be checked carefully for evidence of thrombophlebitis. Anticipatory guidance can be begun regarding weight reduction and an exercise program.

The neonate should have glucose levels monitored carefully for the first 6 hours of life since hypoglycemia is common. Otherwise, neonatal management is normal, with attention given to any problems resulting from maternal disease or delivery complications.

UNDERWEIGHT

Definition

Underweight is defined as a prepregnancy weight lower than 10% below the standard weight for height. Alternatively, it may be defined as a prepregnancy weight less than 120 pounds. Using the latter definition, the incidence has been reported to be 37.2% in white women and 29.2% in black women (21).

Etiology

The etiology of underweight, like that of obesity, probably is multifactorial, with both physiological and psychological components. Some women seem to be normally thin. Others may be striving through dieting for "emaciated model thinness" (26), the standard of beauty in our culture.

Maternal size may reflect long-term nutritional intake (6, p 321). Since women in our society usually increase their weight for height with age and parity, underweight is more common in young women (6, p 323). In multiparas underweight may reflect cumulative depletion, resulting from inadequate weight gain and poor nutritional status in previous pregnancies (26).

Maternal and Fetal Outcome

The major effects of low prepregnancy weight are an increased incidence of prematurity (27–30) and intrauterine growth retardation (6, 31). Table 26.7 lists the incidence of selected perinatal outcomes in underweight and normal weight women.

Eastman and Jackson in their classic study demonstrated that for both races and for all weight gain groups, there was an almost linear correlation between prepregnancy weight and birth weight. That is, as prepregnancy weight increased, so did birth weight, and this is independent of weight gain during pregnancy (21). Weight gain during pregnancy, however, is of crucial importance in determining the outcome of pregnancy in the underweight woman (see below, Weight Gain in Pregnancy).

It has been suggested that there may be an increased incidence of spontaneous abortions, neural tube defects and other anomalies, decreased mental and motor development, and even neonatal death in infants of underweight women (29).

There is an increased incidence of anemia in underweight women (30), suggesting that the nutritional deficit may be a deficit in many nutrients—not just body fat. Hunscher and Tompkins (28) also report an increased incidence of preeclampsia/eclampsia in underweight women.

Medical Management

The best management of underweight is to prevent it by achieving good nutritional status (i.e., sound dietary intake and adequate weight) prior to conception.

Several studies have indicated that the adverse effects of a low prepregnancy weight can be offset largely by an adequate weight gain during pregnancy (21, 32). Naeye reports optimal outcome

Table 26.7.

INFANT OUTCOME IN WOMEN WITH LOW PREPREGNANCY WEIGHT[a]

INFANT MORBIDITY	LOW PREPREGNANCY WEIGHT WOMEN[b]	NORMAL WEIGHT CONTROLS
	% of births	% of births
Low birth weight	15.3	7.6
Prematurity	23.0	14.0
Low Apgar Score	19.0	12.0

[a]Reproduced with permission from Worthington-Roberts BS, William SR: *Nutrition in Pregnancy and Lactation*, ed. 4, St. Louis, Times Mirror/Mosby College Publishing, 1989; Based on data from Edwards LE, et al.; Pregnancy in the underweight woman: course, outcome, and growth patterns of the infant *Am J Obstet Gynecol* 135:297, 1979.
[b]Ten percent or more below standard weight for height.

when the underweight woman gains about 30 pounds (5).

Weight gain is correlated with caloric intake (5). Eastman and Jackson (21) recommend that underweight women be encouraged to "eat to appetite" during the early part of pregnancy. Most will have an increased appetite after the first trimester and will gain sufficiently. The advice to "eat to appetite" should not be taken as a license to eat empty calorie foods, since the underweight woman may be deficient in a number of nutrients.

At approximately 20 weeks' gestation, the patient who began pregnancy underweight should be reevaluated. If she has not gained at least 10 pounds, she should be regarded as "high risk" nutritionally. A diet history and individual nutrition counseling should be done to help her maintain her weight gain at approximately 1 pound each week during the remainder of her pregnancy. Since fetal growth is much more rapid in the second half of pregnancy, this approach should allow adequate intake to support the fetus's growth.

The underweight woman should be screened for complications associated with low prepregnancy weight, and she should be cautioned about the dangers of cigarette smoking and drug and alcohol abuse since they, too, are associated with IUGR (see Chapter 27). Serial sonograms can be used to monitor fetal growth if there is a suspicion of IUGR clinically. The patient should be counseled about signs and symptoms of preterm labor and evaluated for them at each prenatal visit (see Chapter 28), and she should be screened carefully for anemia and preeclampsia and treated as necessary (see Chapters 8 and 13).

WEIGHT GAIN IN PREGNANCY

Some of the research regarding weight gain during pregnancy is conflicting; for example, one study reports that weight gain is correlated negatively with prepregnancy weight (21), while another reports there is no correlation (except for a decrease in weight gain in women over 160 pounds) (33). However, it does seem clear that birth weight is associated positively with both maternal weight gain in pregnancy and maternal prepregnancy weight, that each of these factors exerts an effect that is independent of the other, and that maternal weight gain is a stronger determinant of birth weight than prepregnancy weight.

Much research has centered on determining the optimal weight gain for pregnant women. Most studies conclude that women who are underweight at the beginning of pregnancy need to gain more than the average, and women who are overweight prior to pregnancy have more adipose (and perhaps nonadipose) reserves so that they do not need to gain as much. For example, Naeye, after analyzing data from the Collaborative Perinatal Project of the National Institute of Neurological and Communicative Disorders and Stroke (1959–1966), concluded that the lowest perinatal mortality occurred when underweight women gained 30 pounds, normal weight women gained 20 pounds, and overweight women gained 16 pounds by term. Perinatal mortality rates rose when women in any of the weight gain groups gained significantly (i.e., 5–10 pounds) more or less than the optimum (5).

Rosso (34) has proposed a new chart to monitor weight gain in pregnancy (Fig. 26.3). The goal for women who start pregnancy underweight or at normal weight is to reach 120% of their standard weight by term. This averages a gain of 12 kg (26.4 pounds). For women starting pregnancy at greater than 120% of their standard weight, the recommendation varies, but a minimal gain of 7 kg (15.4 pounds) to account for the weight of the products of conception and necessary maternal growth is recommended. Women who meet the recommendations have babies with significantly higher birth weight and lower perinatal mortality than women

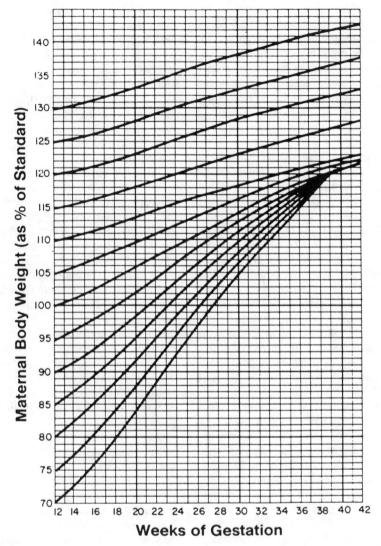

Figure 26.3. Chart to monitor weight gain during pregnancy considering prepregnancy weight and height. Reprinted with permission from Rossi P: A new chart to monitor weight gain during pregnancy. Am J Clin Nutr 41:645, 1985.

who do not. This chart, although slightly more difficult to use than the commonly used weight gain grid, has the following advantages: it takes into consideration very short and very tall women who need to gain more or less than the average, and it can be used for women, especially late registrants for prenatal care, who cannot accurately recall their prepregnancy weight.

Tompkins et al. found that an average or greater weight gain in the first two trimesters of pregnancy is associated with a lower incidence of preterm delivery (27). Weight gain in the third trimester has been found to be of great importance in determining birth weight. During the Dutch fam-

ine in the mid 1940s, it was found that good nutrition beginning in the early third trimester following two trimesters of hunger resulted in delivery of normal weight infants (35). Thus, it is evident that good nutritional status is important at all stages of pregnancy.

Inadequate Weight Gain

It is impossible to define inadequate maternal weight gain precisely in the number of pounds gained since it depends upon prepregnancy weight, body build, and special circumstances, such as adolescence or multiple gestation.

The causes of inadequate weight gain are varied; it may be due to social pressure from family and friends (i.e., pressure to achieve weight loss ultimately if she does not gain too much weight during the pregnancy); it could be due to poor dietary habits or unavailability of adequate amounts and types of food; it may be due to dietary restrictions by medical personnel; or it could be the result of chronic ill health of the mother or fetus, resulting in poor intake.

Picone et al. found that smokers gained less weight than nonsmokers in spite of a higher caloric intake, perhaps because nicotine stimulates release of epinephrine. Epinephrine causes a higher heart rate, blood pressure, basal metabolic rate, and rate of lipolysis. Calories thus may be used by the body rather than stored as adipose tissue. Interestingly, lower maternal weight gain accounts for three-quarters of the decrease in birth weight caused by smoking. Obesity has a protective effect, eliminating the negative effects of smoking on birth weight (36). Adequate weight gain in pregnancy can counteract the effects of smoking partially (37), so it may be suggested that women who cannot or will not stop smoking during pregnancy should be advised to increase their weight gain by an even greater caloric intake.

Picone et al. noted also that women under a great deal of stress also tended to gain less weight than normal. The stress, they found, did not decrease caloric intake, as might be supposed. They hypothesized that the mechanism might be as follows: stress causes an increase in secretion of corticoids, catecholamines, growth hormone, and prolactin. These hormones impair release of insulin and stimulate glycogenolysis, lipolysis, gluconeogenesis, and an increase in the basal metabolic rate, which may utilize the calories rather than allowing them to be available for weight gain. Stress before and during pregnancy also was demonstrated to be associated with an increase in pregnancy complications, which may also affect weight gain (36).

Inadequate weight gain in pregnancy is associated with poor perinatal outcome. Winick suggested that inadequate nutrition results in a poor maternal adaptation to pregnancy, such as inadequate blood volume expansion (38). Brown et al. reported that underweight and normal weight women who gained less than 9 kg (19.8 pounds) had 27.8% low birth weight infants, whereas those who gained greater than 9 kg had an incidence of only 7.2% low birth weight infants (31). Naeye found an increased incidence of placenta previa and chorioamnionitis in women with poor weight gain. He also found excess perinatal morbidity and mortality in women with poor weight gain (or weight loss). Even among overweight women, those with low weight gain had twice the perinatal mortality of overweight women with optimal weight gain. He suggests that the quantity or balance of nutrients from maternal reserves is not as beneficial to the fetus as those from dietary intake. Alternatively, he suggests that the poor perinatal outcome may be associated with acetonuria, resulting from utilization of maternal fat stores when caloric intake is inadequate (5).

On the other hand, some experts question whether there is any adverse effect from acetonuria (4). Also, Tavris et al., in a study that did not control for prepregnancy weight, concluded that in pregnancies lasting longer than 35 weeks, maternal weight gain had no effect on fetal, neonatal, or childhood mortality rates. They did *not* focus on birth weight as an outcome related to maternal weight gain—only mortality rates. These researchers questioned whether women with poor outcomes owing to inadequate weight gain in pregnancy had a poor total gain because of shortened duration of gestation (i.e., prematurity) or whether poor nutritional status might have caused preterm delivery. They imply that increased mortality in infants of women with inadequate weight gain is due entirely to prematurity. However, children of women who gained very little weight (less than 5 pounds) or an excessive amount of weight (greater than 29 pounds) had lower scores at age 5 on a nonverbal test of cognitive ability (39).

The management of low weight gain in pregnancy is to prevent it through sound nutrition counseling beginning early in the pregnancy. Weight gain should be monitored throughout the pregnancy, with additional nutritional assessment and counseling when needed. Because the effects of prepregnancy weight and weight gain during pregnancy are independent of each other and are additive in effect, particular attention should be focused on the woman who begins the pregnancy underweight. She should be encouraged to gain more than the average—approximately 30 pounds (5), or enough to reach 120% of her standard weight for height (34). The National Academy of Sciences recommends an average weight gain of 24–27 pounds for normal women. Overweight women may have a more modest weight gain goal, but most experts agree currently that it should be around 7 kg (15–16 pounds) to provide sufficiently for the growth of pregnancy.

Of course, other potential causes of poor weight gain should be addressed: maternal and fetal illness should be diagnosed and treated as appropriate; the woman should be counseled to stop smoking; psychosocial stress should be dealt with and alleviated as much as possible through professional counseling, financial assistance, referral to food assistance programs, and so on, as appropriate; the woman should be counseled about the desirability of weight gain during pregnancy, regardless of pressures from family and friends; and, of course, the woman should understand fully any medical recommendations concerning her diet so that she does not believe erroneously that she should severely limit her weight gain or diet prior to prenatal appointments.

Excessive Weight Gain

Excessive weight gain in pregnancy may be the result of the woman giving herself license to eat whatever she wants, regardless of the quantity or nutritional value. Some women may overeat for psychological reasons (e.g., ambivalence regarding the pregnancy, poor body image, changes in relationships among family and friends). Some women who were very active prior to pregnancy may not compensate for decreased activity levels during pregnancy by decreasing their intake.

Naeye's study of perinatal outcome indicated that perinatal mortality increased with a weight gain of greater than 32 pounds, regardless of prepregnancy weight for height. He found that there was very little increase in the incidence of fetal and placental abnormalities in women who gained an excessive amount of weight, but once such a problem existed, it had a much greater chance of ending in perinatal death than in the woman with normal weight gain (5).

As previously stated, Tavris et al. found that there was no increased fetal, neonatal, or childhood mortality in women who gained more than 29 pounds, but their children at age 5 did have lower scores on a nonverbal test of cognitive ability. Of course, a cause-effect relationship could not be established (39).

Since birth weight is influenced strongly by maternal weight gain in pregnancy, macrosomia is a potential result of excessive gain. With macrosomia, of course, are the associated risks of birth trauma, operative delivery, asphyxia, and neonatal hypoglycemia.

Excessive weight gain during pregnancy may result in postpartum obesity. If the weight is not lost, the woman will have all of the associated problems of obesity, including the risk of diabetes mellitus, hypertension, cardiovascular disease, and a shortened life expectancy.

The best management of excessive weight gain is, again, to prevent it through nutritional counseling early in the pregnancy. Weight gain should be monitored at each prenatal visit, and nutritional assessment and counseling should be initiated as soon as a deviation from the normal is noted. The woman should also be assisted with any associated needs—foods assistance program or financial assistance so she is able to make wise food choices, counseling regarding desirable activity levels during pregnancy, or professional counseling for the psychosocial needs she may have.

NURSING MANAGEMENT

Nursing care specific for the patient with inadequate or excessive weight gain:

☐ Whenever possible, provide preconception counseling regarding the following:
— Sound dietary habits, including intake of a variety of foods from each of the food groups; and intake of supplemental vitamins prior to conception;
— Standard weight for height, including a diet and exercise plan to achieve that weight prior to conception;
— An exercise program that can be maintained (or altered as needed) during pregnancy; and
— Cessation of smoking.

☐ Screen all pregnant women by eliciting a baseline dietary evaluation (24-hour recall) and by monitoring incremental and total weight gain at each prenatal visit; use of a standard weight gain chart will assist in identifying deviations from the norm.

☐ When a deviation is identified, provide appropriate intervention, e.g.:
— Nutrition counseling;
— Referral for psychological assessment/counseling as needed; and
— Referral for financial assistance programs as needed.

☐ Encourage patients to stop smoking, or to cut down as much as possible during pregnancy.

Nursing care specific for the underweight gravida:

☐ Consider a weekly nursing visit either in the home or in the care setting for a weight check until a consistent pattern of weight gain is achieved.

NURSING MANAGEMENT

☐ Screen the underweight patient for associated complications (e.g., anemia, pre-eclampsia, IUGR).

☐ Teach signs/symptoms of preterm labor; screen for preterm labor at each prenatal visit.

Nursing care specific for the obese gravida:

☐ Encourage normal eating habits, and encourage appropriate weight gain for pregnancy.

☐ Screen the obese patient for associated complications (e.g., diabetes mellitus, hypertension).

☐ Be alert to labor and delivery complications (e.g., dysfunctional labor, shoulder dystocia, birth injury, birth asphyxia); provide nursing care for complications that arise.

Nursing diagnoses most frequently associated with *inadequate or excessive weight gain* (see Section V):

☐ Altered nutrition: less than body requirements.

☐ Altered nutrition: more than body requirements.

☐ Knowledge deficit regarding etiology, disease process, treatment, and outcome.

☐ Ineffective individual coping.

☐ Disturbance to body image, self-esteem.

REFERENCES

1. Henley EC, Bahl S: Nutrition across the woman's life cycle. *Nurs Clin N A* 17:99–109, 1982.
2. Oakes GK, Chez RA: Nutrition during pregnancy with emphasis on overweight and underweight patients. *Contemp OB/GYN* 4:147–150, 1974.
3. Travers CK: Obesity and pregnancy: a review. *Obesity/Bariatric Med* 5:172–177, 1976.
4. Kliegman RM, Gross T: Perinatal problems of the obese mother and her infant. *Obstet Gynecol* 66:299–305, 1985.
5. Naeye RI: Weight gain and the outcome of pregnancy. *Am J Obstet Gynecol* 135:3–9, 1979.
6. Beal VA: Nutritional studies during pregnancy. *J Am Diet Assoc* 58:321–326, 1971.
7. Higgins AC: Nutritional status and the outcome of pregnancy. *J Can Diet Assoc* 37:17–34, 1976.
8. Curda LR: What about pica? *J Nurse-Midwifery* 22:7–11, 1977.
9. Lackey CJ: Pica—pregnancy's etiological mystery. In Committee on Nutrition of the Mother and Preschool Child: *Alternative Dietary Practices and Nutritional Abuse in Pregnancy*. Washington, DC, National Academy Press, 1982, pp 84–96.
10. Bullough VL, Bullough B: *Health Care for the Other Americans*. New York, Appleton-Century-Crofts, 1982.
11. O'Rourke DE, Quinn JG, Nicholson JO, Gibson HH: Geophagia during pregnancy. *Obstet Gynecol* 29:581–584, 1967.
12. Blum M, Orton CG, Rose L: The effect of starch ingestion on excessive iron absorption. *Ann Intern Med* 68:1165, 1968.
13. Talkington KM, Gant NF, Scott DE, Pritchard JA: Effects of ingestion of starch and some clays on iron absorption. *Am J Obstet Gynecol* 108:262–267, 1970.
14. Gold M: The practice of pica during pregnancy. Unpublished, 1982.
15. Edwards CH, McDonald S, Mitchell JR, Jones L, Mason L, Kemp AM, Laing D, Trigg L: Clay and corn starch eating women. *J Am Diet Assoc* 35:810–815, 1957.
16. University of California, Berkeley: *Wellness Letter*. 2:4–5, 1986.
17. Calandra C, Abell DA, Beischer NA: Maternal obesity in pregnancy. *Obstet Gynecol* 57:8–12, 1981.
18. Kemp R: The overall picture of obesity. *Practitioner* 209:654, 1972.
19. Tracy TA, Miller GL: Obstetric problems of the massively obese. *Obstet Gynecol* 33:204, 1969.
20. Gross T, Sokol RJ, King KC: Obesity in pregnancy: risks and outcome. *Obstet Gynecol* 56:446–450, 1980.
21. Eastman NJ, Jackson E: Weight relationships in pregnancy. I. The bearing of maternal weight gain and pre-pregnancy weight on birth weight in full term pregnancies. *Obstet Gynecol Survey* 23:1003–1024, 1968.
22. Sullivan N. Early determinants of obesity: maternal, prenatal, genetic and environmental factors. Unpublished, 1982.
23. Worthington-Roberts BS, Vermeersch J, Williams SR: *Nutrition in Pregnancy and Lactation*, ed 2. St. Louis, Mosby, 1981.
24. Churchill JA, Berendes HW, Nemore J: Neuropsychological deficits in children of diabetic mothers. A report from the Collaborative Study of Cerebral Palsy. *Am J Obstet Gynecol* 105:257, 1969.
25. Naeye RL, Chez RA: Effects of maternal acetonuria and low pregnancy weight gain on children's psychomotor development. *Am J Obstet Gynecol* 139:189, 1981.
26. Luke B: *Maternal Nutrition*. Boston, Little, Brown, and Co., 1979, p 8.
27. Tompkins WT, Mitchell, Wiehl DG: The underweight patient as an increased obstetrical hazard. *Am J Obstet Gynecol* 69:114, 1955.
28. Hunscher HA, Tompkins WT: The influence of maternal nutrition on the immediate and long-term outcome of pregnancy. *Clin Obstet Gynecol* 13:130, 1970.

29. Wynn M, Wynn A: The importance of maternal nutrition in the weeks before and after conception. *Birth* 9:39–45, 1982.

30. Edwards LE, et al.: Pregnancy in the underweight woman: course, outcome, and growth patterns of the infant. *Am J Obstet Gynecol* 135:297, 1979.

31. Brown JE, Jacobson HN, Askue LH, Peick MG: Influence of pregnancy weight gain on the size of infants born to underweight women. *Obstet Gynecol* 57:13–17, 1981.

32. Lechtig et al.: Effect of food supplementation during pregnancy on birth weight. *Pediatrics* 56:508, 1975.

33. Rush D, Stein Z, Susser M: Another viewpoint. *Birth* 9:43–45, 1982.

34. Rosso P: A new chart to monitor weight gain during pregnancy. *Am J Clin Nutr* 41:644–652, 1985.

35. Smith CA: The effect of wartime starvation in Holland upon pregnancy and its product. *Am J Obstet Gynecol* 53:599, 1947.

36. Picone TA, Lindsay HA, Schramm MM, Olsen N: Pregnancy outcome in North American women. Effects of diet, cigarette smoking, and psychological stress on maternal weight gain. *Am J Clin Nutr* 36:1205–1213, 1982.

37. Luke B, Hawkins MM, Petrie RH: Influence of smoking, weight gain, and pregravid weight for height on intrauterine growth. *Am J Clin Nutr* 34:1410–1417, 1981.

38. Winick, M: Weight gain during pregnancy. *Nutr Health* 4:1–6, 1979.

39. Tavris DR, Read JA: Effect of maternal weight gain on fetal, infant, and childhood health and on cognitive development. *Obstet Gynecol* 60:689–694, 1982.

Chapter 27
Intrauterine Growth
Retardation

Nola Geraghty Snyder, R.N., M.S.N.

INTRODUCTION

Intrauterine growth retardation (IUGR) is a major cause of medical morbidity in the neonatal period. Growth-retarded fetuses are five times as likely to suffer from perinatal asphyxia. There is also an eight times higher risk of neonatal death in this group, making identification of these infants in the prenatal period particularly important (1). IUGR complicates between 3–7% of all pregnancies, but 50–80% of these cases are not diagnosed until delivery (2). Various indices of fetal growth are used to determine IUGR antenally, including clinical assessment, ultrasound, and biochemical testing. The antenatal identification of these at-risk fetuses may enable providers to intervene, thereby reducing complications and improving overall pregnancy outcome.

Normal fetal development is dependent upon factors such as fetal ability to maintain normal growth, lack of growth-retarding factors in the environment, adequate placental function to transport oxygen and nutrients to the fetus, adequate maternal nutrient intake, and sufficient maternal blood volume. Each trimester of pregnancy is characterized by significant developmental progress.

The first trimester is the time of organogenesis, which follows a cephalocaudal progression. At this time there is an increase in cell numbers referred to as the *hyperplastic stage* (3).

The second trimester is marked by more rapid fetal growth. This stage of growth is called *hyperplastic/hypertrophic*, because while cell numbers are still increasing, the cells also are getting larger in size. Tissue weight and protein content increase in this stage (3, p 503).

The third trimester is characterized by significant increase in fetal size, particularly weight, as subcutaneous fat is laid down. This is referred to as the *hypertrophic* stage since the cells increase in size at this time relative to the increase in DNA content. Brain and muscle tissue continues hyperplastic growth during this time as well as after birth (3, p 503).

The growth of the normal fetus is dependent on placental growth, which occurs linearly during pregnancy until about 36 weeks' gestation. Placental growth and increases in maternal blood volume precede fetal growth. After 36 weeks' gestation, the placental surface area remains the same, while fetal growth demands are maximal. This may account for a normal slowing of the rate of weight gain in fetuses between 36–38 weeks or in the postdate fetus (P. Rosso, unpublished observations).

DEFINITION

The definition of IUGR lacks uniformity, which complicates early identification and epidemiological studies (2, 4). The most common definition is that birth weight is below the tenth percentile of mean birth weight for gestational age (1). Some babies will normally be below the tenth percentile because of a genetically small body type. Frequently used measures of size for gestational age were developed by Lubchenco (Figs. 27.1 and 27.2). While these growth curves remain in use universally, there are those investigators who state that they are only applicable to populations living at least 6000 feet above sea level, as they were based on birth weights of infants in the Denver area. This

Cm

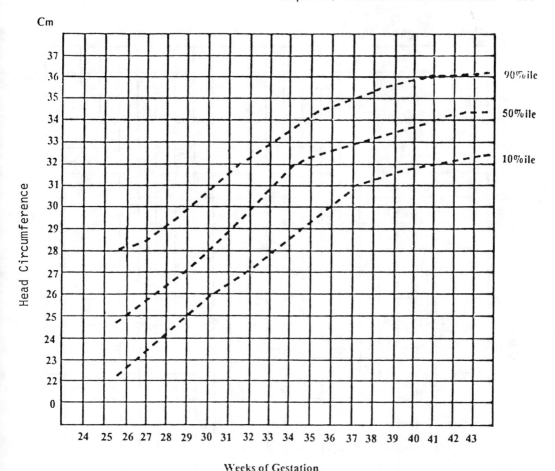

Weeks of Gestation

Figure 27.1. Classification of newborns by head circumference and gestational age. (*Note:* Adapted from Lubchenco LO, Hansman C, Boyd E: Intrauterine growth in length and head circumference as estimated from live births at gestational ages from 26 to 42 weeks. *Pediatrics* 37(3):403–416, 1966. Copyright 1966 by the American Academy of Pediatrics. Reprinted with permission. This form may be reproduced. The March of Dimes Birth Defects Foundation, 1982.)

means that infants born at lower altitudes may be assessed incorrectly because high altitude causes a decrease in birth weight. In some areas IUGR is diagnosed only when birth weight is below the fifth or third percentile (5).

The term *small for gestational age* (SGA) sometimes is used synonymously with IUGR. It is useful to consider IUGR as a term describing antenatal fetal status and reserve SGA for describing the assessment of the infant after delivery. IUGR is a diagnostic term made by indirect observations of the fetal status, whereas SGA is a determination made after actual measurements of the infant. Depending upon the cutoff point on the growth curve that is used, an infant is said to be growth retarded or SGA. Ideally, a growth curve should be based on the maternal population in a given geographic area

to identify SGA most reliably. Since this is not always possible, adjustment of the Lubchenco curve may be necessary, as well as use of several indicators of fetal growth other than weight.

Growth retardation can occur at any gestational age, and accurate determination of gestational age is crucial in identifying growth retardation. There have been two types of IUGR described in the literature. The first type is called *symmetrical* or proportional IUGR, since it is characterized by overall diminished growth. This means that all fetal parameters that can be measured are smaller than normal and, if severe enough, can lead to fetal wastage (3, p 503, 6). Symmetrical IUGR results from an early insult in fetal development. This occurs in the hyperplastic phase of growth and results in fewer numbers of cells. Women who are chroni-

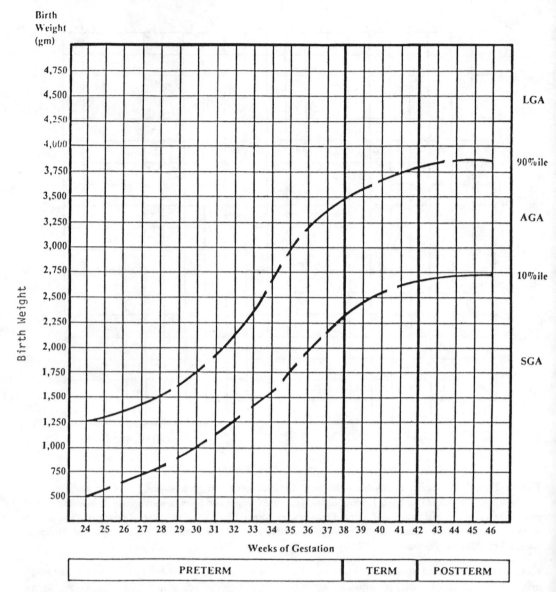

Figure 27.2. Classification of newborns by birth weight and gestational age. (*Note:* Adapted from Lubchenco LO, Searls DT, Brazie JV: Neonatal mortality rate: relationship to birth weight and gestational age. 81(4):814–822, 1972. Copyright 1972 by Mosby. Reprinted by permission. This form may be reproduced. The March of Dimes Birth Defects Foundation, 1982.)

cally malnourished and/or who smoke during this phase are at risk for this type of IUGR (7, 8). Other potential causes are intrauterine infection, congenital anomalies, and familial short stature. Because of the reduced numbers of cells in this type of IUGR, the impairment may not be reversible.

Asymmetrical IUGR is the second type of growth retardation and pertains to the period of hyperplastic/hypertrophic and hypertrophic growth. Asymmetrical IUGR is characterized by normal head growth but a smaller abdominal circumfer-

ence. The infant appears to have little subcutaneous fat, with loose skin folds. Pregnancies complicated by pregnancy-induced hypertension are at risk for this type of IUGR (3, p 503). Asymmetrical IUGR usually is related to a uteroplacental abnormality or decreased uteroplacental circulation, causing a decrease in exchange of nutrients and oxygen to the fetus. This "brain-sparing" growth pattern may result from fetal carotid artery receptor stimulation, which in turn dilates the vessels to enhance oxygen perfusion to the brain. The potential

Table 27.1.
ETIOLOGICAL FACTORS OF IUGR.[a]

FETAL	MATERNAL	ENVIRONMENTAL
Chromosomal abnormalities	Low prepregnancy weight	Maternal drug abuse
Familial short stature	Poor prenatal weight gain	Alcohol abuse
Sex	Anemias	Tobacco
Race	Placental abnormalities	High altitude
Congenital malformations	Diabetes mellitus	Chemicals
Intrauterine infection	Extrauterine pregnancy	Ionizing radiation
Multiple gestation	Pregnancy-induced hypertension	Decompression illness
Hormonal abnormalities	Chronic hypertension	
	Renal disease	
	Cyanotic heart disease	
	Pulmonary insufficiency	
	High parity	
	Previous history of IUGR	
	Uterine malformations	

[a]Modified from Crawford CS: In Bologhese RJ, Schwartz RH, Schneider J (eds.): *The Growth Retarded Newborn in Perinatal Medicine: Management of the High Risk Fetus and Neonate*, ed 2. Baltimore, Williams & Wilkins, 1982.

for catching up in growth is greater for this type of growth retardation, provided the condition is discovered in the prenatal period.

ETIOLOGY

Many factors have been associated with increased incidence of IUGR. These factors can exert independent and interdependent influences on fetal growth. The probable multifactorial pathophysiology complicates the understanding of IUGR and its identification and the potential for intervention. Table 27.1 and Figure 27.3 depict these multiple factors.

Such fetal factors as congenital malformations, race, sex, familial short stature, and multiple gestation cannot be changed. The risk of intrauterine infection can be affected by good patient education and prenatal screening for common infections related to IUGR, such as malaria and the TORCH diseases.

Maternal factors can be divided into personal, placental, or preexisting disease categories. Personal characteristics are those such as low prepregnancy weight; poor nutritional status during pregnancy; maternal age less than 15 years; high parity; previous birth of IUGR infant; and maternal alcohol, drug, or tobacco use. All of these have been associated with retarded fetal growth (6). Some of these can be altered by patient education, follow-up, and, in the case of nutrition, an active intervention to supplement the diet.

Maternal smoking is shown to have a dose related response in the fetus. The cotinine (nicotine derivative) causes decreased oxygenation of uteroplacental blood flow (17). This effect of nicotine

often is combined with a simultaneous food intake reduction in smoking women to complicate fetal growth even further (7). Reduction of smoking by the mother during pregnancy has been shown to increase birth weight for single live births (19). The abuse of other drugs such as heroin and alcohol also are implicated in IUGR and are covered in detail in Chapter 19.

Placental factors related to growth retardation, such as abnormal placental size, previa, and minor abruption, cause reduced nutrient and oxygen transfer to the fetus, resulting in an IUGR fetus. Such placental pathology often can lead to preterm delivery (see Chapter 31).

Preexisting maternal disease also is significant in the development of IUGR. Vascular diseases, such as chronic hypertension, pregnancy-induced hypertension, and advanced diabetes, result in impaired uteroplacental blood flow (11, 12). Chronic maternal hypoxia resulting from cystic fibrosis, asthma, cyanotic heart disease, and hemoglobinopathies such as sickle cell anemia may, in turn, negatively affect fetal growth (13). Renal and gastrointestinal disorders (e.g., Crohn's disease, colitis, anorexia nervosa) are other factors. Rare or unusual endocrine and connective tissue diseases such as pseudoxanthoma elasticum or Addison's disease have been related to IUGR in a few cases (14, 15).

Hazards such as radiation, toxic chemicals, and high altitude hypoxia are environmental factors that should be evaluated when caring for pregnant patients. Related to this are the effects of decompression sickness in women who scuba dive for recreation or for their work (16).

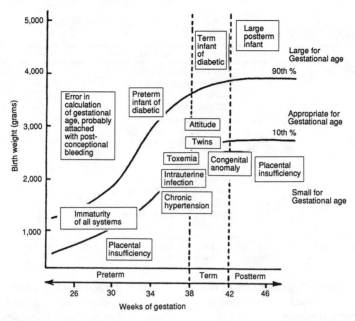

Figure 27.3. Representation of birth weight relationship to gestational age, with associated conditions. Note that a newborn is considered growth retarded if the birth weight is below the tenth percentile for gestational age. (Adapted from Lubchenco LO, Hausman C, Backstrom L: Factors influencing fetal growth. In: *Nutricia Symposium: Aspects of Prematurity and Dysmaturity*. Leiden, The Netherlands. H.E. Stenford Kroese B.V., 1968.)

DIAGNOSIS

The presence of etiological risk factors in a given patient's history should be considered during the initial visit. Subsequent prenatal visits should include reassessment for the development of any of these factors as pregnancy progresses. In the case of previous SGA births, the old records should be examined.

The physical examination can reveal clinical findings suspicious of IUGR. After careful pregnancy dating (see Chapter 6), a size-dates discrepancy may be the first indication of IUGR. The usual protocol is to consider ultrasound examination or further diagnostic studies if the fundal height measurement is more than 2 cm behind dates on two occasions or more than 3 cm on one occasion. Abdominal palpation for estimating fetal size can be done as well. Other signs such as a low maternal weight gain should be noted (3, p 514).

The use of ultrasound has advanced the diagnosis of IUGR tremendously. It is an integral tool in the follow-up of those patients who are at risk or who demonstrate clinical signs of IUGR. The nature of IUGR necessitates the use of serial measures to evaluate changes in growth patterns. For greatest accuracy, a scan should be done early in pregnancy.

A crown-rump length measurement in the first trimester can provide accurate data regarding the correct estimated date of confinement (EDC). Other measures can be taken beginning early in gestation or between 20–24 weeks' gestation and at other intervals if indicated (6, p 240, 17).

Biparietal diameter (BPD) measurements are common measures of fetal growth and aid in confirming EDC. Serial measures are required for any predictive capacity for IUGR. Alone, BPD is not a sensitive indicator of IUGR since it fails to detect asymmetrical IUGR and can be unreliable when side-to-side flattening of the head is present (32) (5). Abdominal circumference is measured at the level of the umbilical vein. When this measurement is small in comparison with a normal BPD, it will detect asymmetrical IUGR. In a normal fetus the abdominal circumference becomes greater in the last few weeks of gestation secondary to liver enlargement. This is not the case in IUGR.

Total intrauterine volume (TIUV) uses a formula to determine an overall intrauterine measurement. If TIUV is within two standard deviations of the mean for gestational age, the chance of IUGR is less than 1% (1, p 183). Conversely, amniotic fluid volume measures indicate possible IUGR if there is severe oligohydramnios.

Fetal femur length can be used in the second and third trimesters to estimate fetal length. When this length measure is used with weight determinations, it can be useful in the diagnosis of IUGR and in detection of dwarfism.

Other uses of ultrasound include measurement of umbilical blood flow and real-time observation of fetal breathing, heart rate, fetal tone, and movement. These observations make up the *biophysical profile*, which can be used as an additional assessment tool (5). Accuracy of these measurements depends upon the number of parameters used, timing of scan, accuracy of EDC, skill of the examiner, and quality of the equipment. In the future new methods of assessment may be possible with nuclear magnetic resonance (NMR) (18).

Biochemical testing sometimes can indicate impaired fetal growth. Maternal urinary estriol levels usually are low with IUGR. Since this is an inaccurate form of diagnosis, serial estriol levels should be used in conjunction with ultrasound (1, p 183). Human placental lactogen (HPL) levels can be used to estimate placental mass. They have been used to detect IUGR but are highly unreliable.

MATERNAL AND FETAL OUTCOME

Maternal implications predominantly are related to the maternal etiological factors associated with IUGR. The woman may need treatment for preexisting disease and a more closely monitored pregnancy in general. Life-stye changes such as bed rest, dietary changes, limited exercise, and cessation of drug, alcohol, and cigarette consumption may be indicated. Timing of the delivery is based upon evaluation of the benefits versus the risks of the fetus remaining in the intrauterine environment. Severe IUGR may require induced labor and an increased incidence of cesarean delivery if induction fails or if the fetus is too compromised to withstand the stress of labor.

Fetal outcome is related to abnormal growth or concomitant anomalies discussed previously. The growth-retarded fetus is susceptible particularly to perinatal asphyxia, meconium aspiration,

and persistent fetal circulation (3, p 518). In the presence of oligohydramnios, the incidence of cord compression during labor is increased. These fetuses, however, are protected somewhat from respiratory distress owing to a hastened pulmonary maturation secondary to chronic intrauterine stress (hypoxia).

In the neonatal period the IUGR infant is at risk for polycythemia, hypothermia, hypoglycemia, and sepsis. Polycythemia may be due to increased erythropoiesis secondary to chronic stress. Hypothermia and hypoglycemia can be caused by the infant's increased metabolic rate and decreased glycogen stores. Susceptibility to infection may be related to decreased thymic hormone and T-cell activity. The long-term prognosis for these infants depends upon the type, severity, and duration of the growth-retarding insult; how soon it was identified and treated; and the immediate care of the infant (19). Delayed head growth before the third trimester as evidenced by serial ultrasonography results in a subsequent delay in neurologic and intellectual development.

MEDICAL MANAGEMENT

Management consists of prevention of potential causative factors by careful prenatal assessment, early and accurate diagnosis of altered fetal growth, and identification and treatment of causative factors. Some direct interventions include decreased activity and bed rest to facilitate uteroplacental blood flow; a high protein diet; and fetal surveillance through ultrasound, antepartum nonstress testing, and fetal movement counts (6, p 242). Timing of delivery to enhance neonatal outcome must weigh the risks of prematurity against the risks associated with remaining in utero. During labor, fetal status must be monitored by electronic fetal monitoring and scalp pH sampling as necessary, since the incidence of fetal distress is increased. The pediatric team should be present at delivery and prepared for full-scale resuscitation.

NURSING MANAGEMENT

Nursing care specific for a patient with intrauterine growth retardation:

☐ Teach all patients (preconceptionally or as early in the pregnancy as possible) health behavior to prevent IUGR (e.g., avoid smoking, alcohol, and drug use; maintain good nutri-

tion; avoid environmental hazards such as radiation and toxic chemicals).

☐ Identify patients at risk for IUGR (e.g., patients with diabetes, hypertension, TORCH diseases, low prepregnancy weight, poor nutritional status during pregnancy, alcohol/drug/tobacco

NURSING MANAGEMENT

use); monitor fetal growth at each prenatal visit.

☐ Educate the patient regarding the following:
- Fetal assessment (risks, benefits, frequency of tests): NSTs (weekly or biweekly); serial ultrasound examinations; fetal activity record;
- Treatment regimen:
  * Bed rest in left lateral position (may require homemaker services or discontinuation of employment);
  * high protein, high iron, high calorie diet, with vitamin and mineral supplements, as needed; and
  * management specific to preexisting conditions.

☐ Observe for fetal distress during labor:

- Use continuous electronic fetal monitoring and
- Observe for meconium staining.

☐ Prepare for emergency cesarean section and/or neonatal resuscitation.

Nursing diagnoses most frequently associated with IUGR (see Section V):

☐ Anxiety/fear.

☐ Grieving related to potential/actual loss of infant or birth of an imperfect child.

☐ Knowledge deficit regarding condition, treatment, and expected outcome.

☐ Altered nutrition: less than body requirements.

☐ Altered fetal cardiac and cerebral tissue perfusion.

REFERENCES

1. Hobbins JC: Intrauterine growth retardation. In Queenan JR, Hobbins JC (eds): *Protocols for High Risk Pregnancies*. Oradell, NJ, Medical Economics, 1982, p 182.
2. Read MS, Catz C, Grave G, McNellis D: Intrauterine growth retardation: identification of research needs and goals. *Semin Perinatol* 8:2–5, 1984.
3. Crawford CS: The growth-retarded newborn. In Bologhese RJ, Schwarz RH, Schneider J (eds): *Perinatal Medicine: Management of the High Risk Fetus and Neonate*, ed 2. Baltimore, Williams & Wilkins, 1982, p 502.
4. Stein ZA, Susser M: Intrauterine growth retardation: epidemiological issues and public health significance. *Semin Perinatol* 8:5–13, 1984.
5. Sabbagha RE: Intrauterine growth retardation: avenues of future research in diagnosis and management by ultrasound. *Semin Perinatol* 8:31–36, 1984.
6. Haesslein HC: Diseases of fetal growth. In Niswander KR (ed): *Manual of Obstetrics*. Boston, Little, Brown, 1980, p 239.
7. Fielding JE: Smoking in pregnancy. *N Engl J Med* 298:537–539, 1978.
8. Brasel JA, Winick M: Maternal malnutrition and prenatal growth. Experimental studies of effects of maternal undernutrition on fetal and placental growth. *Arch Dis Child* 47:479–485, 1973.
9. Machizuki M, Maruo T, Masuko K, Ohtsu T: Effects of smoking on fetoplacental maternal system during pregnancy. *Am J Obstet Gynecol* 149:413–420, 1984.
10. Sexton M, Hebel JR: Clinical trial of changes in maternal smoking and its effect on birth weight. *JAMA* 251:911–915, 1984.

11. Sibai BM, Watson DL, Hill GA, Spinnato JA, Anderson GD: Maternal-fetal correlations in patients with severe preeclampsia. *Obstet Gynecol* 62:745–749, 1983.
12. Eriksson UJ: Diabetes in pregnancy: retarded fetal growth, congenital malformations and feto-maternal concentrations of zinc, copper and manganese in the rat. *J Nutr* 114:477–484, 1984.
13. Palmer J, Dillon-Baker C, Tecklin J, Wolfson B, Rosenberg B, Burroughs B, Holsclaw DS, Scanlin T, Huang NN, Sewell EM: Pregnancy in patients with cystic fibrosis. *Ann Intern Med* 99:596–600, 1983.
14. Broekhuizen F, Hamilton P: Pseudoxanthoma elasticum and intrauterine growth retardation. *Am J Obstet Gynecol* 148:112–114, 1984.
15. Drucker D, Shumak S, Angel A: Schmidt's syndrome presenting with intrauterine growth retardation and post partum Addisonian crisis. *Am J Obstet Gynecol* 149:229–230, 1984.
16. Gilman S, Bradley M, Greene K, Fischer G: Fetal development: effects of decompression sickness and treatment. *Av Sp Environ Med* 54:1040–1042, 1983.
17. Sabbagha RE: Intrauterine growth retardation: antenatal diagnosis by ultrasound. *Obstet Gynecol* 52:252–256, 1978.
18. Johnson I, Symonds E, Kean D, Worthington B, Pipkin F, Hawkes R, Gyngell M: Imaging the pregnant uterus with nuclear magnetic resonance. *Am J Obstet Gynecol* 148:1136–1139, 1984.
19. Allen MC: Developmental outcome and followup of the small for gestational age infant. *Semin Perinatol* 8:123–151, 1984.

Chapter 28
Preterm Labor
Nancy W. Kulb, C.N.M., M.S.

INTRODUCTION

Preterm labor is the greatest problem facing obstetrics today. The 6–8% of babies born prior to term account for 75–85% of neonatal deaths not due to congenital anomalies (1). A number of strategies for preventing and treating preterm labor are being investigated with some degree of success, but much is yet to be learned about its physiology and clinical management.

Although many aspects of the physiology of human labor are understood, its initiation is a complex phenomenon that has not yet been elucidated clearly. The fact that factors known to initiate labor vary from species to species means that animal studies cannot be applied necessarily to human labor, making the study more difficult.

In the past there were a number of theories concerning the onset of labor at term (2, 3):

1. Uterine stretch theory: Once the uterus is stretched to a certain point, it contracts in order to empty itself. This theory is supported by the fact that labor tends to begin earlier in cases of multiple gestation and polyhydramnios.
2. Progesterone deprivation theory: The level of progesterone decreases just before the onset of labor. In some animals administration of progesterone has been demonstrated to prolong gestation.
3. Oxytocin theory: The uterus becomes sensitive increasingly to oxytocin as gestation advances, and it is well known that oxytocin can induce labor near term. Also, blood levels of oxytocin increase markedly as labor advances. However, normal labor may occur in women in whom the hypophysis—the source of oxytocin—has been removed or destroyed.
4. Fetal endocrine control theory: Pregnancy tends to be prolonged when the fetus is anencephalic. In these babies the hypophysis is absent or small, and the adrenal glands also are quite small, suggesting that some hormonal signal from the fetus is absent.
5. Pressure theory: Pressure on the cervix and lower uterine segment as well as on nearby nerve plexuses may stimulate labor.
6. Cycle theory: The menstrual cycle occurs every 4 weeks. Labor usually begins at 40 weeks, after 10 menstrual cycles.
7. Shock theory: Emotional or physical shock, trauma, or stress may precipitate labor.

Currently, it is known that the conceptus participates in determining the timing of the onset of normal labor and that the release of prostaglandins (PGs), probably from the endometrium, is the final major event leading to labor (4). The critical role of PGs in the initiation of labor is supported by the following facts (4, p 131):

1. There is a sharp rise in PGs and their metabolites in both maternal blood and amniotic fluid during labor.
2. PGs will induce labor at any time during gestation. Oxytocin, on the other hand, will stimulate uterine activity but not necessarily effacement and dilatation until near term.
3. PG inhibitors also inhibit uterine activity.

Arachidonic acid (AA) is the precursor for PGs. AA is found in the lipid stores of cells; probably, AA from the amnion and chorion supplies the endometrium with the substrate to make PGs. A group of enzymes called prostaglandin synthetase convert AA to PGs. PGs then act locally, causing uterine contractions, perhaps by raising the level of calcium within smooth muscle cells. PGs are known to soften the cervix. Since there is little smooth muscle in the cervix, the effect probably is due to a decrease in collagen production.

Phospholipase A is probably the factor that controls the rate of PG synthesis, because it is responsible for releasing AA from the phospholipid stores in the cells. The stimulus for initiating this process is as yet unknown, although several ways to activate the system are known. Passing a finger through the cervix to "strip" the membranes may initiate labor, perhaps by stimulating PG production. Infection and hemorrhage may activate the process. But what normally starts it in the term uterus is not clear. Gap junctions, connections that transmit electrical impulses from one cell to the next, are more abundant near term, perhaps because of the increasing concentration of $PGF_2\alpha$. Oxytocin stimulates the release of PG. It may do this by stimulating PG synthesis or by removing a PG inhibitor. At any rate, oxytocin receptors increase in the myometrium and endometrium as term approaches (4, pp 133, 137, 141). In some animals phospholipase A, which controls the rate of PG synthesis, is controlled by the estrogen/progesterone ratio (a higher ratio results in greater PG production). The role of progesterone in human parturition is not clear; there is a wide range in normal serum values just prior to and during labor.

It seems that the signal for initiation of labor normally comes at a time when the needs of the fetus are no longer being met in utero. When labor occurs prematurely and no other cause can be identified, it may be that the normal "timing mechanism" is overruled by some strong, but as yet unidentified, stimulus (5).

DEFINITION

Because in the past different definitions were used for the same terms, literature regarding "premature" birth was confusing. In order to use accurate and precise terminology, pertinent terms are defined below.

Low birth weight: Birth weight less than 2500 g (5.5 lb). Because gestational age is difficult to assess accurately and consistently but birth weight is precise, easy to determine, and routinely recorded, in 1961 the World Health Organization defined a "premature" baby as one weighing less than 2500 g. It is now known, however, that low birth weight babies may be born prior to term, may be small for gestational age, or both. This chapter discusses preterm labor. See Chapter 27 for information on intrauterine growth retardation (IUGR).

Preterm (premature) birth: Birth occurring after less than 37 completed weeks (259 days) of gestation since the start of the last normal menstrual period.

Term birth: Birth occurring from 37 to less than 42 completed weeks (259–293 days) of gestation.

Postterm birth: Birth occurring at 42 completed weeks (294 days) of gestation or more.

Labor: The physiological process by which the mature or nearly mature products of conception are expelled from the uterus.

False labor: Uterine activity (contractions) that may be regular and strong but do *not* lead to progressive cervical effacement and dilatation.

Premature baby: Baby born from 28 to less than 37 weeks of gestation.

Immature baby: Baby born from 20–28 weeks of gestation.

Preterm (premature) labor: Labor occurring from 20 to less than 37 weeks of gestation.

Although the definitions seem clear enough, often they are problematic clinically. Labor occurs normally within a 4-week time period—2 weeks before to 2 weeks after the expected date of confinement. A bigger problem is in defining labor, especially in differentiating false labor from preterm labor. The diagnosis of preterm labor requires cervical change—the very thing treatment is designed to prevent or arrest. The earlier preterm labor treatment is begun, the greater the likelihood of success. However, erroneously labeling false labor as preterm labor leads to unnecessary treatment of a large number of women (6).

The incidence of preterm delivery in the United States is approximately 8%. Although much has been done to improve survival rates of babies born prior to term, so far little impact has been made on the incidence of preterm birth. The United States' overall low birth weight rate has decreased only from 7.5% in 1951 to 6.8% in 1986. Conventional prenatal care, nutritional support, and tocolytic drugs thus far have done little to reduce prematurity or low birth weight. Similarly, international statistics show that al-

Table 28.1.

FACTORS ASSOCIATED WITH PRETERM LABOR[a]

Demographic status
  Nonwhite
  Unmarried
  Low socioeconomic status
  Maternal age less than 20 years
  Place of residence (the larger the city, the greater the risk of preterm labor)
Obstetrical history
  Prior induced abortions[b]
  Prior low birth weight baby
  Prior preterm delivery
  Prior second trimester spontaneous abortion
  History of infertility
  Close pregnancy spacing (less than 1 year between last birth and conception of present pregnancy)
Medical status
  Heart disease
  Small heart volume relative to body size (maternal)
  Anemia
  Urinary tract infection in third trimester
  DES exposure in utero
Current pregnancy factors
  Lack of or late prenatal care[b]
  Low prepregnancy weight
  Poor weight gain during pregnancy
  Vaginal spotting
  Colonization with gonorrhea, β-streptococcus, or *Mycoplasma*
  Male fetus
  Abnormal placental implantation
Life-style
  Poor nutrition
  Lack of exercise before pregnancy
  Lack of leisure time physical activities
  Smoking
  Alcohol consumption prior to the third trimester
  Use of illicit drugs
  Exposure to toxins
  Coitus during pregnancy
  Employment, especially in a repetitive or physically demanding job
  Commuting a long distance
  Strenuous physical activity or exercise during pregnancy
Psychological factors
  Negative attitude toward the pregnancy
  Psychic trauma
  Stress

[a]Sources include references 5, 6, 10–12, 14, 16, 27, and 28.
[b]Positive association in some studies, not in others.

though there is wide variation in rates of low birth weight from country to country, there has been little change over time within an individual country (7). In fact, the incidence of preterm delivery actually may be increasing owing to socioeconomic factors, the increased incidence of induced abortions, and the shift of the population from rural to urban areas (5, p 208).

ETIOLOGY

In only 20% (8) to 40% (9) of cases of preterm birth is the cause due to obstetrical complications. In some cases the preterm birth is due to appropriate obstetrical intervention, when the risk to mother or baby is greater if gestation is allowed to continue than if delivered. Among the identifiable pathological causes of spontaneous preterm labor are: severe IUGR, premature rupture of the membranes, uterine anomalies (e.g., septate uterus, myomas, Asherman's syndrome), preeclampsia, severe hypertension, chorioamnionitis, congenital anomalies, cervical incompetence, placental malformations (e.g., circumvallate), antepartum hemorrhage (e.g., placenta previa, abruptio placentae, unexplained bleeding), overdistention of the uterus (e.g., multiple gestation, polyhydramnios), oligohydramnios, cholestasis, abdominal surgery, systemic febrile illness (10), insufficient progesterone secretion (11), fetal death, and retained intrauterine device (2, p 750).

In addition, there is a multitude of factors associated with preterm labor, although they probably are not direct causative factors. Table 28.1 lists the factors that have been identified by various studies. Note that many of these factors tend to occur in clusters, adding to the difficulty of determining the effect of any one of them. For example, in Berkowitz's study, the effects of age and marital status lost significance if socioeconomic status was controlled (12).

Uterine activity has been shown to increase when uterine blood flow is compromised, as with hypertension, heavy smoking, multiple pregnancy, poor nutrition, and supine position of the mother. Uterine activity decreases with increased uterine perfusion. Indeed, hydration and bed rest often have been shown to stop preterm labor (13).

Since women frequently are employed during pregnancy, the effect of employment on prematurity has been studied. Sources of occupational fatigue have been identified (Table 28.2) and have been demonstrated to be associated positively with prematurity. According to one study, the presence of several sources of occupational fatigue has an additive effect on prematurity rates. Medical risk factors and occupational risk factors present simultaneously have a synergistic effect on prematurity rates (14).

It is postulated that maternal stress has a strong bearing on pregnancy outcome, although this has not yet been proven. Stress is defined as mental, emotional, or physical tension, strain, or distress. Many disparate factors can contribute to

Table 28.2.
OCCUPATIONAL FATIGUE[a]

SOURCE OF OCCUPATIONAL FATIGUE	DESCRIPTION (SCORE "HIGH" IF ONE OR MORE ELEMENTS OF THE JOB LISTED IS PRESENT)
Posture	Posture in standing position more than 3 hours/day.
Work on industrial machine	Work on industrial conveyor belt. Independent work on industrial machine with strenuous effort or vibrations.
Physical exertion	Continuous or periodical physical effort. Carry load of more than 10 kg.
Mental stress	Routine work. Varied tasks requiring little attention without stimulation.
Environment	At least two of the following: Cold temperature Significant noise level Very wet atmosphere Manipulation of chemical substances.

[a]From Mamelle N, Laumon B, Lazar P: Prematurity and occupational activity during pregnancy. *Am J Epidemiol* 119:311, 1984.

stress. A multifactorial etiology of preterm labor based on maternal behaviors, personal characteristics, and inadequate social supports has been postulated.

Some studies have attempted to determine the magnitude of the risk of preterm delivery for individual factors. For example, Berkowitz found that a history of infertility tripled the incidence of preterm birth (12, p 83). After one preterm birth, the risk of recurrence is 25–50% (38% in Creasy's population (10, p 296)), but after two or more preterm births, the risk of another is 70% (15).

Although the precise physiology for the initiation of preterm labor is not known, it is possible to develop a risk assessment scale to identify patients at high risk of preterm labor (see Medical Management). Whether the mechanism is the same as that for term labor with merely an alteration in timing, whether the mechanism is different for preterm labor, or whether the particular mechanism varies from patient to patient still is not known (16).

SIGNS AND SYMPTOMS

The early signs and symptoms of preterm labor often are subtle and difficult to differentiate from false labor or from discomforts that are normal and common during late pregnancy. Possible early signs and symptoms are menstrual-like cramps; pelvic pressure; abdominal or intestinal cramps; diarrhea; low backache, especially of a character different from that previously experienced; and a change in character or an increase in amount of vaginal discharge (10). Of course, regular uterine contractions, bloody show, and rupture of membranes are signs of labor, regardless of gestational age.

Interestingly, of the patients who experience regular, painful uterine contractions prior to term, only 25–50% progress to delivery if no treatment is instituted (17). The remainder, in retrospect, were experiencing false labor.

DIAGNOSIS

The accurate diagnosis of preterm labor is of paramount importance but, as emphasized before, is difficult to confirm. It requires both documentation of gestational age and diagnosis of labor. The usual parameters are used to document gestational age: date of last menstrual period; length of menstrual cycles; recent history of pregnancy, lactation, or hormonal contraceptives; uterine size at first visit and growth pattern throughout gestation; date of quickening; date of first hearing fetal heart tones with a stethoscope; date of positive pregnancy test; and results of sonogram, if available.

The diagnosis of labor is based upon uterine activity and cervical change. Uterine contractions are normal in the third trimester, and, as previously stated, regularity, frequency, or association with pain does not differentiate normal activity from preterm labor (17, p 256). A single cervical examination may not be diagnostic either. A 1961 study by Floyd demonstrated that of patients who delivered at term (after 36 weeks), 15% of primigravidas and 36% of multigravidas were at least 1 cm dilated at 6 months' gestation (18). Parikh and Mehta found that 16% of primigravidas and 17% of multiparas were dilated 1.5–2 cm at 21–28 weeks' gestation. With no intervention their preterm delivery rate was 13.9%, compared with 11.1% of those who had a closed cervix (19). Schaffner and Schanzer found that 27.4% of patients were 2–3 cm dilated at 28–32 weeks, but birth weights and gestational ages were similar to patients whose cervices were closed at 28–32 weeks (20).

Because treatment of preterm labor is more effective if begun early but should be avoided unless the patient really is in labor, the following criteria are suggested by Creasy and Herron for the diagnosis of preterm labor (10, p 174):

1. Gestational age 20–36 weeks.
2. Documented regular contractions (at least four in 20 minutes or eight in 60 minutes).
3. At least one of the following:
    a. Ruptured membranes;
    b. Documented cervical change; or
    c. Cervix at least 2 cm dilated or 80% effaced.

Even with preterm labor diagnosed by these criteria some patients would go on to term with placebo intervention (8, p 179). The high effectiveness of placebo treatments may be due to imprecise diagnosis or to bed rest, hydration, and hospitalization that usually accompany treatment (8, p 174).

MATERNAL AND FETAL OUTCOME

The maternal outcome depends upon accompanying medical or obstetrical complications. For the majority of cases where no complication contributes to preterm labor, the outcome is quite good, although the rate of cesarean section for fetal indications is higher than in patients that deliver at term.

The impact on the baby can be severe, depending primarily upon the birth weight and gestational age at delivery (rather than the *reason* for preterm delivery). The mortality rate is high: as previously stated, the 6–8% of births that are preterm account for 75% of neonatal deaths not attributable to anomalies (8, p 173). In recent years the United States neonatal mortality rate, which is largely due to prematurity, has decreased dramatically because of improved neonatal care. Neonatal deaths per 1000 live births have decreased from 15.1 in 1970 to 7.4 in 1983 (2, p 4). Indeed, the birth weight-specific neonatal mortality rate in the United States may be lower than in any other country (21). However, neonatal death still is too often the outcome for the very small premature baby.

There also is significant morbidity accompanying the high mortality rate. Among the immediate problems encountered by preterm babies are respiratory distress, central nervous system damage, patent ductus arteriosus, necrotizing enterocolitis, hy-

perbilirubinemia, infections, nutritional problems, coagulopathies, and the developmental difficulties associated with prolonged hospitalization (1, p 98). A 1977 study by Stewart demonstrated that of babies less than 1000 g at birth, 13% had significant handicaps at 18 months of age, and of those 1000–1500 g, 8% were handicapped (22).

In addition to medical complications experienced by premature babies, there is a high incidence of "mothering disorders" that may contribute to emotional and developmental problems later in life (16, p 238). The importance of the development of a maternal-infant bond soon after birth has been demonstrated (23). With a small or sick premature baby, there may not be the opportunity to develop this special relationship immediately. The incidence of child abuse is increased in children born prematurely. The emotional cost of having a sick or very small baby who does not meet the family's expectations or fantasies cannot be quantified.

MEDICAL MANAGEMENT

W. H. Clewell states "Since premature delivery is not a disease, but a single symptom of many diseases, solution of this problem depends on improvements in the treatment of many conditions and a basic understanding of the mechanisms of parturition" (16, p 238). A. B. M. Anderson agrees, stating that prevention of preterm labor seems to require "finding a solution to almost all the major problems in obstetrics" (9, p 235).

In general, the approach to preterm labor is twofold: first, to attempt to prevent its occurrence and, second, to identify preterm labor promptly when it occurs so it can be treated adequately and preterm delivery can be prevented.

Prevention

The Institute of Medicine of the National Academy of Sciences issued a report in 1985 on prevention of low birth weight—both prematurity and IUGR. In it they recommended a variety of strategies to attack low birth weight, cautioning that no single approach is likely to solve the problem. They suggested the following:

1. Reducing risks of low birth weight prior to conception by risk identification and appropriate counseling, expanding the scope of general health education relating to reproduction, and expanding and improving family planning services.

2. Increasing the accessibility and quality of prenatal care to all women and removing barriers to receiving this care early in the pregnancy.
3. Expanding the content and flexibility of prenatal care for all women and providing additional components of care designed to lessen the risk and detect problems early for women at high risk for IUGR or prematurity.
4. Providing long-term, extensive public education about the problem of low birth weight and conveying certain messages about reproductive health.
5. Conducting comprehensive research on low birth weight (24).

Because only a portion of all preterm deliveries is likely to respond to improvements in medical care and public health measures, it seems that attention also should be focused on amelioration of sociodemographic factors. Unfortunately, currently we do not understand how these factors affect prematurity, nor do we have proof that rectifying those factors will result in a reduction of prematurity (7, p 115).

Since maternal physical and/or emotional stress *may* contribute to preterm labor, some investigators are attempting to assess sources of stress in the patient's life and assist in alleviating them when possible. Table 28.3 is a sample tool for assessing stress factors. Of course, many stresses are not amenable to intervention from the outside. Examples of interventions that may assist in alleviating certain stresses are:

1. Social services to assist with financial and housing concerns.
2. Counseling regarding activities that may be physically stressful, with specific suggestions for minimizing those activities.
3. Initiation of medical disability for working patients who are at high risk of preterm delivery, particularly if the job requires a long commute or involves sources of occupational fatigue (see Table 28.2).
4. Provision of homemaker services, when necessary, for patients at high risk.

It is recommended that during or before pregnancy, patients should be counseled regarding health behaviors that will maintain general good health while minimizing the risk of preterm labor (e.g., exercise; good nutrition; avoidance of smoking, alcohol, street drugs, or unnecessary medication; and adequate amounts of rest and sleep). In addition, counseling or referral for help with finan-

cial, social, or psychological problems should be available.

During, or even before pregnancy if possible, obstetrical complications that might cause or contribute to preterm labor should be evaluated and treated (e.g., chronic hypertension, maternal infection such as β-streptococcus and *Chlamydia*, maternal anemia, and hypovolemia).

Several preterm prevention strategies that are being studied but have not yet been proven successful include:

1. Prohibiting coitus, or at least recommending use of a condom to prevent vaginal or cervical infection.
2. Increasing bed rest.
3. Minimizing strenuous physical activity.
4. Using a pessary to keep the cervix in a posterior position and to keep pressure of the fetal head off the cervix (10, pp 299–300).

Studies also are being conducted regarding the weekly injection of progesterone compounds to prevent preterm labor. To be effective, progesterone must be used before contractions develop. Since the criteria for patient selection are not clear, many patients may be treated unnecessarily. There is concern that progesterone might have teratogenic effects on the fetus, so this prevention strategy is being evaluated carefully (5, p 213).

Use of cerclage to prevent preterm labor has not been found to be of benefit except for patients with cervical incompetence. Specifically, it has not improved outcome in patients with a history of first or second trimester loss due to any other cause or in patients with multiple gestation (9, p 242). Actually, it may be detrimental because cervical infection or irritation might stimulate prostaglandin production (10, p 300).

Treatment

The second aspect of medical management is treatment of preterm labor in an attempt to prevent preterm delivery. As emphasized before, treatment must be instituted early in preterm labor to be effective. Prematurity prevention programs provide special services to clients identified as being at high risk for preterm labor in order to facilitate early diagnosis of preterm labor. In order to utilize resources effectively, several scoring systems have been developed to identify clients at risk. Table 28.4 is an example of one such risk-scoring system.

The scoring systems are not perfect. The scoring system in Table 28.4 indicated that about 10% of patients in the population studied were at high

Table 28.3.
ASSESSMENT OF MATERNAL STRESS FACTORS[a]

Patient's name _____ Date _____

During this week, was there anything particularly tiring or stressful that you had to do or that happened to you? What? Can it be avoided?

_____

_____

Stressful events during the past week:
  1. Less than usual
  2. Same as usual
  3. More than usual

Physical stress
  Domestic _____
  Work-related _____

Emotional
  Domestic _____
  Work-related _____

Comment _____

_____

_____

Has anything *changed* this week in your routine or the things you do? _____

Comment _____

_____

Is there anything we can help you with? _____

Comment _____

Changes in habits this week:

Smoking	Average # cigarettes/day	_____
Housework	Average # hours/day	_____
Child care	Average # hours/day	_____
Rest	Average # hours/day	_____
Stairs	Average # flights/day	_____
Heavy lifting	# times/week	_____
Standing >30 minutes	# times/week	_____
Commute >30 minutes	# times/week	_____
Employment	# hours/week	_____
Help from others	yes/no	_____
Sexual intercourse	# times/week	_____
Alcohol	# drinks/week	_____
Drug use _____	# times/week	_____

Other _____

Other _____

Other _____

[a]Adapted from Weekly Activity Form, New York State Department of Health, Prevention of Low Birth Weight Program. Harlem Hospital, 1984.

Table 28.4.
PRETERM LABOR RISK ASSESSMENT TOOL[a, b]

SCORE[c]	SOCIOECONOMIC	PAST HISTORY	DAILY HABITS	CURRENT PREGNANCY
1	Two children at home; low socioeconomic status	One abortion; <1 year since last birth	Work outside home	Unusual fatigue
2	<20 years old; >40 years old; single parent	Two abortions	More than 10 cigarettes per day	12 pounds by 32 weeks; albuminuria; hypertension; bacteriuria
3	Very low socioeconomic status; <5 feet tall; <100 pounds	Three abortions	Heavy work; long, tiring trip	Breech at 32 weeks; weight loss of 5 pounds; head engaged; febrile illness
4	<18 years old	Pyelonephritis		Metrorrhagia after 12 weeks; effacement; dilatation; uterine irritability
5		Uterine anomaly; second trimester abortion; DES exposure		Placenta previa; hydramnios; uterine myoma
10		Premature delivery; repeated second trimester abortion		Twins; abdominal surgery

EDC _____

HIGH RISK   Yes   No

[a]From Creasy RK, Herron MA: Prevention of preterm birth. *Semin Perinatol* 5:297, 1981.
[b]This preterm risk assessment tool is used at the initial prenatal visit and again at 26–28 weeks' gestation.
[c]0–5 = low risk; 6–9 = medium risk; ≥10 = high risk.

risk for preterm labor. Only about one-third of them went into preterm labor, accounting for about two-thirds of the cases of preterm labor. Thus, one-third of the cases of preterm labor were from the low risk population, and two-thirds of the high risk population had no preterm labor. The score is more accurate when evaluated at 26–28 weeks than at the first prenatal visit, and it is more accurate for multiparas than for primigravidas (25).

One preterm prevention program in California (10, p 297) identified high risk clients by using the risk assessment system given in Table 28.4. They taught those patients the subtle signs and symptoms of preterm labor. They also taught them to palpate for uterine contractions twice daily (Fig. 28.1). Patients were followed in a prenatal clinic weekly, with pelvic examinations at each visit to detect cervical change. Doctors and nurses were sensitized through an educational program to the need to evaluate seriously even minor complaints that might indicate preterm labor. As a result of this program, preterm labor was detected early enough for treatment to be instituted in 93% of their high risk patients and 79% of their low risk patients. Their preterm delivery rate was cut approximately in half.

The usefulness of weekly cervical examinations still is being studied. Since some cervical dilation and effacement may occur in normal patients, the examination's significance is unclear. There is evidence that prostaglandin levels increase in maternal blood after a cervical examination. There is also concern that the examination might introduce infection, which may actually make the examination harmful.

Home monitoring of uterine contractions also is being investigated in some centers to determine whether it contributes to the early recognition of preterm labor. Patients who are at high risk for preterm labor are given a small, portable monitoring unit with a tocodynamometer. (There is no Doppler transducer for fetal heart rate monitoring.) The patient is instructed to lie down at a 45° angle with slight left tilt, place the tocodynamometer over the fundus firmly with a belt, and record for 30–60 minutes once or twice daily. The recording then is transmitted via telephone to the perinatal center where it is read and interpreted. Instructions based on the recording can be given to the patient over the telephone. The home monitor currently is being studied to determine whether it identifies contractions that would not have been recognized by the patient, even after education regarding signs and symptoms of preterm labor and self-palpation of contractions.

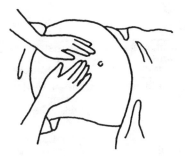

Figure 28.1. Self-palpation of contractions. The patient is instructed to lie down, tilted toward one side, and to place her fingers wide apart over the uterus. She is to note whether she is able to detect tightening and relaxation ("hardening" and "softening") of the uterus under her fingertips. She is taught to differentiate contractions, involving the whole uterus, from palpation of fetal parts, which may feel "hard" over a portion of the uterus. It is often possible to teach a woman how to feel for contractions in the examining room—often a woman in the third trimester will experience a mild contraction immediately upon lying down. If she does detect tightening of the uterus, the patient should be instructed to note how long it lasts, how often it occurs (either timing from the beginning of one contraction to the beginning of the next, or how many contractions occur in 30 minutes), and whether she believes it is mild or strong. She should be instructed where to call to report her contractions. The patient is instructed to palpate for contractions twice daily, and more often if she is experiencing any of the subtle signs and symptoms of preterm labor.

Tocolytic Therapy

Once preterm labor is diagnosed, the next step is treatment. When evaluating studies of the effectiveness of various treatment regimens, it must be remembered that placebos have a high rate of effectiveness (35–50%). It may be that bed rest, hydration, or the psychological effects of hospitalization, all of which accompany tocolytic therapy, are more effective than the tocolytics themselves. Alternatively, the high effectiveness rate for placebos merely may reflect the faulty diagnosis of preterm labor. See Table 28.5 for a suggested management plan for early preterm labor. Because of the indications and contraindications for tocolytic therapy, in most institutions only about 10–15% of patients presenting in preterm labor are candidates for tocolytic therapy (Table 28.6).

Most studies show little if any benefit from the use of tocolytic drugs, and so far they have made little impact on the rate of premature delivery. Overall, delivery may be delayed an average of 3–7 days in the small number of patients who receive tocolytic therapy. The possible explanations are as follows: most studies have no strict diagnostic criteria for preterm labor; tocolytics are evaluated using different protocols, such as being initiated at various stages of labor; only a small percentage of patients in preterm labor are candidates for tocolysis upon admission to the hospital; and placebos have a high rate of effectiveness.

There are several tocolytic agents available. In the past, ethanol was the drug of choice. Its action was to inhibit release of oxytocin and vasopressin from the posterior pituitary (16, p 242). Its side effects were unpleasant and presented a challenge for nursing care. There is some concern that ethanol, even in the third trimester, might affect fetal neurological development. Therefore, ethanol is seldom used today for tocolysis.

Prostaglandin synthetase inhibitors have been found to be effective in arresting preterm labor, but the side effects in the baby are unacceptable (e.g., premature closure of the ductus arteriosus and pulmonary hypertension in the neonate) (5, p 213).

Magnesium sulfate ($MgSO_4$) acts by interfering with the availability of calcium, which is necessary for muscle contraction. It has three major advantages:

1. Labor and delivery personnel already are familiar with the drug, its side effects, and how to monitor its administration because of its frequent use in treating preeclampsia.
2. Calcium gluconate and calcium chloride are readily available antagonists.
3. It can be used in many patients for whom ritodrine (or other β-adrenergic drugs) is contraindicated.

Table 28.7 gives a sample protocol for administration of $MgSO_4$ for treatment of preterm labor.

Pharmacology of Magnesium Sulfate ($MgSO_4$)

Magnesium is abundant in the body, with approximately 12 g stored in bone and another 12 g in the intracellular compartment. A small amount is available in extracellular fluids. Normal serum magnesium levels in the pregnant patient range from 1.8–3.0 mg/dl. During early pregnancy, the levels fall and then gradually rise toward normal near term. During both normal and preterm labor, the serum level of magnesium falls.

How magnesium inhibits uterine contractions is not understood completely. It does decrease the release of ac-

Table 28.5.

TREATMENT OF EARLY PRETERM LABOR[a]

CATEGORY OF PRETERM LABOR	ARRESTED UTERINE ACTIVITY WITHOUT CERVICAL CHANGE	PERSISTENT UTERINE ACTIVITY WITHOUT CERVICAL CHANGE	PERSISTENT UTERINE ACTIVITY WITH CERVICAL CHANGE
Definition	Uterine activity that ceases with bed rest and results in no cervical change.	Uterine activity that does not cease with bed rest but results in no cervical change.	Uterine activity that does not cease with bed rest and results in cervical change.

Immediate treatment	1. Bed rest.
	2. Baseline cervical examination.
	3. Monitor uterine activity and woman's symptoms for:
	  a. 1–2 hours.
	  b. 3–4 hours.
		1. Bed rest.
		2. Baseline cervical examination.
		3. Monitor uterine activity and woman's symptoms for approximately 1 hour.
		4. Reexamine cervix, and if no cervical change:
		  a. Continue to monitor for 24 hours.
		  b. Note uterine activity every 30 minutes to 1 hour.
		  c. Sedate.
			1. Bed rest.
			2. Baseline cervical examination. (If cervix is 2 cm dilated or 80% effaced, drug therapy should be started.)
			3. Monitor uterine activity and woman's symptoms for about 1 hour.
			4. Reexamine cervix, and if there is cervical change:
			  a. Continue to monitor.
			  b. Start drug therapy.
			5. Reexamine cervix about 1–2 hours after drug therapy started, and if no cervical change and uterine activity remains suppressed:
			  a. Continue drug therapy and monitoring.
			  b. Limit cervical examinations to every 12 hours.
			6. Reexamine cervix 12 hours after oral drug therapy started, and if no cervical change and uterine activity remains suppressed:
			  a. Institute modified bed rest.
			  b. Observe woman's uterine activity and symptoms for 24–48 hours on modified bed rest.

Follow-up plan	If no cervical change: 1. Discharge home on modifed bed rest. 2. Instruct woman to call hospital or health care provider if symptoms of preterm labor recur. 3. Follow with weekly visits and cervical examinations until 37 weeks' gestation. 4. Activity level may be increased depending on woman's symptoms and cervical examination.	If no cervical change: 1. Discharge home on modified bed rest. 2. Instruct woman to call hospital or health care provider if symptoms of preterm labor recur or intensify. 3. Follow with weekly visits and cervical examinations until 37 weeks' gestation. 4. Activity level may be increased depending on woman's symptoms and cervical examination.	If no cervical change and uterine activity is suppressed: 1. Discharge home on oral medications and modified bed rest until 37 weeks' gestation. 2. Instruct woman to call hospital or health care provider if signs and symptoms of preterm labor recur. 3. Follow with weekly visits and cervical examinations until 37 weeks' gestation.

[a]From Herron MA, Dulock HL: *Preterm Labor.* White Plains, NY, March of Dimes Birth Defects Foundation, 1982, pp 22–23.

Table 28.6.

CRITERIA FOR TOCOLYTIC THERAPY

1. Gestational age 20–36 weeks.
2. Estimated fetal weight less than 2500 g.
3. Labor is diagnosed:
   a. Documented regular uterine contractions, at least four in 20 minutes or eight in 60 minutes, lasting at least 30 seconds each, and
   b. Documented cervical change *or* cervix at least 2 cm dilated or 80% effaced.
4. None of the following contraindications:
   a. Ruptured membranes.
   b. Labor too far advanced (i.e., dilation greater than 4 cm).
   c. Medical or obstetrical complication in which early delivery is the treatment of choice (e.g., active vaginal bleeding, severe preeclampsia, severe intrauterine growth retardation, intrauterine infection, fetus that is dead or has an anomaly incompatible with life.)
   d. Contraindications specific to the tocolytic agent:
      1. Ritodrine: Uncontrolled diabetes mellitus, hypertension, hyperthyroidism, fever of unknown origin, maternal cardiac disease, patient already being treated with a β-adrenergic drug (e.g., for asthma).
      2. Magnesium sulfate: myasthenia gravis, impaired renal function, history of recent myocardial infarction.
5. Informed consent.

Table 28.7.

SAMPLE PROTOCOL FOR ADMINISTRATION OF MAGNESIUM SULFATE (MgSO$_4$)[a]

1. Begin i.v. infusion as soon as preterm labor is diagnosed and contraindications are ruled out.
2. Maintain bed rest in the left lateral position.
3. Initially, provide moderate hydration, approximately 400 cc of fluid i.v., in the first 2 hours. Decrease the rate of infusion subsequently so that no more than 3500 cc is given in 24 hours to reduce the chance of developing pulmonary edema.
4. Administer a bolus of 4–6 g MgSO$_4$ i.v. in 15 minutes.
5. During infusion of the MgSO$_4$ bolus, 0.25 mg terbutaline may be given subcuticularly to stop contractions immediately.
6. After the bolus of MgSO$_4$, begin a constant infusion of MgSO$_4$ at the rate of 3 g/hour. The standard solution for the maintenance dose is 20 g MgSO$_4$ in 1000 cc i.v. fluid. An i.v. infusion pump should be used to administer the MgSO$_4$ solution.
7. Monitor vital signs, including reflexes and respirations every hour. Keep an accurate record of intake and output.
8. Stop infusion of MgSO$_4$ if urine output is less than 25 cc/hour or patellar reflexes are absent. Have antidote (calcium gluconate or calcium chloride) available at the bedside. Have resuscitation equipment readily available.
9. Monitor fetal heart rate and uterine contractions continuously via external fetal monitoring.
10. Obtain a serum level of magnesium 6 hours after beginning the infusion. Alter the infusion rate, if necessary, to maintain the serum magnesium level in the therapeutic range of 5.5–7.5 mg/dl.
11. Maintain the lowest effective dosage.
12. Oral tocolytic therapy may be used, when indicated, after labor has been arrested.

[a]Adapted from Elliott JP: Magnesium sulfate as a tocolytic agent. *Contemp OB/GYN* 25:58, 1985.

etylcholine from the motor end plate at the neuromuscular junction. Excess extracellular magnesium from intravenous infusion is diffused passively into the intracellular compartment. There it decreases the concentration of cAMP, which is required for muscle contraction. It also stimulates transport of calcium outside of the cell. The intracellular magnesium thus may reduce available calcium so that actin and myosin cannot interact normally, thereby inhibiting muscle contraction.

MgSO$_4$ is excreted via the kidneys, with the urinary clearance reflecting the serum concentration.

The efficacy of MgSO$_4$ in inhibiting labor is similar to that of terbutaline. However, its low cost, relative safety, and lack of side effects make it an attractive tocolytic agent. Side effects include nausea and vomiting, muscle weakness and fatigue, and transient hypotension.

There is a fairly wide margin of safety before toxic effects occur. The therapeutic serum level of MgSO$_4$ is 5.5–7.5 mg/dl. Above 12 mg/dl, electrocardiogram abnormalities, cardiac arrhythmias, and cardiac arrest may occur. Respiratory depression may occur with levels over 18 mg/dl. Calcium gluconate or calcium chloride is a ready antidote.

Magnesium easily crosses the placental barrier. Effects on the baby of MgSO$_4$ given for tocolysis have not yet been studied. Studies of the effects of MgSO$_4$ used to treat preeclampsia in term babies indicate that there is an elevated magnesium level for 24–48 hours after birth but no hypocalcemia, and the magnesium level is not related to Apgar score or neonatal mortality. Infants of mothers being treated for preeclampsia may experience lethargy and a decrease in muscle tone, although not all studies con-

Table 28.8.

SAMPLE PROTOCOL FOR USE OF RITODRINE[a]

1. Begin i.v. infusion as soon as preterm labor is diagnosed and contraindications to tocolysis are ruled out.
2. Auscultate breath sounds as baseline assessment. Obtain a baseline electrocardiogram, as ordered.
3. Administer ritodrine via an i.v. infusion pump. The ritodrine line should run through a "keep open" line. The total fluid volume to the patient should not exceed 150 ml/hour.
4. Ritodrine is diluted in i.v. fluids. A suggested protocol is 150 mg ritodrine hydrochloride (3 ampules) in 500 cc i.v. fluids.
5. Begin the infusion at 50 μg/minute of ritodrine. Increase the dose every 10 minutes by 50 μg/minute until contractions cease or unacceptable side effects occur. Do not exceed 350 μg/minute.
6. Monitor maternal heart rate and blood pressure frequently, at least every 10 minutes while increasing the dosage, and every 15 minutes thereafter. Do not increase the dosage further if the maternal heart rate reaches 140 beats/minute. A maternal cardiac monitor may be used during i.v. administration of ritodrine.
7. Assist the patient to maintain bed rest, preferably in the left lateral recumbent position, during the infusion.
8. Monitor fetal status and uterine contractions with continuous external electronic monitoring.
9. Assess pulmonic status for presence of rales and rhonchi, suggestive of pulmonary edema (see Chapter 16).
10. Reduce the dose if side effects occur. Discontinue the infusion if unacceptable side effects occur of if labor continues at the maximum dose.
11. Have antidote (propranolol hydrochloride) available if required for life-threatening arrhythmias. The rate of administration of the antidote should not exceed 1 mg/minute.
12. When labor is arrested, continue the i.v. infusion for at least 12 hours, when oral therapy may be started. The i.v. dose gradually may be weaned down.
13. Administer the first oral dose of ritodrine 30 minutes before stopping the i.v. infusion. The oral dose is 10 mg every 2 hours (or 20 mg every 4 hours) for the first 24 hours, followed by 10–20 mg every 4–6 hours. The maintenance dose may be continued until inhibition of labor is indicated no longer.
14. Inform the patient to take oral ritodrine with food, as it may be better tolerated. Advise her not to use over-the-counter drugs unless the physician approves since use concurrent with ritodrine may have deleterious effects.
15. If labor recurs while the patient is on oral ritodrine, the i.v. infusion may be restarted as long as the patient is still eligible for treatment (see Table 28.6).

[a]Adapted from Barden TP, Peter JB, Merkatz IR: Ritodrine hydrochloride: a betamimetic agent for use in preterm labor. *Obstet Gynecol* 56:4, 1980.

firm that effect. It seems likely that $MgSO_4$ would cause lethargy in the preterm infant, but that has not yet been documented.

The effective dosage of $MgSO_4$ is difficult to determine since there are large variations from person to person. However, the therapeutic serum level appears to be around 5.5–7.5 mg/dl. The dosage often is higher than that used for preeclampsia. Table 28.7 gives a suggested protocol for administration of $MgSO_4$ for tocolysis.

The fact that $MgSO_4$ does not have Federal Food and Drug Administration approval as a tocolytic does not mean that it is illegal or that using it constitutes substandard care. Indeed, $MgSO_4$ often is the drug of choice for patients for whom ritodrine is contraindicated. (Adapted from Elliott JP: Magnesium sulfate as a tocolytic agent. *Contemp OB/GYN* 25:49–61, 1985.)

The β-adrenergic drugs (also called β-sympathomimetic drugs or β-agonists) are the drugs most commonly used for treatment of preterm labor today. Ritodrine is the only one currently approved by the Food and Drug Administration for treatment of preterm labor. See Table 28.8 for a sample protocol for administration of ritodrine.

Pharmacology of β-Adrenergic Drugs

The sympathomimetic drugs are epinephrine-like derivatives. They exert their various and contradictory effects in the body by stimulating one of two different types of receptors: the α-adrenergic and β-adrenergic receptors. The α-adrenergic receptors stimulate the uterus to contract, whereas β-adrenergic receptors have the opposite effect. The β-adrenergic receptors are differentiated further into β_1 receptors, which, when stimulated, result in an increase in heart rate and force, lypolysis, and a decrease in intestinal motility, and β_2 receptors, which result in glycogenolysis and relaxation of arterioles, the bronchi, and the uterus. A drug may be primarily a β_1 or β_2 stimulant, but ordinarily there is some cross-over in effect.

Ritodrine hydrochloride is a β-adrenergic stimulant, primarily affecting β_2 receptors. Thus, it is effective in producing uterine relaxation, while having only minor effects on the cardiovascular system.

When given intravenously, serum levels rise quickly—to 60–75% of maximum within 20 minutes. An infusion rate of 150 μg/minute will result in a serum level of 32–52 ng/ml. After stopping intravenous infusion, the levels fall rapidly: the first half-life is 6–9 minutes, the second is 1.7–2.6 hours, and the third is longer than 10 hours.

The administration of oral ritodrine results in a serum level only 30% of what it would be if the same dose were administered intravenously. Presumably, the ritodrine is metabolized as it is absorbed and passed through the liver. The serum level peaks at 30–60 minutes after oral administration. The maximum serum level after administering 10 mg of ritodrine orally is 5–15 ng/ml. The first half-life of the drug is about 1.3 hours, and the second one is about 12 hours.

Ritodrine and its metabolites pass freely across the placental barrier, but fetal levels generally are only about 20% of maternal levels.

Most ritodrine is finally excreted in the urine; some of it is excreted unaltered, and some is excreted as inactive metabolites.

The side effects of ritodrine result from the fact that it exerts some effect on β_1 receptors and on receptors in organs other than the uterus. Among the side effects are a dose-related increase in maternal heart rate, a widening of pulse pressure, a moderate decrease of serum potassium, a small decrease in maternal pH, and a transient increase in blood glucose and plasma insulin. The mother may feel "nervous" or experience tremors, nausea, vomiting, palpitations, headache, erythema, anxiety, or chest pain. Rarely, pulmonary edema may occur in patients who also are receiving corticosteroids.

Ritodrine may cause a mildly increased heart rate in the fetus and neonate. Other possible side effects are ileus, hypocalcemia, and hypoglycemia.

The proper patient selection for use of ritodrine, including contraindications to its use, are listed in Table 28.6.

Ritodrine currently is the only drug approved by the Food and Drug Administration for tocolysis. Other β_2 stimulants—isoxsuprine and terbutaline—have been used extensively and seem to be similar to ritodrine in effectiveness and side effects. Further investigation of subtle differences is continuing. Terbutaline is much less expensive than ritodrine and is therefore attractive as an alternative.

Corticosteroids

If preterm labor cannot be stopped, the goal of management is to minimize the adverse effects of prematurity on the neonate. Respiratory distress syndrome (RDS) is the major cause of death in premature babies. The best way to prevent RDS is to prevent preterm birth; however, when it is clear that preterm delivery will occur, one approach is to try to induce fetal lung maturity prior to delivery. RDS occurs when there is insufficient surfactant in the lungs. Surfactant production begins at 24–26 weeks and by 36 weeks normally is adequate to prevent RDS.

It has been shown that administration of corticosteroids to pregnant women 24 hours to 7 days before preterm delivery will reduce the incidence of RDS (26). The mechanism of action is not known, other than that they stimulate surfactant production (5, p 216). Several corticosteroids have been used (e.g., betamethasone, dexamethasone, hydrocortisone). It is not clear yet which drug or what dose is best. Appropriate patients for corticosteroid treatment must meet the criteria listed in Table

Table 28.9.

CRITERIA FOR USE OF CORTICOSTEROIDS[a]

1. The lecithin:sphingomyelin (L:S) ratio is immature. (Up to one-fourth of patients have a mature L:S ratio by 32 weeks. See Chapter 6.)
2. It is anticipated that delivery can be delayed for at least 24 hours.
3. Gestational age is well documented and is between 28 and 34 weeks.
4. None of the contraindications to corticosteroid administration is present: active tuberculosis, viral hepatitis, active peptic ulcers. (Patients already taking corticosteroids for other indications will not benefit from more.)

[a]Adapted from Morrison JC, Martin JN: Selecting patients for antenatal steroid treatment. *Contemp OB/GYN* 20:214, 1982.

28.9. If delivery occurs more than 7 days after treatment but still preterm, the treatment has to be repeated to be effective. Interestingly, in one study corticosteroids were more effective for girl babies than for boys and for black patients rather than white (26, p 212).

Possible adverse effects from corticosteroid treatment still are being studied. It is known that it alters adrenal function in the neonate, and that there is an increase in both maternal and neonatal infections after corticosteroids are used. In animals adverse effects include an altered immune response, decreased intelligence, a decrease in weight of the brain and other organs, and neurologic retardation.

Corticosteroids should be used only in a tertiary care center where the anticipated preterm baby can be cared for properly; they should not be relied upon to prevent all complications of prematurity. If the baby is not immature enough to need special care, it probably does not need corticosteroids. Also, corticosteroids should be used with informed consent since long-term effects are still unknown.

Preterm Delivery

When preterm labor is going to end in a preterm delivery, the management must focus on carefully and continuously observing the baby's status. Fetal monitoring is indicated. Cesarean section should be done if fetal distress occurs. Systemic analgesics or sedation should be avoided since they might depress the baby at birth and for days afterwards. Regional analgesia or anesthesia is preferred if any is needed. Since the preterm baby is more susceptible to intracranial hemorrhage, the delivery should be gentle—between contractions, with a generous episiotomy. Some obstetricians may prefer to use forceps to ensure a slow, gentle delivery of the head. However, recent studies indicate that there is no advantage to the use of forceps and that their use actually may increase neurological damage. If the baby is breech, many obstetricians would elect to deliver by cesarean section because of the increased risk of intracranial hemorrhage, asphyxia, and cord prolapse. Once the baby is delivered, it should be handed quickly to the pediatrician, who can resuscitate it as quickly as possible. Maintaining warmth of the premature baby is of utmost importance.

NURSING MANAGEMENT

Nursing care specific for a patient *at risk* for preterm labor:
- [ ] Teach behaviors to minimize the risk of preterm labor:
  - Minimize strenuous physical activity;
  - Increase rest periods;
  - Stop smoking;
  - Maintain good nutrition;
  - Utilize stress management techniques; and
  - Avoid prenatal preparation for breastfeeding.
- [ ] Using a standardized tool screen all prenatal patients for preterm labor risk status
- [ ] Teach signs/symptoms of preterm labor.
- [ ] Teach self-palpation for contractions.
- [ ] Advise patient to have weekly prenatal clinic visits.
- [ ] Teach procedure for notifying health care team at once if signs/symptoms of preterm labor occur.
- [ ] Question the patient at each prenatal visit after 20 weeks' gestation if she has experienced the subtle signs/symptoms of preterm labor; encourage the patient who calls in between visits to come in for evaluation if she is experiencing signs or symptoms of preterm labor.
- [ ] Evaluate the physical and emotional stress level changes using a standardized tool (Table 29.3); make appropriate interventions and referrals e.g., public health nursing referral.

For the patient in *preterm labor*:
- [ ] Ensure maximum uterine perfusion to attempt to decrease uterine activity:
  - Position the patient in a left lateral position and
  - Assess hydration status, administering intravenous fluids as ordered.
- [ ] Assist with any examinations/procedures required for thorough evaluation (e.g., ultrasound, amniocentesis, urine culture).
- [ ] Administer tocolytics and/or corticosteroids as ordered (see Tables 28.7, 28.8, and 28.9) and observe the patient for desired effects or adverse effects.

Nursing diagnoses most frequently associated with *preterm labor* (see Section V):
- [ ] Grieving related to potential/actual loss of infant or birth of an imperfect child.
- [ ] Potential altered parenting.
- [ ] Knowledge deficit regarding etiology, disease process, treatment, and outcome.
- [ ] Knowledge deficit regarding medication regimen.
- [ ] Anxiety/fear.
- [ ] Disturbance in body image, self-esteem.

REFERENCES

1. Creasy RK: Prevention of preterm birth. *Birth Defects: Original Article Series* 19:97–102, 1983.
2. Pritchard JA, MacDonald PC, Gant NF: *Williams Obstetrics,* ed 17. Norwalk, CT, Appleton-Century-Crofts, 1985, pp 295–299.
3. Oxorn H, Foote WR: *Human Labor and Birth,* ed 3. New York, Appleton-Century-Crofts, 1975, pp 101–102.
4. Liggins GC: New concepts of what triggers labor. *Contemp OB/GYN* 19:131–141, 1982.
5. Fuchs F, Ylikorkala O: Preterm birth. In Caplan RM (ed): *Principles of Obstetrics.* Baltimore, Williams & Wilkins, 1982, p 210.
6. Keirse MJNC: Epidemiology of preterm labor. In Keirse et al. (eds): *Human Parturition.* The Hague, Martinus Nijhoff, 1979, pp 221–223.
7. Lee K, Gartner LM: What mortality statistics tell us about perinatal care. *Contemp OB/GYN* 25:111–138,1985.
8. Creasy RK: Ways of preventing preterm labor. *Contemp OB/GYN* 32:64–67, 1988.
9. Anderson ABM: Prevention of pre-term labor. In Keirse et al. (eds): *Human Parturition.* The Hague, Martinus Nijhoff, 1979, pp 235–245.
10. Creasy RK, Herron MA: Prevention of preterm birth. *Semin Perinatol* 5:295–301, 1981.
11. Hemminki E, Starfield B: Prevention of low birthweight and pre-term birth. *Health Soc:*

Milbank Memorial Fund Quarterly 56:339–361, 1978.

12. Berkowitz GS: An epidemiologic study of preterm delivery. *Am J Epidemiol* 113:81–92, 1981.

13. Barden TP: Premature labor. In Queenan JT (ed): *Management of High-Risk Pregnancy.* Oradell, NJ, Medical Economics, 1980.

14. Mamelle N, Laumon B, Lazar P: Prematurity and occupational activity during pregnancy. *Am J Epidemiol* 119:309–321, 1984.

15. Keirse MJNC, Rush RW, Anderson ABM, Turnbull AC: Risk of pre-term delivery in patients with previous pre-term delivery and/or abortion. *Br J Obstet Gynaecol* 58:81–85, 1978.

16. Clewell WH: Prematurity. *J Repro Med* 23:237–244, 1979.

17. Lipshitz J: Beta-adrenergic agonists. *Semin Perinatol* 5:252–265, 1981.

18. Floyd WE: Cervical dilation in the mid-trimester of pregnancy. *Obstet Gynecol* 18:380, 1961.

19. Parikh MN, Mehta AC: Internal cervical os during the second half of pregnancy. *J Obstet Gynaecol Br Commonw* 68:818, 1961.

20. Schaffner F, Schanzer SN: Cervical dilation in the early third trimester. *Obstet Gynecol* 27:130, 1966.

21. Guyer B, Wallach LA, Rosen SL: Birthweight-standardized neonatal mortality rates and the prevention of low birthweight: how does Massachusetts compare with Sweden? *N Engl J Med* 301:1230, 1982.

22. Stewart A: Follow-up of pre-term infants. In Anderson ABM, Beard RW, Brudenell JM, Dunn PM (eds): *Pre-term Labor.* London, Royal College of Obstetricians and Gynaecologists, 1977, pp 372–384.

23. Klaus M, Kennell

24. Committee to Study the Prevention of Low Birthweight: *Preventing Low Birthweight.* Washington, DC, Institute of Medicine, National Academy Press, 1985.

25. Creasy RK, Gummer BA, Liggins GC: System for predicting spontaneous preterm birth. *Obstet Gynecol* 55:692–695, 1980.

26. Morrison JC, Martin JN: Selecting patients for antenatal steroid treatment. *Contemp OB/GYN* 20:211–215, 1982.

27. Reagan JA, Chao, S, James LS: Premature rupture of membranes, preterm delivery, and group B streptococcal colonization of mothers. *Am J Obstet Gynecol* 141:184–186, 1981.

28. Terris M, Gold EM: An epidemiologic study of prematurity. *Am J Obstet Gynecol* 103:371–379, 1969.

Chapter 29
Maternal-Fetal Blood Incompatibility
Kathleen Buckley, M.S.N., C.N.M.

INTRODUCTION

Prior to the 1960s, the reproductive outlook for Rh-negative women was bleak. Risk of sensitization was 2–3% after abortion and 14% after pregnancy (1). Once sensitized, the Rh-negative woman's potential to deliver a living child decreased with every subsequent pregnancy. In the face of this tragedy, many families chose to limit childbearing rather than to risk delivery of a dead or dying infant.

During the last 25 years, much has been learned about the identification and treatment of blood incompatibilities. The outcome of both the Rh- and the ABO-incompatible infant has improved dramatically.

Many blood factors have been discovered. Some, such as C and c and E and e, are closely related to Rh, but they seldom are responsible for development of an antigen/antibody reaction. This chapter focuses on the two major incompatibilities, Rh and ABO.

An understanding of the terminology given in the Glossary to the chapter will aid in clarification of the etiology, diagnosis, and treatment of blood incompatibilities (2).

Rh DISEASE

Definition/Etiology

Rh blood types are determined genetically. From each of his parents an individual receives one of a pair of genes that gives rise to a particular blood factor. Many clinicians now use the letter D

instead of the original term Rh. Thus, a D cell is Rh positive, which is a dominant characteristic. A cell lacking D is termed d (Rh negative). The homozygous Rh-positive father (DD) and Rh-negative (dd) mother can produce only Rh-positive (Dd) children. The heterozygous father (Dd) and Rh-negative (dd) mother have a 50% chance of producing Rh-posi-

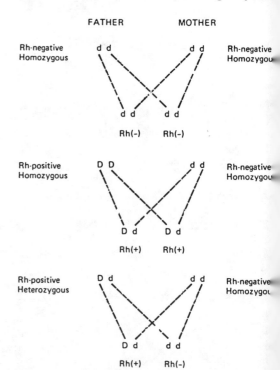

Figure 29.1. Illustration of inheritance of the Rh genes D and d. The C and c and E and e genes are inherited in the same manner.

How Rh disease develops...

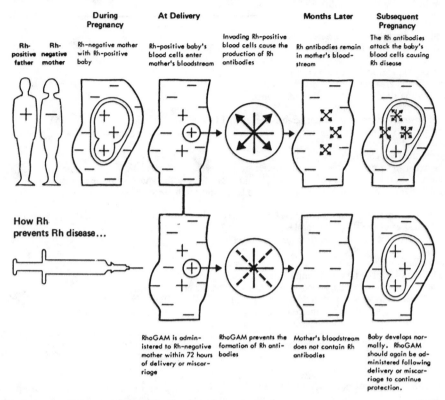

Figure 29.2. The etiology of Rh sensitization and the physiology of Rh isoimmunization. (Adapted from *How RhoGAM Prevents Rh Disease. Ortho Diagnostics, 1968.*)

tive offspring and a 50% chance of an Rh-negative (dd) baby (Fig. 29.1) (3).

While there is no difference in incidence of the Rh factor according to sex, certain racial groups do have significant differences (4):

1. 1% of American Indians, Chinese, and Asian populations are Rh negative.
2. 7% of black Americans are Rh negative.
3. 13% of white Americans are Rh negative.
4. The highest Rh-negative incidence occurs in the Basques (Spanish) (34%).

Rh isoimmunization primarily is a disease of the fetus and neonate (4). It occurs when Rh-positive fetal blood cells cross over into the maternal bloodstream at birth and stimulate maternal antibody production. In subsequent pregnancies, if the fetus is Rh positive, maternal antibodies may cross back into fetal circulation and destroy fetal red blood cells. Maternal antibodies destroy fetal red blood cells by coating them, altering their proper-

ties, and making them destroyed more easily by phagocytes. As the phagocytes destroy the fetal red blood cells, hemoglobin is broken down and bilirubin, a biproduct, is produced. Figure 29.2 details the etiology and the physiologic basis for Rh isoimmunization.

Isoimmunization also may occur if an Rh-negative woman inadvertently receives transfusion of Rh-positive blood. Failure to receive Rh immunoglobulin after spontaneous abortion or ectopic pregnancy also is another iatrogenic cause of isoimmunization (see Chapter 24).

Diagnosis

Every pregnant woman should be tested to determine her blood type and the presence or absence of the Rh factor. If the mother is Rh negative, periodic screening for the presence of circulating antibodies to red cell antigens is necessary. The indirect Coombs' test, also called the indirect antiglobulin test, detects 95% of unexpected circulating antibodies (5). A test result above a titer

Table 29.1.
TYPES OF ERYTHROBLASTOSIS FETALIS[a]

1. Hydrops fetalis—most severe type
   a. Usually stillborn but may survive a few hours
   b. Variable degree of maceration
   c. Generalized edema
   d. Pallor of skin and mucous membranes
   e. Petechiae and areas of purpura may be present
   f. Facial edema suggests a mongoloid appearance
   g. Marked hepatosplenomegaly
   h. Severe anemia—erythrocyte count often is less than 1,000,000/mm^3 of blood
   i. Great numbers of immature or nucleated red blood cells present in circulation—counts as high as 100,000/mm^3 of blood
   j. Lowered plasma protein
2. Icterus gravis neonatorum—second most severe type
   a. Jaundice of skin and sclerae appears within the first 24 hours of life and reaches its maximum in 3–7 days
   b. High bilirubin levels in the first 5 days of life, often leading to brain damage or kernicterus
   c. Progressive anemia
   d. Ecchymotic hemorrhages on the face and upper parts of the body appearing at or shortly after birth
   e. Variable degree of hepatosplenomegaly
   f. Nucleated red blood cells range from 10,000–100,000/mm^3
   g. Lethargy
   h. Poor feeding
3. Congenital anemia of the newborn—mild type
   a. Varying degree of anemia appearing within the first 3 weeks of life
   b. Faint jaundice may appear within 24–36 hours of life but fades within a few days
   c. Pallor becomes noticeable as jaundice fades
   d. Nucleated red blood cells are few or absent in the circulation

[a]Adapted from Ross Laboratories: *Erythroblastosis Fetalis*. 1960, pp 14–16.

of 1:16 indicates sufficient antibody production to cause hemolytic disease of the newborn (4, p 772).

Signs and Symptoms

Signs of isoimmunization are few. A sinusoidal fetal heart rate pattern is thought by some to indicate maternal-fetal transfusion (4, p 772).

Maternal and Fetal Outcome

Prognosis for the Rh-positive infant of a sensitized mother is poor. Destruction of fetal red blood cells may be severe enough to cause not only anemia but also generalized edema and circulatory collapse (hydrops fetalis) (see Table 29.1). In fact, the term "erythroblastosis fetalis" is derived from the physiological fetal mechanism that attempts to compensate for the anemia. The fetal bone marrow produces many immature red blood cells (erythroblasts). An affected fetus/newborn has a high percentage of erythroblasts in the circulating blood compliment. Thus, the condition is termed erythroblastosis (6).

High bilirubin levels result in staining and deposit of unconjugated bilirubin within neurons, causing irreversible necrosis. Survivors of very high levels (≥20 mg/dl) may have cerebral palsy, sensory deafness, loss of vertical gaze, dental enamel dysplasia, and visual motor defects. Less severe elevations of bilirubin may produce short-term memory loss or shortened attention span. Preterm infants may be affected significantly by lower levels of bilirubin (7).

The risk of stillbirth in the first pregnancy is 8%. Risk increases with each subsequent pregnancy. History of a previous severely affected infant increases the risk to 50% (8).

Maternal physical health is not affected. However, the grief and guilt of producing a severely ill child may be overwhelming. If the child dies, the emotional sequelae are intensified.

Medical Management

Screening

The cornerstone of management is careful, conscientious screening of every prenatal patient. A successful Rh prophylaxis screening program includes the following procedures (1, p 289):

1. After the initial prenatal visit, every pregnant woman and the father of the baby have blood sent to the blood bank for ABO and Rh determination, as well as an indirect Coombs'.
2. The blood bank determination is available within 2 weeks, and the blood type and Rh fac-

tor are posted in a prominent place in the patient's chart.

3. Patients identified as sensitized are referred immediately to a tertiary center for intensive follow-up.

Use of Prenatal Rh-Immune Globulin to Prevent Isoimmunization

It has been demonstrated that use of Rh-immune globulin can reduce the incidence of isoimmunization during pregnancy from 1–2% to 0.1%. However, prenatal use is controversial (9). While maternal side effects are rare, and fetal side effects have not been reported, the cost-effectiveness of preventing prenatal sensitization approximately is 50 times less than the cost of preventing postnatal sensitization. On the other hand, the cost of comprehensive, intensive services to save a hydropic infant is staggering.

Protocols for Rh immunoglobulin use in the Rh-negative, unsensitized gravida are as follows (1, pp 289–292):

1. In the event of a first trimester abortion or an ectopic pregnancy, 50 micrograms of Rh-immune globulin is administered.
2. Unsensitized patients are screened on a routine basis at 24, 32, 36, 38, and 40 weeks' gestation for a change in indirect Coombs' titers that would indicate sensitization.
3. If the patient miscarries in the second trimester, 300 mg of Rh-immune globulin is administered.
4. The patient is given an appointment in order that administration of Rh-immune globulin will be given at 28 weeks. The blood bank also monitors the administration at 28 weeks and notifies the care giver if any Rh-negative woman does *not* receive the injection.
5. The patient receives 300 μg of Rh-immune globulin at 28 weeks' gestation.
6. An indirect Coombs' test is performed to verify that the patient still is unsensitized.
7. Maternal-fetal hemorrhage should be suspected in cases of abruptio placentae, bleeding from placenta previa, fetal demise, or nonimmune hydrops fetalis. In such cases a quantitative laboratory test should be used to determine incidence and amount of hemorrhage. Dosage of immune globulin should be titered to amount of hemorrhage.
8. In addition to the dose at 28 weeks, every diagnostic amniocentesis requires an additional dose of 300 μg of Rh-immune globulin.
9. If amniocentesis is done near term and the baby is sure to be born within 28 hours, the dose may be withheld. If the 300 mg dose is given after amniocentesis in the third trimester and the baby is delivered within 30 days, the postpartum dose may be omitted if the quantitative blood test demonstrates minimal maternal-fetal hemorrhage.
10. All other Rh-negative women who deliver an Rh-positive infant should receive a routine dose of 300 μg of Rh-immune globulin within 72 hours after delivery. The dose should be adjusted upward if a quantitative blood test demonstrates large fetal-maternal hemorrhage.

Management of the Rh-Sensitized Mother

Intensive management of the maternal-fetal unit should include the following key information (4, p 774):

1. Past obstetric history, with emphasis on details of management and fetal outcome.
2. Accurate documentation of gestational age of present pregnancy.
3. Documentation of the Rh status of the father of the baby.
4. Serial maternal antibody titers throughout pregnancy.
5. Spectrophotometric analysis of amniotic fluid.
6. Identification and treatment of other coexisting maternal complications.

The indirect Coombs' test is used for screening the isoimmunization status of the sensitized mother. Titers of 1:64 or consistently rising titers suggest current sensitization. A titer of 1:16 is suspicious, and serial amniocentesis should begin in order to assess accurately amniotic fluid bilirubin levels. Determinations should be initiated at 18–20 weeks and repeated every 2 weeks for mothers with titers greater than 1:16 or who have a prior history of fetal erythroblastosis (8, p 94).

Spectrophotometric analysis of amniotic fluid bilirubin levels has been proven to accurately reflect the severity of the disease (Fig. 29.3) (10):

1. Low levels (zone 1)—the fetus is unaffected; no treatment required.
2. Moderate levels (zone 2)—the fetus is affected but will not have hydrops.
3. High levels (zone 3)—the fetus is affected severely with the prognosis of severe hemolytic anemia, hydrops, and death.

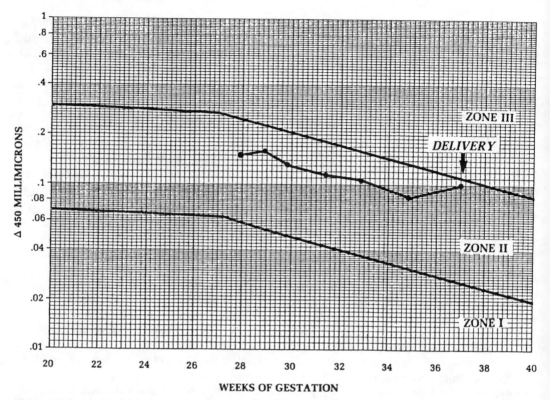

Figure 29.3. Modified Liley graph of zones to predict severity of fetal disease with lines extended to 20 weeks. Zone 1 includes infants who are virtually unaffected; zone 2 includes mild to moderately affected newborns; and zone 3 includes infants who died in utero or were born hydropic or severely anemic. In this example serial ΔOD 450s of a patient in mid-zone 2 are shown. A rise in ΔOD 450 at 37 weeks precipitated delivery. The baby was moderately affected and required neonatal exchange transfusions. Cord hematocrit was 35% and the infant did well. (Reprinted with permission from Perry S, et al: Intrauterine transfusion for severe isoimmunization. *MCN.* 11:183, 1986.)

If levels are in zone 3, amniotic fluid should be evaluated weekly. Risks of fetal transfusion must be weighed against the alternative of preterm delivery. Zone 3 levels warrant intensive management and delivery as soon as the fetus is viable. Between 23 and 32 weeks' gestation, biweekly intrauterine transfusions of O-negative packed red blood cells (into the fetal peritoneal cavity) can be done. The red cells are absorbed into the fetal circulation through the subdiaphragmatic lymphatic vessels at a rate of approximately 12% per week. This procedure is done under fetoscopy and has an inherent 2–5% risk of fetal loss (10). The transfusion provides some amelioration of the hemolytic anemia. A new technique developed at Yale University Hospital provides for intravascular exchange directly through the percutaneous umbilical vein under ultrasound examination. It may become a safer,

more accurate alternative to peritoneal transfusion when clinicians become skilled in the technique (11).

At 32 weeks' gestation an amniotic fluid analysis of fetal surfactant levels (e.g., lecithin/sphingomyelin or L:S ratio) is performed. If levels are above 1.5:1, the fetus is delivered (see Chapter 6). If they are below that level, the fetus once again is transfused. Regardless of L:S ratio at 34 weeks, the fetus is delivered (10, p 184). Table 29.2 details the management of Rh-sensitized patients.

Delivery of an affected infant is managed best with minimum use of analgesia and anesthesia. If the infant is compromised severely, cesarean section should be performed to alleviate the stress of labor (2, p 24).

In less severely affected infants, induction of labor may be attempted. However, the fetus should be monitored continuously, and any fetal

Table 29.2.

MANAGEMENT OF THE ISOIMMUNIZED PATIENT[a]

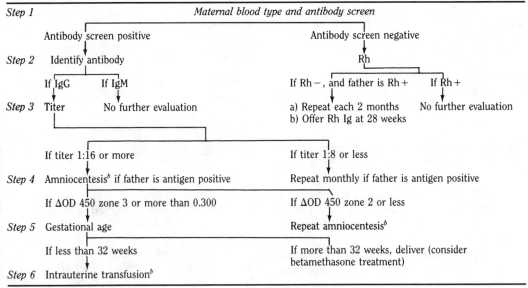

[a]Reprinted with permission from Perry S, et al.: Intrauterine transfusion reaction for severe isoimmunization. *MCN*, 11:184, 1986.
[b]Initial and repeat procedures individually determined.

distress requires emergency cesarean section. At birth the following procedures are recommended (2, p 24):

1. Clamp umbilical cord as soon as possible to prevent increase of blood volume, which would otherwise result from "transfusion" of affected erythrocytes from the placenta.
2. Cut long length of cord (allow at least 3 inches between the umbilicus and the tie) to facilitate use of umbilical vein if exchange transfusion is necessary. Wrap cord with gauze soaked in warm saline solution to prevent drying of tissue.
3. Collect specimen(s) of cord blood for Rh typing, Coombs' test, hemoglobin level, and serum bilirubin.
4. Perform thorough physical examination of infant.

The pediatrician and the anesthesiologist should be present and ready to resuscitate a severely depressed infant. Following the physical examination and laboratory tests, the severity of the incompatibility and resulting anemia should be determined and appropriate treatment initiated as soon as possible. Treatment must be initiated promptly, not only to relieve congestive heart failure but also to prevent brain damage (kernicterus)

from high bilirubin levels. Once brain damage does occur, it is irreversible.

For severely affected infants, exchange transfusions are the treatment of choice (Table 29.3). Exchange transfusion has the following benefits (2, p 24):

1. It removes sensitized red blood cells, thus reducing phagocytosis and hemolysis.
2. It corrects the blood volume, thus relieving heart failure.
3. It improves the blood's oxygen-carrying capacity, thus relieving hypoxia.
4. It decreases serum bilirubin, thus preventing kernicterus.

Risks of transfusion are hemosiderosis, transfusion reaction, and hepatitis or AIDS infection.

The exchange requires compatible fetal blood with low titers of anti-A and anti-B antibodies. In an emergency O Rh-negative blood can be administered safely regardless of the infant's blood type. The blood should be warmed to body temperature (37°C) before the exchange. Blood then is alternately withdrawn and introduced through the umbilical vein—20 ml at a time until approximately 500 cc or 75 ml/pound have been exchanged. During the exchange, the health care team should monitor vital signs closely, observ-

Table 29.3.

INDICATIONS FOR NEWBORN EXCHANGE TRANSFUSION[a]

Cardiac failure
Severe anemia
Jaundiced premature infants
Cord blood bilirubin of 4 mg/100 ml
Serum bilirubin of 20 mg/100 ml

[a]Adapted from Ross Laboratories: *Erythroblastosis Fetalis*, 1960, p 25.

Table 29.4.

DELETERIOUS EFFECTS OF PHOTOTHERAPY[a]

Retinal damage
Dehydration
Diarrhea
Skin rash
Priapism
Hyperthermia
Hemolysis
Lethargy
Poor feeding
Delayed growth rate in later childhood

[a]Adapted from Perez R: *Protocols for High Risk Nursing*, St. Louis, Mosby, 1981, pp 95–96.

ing for shock and/or transfusion reaction. After each 100 ml of blood, the physician transfusing the infant is notified so that calcium gluconate can be administered, because the preservative in the donor blood (potassium citrate) will capture the newborn's serum calcium and significantly lower the level.

For infants less severely affected at birth (2, p 24) a smaller transfusion may be able to stabilize the hematocrit. In mildly affected infants repeated single transfusions may correct anemia satisfactorily. Others may need only phototherapy to decrease bilirubin levels effectively. Although the exact physiologic mechanism still is unknown, phototherapy increases bilirubin breakdown by providing an alternate pathway for metabolism. Phototherapy is not without risk. Table 29.4 lists the deleterious effects of phototherapy (7, p 95).

Brain damage most often occurs within the first 5 days of life and is manifested by lethargy, opisthotonos, poor sucking, high pitched cry, depressed Moro's reflex, vomiting, muscular flaccidity or rigidity, and downward rolling of eyes. Any signs and symptoms of kernicterus call for immediate, intensive treatment (7, p 95).

Hemoglobin/hematocrit levels should be followed closely for the first 6 weeks of life. Falling levels warrant exchange transfusion. The infant should be stabilized by 6 weeks of age.

ABO INCOMPATIBILITY

Definition/Etiology

The ABO groups are genetically determined characteristics, and their presence or absence determines the four basic blood groups of A, B, AB, and O.

Antibodies to the blood group A or B develop naturally when the corresponding blood group is absent. Blood "typing" is based on this factor. For example, group O women may have both anti-A and anti-B antibodies. Thus, ABO incompatibility usually develops when a group O woman with significant anti-A/anti-B agglutinins carries a fetus who is group A, B, or AB. The anti-A/anti-B agglutinins cause hemolytic disease in the fetus and newborn. This condition differs from Rh disease in that prior sensitization is not required because the antibodies are present naturally prior to pregnancy. Thus, hemolytic anemia commonly occurs in the *first* pregnancy. ABO incompatibility is more common but less severe than Rh isoimmunization. While 20% of infants have a major ABO incompatibility as documented by laboratory testing, only 5% become symptomatic. Black infants tend to be affected more often than white infants. However, the disease does not appear to be any more severe in the black infant than the white (4, p 778).

Signs and Symptoms

The major sign is jaundice developing within the first 24 hours of life.

Diagnosis

Diagnosis is made after the fact when jaundice is observed in the newborn (4, p 778).

Criteria for diagnosis include:

1. Maternal blood group O.
2. Newborn blood group A, B, or AB.
3. Newborn anemia, mild to moderate.
4. Elevated bilirubin levels within the first 24 hours of life.
5. Exclusion of other possible diagnoses.
6. Positive Coombs' test.

Maternal and Fetal Outcome

The mother is unaffected physically. However, the anxiety and fear for her newborn's condition may be overwhelming emotionally. The mother has an 87% chance of producing another affected infant (4, p 778).

The newborn and/or fetus will have varying degrees of hemolytic anemia and elevated bilirubin levels. Incidence of stillbirth is *not* elevated in ABO incompatibility. Anemia and bilirubin levels usually are mild to moderate—not severe.

Medical Management

Principles of management are the same as for the Rh-sensitized infant. Exchange tranfusion rarely is necessary and phototherapy is the treatment of choice. However, a recent study documents that ABO-incompatible infants can be managed safely without phototherapy with higher bilirubin levels than previously thought.

NURSING MANAGEMENT

Nursing care specific for *maternal fetal blood incompatibilities:*
- ☐ Screen every pregnant woman for blood type and Rh factor at the first prenatal visit.
- ☐ Post the laboratory evaluation of blood type and Rh in a prominent place in the patient's chart within 2 weeks after the first prenatal visit.
- ☐ Report abnormal findings to the physician immediately. Alert all other members of the health care team to findings.
- ☐ Inform every pregnant patient of her blood type and Rh factor.

If the patient is Rh negative:
- ☐ Explain the significance of the Rh factor:
  - — Genetic determination of blood factors;
  - — Impact on fetal health;
  - — Purpose of Rh immunization during pregnancy and in the postpartum period; and
  - — Importance of routine periodic screening of Rh titers during pregnancy and significance of results.
- ☐ Obtain paternal blood type and Rh factor.
- ☐ Schedule the Rh-negative unsensitized patient for a prenatal visit at 26 weeks' gestation and perform another antibody screen (indirect Coombs' test).
- ☐ If titers are ≤1:8 at 28 weeks' gestation, administer 300 µg of Rh-immune globulin as ordered.
- ☐ Be aware that antibody titers may be normally slightly higher at delivery if Rh-immune globulin was given at 28 weeks' gestation.
- ☐ At delivery collect cord blood for blood type, Rh factor, and direct Coombs' test.
- ☐ If the infant is Rh positive, administer 300 µg of Rh-immune globulin to the mother within 72 hours after delivery.

- ☐ Be prepared to administer multiple doses if laboratory tests indicate that a large fetal-maternal hemorrhage has occurred.
- ☐ Observe the newborn for jaundice. Be aware that jaundice occurring within the first 24 hours after birth always is abnormal and may indicate blood incompatibility.

If the patient is Rh sensitized:
- ☐ Explain diagnostic procedures (e.g., amniocentesis, L:S ratio) and their results in relation to fetal status.
- ☐ Explain the risks/benefits and the procedures involved in fetal transfusion, if appropriate.
- ☐ Encourage the patient to verbalize concerns about fetal outcome.
- ☐ Prepare the patient for the possibility of preterm cesarean section.
- ☐ If the mother is Rh sensitized, be prepared for exchange transfusion immediately at delivery.
- ☐ For less severely Rh sensitized or ABO incompatible infants, counsel the parents about phototherapy, including:
  - — The cause and effects of jaundice;
  - — Rationale for phototherapy;
  - — The need to uncover the infant;
  - — The need for eye patches; and
  - — The importance of continued maternal/paternal contact (including touch and bonding).

Nursing diagnoses most frequently associated with *blood incompatibility* (see Section V):
- ☐ Grieving related to potential/actual loss of infant or birth of an imperfect child.
- ☐ Knowledge deficit regarding etiology, disease process, treatment, and expected outcome.
- ☐ Altered fetal cardiac and cerebral tissue perfusion.
- ☐ Anxiety/fear.

GLOSSARY

Agglutination——Collection of cells into clumps.

Agglutinin——Antibodies that cause agglutination of cells.

Antibody——A specifically reacting gamma globulin synthesized by the body in response to the introduction of an antigen.

Antigen——A substance that, when introduced into a person, stimulates the formation of specific antibodies.

Bilirubin——Bile pigment that is formed from the hemoglobin. When red blood cells are destroyed, bilirubin appears in the blood tissues as an end product of hemoglobin destruction.

Blood group factor——One of a number of substances, usually a complex carbohydrate, occurring on the red cell surface that is responsible for the blood group or type of the red cell (e.g., A substance or Rh substance).

Blood grouping——Classification of blood into groups according to the blood factors or agglutinins found on the surface of the red blood cell.

Coombs' or Antiglobulin test——Laboratory test used to demonstrate the presence of antibody absorbed or bound to red blood cells. Direct Coombs' test: test used to detect coating of red blood cells by antibodies. Indirect Coombs' test: test used to detect circulating antibodies that coat red blood cells.

Genotypes——Constitution of an individual as determined by the genes inherited from both parents.

Heterozygous——Refers to the inheritance of dissimilar genes for a certain trait from each parent.

Homozygous——Refers to the inheritance of similar genes for a certain trait from each parent.

Isoimmunization——Immunization resulting from the injection of an antigen into a member of the same species who lacks this particular antigen.

Kernicterus——Postnatal complication of hyperbilirubinemia in which there are degenerative changes and pigmentation of the nuclear masses of the brain with bile pigments; common complication of erythroblastosis.

Normal or Naturally occurring antibodies——Antibodies present in serum that are not known certainly to result from exposure to the antigen concerned. Examples of such antibodies are anti-A and anti-B antigen.

Phagocytosis——Engulfing of cells and foreign particles by scavenger cells of the body, referred to as phagocytes. The ingested material often is digested within the phagocyte.

Rhesus or Rh or D factor——Antigen present on the erythrocytes of 85% of humans. It is similar to an antigen first discovered on the red cells of the rhesus monkey. The significance of this factor is its ability to cause hemolytic reactions in sensitized Rh-negative recipients and its casual relationship to erythroblastosis.

Titer——Measurement of the amount of antibody determined by measuring the highest dilution of a serum that can agglutinate cells.

REFERENCES

1. Kochenour N, Beeson J: The use of Rh-immune globulin. *Clin Obstet Gynecol* Volume 25:253, 1982.
2. Ross Laboratories: *Erythroblastosis Fetalis*, 1960.
3. Ziegal, E. and Cranley, M. *Obstetric Nursing*, New York, MacMillan Publishing Company (1984) p.
4. Pritchard J, et al.: *Williams Obstetrics*, ed 17. Norwalk, CT, Appleton-Century-Crofts, 1985, p 772.
5. Nursing Reference Library: *Diagnostics*. Springhouse, PA, Springhouse Publishing, 1986, p 283.
6. Miller B, Keane C: *Encyclopedia and Dictionary of Medicine, Nursing and Allied Health*. Philadelphia, WB Saunders, 1983, p 392.
7. Perez R: *Protocols for Prenatal Nursing Practice*. St. Louis, Mosby, 1981, p 94.
8. Freedman E: *Obstetric Decision Making*. St. Louis, Mosby, 1982, p 94.
9. Hammer R, et al.: The prenatal use of Rh immune globulin. *MCN*. 9:30, 1984.
10. Perry S, et al.: Intrauterine transfusion for severe isoimmunization. *MCN* 11:183–184, 1986.
11. Queenan J: Erythroblastosis fetalis: closing the circle. *N Engl J Med* 314:1448–1449, 1986.

Chapter 30
Abnormalities of the Amniotic Fluid
Nancy W. Kulb, C.N.M., M.S.

INTRODUCTION

Amniotic fluid surrounds the embryo and fetus from the second week after conception until birth. Early in pregnancy the composition is similar to maternal plasma except for a lower protein content and probably results from transudation of water, electrolytes, and other small molecules across the amniotic membranes and fetal skin. The composition of the fluid changes throughout pregnancy, reflecting the contributions of other sources of fluid as the fetus matures.

Amniotic fluid is not static. Its water content is exchanged approximately every 3 hours. The volume of fluid at any given time reflects the balance between production and removal of fluid. Fluid continues to be secreted from cells of the amnion or as a transudate from maternal blood throughout pregnancy. Starting at around the fourth month of gestation, fetal urine makes an increasingly important contribution to amniotic fluid. By late pregnancy fetal urine volume is approximately 500 ml/day. Secretions from the respiratory and gastrointestinal tracts make smaller contributions. Fetal swallowing seems to be a major factor in controlling the volume of fluid. Interestingly, the amount of fluid swallowed every day approximates the amount contributed by fetal urine.

Amniotic fluid consists primarily of water but also contains fetal squamous and fat cells, uric acid, urea, creatinine, electrolytes, protein, enzymes, respiratory secretions, lanugo, and vernix caseosa. As gestation advances, the osmolality decreases about 1 mOsm/liter/week beginning about the 20th week. This is thought to reflect the contribution of fetal urine, which is hypotonic because of its low

Table 30.1.
AVERAGE AMNIOTIC FLUID VOLUME[a]

WEEKS GESTATION	AVERAGE FLUID VOLUME
10 weeks	50 ml
16 weeks	200 ml
20 weeks	350 ml
38 weeks	1000 ml

[a]Adapted from Butnarescu GF, Tillotson DM: *Maternity Nursing Today: Theory to Practice.* New York, John Wiley & Sons, 1983, p 184.

electrolyte concentration. Fetal urine does contain more urea, creatinine, and uric acid than does plasma, and this is reflected in rising levels of these substances as gestation advances.

The volume of fluid generally increases until term, with a slight decrease between 38 and 40 weeks and a significant decrease after 42 weeks. The range of normal volume is wide, but average volume by weeks gestation is given in Table 30.1.

Amniotic fluid has several important functions. It cushions the fetus from external pressure and trauma, and it helps to maintain a stable thermal environment. During labor, while fetal membranes are intact, its hydrostatic pressure may aid in cervical dilatation. At the same time, it may protect the fetal presenting part from excessive pressure of uterine contractions by equalizing pressure throughout the amniotic sac. This effect is thought to prevent excessive molding or other trauma to the fetus's head.

Components of amniotic fluid are very useful clinically as a source of information about fetal status. Amniocentesis—withdrawal of small amounts of amniotic fluid—in the second trimester of preg-

335

Table 30.2.

POLYHYDRAMNIOS: CHRONIC VERSUS ACUTE[a]

CHARACTERISTICS	CHRONIC	ACUTE
Week of diagnosis	28–38	20–24
Fundal height by 24 weeks' gestation (cm)	20–26	29–32
Weight gain per 4-week interval at diagnosis (pounds)	2–8	10–12
Week of delivery	32–40	24–27
Outcome	Varies according to cause	Perinatal death
Maternal symptoms	Mild to severe	Severe

[a]Reprinted from Queenan JT, Gadow EC: Polyhydramnios: chronic vs acute. *Am J Obstet Gynecol* 108:349, 1970.

Table 30.3.

COMPLICATIONS OF PREGNANCY ASSOCIATED WITH POLYHYDRAMNIOS[a]

COMPLICATION OF PREGNANCY	PERCENTAGE OF CASES OF POLYHYDRAMNIOS ASSOCIATED WITH EACH COMPLICATION
Diabetes mellitus	22–26%
Congenital anomalies (especially of the CNS or GI tract)	20–24%
Multiple gestation	8–10%
Erythroblastosis fetalis	4–11%
None	34–40%

[a]Adapted from Queenan JT, Kubarych SF: Detecting and managing polyhydramnios. *Contemp OB/GYN* 16:113–125, 1980.

nancy allows for evaluation of a limited but ever-growing number of genetic abnormalities (see Chapter 25). In the third trimester it may be used to assess fetal maturity (see Chapter 6) or for management of Rh sensitization (see Chapter 29). During labor, the presence or absence of meconium or blood in the amniotic fluid gives information about fetal status (see Chapter 39).

POLYHYDRAMNIOS

Definition

Polyhydramnios, or hydramnios, is the pathological accumulation of an excessive amount of amniotic fluid. It is defined as a volume greater than 2000 ml (the normal volume at term is 1000 ml). Volumes can be quite large; as much as 15,000 ml has been recorded (1). The appearance and composition of the fluid are very similar to normal fluid.

Polyhydramnios occurs in approximately 1:150 to 1:280 pregnancies (2). Because accurate measurement of fluid is very difficult, the diagnosis is rather subjective and an even wider range may be reported. Usually , there is a gradual, slow accumulation of fluid that becomes evident in the third trimester. In about 2% of the cases of polyhydramnios, however, the onset is rapid and occurs in the

second trimester. Table 30.2 contrasts acute versus chronic polyhydramnios.

Etiology

The etiology of polyhydramnios is not always clear, but it is associated with other complications of pregnancy (Table 30.3).

Polyhydramnios occurs more often with monozygotic than dizygotic twins. It is proposed that polyhydramnios develops when one twin usurps a greater part of the circulation, resulting in polycythemia, cardiac hypertrophy, and greater urine volume. Indeed, the fetus with polyhydramnios often has dilated renal tubules and an enlarged bladder, while the other often has contracted renal tubules and oligohydramnios.

The explanation of polyhydramnios associated with certain fetal anomalies is more satisfactory. Anomalies of the gastrointestinal system that interfere with fetal swallowing allow fluid to accumulate. Approximately three-quarters of babies with tracheoesophageal fistula have polyhydramnios (2, p 115). There is also a high rate of polyhydramnios associated with central nervous system (CNS) abnormalities, such as spina bifida or anencephaly. It is possible that there is some excess fluid production as a transudate from exposed meninges. It is more likely that excessive urine is produced because of the lack of antidiuretic hormone or from direct stimulation of the CNS. A fetus with a CNS anomaly also may have impaired swallowing ability.

The reason polyhydramnios is associated with diabetes mellitus and erythroblastosis fetalis is not clear. Fetal urine production in those cases appears normal. It may be that large placental size contributes in some way to excessive fluid (1, p 463).

Signs and Symptoms

The signs and symptoms of polyhydramnios depend to a great extent on the amount of fluid present. There may be no symptoms at all until a volume of 3000 ml is reached (1). At that point, the patient may feel that she is "bigger" than she should be. She may have gained an excessive amount of weight. Because of the increased pressure from the distended uterus, she may have more edema, especially of the legs, vulva, and abdomen. She may experience shortness of breath, especially after exertion, or orthopnea.

Upon examination, the fundal height will be larger than expected at that point in gestation. This discrepancy may be sudden or slowly increasing. Upon palpation, the examiner may get the sensation that there is an excess of fluid between his hands and the fetus. The entire fetus may be ballotable. The examiner may be able to detect a tremor called a "fluid thrill" upon palpation of the abdomen. Serial abdominal girth measurements, which normally increase about 1 inch/week in the third trimester, may increase more rapidly with polyhydramnios. The maternal abdomen may feel tense, even to the point where it is difficult to palpate the fetus, and it may appear shiny. Fetal heart tones may sound distant and muffled.

With severe or acute polyhydramnios, the symptoms usually are more severe. The mother may experience pain, difficulty breathing, oliguria from obstruction of the urinary tract, and/or nausea and vomiting. Often, the patient will go into premature labor because of the overdistended uterus.

Diagnosis

The diagnosis of polyhydramnios is suspected clinically and confirmed by ultrasound. Occasionally, an ultrasound performed for other reasons will reveal polyhydramnios, or at least a tendency toward it. Although it is possible to measure the amount of amniotic fluid by injecting a known amount of a marker into the amniotic fluid and measuring its concentration after being dispersed through the fluid, that information does not aid in clinical management. Management depends upon maternal condition and complications associated with the polyhydramnios rather than on the absolute volume of fluid.

Of much greater importance is a diagnostic workup of the patient to detect conditions associated with polyhydramnios. Presence of these conditions might alter clinical management and outcome significantly. While a sonogram is being done, a careful search should be made for fetal anomalies, especially of the CNS and gastrointestinal (GI) tract, and for multiple gestation. A glucose tolerance test to diagnose diabetes mellitus and a serologic test for irregular antibodies also should be done.

Maternal and Fetal Outcome

The prognosis depends upon the cause and severity of the polyhydramnios. The high incidence of fetal anomalies means the prognosis is guarded for the baby, even if anomalies were not evident upon ultrasound examination. The presence of multiple gestation, diabetes mellitus, or erythroblastosis also adversely affects the prognosis (see Chapters 10, 29, and 33).

In addition, there are risk factors from the polyhydramnios itself. Because of the overdistended uterus, premature labor is more common; indeed, with polyhydramnios, the rate of prematurity is doubled (1, p 464). The incidence of malpresentations or malpositions is high because of the excess fetal mobility allowed by the distended uterus. Uterine contractions during labor may be of poor quality, also because of the overdistention. Rupture of the membranes, especially if not slow and controlled, can cause prolapse of the umbilical cord or placental abruption (see Chapters 31 & 39). Thus, the need for operative delivery is greater than normal.

In general, then, the fetal prognosis is poor if polyhydramnios is associated with malformations, erythroblastosis, or extreme prematurity. If it is idiopathic, the prognosis is fairly good, with prematurity and malpresentation presenting the major problems (2, p 123).

The problems for the mother are significant; acute or severe polyhydramnios may even threaten her life because of excessive pressure on her organs, leading to difficulty breathing, and impeding the circulatory system. More common are abruptio placentae, uterine dysfunction, and postpartum hemorrhage, resulting from overdistention of the uterus. In general, however, the threats to the mother can be treated effectively, thereby preventing serious sequelae.

Medical Management

The management of polyhydramnios depends upon its cause and severity. If fetal anomalies incompatible with life are found, the appropriate treatment is to terminate the pregnancy. Membranes should be ruptured slowly and carefully, preferably by the needle prick of a pudendal or paracervical needle. Slow release of fluid helps to prevent abruption from sudden decompression of the uterus. Induction of labor may be required.

If diabetes or erythroblastosis is associated, it should be treated as usual (see Chapters 10 and 29). The fetal prognosis is rather poor, especially with acute polyhydramnios. The patient and her family should be involved in deciding whether aggressive steps should be taken to save the fetus (e.g., whether intrauterine transfusion is warranted to treat erythroblastosis).

When polyhydramnios is idiopathic, whether acute or chronic, management is conservative, with the goal of achieving fetal maturity before delivery is required. If polyhydramnios is mild, hospitalization prior to labor may not be necessary. If the patient experiences dyspnea, abdominal pain, or difficulty walking, hospitalization is required.

Once hospitalized, the patient is placed on partial or total bed rest, depending upon her condition. Sedation may be required to maintain bed rest and alleviate stress. Because of the likelihood of hypoproteinemia owing to the increased loss of protein into the amniotic fluid, a high protein diet is given, and serum protein levels are monitored. The patient is observed for symptoms of congestive heart failure. The fetus is observed by serial ultrasound for normal growth and development.

Diuretics may help excessive edema but will not affect amniotic fluid volume. Because they alter fluid dynamics throughout the body, diuretics should be used with extreme care if they are used at all. Antibiotics are not recommended since they might mask early amnionitis.

If maternal distress (e.g., pain, difficulty breathing) develops before the fetus is mature, dramatic relief can be obtained by amniocentesis. Amniocentesis is performed under strict asepsis to minimize risk of infection and under ultrasound to guide placement of the needle. By either slow continuous suction or gravity drainage, 500–1000 cc of fluid is slowly removed. The procedure may need to be repeated as often as every 2–3 days. Frequent removal of a small amount of fluid is less likely to initiate premature labor than less frequent removal of a large amount. However, if labor is initiated by amniocentesis, tocolytics can be used as necessary to inhibit the labor.

Once the fetus is mature, delivery is allowed. Labor may be initiated spontaneously or may be induced because of maternal distress. Because of the risk of placental abruption from rapid decompression of the uterus and of postpartum hemorrhage resulting from overdistention of the uterus, the following blood work should be performed: type and cross-match and baseline coagulation studies, including complete blood count, platelets, and fibrinogen. Artificial rupture of membranes by a needle prick with very slow, controlled release of fluid is performed. The fetal heart rate is auscultated throughout the procedure, and the examining fingers check to rule out prolapsed cord. The patient is observed for abruptio placentae. Cesarean section is performed when necessary for obstetric indications, especially malpresentation, multiple gestation, cephalopelvic disproportion, cord prolapse, abruptio placentae, or fetal distress. After delivery the patient should be observed for postpartum hemorrhage and treated for it as necessary (see Chapter 42).

NURSING MANAGEMENT

Nursing care specific for the patient with
polyhydramnios:

☐ Assess for signs/symptoms of polyhydramnios at each prenatal visit (e.g., tense, shiny abdomen, excessive fundal height, fluid thrill).

☐ Assist in the diagnostic workup for etiology, including glucose tolerance test, antibody titers, and sonogram(s).

☐ Explain the purpose of the tests and their results to the patient.

☐ Observe for signs/symptoms of complications (congestive heart failure, compromised respiratory function, chorioamnionitis, preterm labor, increasing abdominal pressure): e.g., fever; tachycardia; weakness; abdominal discomfort; dyspnea; shortness of breath; edema of legs, vulva, or abdomen.

☐ Teach the patient to report any increase in shortness of breath immediately. Give her an emergency telephone number to call.

☐ Teach the patient the following:

NURSING MANAGEMENT

— Signs/symptoms of preterm labor;

— Importance of bed rest;

— Importance of high protein diet; and

— Methods to prevent/relieve discomfort (e.g., use pillows for support, sitting up to improve respirations).

☐ Assist with amniocentesis, if necessary.

☐ After artificial rupture of membranes:

— Monitor fetal heart rate to rule out prolapsed cord and

— Observe for signs/symptoms of abruptio placentae (e.g., vaginal bleeding, uterine pain or tenderness , tetanic contractions, shock, fetal distress).

☐ Be prepared for emergency cesarean section and postpartum hemorrhage.

☐ When a fetal anomaly is associated with polyhydramnois, provide accurate information about the anomaly, prognosis, and treatment. When an anomaly is present, if the baby is premature, or if the baby dies, provide counsel-ing, anticipatory guidance, referrals, and follow-up visits or telephone calls as needed.

Nursing diagnoses most frequently associated with *polyhydramnios* (see Section V):

☐ Grieving related to potential/actual loss of infant or birth of an imperfect child.

☐ Anticipatory grieving related to actual/perceived threat to self.

☐ Disturbance to body image, self-esteem.

☐ Knowledge deficit regarding etiology, disease process, treatment, and outcome.

☐ Fluid volume deficit.

☐ Altered maternal tissue perfusion.

☐ Altered fetal cardiac and cerebral tissue perfusion.

☐ Pain.

☐ Impaired gas exchange.

☐ Self-care deficit—feeding, bathing/hygiene, dressing, grooming, toileting.

☐ Spiritual distress.

OLIGOHYDRAMNIOS

Definition

Oligohydramnios, as the name suggests, is the condition in which the volume of amniotic fluid is far below normal limits. Since the volume of fluid generally increases with gestational age, the specific volume indicating oligohydramnios also will vary with gestational age. However, a volume of less than 300 ml near term indicates oligohydramnios. Since there is no safe and reliable method of determining amniotic fluid volume, the reported incidence varies with diagnostic criteria but has been reported to range from 0.43–3.9% (3).

Etiology

The etiology of oligohydramnios is poorly understood. It is almost always present when the fetus has renal agenesis or urinary tract obstruction, both of which cause anuria. Since fetal urine is an important source of amniotic fluid, the cause seems clear. Indeed, with urinary tract obstruction, the degree of hydronephrosis seems to correlate fairly well with the degree of oligohydramnios (4). But there have been cases in which the fetus had renal agenesis and amniotic fluid volume was normal or even excessive (2, p 118).

Occasionally, with monozygotic twins, one twin will "usurp" a greater part of the circulation, causing cardiac hypertrophy and greater urine volume. The "disadvantaged" twin has a smaller portion of the circulation, resulting in less urine output and, therefore, oligohydramnios (1, p 463).

Rarely, a small, chronic leak in the fetal membranes may cause oligohydramnios. Usually, however, spontaneous labor ensues, chorioamnionitis develops, or rarely, the leak spontaneously "seals" and volume readjusts to normal.

Since fetal pulmonary fluid is a component of amniotic fluid, it is possible that a defect in pulmonary function causes failure of the lungs to secrete fluid, resulting in oligohydramnios.

Amniotic fluid volume tends to rise slowly or remain constant near term and actually to decrease after term. By several weeks after the due date, the fluid volume may be reduced markedly. The mechanism is not clear but may be related to poor perfusion of the aging placenta. Oligohydramnios, especially in conjunction with meconium passage, is associated with a high incidence of poor fetal outcome after term (4, pp 204–205).

There also is a strong association between oligohydramnios and intrauterine growth retardation (IUGR). The reason is unclear but again may be related to uteroplacental blood flow. It is postulated that decreased placental circulation causes reduced fetal cardiac output and therefore reduced urinary output. Indeed, many factors associated with IUGR, such as hypertension and cigarette smoking, are associated with oligohydramnios (3, p 271).

Signs and Symptoms

The clinical signs and symptoms of oligohydramnios are rather vague. Generally, the mother experiences no subjective symptoms. Upon abdominal examination, the care provider may find the fundal height low for gestational age because of small fluid volume, IUGR, or both, and the fetus may feel easily palpable. Often, the diagnosis is made during an ultrasound examination being done for suspected IUGR or for an unrelated indication. Finally, it may not be suspected until amniotic fluid volume is low when the membranes rupture; unfortunately, estimates of fluid volume often are grossly inaccurate.

Diagnosis

Clinical diagnosis of oligohydramnios is difficult because of the difficulty in estimating fluid volume accurately. Misdiagnosis at amniotomy also may occur when only forewaters leak out and fluid is retained behind a tightly fitting presenting part, masking the true volume.

It is possible to assess amniotic fluid volume accurately by injecting a dye, allowing it to be distributed uniformly throughout the fluid, and then withdrawing some fluid and measuring the concentration of the dye. Clinically, this procedure is neither safe nor efficient enough to be used except in research protocols. The diagnosis of oligohydramnios usually is based upon ultrasound examination. The diagnostic criteria vary. One commonly used criterion is the absence of a pocket of amniotic fluid greater than 1 cm in its longest diameter (15). An alternative and less strict definition is:

1. Obvious lack of amniotic fluid,
2. Poor fluid/fetal interface; or
3. Marked crowding of fetal small parts (3, p 272).

Experienced sonographers may have a subjective impression that fluid volume is decreasing before it meets criteria for oligohydramnios, and they may suggest follow-up sonograms to see whether oligohydramnios develops.

Maternal and Fetal Outcome

There are no known maternal sequelae resulting from oligohydramnios itself, although there may be sequelae from associated conditions, such as hypertension and cigarette smoking.

Effects on the fetus, however, can vary widely, with more profound effects the earlier in gestation it develops. Adhesions between the amnion and fetal small parts can cause skeletal deformities or even amputation of limbs. Excessive pressure from the uterine wall can result in facial and other skeletal malformations. The skin of the newborn may appear dry, wrinkled, and leathery (1, p 465).

Oligohydramnios occurring before or during the time of fetal lung development is associated with pulmonary hypoplasia. The mechanism is not known but is suspected to be one or a combination of the following:

1. A pulmonary defect causes oligohydramnios. It is responsible for failure of the lungs to secrete pulmonary fluid necessary to maintain amniotic fluid volume.
2. Oligohydramnios allows constant pressure on the fetal thorax by the uterine wall, thus preventing lung expansion.
3. With oligohydramnios there is insufficient fluid to be inhaled into the alveoli, resulting in faulty lung growth (1, p 465).

The fact that a significant amount of fluid normally is drawn into the lungs during fetal breathing movements suggests that the fluid is important in pulmonary development and function. The severity of pulmonary hypoplasia is related to the degree of oligohydramnios, suggesting that external chest compression also plays a significant role (6).

In addition to the effects of oligohydramnios itself, the baby also will be affected by the causative or associated factor(s). Congenital anomalies resulting in oligohydramnios may be relatively mild and amenable to treatment or they may be lethal before or after birth. Postmaturity, multiple gestation, and IUGR carry their own risks for the fetus and newborn (see Chapters 27, 32, and 33). Compression of the umbilical cord because of insufficient "cushioning" by fluid may contribute to fetal distress.

The relationship between oligohydramnios and IUGR is under investigation. In one study patients who were suspected of having IUGR by clinical parameters and who had oligohydramnios on ultrasound examination (no pocket of fluid greater than 1 cm in the longest diameter), had six to tenfold increase in perinatal morbidity and mortality: increased fetal distress in labor, increased number of low Apgar scores at 5 minutes after birth, and a cesarean section rate of 44%. Those found to be small for gestational age at delivery but with normal fluid volume had low perinatal morbidity and no mortality—perhaps because they were normal, genetically small babies (5, pp 254–257). Another study using a general obstetric population and less strict criteria for the diagnosis of oligohydramnios showed an increase in IUGR among the patients with oligohydramnios, but there was no adverse fetal outcome (i.e., Apgar scores were not significantly lower in the group with oligohydramnios, nor were there any severe congenital anomalies) (3, pp 273–275). Differences in study design may account for the discrepancies, and investigation of the problem is continuing.

Medical Management

There is nothing that can be done to directly treat oligohydramnios itself. Once oligohydramnios is diagnosed, however, a careful sonogram should be done, looking for congenital anomalies, especially of the urinary tract, and for evidence of IUGR. Some urinary tract obstructions now can be treated by fetal surgery (6).

Delivery may be required because of the associated condition, such as IUGR or postmaturity. Oligohydramnios itself may be an indication for early delivery, because it may result from poor uteroplacental perfusion and it may cause limb or facial defects or pulmonary hypoplasia.

When the patient is in labor, the fetus should be monitored carefully by electronic fetal monitoring and fetal blood gas sampling as necessary because of the potential for fetal distress. Cesarean section should be performed when indicated because of the fetus's condition or because of another obstetric reason.

NURSING MANAGEMENT

Nursing care specific for the patient with oligohydramnios:

☐ Assist with diagnostic tests, such as sonograms and fetal monitoring.

☐ Provide care for any conditions associated with oligohydramnios, such as hypertension, intrauterine growth retardation, multiple gestation, or postmaturity.

☐ During labor, monitor the fetus carefully, observing for fetal distress and meconium staining.

☐ Assist with oxytocin induction of labor if indicated (see Chapter 37).

☐ Be prepared for emergency cesarean section.

Nursing diagnoses most frequently associated with oligohydramnios (see Section V):

☐ Grieving related to potential/actual loss of infant or birth of an imperfect child.

☐ Knowledge deficit regarding etiology, disease process, treatment, and outcome.

☐ Altered fetal cardiac and cerebral perfusion.

☐ Spiritual distress.

PREMATURE RUPTURE OF THE MEMBRANES

Definition

Premature rupture of the membranes (PROM) is spontaneous rupture of the membranes at any time in gestation before the onset of labor. The term "preterm rupture of the membranes" should be used to indicate rupture of membranes prior to term. In the past, the definition of PROM often has included a "latent" interval of from 1–24 hours between rupture and onset of uterine contractions. This variation in definitions has led to confusion in reported management and outcome. Many experts today agree that PROM should be defined as rupture at any time prior to the onset of labor and that alternate definitions should be taken into consideration when reading obstetric literature.

PROM occurs in approximately 10% of all deliveries; 20% of these occur before 36 weeks' gestation (7), and 20–30% of all premature infants are delivered because of PROM. In some institutions PROM may occur more frequently than idiopathic preterm labor (8).

Etiology

The etiology of PROM is unknown. However, recent studies indicate that there is not only an association between PROM and infection but that intrauterine or cervical infection may precede and actually cause PROM. Organisms implicated in causing PROM include β-streptococcus, *Chlamydia*, and *Listeria*.

Signs and Symptoms

PROM is manifested by a gush of fluid from the vagina or by a slow, steady leaking of watery fluid from the vagina.

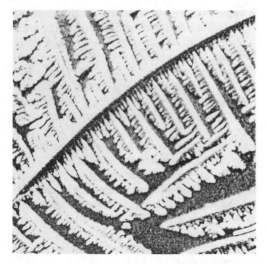

Figure 30.1. Ferning of amniotic fluid. Microscopic appearance of dried amniotic fluid, showing the characteristic fern-like pattern. Reprinted with permission from The American College of Obstetricians and Gynecologists. From Zaneveld, Tauber, Port, Propping. *Obstet Gynecol* 46:424, 1975.

Diagnosis

The diagnosis is confirmed by a sterile speculum examination. Amniotic fluid in the posterior vaginal vault is tested for pH by dipping a sterile cotton-tipped swab in the fluid and then placing it on nitrazine paper. The sudden change of nitrazine paper from orange to dark blue indicates the alkaline pH of amniotic fluid. Blood and vaginal secretions may cause a false-positive nitrazine test.

Another cotton-tipped swab is dipped in the pooled fluid and rolled across a slide. After air drying, the slide is observed under a microscope for the characteristic fern-like pattern indicative of amniotic fluid. The pattern develops from crystallization of sodium chloride in the amniotic fluid as it dries (Fig 30.1). Blood and cervical or vaginal secretions disrupt the pattern. Fluid from the cervix or perineum should *not* be tested since it may confuse the picture. Fluid pooled in the vaginal vault also may be examined for vernix caseosa or bits of lanugo. While the speculum is in place, the cervix is checked visually for an approximation of dilatation. Occasionally, the cervix will be dilated sufficiently to see the fetal scalp, confirming the rupture of membranes.

When the diagnosis still is uncertain, ultrasound can be used to show a decreased amount of fluid but can only *suggest*, not *confirm*, rupture of membranes (9). The patient can be asked to walk

for a few hours with a perineal pad in place, which then can be checked with nitrazine paper.

Maternal and Fetal Outcome

The maternal outcome in cases of PROM is good. The greatest risks to the mother are chorioamnionitis, which is treated effectively with antibiotics, and operative delivery. The reported incidence of chorioamnionitis varies widely from one population to another but generally increases as the time between rupture of membranes and delivery increases. As many as 75% of cultures obtained by amniocentesis are positive after 24 hours, although the rate of clinically apparent infection is less (10).

The risk to the fetus depends upon the gestational age at the time of PROM. After 36 weeks, the greatest risk is from sepsis since respiratory distress syndrome (RDS) is rare. Before 36 weeks, prematurity is the greatest risk: 50% of babies will deliver within 24 hours of preterm PROM and 85% within 1 week (8, p 178). Most of the mortality in premature infants is from RDS, although it is possible that prolonged PROM *may* accelerate fetal lung maturity. In addition, fetal distress due to malpresentation, prolapsed cord, or cord compression in the absence of prolapse (from insufficient fluid to "cushion" the cord) may contribute to perinatal morbidity and mortality. When chorioamnionitis accompanies PROM, the additional risks of infection, especially pneumonia, meningitis, and septicemia, arise (8, p 179). There is some evidence that prolonged PROM in the absence of infection may cause pulmonary hypoplasia secondary to prolonged oligohydramnios.

Medical Management

The management of PROM depends primarily upon gestational age. Regardless of gestational age, however, the following principles apply:

1. No digital vaginal examination is performed unless a decision has been made to deliver the patient since examination may increase the risk of infection.
2. The fetus should be monitored initially upon diagnosis of PROM and while the patient is in labor to rule out cord compression.
3. The patient should be observed constantly for signs and symptoms of chorioamnionitis.

Gestational age is evaluated by the usual parameters (see Chapter 6). After 34–36 weeks' gestation, the risk of infection is greater than the risk of RDS from prematurity. Once PROM is diagnosed and the gestational age is confirmed, delivery is the treatment of choice. If labor does not ensue spontaneously, it should be induced (or cesarean section should be done if there is an obstetric indication). How long to await spontaneous labor before initiating induction is controversial. Some experts wait only 5–6 hours, others wait 12 hours, and yet others wait much longer (9, p 232). Probably the decision should be based on the incidence of chorioamnionitis in that particular population and on whether or not a digital vaginal examination (which increases the risk of infection) has been done.

Between 33 and 36 weeks' gestation, there is some risk of prematurity. Even so, if there is clinical evidence of chorioamnionitis, active labor, or fetal distress, the baby is delivered. If not, it is sometimes possible to obtain fluid from the posterior vaginal pool, which can be used to evaluate fetal maturity by doing a lecithin:sphingomyelin (L:S) ratio and/or phosphatidylglycerol (PG) level. If fluid cannot be obtained vaginally, amniocentesis is attempted. If amniocentesis is attempted, the patient first is placed in the Trendelenburg position to try to accumulate fluid within the uterus. The amniocentesis is done under ultrasound to guide placement of the needle. The fluid is checked for lung maturity (by PG or L:S ratio) and for evidence of infection (white blood cells, Gram's stain, cultures). If the fetus is mature or if there is evidence of infection, labor should be induced. If the fetus is immature and there is no evidence of infection, the pregnancy should be allowed to continue, but delivery is indicated if signs or symptoms of infection become evident or if there is fetal distress. If fluid cannot be obtained, management should be based on the incidence of infection in that population. Again, no digital vaginal examination should be done until the decision has been made to deliver the patient. The fetus should be monitored initially when the diagnosis of PROM is made, when the patient is in labor, and periodically (perhaps daily if the fetus is breech or transverse lie) while awaiting maturity or labor.

Between 28 and 33 weeks' gestation, the management becomes even more difficult and controversial. Some experts would perform amniocentesis (as above) to determine fetal maturity and to look for evidence of infection. Amniocentesis would only be indicated, however, in patients at 28–33 weeks' gestation who are not in active labor, who have no evidence of fetal distress, and who have no clinical evidence of infection (or perhaps for those who have evidence of some infection when the source is not clear).

Others would *not* perform amniocentesis in these patients. The benefit of delivering patients of less than 33 weeks' gestation with a mature L:S ratio is not clear since CNS sequelae such as intracranial hemorrhage still may occur. Also, it is unclear whether there is any benefit in delivering these preterm babies when the amniotic fluid shows evidence of infection but infection is not *clinically* apparent. These practitioners feel that the risks of amniocentesis outweighs the benefits, which are uncertain at best (7, p 211).

When the fetus is less than 34 weeks' gestation or has evidence of immature lungs after amniocentesis, some would administer glucocorticoids to try to hasten fetal lung maturity. However, the benefits to the baby are not proven, and there is some evidence that glucocorticoids may increase the incidence of neonatal septicemia and maternal endometritis.

The usefulness of tocolytics for patients with PROM and no evidence of infection is as yet unknown. Also controversial is the use of prophylactic antibiotics.

In general, however, once PROM is diagnosed in a patient who is 28–33 weeks' gestation, most experts would agree that delivery is indicated in patients with clinical evidence of infection, fetal distress, or active labor. Some might also deliver if there is amniotic fluid evidence of fetal lung maturity or of infection. If expectant management is decided upon, the patient is hospitalized, her temperature is taken frequently (at least every 4–6 hours), daily CBCs are done to follow the white blood cell count, a daily C-reactive protein test may be done for evidence of infection, and the fetal heart rate is frequently auscultated or monitored electronically. Sonograms should be done weekly to document fetal growth. Depending upon the physician's belief about the value of amniocentesis, it might be done weekly to check for evidence of infection or maturity. Depending upon the gestational age and the facilities of the hospital where PROM is diagnosed, transfer to a tertiary care center might be in order, as the majority of patients will deliver within a few days to 1 week.

When PROM occurs in the patient less than 28 weeks' gestation, the outlook is more bleak; 80% of these patients will deliver within 1 week of PROM (9, p 235). Although the point in gestation before which one can say there is absolutely no hope for salvaging the baby is debatable, some experts would advocate terminating the pregnancy if the estimated fetal weight is less than 750 g and there is oligohydramnios on ultrasound (9, p 236). When fluid has not begun to reaccumulate after 2–3 days of PROM, it probably will not, and the fetus is at risk for pulmonary hypoplasia and musculoskeletal deformities. After delivery of a patient who experienced early PROM, possible causes should be investigated by fetal cultures, autopsy, cytogenetic studies, maternal serologic test for syphilis, and maternal cultures for possible causative organisms, including β-streptococcus, *Chlamydia, Listeria,* and cytomegalovirus.

The need for informed consent is evident in the management of PROM at all points in gestation since there are so many controversial aspects of management. It is especially crucial in the management at an early gestational age when the risks and benefits of many procedures are unknown and the potential for good outcome is unpredictable. Garite summarizes the dilemma well:

> Controversy surrounds the place of corticosteroids, the influence of duration of PROM on neonatal morbidity, the place of tocolytic and antibiotic therapy, the usefulness of amniocentesis, the necessity for delivering mature fetuses, and even the basic impact of PROM on perinatal morbidity and mortality. (8, p 187).

It is probably appropriate that at this point management of PROM varies from one institution to another since the outcome varies from one population to another.

NURSING MANAGMENT

Nursing care specific for the patient with
premature rupture of the membranes
(PROM):
- [ ] Teach all pregnant patients signs/symptoms of ruptured membranes and how to report them if they occur.
- [ ] Observe for signs/symptoms of chorioamnionitis:
  - — Take maternal temperature and pulse hourly;
  - — Assess for foul-smelling/purulent discharge and uterine tenderness hourly;
  - — Obtain complete blood count with differential upon diagnosis of PROM;
  - — Obtain maternal cultures as necessary; and
  - — Observe for fetal tachycardia.
- [ ] Assist with diagnostic tests as necessary (e.g., sterile speculum examination, nitrazine test, fern test, ultrasound, amniocentesis); ensure that a strict sterile technique is maintained. (Unsterile nitrazine paper should not be introduced into the vagina).
- [ ] Do *not* perform a digital vaginal examination before labor is established; ensure that a minimal number of examinations is performed and that strict sterile technique is used to prevent infection.

- [ ] Assist with oxytocin induction of labor as necessary (see Chapter 37)
- [ ] Maintain comfort and hygiene; keep patient clean and dry; change pads under bottocks every 2 hours or prn.
- [ ] When expectant management is indicated:
  - — Observe for signs/symptoms of chorioamnionitis every 6 hours (e.g., elevated temperature, malodorous vaginal fluid);
  - — Teach signs/symptoms of labor and observe patient for spontaneous onset of labor;
  - — Educate the patient regarding bed rest as required;
  - — Teach the patient to avoid inserting anything into the vagina; and
  - — Administer glucocorticoids, tocolytics, or antibiotics as ordered. Observe for desired effect and adverse effects.

Nursing diagnoses most frequently associated with PROM (see Section V):
- [ ] Grieving related to potential/actual loss of infant or birth of an imperfect child.
- [ ] Knowledge deficit regarding etiology, disease process, treatment, and outcome.
- [ ] Altered fetal cardiac and cerebral tissue perfusion.

CHORIOAMNIONITIS

Definition

Chorioamnionitis, sometimes called amnionitis infection, is acute inflammation of the fetal membranes. It is clinically evident only in 1–2% of pregnancies but is histologically evident in as many as 10–20%. It is most common and most severe after PROM but can occur with intact membranes and may even cause PROM.

Table 30.4.
INCIDENCE OF CHORIOAMNIONITIS VERSUS LENGTH OF LATENT PERIOD AFTER PREMATURE RUPTURE OF THE MEMBRANES[a]

INCIDENCE OF CHORIOAMNIONITIS	TIME BETWEEN RUPTURE OF MEMBRANES AND ONSET OF LABOR
4%	0–11 hours
5%	12–23 hours
15%	24–47 hours
20%	48–71 hours
25%	After 72 hours

[a]Reprinted from Koh KS, Chang FH, Ledger WJ: When chorioamnionitis threatens mother and offspring. *Contemp OB/GYN* 13:148, 1979.

Etiology

There are three routes by which pathogens can get to the fetal membranes:

1. Most commonly, they ascend from the vagina via ruptured or even intact membranes.
2. They may cross over from the maternal circulation to the amniotic sac via the placenta.
3. Rarely, they may descend from the abdominal cavity through the fallopian tubes (11).

The most common pathogens are those most often found in the vagina and cervix: *Escherichia coli, Streptoccus faecalis, Proteus, Klebsiella, Pseudomonas,* α- and β-streptococcus, and *Staphylococcus.* Less often, *Listeria, Vibrio,* T-strain mycoplasma, or gonorrhea may be the causative organism (11, p 147).

Whether infection will develop in a particular patient depends upon pathogenicity of the organism and resistance of the host. The patient's resistance is affected by her nutritional status and gestational age. Patients of lower socioeconomic status tend to have lower resistance (12).

Most commonly, PROM precedes chorioamnionitis. Table 30.4 illustrates the increasing incidence of infection as the time between rupture of membranes and onset of labor increases. However, it must be remembered that intact membranes do not necessarily prevent infection. It may be that impending chorioamnionitis actually causes PROM and/or premature labor.

The role of internal fetal monitors, particularly the pressure catheters, in chorioamnionitis is unclear. Although contamination of amniotic fluid after insertion of internal catheters can be documented in as many as 50% of cases (11, p 148), the incidence of infection after their use is quite low, not much if any higher than in the general population.

Signs and Symptoms

The classic symptoms of chorioamnionitis are maternal fever and tachycardia; foul-smelling, purulent vaginal discharge; uterine tenderness; and leukocytosis. Often, fetal tachycardia precedes maternal fever. Maternal fever, foul amniotic fluid, and uterine tenderness often do not occur until infection is well established. There is often increased uterine activity when chorioamnionitis is present. Fever may not occur at all, but whenever it is present in a patient near term, especially when membranes are ruptured, the presumptive diagnosis is chorioamnionitis until proven otherwise.

Diagnosis

Early diagnosis of chorioamnionitis is difficult because symptoms are vague. Whenever symptoms of infection are present, a general history and physical examination should be done to rule out other sources of infection. Chorioamnionitis cannot be ruled out if membranes are intact because laboratory studies are of limited value. The white blood cell count (WBC) is elevated with chorioamnionitis, but it is normally elevated in pregnancy and labor. A shift to the left (i.e., a relative increase in immature forms of neutrophils reported on the differential of the CBC) may indicate bacterial infection but does not indicate the site of infection. A rise of 50% in the WBC from a baseline established on admission to the hospital also suggests infection. A new test, C-reactive protein, may indicate infection sooner than changes in the WBC. Laboratory studies such as a urinalysis will help to rule out other sources of infection. Cultures are of little value in the diagnosis and management of chorioamnionitis since they take too long to obtain results. However, since they can be used retrospectively to diagnose infection and to ensure appropriate treatment, and they may help with management of the baby later by identifying the site and organism of maternal infection, they should be done. Cultures of the endocervix for β-streptococcus and gonorrhea should be done as well as cultures of urine, throat, blood, or other sites as required by the patient's symptoms.

Amniotic fluid can be examined for evidence of chorioamnionitis. The fluid should be obtained by amniocentesis or from an internal uterine pressure catheter (after discarding the first 10 cc of fluid). Fluid obtained vaginally will be contaminated with normal vaginal flora and will be of no use for diagnosis. Presence of white blood cells in the amniotic fluid means little. The presence of bacteria on Gram's stain of the fluid is of greater diagnostic significance. In general, the diagnosis is assumed to be chorioamnionitis if the patient is febrile and no other cause of infection is found, if the amniotic fluid is purulent or foul smelling, or if bacteria are present in the amniotic fluid.

Maternal and Fetal Outcome

The prognosis for the mother with chorioamnionitis is good. Rarely, septic shock may occur and may lead to acute renal failure. Disseminated intravascular coagulation may be triggered by sepsis. Maternal death is even more rare. More commonly, chronic pelvic inflammatory disease (PID) may ensue if the infection is not totally eradicated. PID subsequently can cause menstrual disturbances, infertility, or ectopic pregnancy (11, p 152).

The impact of chorioamnionitis on the baby is much greater than that on the mother, although perinatal mortality has decreased considerably in recent years. Chorioamnionitis does not necessarily correlate with fetal infection—some babies have no infection after coming from a uterus filled with foul, purulent fluid. Others are infected at birth even though the time since rupture of membranes was very short and there was no clinical evidence of chorioamnionitis. However, infection of the fetus or neonate is likely after chorioamnionitis. Usually, the infection enters the baby's nose and mouth and affects the lungs and gastrointestinal system. If the infection is transplacental, however, it is more likely to spread through fetal blood to the liver, brain, meninges, heart, adrenal glands, and spleen.

Another major effect of chorioamnionitis on the fetus is its impact on prematurity. Since chorioamnionitis may be responsible for PROM and preterm labor, its effects may be greater than commonly realized. For the very premature infant, the risks of RDS may be even greater than the risk of infection. Chorioamnionitis also may be responsible for many perinatal deaths: up to one-third of stillbirths and early neonatal deaths result from an intrauterine infection (11, p 152).

Medical Management

The management of chorioamnionitis is delivery, regardless of gestational age. Usually, spontaneous labor occurs once infection is established, but if it does not, labor can be induced if the fetus is more than 2000 g and vertex presentation. Continuous fetal monitoring with fetal blood gas sampling when indicated will allow for adequate fetal surveillance. Arbitrary time limits for labor are not required as long as progress continues.

Cesarean section increases the risk of spreading maternal infection, so it is reserved for obstetric indications. It is avoided if at all possible if the fetus is not viable. If cesarean section is required, cultures should be taken upon entering the uterus. Attempts should be made to keep the infection from spreading throughout the abdomen. In the past, the extraperitoneal approach was used for cesarean, but now that is not considered necessary because of the availability of antibiotics. Cesarean hysterectomy also is not indicated unless the infection is severe, maternal age is advanced, and future children are not desired. During and after delivery, it is important to observe for signs and symptoms of septic shock (e.g., hypotension, oliguria) and to provide adequate fluid replacement (12, p 217).

Whether to begin antibiotics during labor depends upon severity of the infection. If the infection is mild and delivery is expected soon, antibiotic treatment may be withheld until after delivery. Antibiotics given before delivery may obscure neonatal infection for a time and may cause neonatal cultures to be negative, even though the pathogens are not fully eliminated and have the ability to infect the baby. If maternal infection is well established during labor or delivery is not anticipated imminently, antibiotics are indicated. The selection of antibiotics may be determined by Gram's stain and by the severity of the infection. One suggested protocol is as follows:

For mild infection: ampicillin, 2 g intravenously every 4–6 hours, or penicillin G, 5 million units intravenously every 6 hours.
For moderate infection: add gentamycin, 3–5 mg/ kg body weight/day.
For severe infection: clindamycin, 600 mg intravenously every 6–8 hours, and an aminoglycoside. Cephalosporins may be used as an alternative (12, pp 215–216).

After delivery the newborn should be monitored carefully for signs and symptoms of infection. Cultures and a thorough physical examination are essential. The workup should include CBC with differential; chest x-ray; urine, blood, and cerebrospinal fluid cultures; and gastic aspirate cell count and Gram's stain. Whether to treat the baby immediately with antibiotics is controversial since some babies may not be infected at all, whereas others that are infected may have nonspecific symptoms. If it is decided that treatment is indicated, ampicillin and gentamycin frequently are the drugs of choice because of their usual efficacy and low toxicity.

NURSING MANAGEMENT

Nursing care specific for the patient with *chorioamnionitis:*
- ☐ Be alert to factors predisposing to chorioamnionitis (e.g., PROM, drug abuse, history of multiple sexual partners, history of STDs, immunosuppression, or positive HIV titer.)
- ☐ Assist with diagnostic tests and procedures (e.g., amniocentesis, cultures, fetal monitoring).
- ☐ Prepare for induction/augmentation of labor or cesarean section as needed.
- ☐ Observe for signs/symptoms of septic shock:
  - — Fever and
  - — Hypotension and oliguria that are not improved quickly by a rapid infusion of fluids.
- ☐ Be prepared to assist with cultures of the newborn, placenta, membranes, and umbilical cord.
- ☐ Provide education about the potential sequelae of chorioamnionitis (e.g., chronic PID, menstrual disturbances, ectopic pregnancy, or infertility). Include signs/symptoms and treatment.

Nursing diagnoses most frequently associated with *chorioamnionitis* **(see Section V):**
- ☐ Grieving related to potential/actual loss of infant or birth of an imperfect child.
- ☐ Anticipatory grieving related to actual/perceived threat to self.
- ☐ Disturbance in body image, self-esteem.
- ☐ Knowledge deficit regarding etiology, disease process, treatment, and outcome.
- ☐ Fluid volume deficit.
- ☐ Altered maternal tissue perfusion.
- ☐ Pain.
- ☐ Anxiety/fear.
- ☐ Impaired tissue integrity.
- ☐ Potential for infection.

REFERENCES

1. Pritchard JA, MacDonald PC, Gant NF: *Williams Obstetrics*, ed 17. Norwalk, CT, Appleton-Century-Crofts, 1985, p 462.
2. Queenan JT, Kubarych SF: Detecting and managing polyhydramnios. *Contemp OB/GYN* 16:113–125, 1980.
3. Philipson EH, Sokol RJ, Williams T: Oligohydramnios: clinical associations and predictive value for intrauterine growth retardation. *Am J Obstet Gynecol* 146:271–278, 1983.
4. Freeman RK, Huddleston JF, Petrie RH, Schifrin B: Ensuring optimum outcome for postdate pregnancy. *Contemp OB/GYN* 22:186–211, 1984.
5. Manning FA, Hill LM, Platt LD: Qualitative amniotic fluid determination by ultrasound: antepartum detection of intrauterine growth retardation. *Am J Obstet Gynecol* 139:254–258, 1981.
6. Harrison MR: Progess in managing hydronephrosis. *Contemp OB/GYN.* 22:47–78, 1983.
7. Berkowitz RL: Premature rupture of the membranes. In Queenan JT, Hobbins JC (eds): *Protocols for High Risk Pregnancies.* Oradell, NJ, Medical Economics Books, 1982, p 210.
8. Garite TJ: What's the best care in preterm PROM? *Contemp OB/GYN* 19:178–187, 1982.
9. Queenan JT, Garite TJ, Berkowitz RL, Mead PB: Managing premature rupture of membranes. *Contemp OB/GYN* 21:228–245, 1983.
10. Cavanagh D, Woods RE: Life-threatening infections. In Cavanagh D, Woods RE, O'Connor TCF (eds): *Obstetric Emergencies,* ed 2. Hagerstown, MD, Harper and Row, 1978, p 78.
11. Koh KS, Chang FH, Ledger WJ: When chorioamnionitis threatens mother and offspring. *Contemp OB/GYN* 13:147–161, 1979.
12. Schwarz R: Amnionitis. In Queenan JT, Hobbins JC (eds): *Protocols for High-Risk Pregnancies.* Oradell, NJ, Medical Economics Books, 1982, p 213.

Chapter 31
Abnormalities of the Placenta and Membranes
Nancy W. Kulb, C.N.M., M.S.

INTRODUCTION

The placenta is a unique organ developed from both maternal and fetal components. The fetus is entirely dependent upon a properly functioning placenta until, at birth, the newborn is able to perform independently the functions performed previously by the mother via the placenta. Maternal and fetal blood normally are kept completely separated by a thin membrane, the "placental barrier." However, it is across this barrier that oxygen, water, and nutrients go to the fetus from the mother's blood and that waste products return from the fetus. Thus, the placenta provides for the respiration, nutrition, and excretion of the fetus. Its proper functioning depends upon an adequate supply of both maternal and fetal blood to effect this exchange. The placenta's "barrier" protects the fetus from many harmful substances and infectious agents. It also functions as an endocrine organ, manufacturing many hormones required for the maintenance of a normal pregnancy.

The placenta develops where the blastocyst implants in the decidua lining the uterine cavity. Normally, the site of implantation is on the fundus or corpus of the uterus, well away from the cervix.

The placenta is discoid in shape, normally about 15–20 cm in diameter and about 1.5–3.0 cm thick. It consists of 12–20 cotyledons recognizable on the maternal surface. Fetal blood is transported to the placenta via the umbilical arteries. Large branches of the umbilical arteries are visible on the fetal surface of the placenta. These arteries form many branches, which get smaller and smaller, eventually forming the villi. The body of the placenta consists of these villi suspended in lacunae,

or pools, filled with maternal blood. It is across the trophoblastic layers of the villi that maternal-fetal exchange occurs. Fetal blood returns to the fetus via the umbilical vein. Maternal blood reaches the lacunae of the placenta via uterine spiral arterioles and exits via veins punctuating the maternal surface of the placenta (Fig. 31.1).

It is clear that the placenta is crucial to the health and well-being of the fetus, and it is clear that abnormalities of the placenta have a profound effect upon the fetus. Details of normal placental development, structure, function, and physiology are not discussed here but may be reviewed in a basic nursing or physiology text.

ABRUPTIO PLACENTAE

Definition

Abruptio placentae is the "separation of the normally situated placenta from its uterine site of implantation after 20 weeks' gestation, but before delivery of the fetus" (1).

There are several systems for classifying the types and severity of placental abruption:

Grade 0: The patient is asymptomatic, but a small retroplacental clot is noted after delivery. Some would include a small rupture of the marginal sinus as grade 0.

Grade 1: The patient has vaginal bleeding, perhaps with uterine tenderness and mild tetany, but neither mother nor baby is in distress.

Grade 2: The patient experiences uterine tenderness and tetany, with or without external evi-

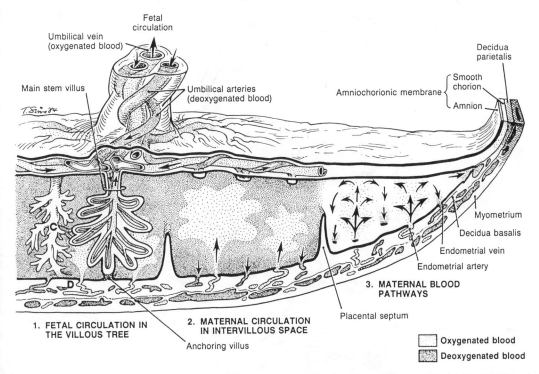

Figure 31.1. Schematic diagram of the placenta. (From Moore: *The Developing Human.* Philadelphia, WB Saunders, 1982, p 116.

dence of bleeding. The mother is not in shock, but there is fetal distress.

Grade 3: Uterine tetany is severe, the mother is in shock, although the bleeding may or may not be revealed, and the fetus is dead. Often, the mother is experiencing coagulopathy (1, p 110).

Following is another system of classifying abruption, based on the signs and symptoms:

1. Revealed: Vaginal bleeding is evident, with the patient's symptoms consistent with the amount of blood lost. Uterine tenderness and tetany, if present, are minor (Fig. 31.2).
2. Concealed: No bleeding is evident. Instead, uterine tenderness and hypertonicity are of primary importance. Often fetal heart tones (FHTs) are not present. (Fig. 31.2).
3. Mixed: Both bleeding and uterine tenderness and tetany are present (2).

The incidence of abruptio placentae varies from report to report, ranging from 1 in 55 to 1 in 250 cases. The incidence is greater with increasing parity (not age) or a history of previous abruption.

Etiology

The etiology of abruptio placentae is unknown. It has been proposed that abruption begins with degenerative changes in the small maternal arterioles that supply the intervillous spaces, resulting in thrombosis, degeneration of the decidua, and, finally, rupture of a vessel. Bleeding from the vessel forms a retroplacental clot. Further bleeding causes increased pressure behind the placenta and results in further separation (1, p 110).

In the past it was thought that compression of the inferior vena cava or folic acid deficiency might play a part in the etiology of abruption, but currently there is little support for the role of either. It is known, however, that the following conditions are associated with abruptio placentae: hypertension, trauma, short umbilical cord, sudden uterine decompression, polyhydramnios, intravenous cocaine use, and uterine leiomyomas or anomalies. Obstetric history plays a role: abruption is more common in women with a history of spontaneous abortion, premature labor, antepartum hemorrhage, stillbirth, or neonatal death. Its incidence is 6 times greater in women of high parity (para 7 or more) and 30 times more common in women with a prior history of abruption (3).

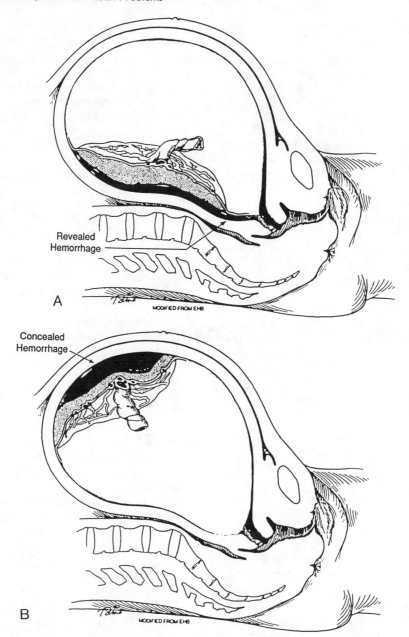

Figure 31.2. Abruptio placentae. **A**, Revealed hemorrhage. **B**, Concealed hemorrhage. (Adapted from Pritchard JA, MacDonald PC, Gant NF (eds): *Williams Obstetrics*, ed 17. Norwalk, CT, Appleton-Century-Crofts, now Appleton & Lange, 1985, p 396.)

Signs and Symptoms

The signs and symptoms of abruptio placentae depend to a great extent on the amount of separation of the placenta and the type of abruption. With mild abruption the mother may complain of "labor pains," and there may be only slight uterine irritability, with no bleeding or a small amount of dark,

old blood. With severe abruption the patient may complain of sudden, knife-like, tearing pain. The uterus may be tender only over the point of placental separation, or tenderness may be generalized over the whole uterus. The uterus may be rigid or "board-like," with little or no relaxation between contractions. External bleeding may be minimal or profuse—15–20% of cases exhibit no external bleeding. The mother's symptoms will be based on the amount of blood lost to her systemic circulation and may be out of proportion to the amount of bleeding that is evident. Even when bleeding is seen, there also can be a significant amount of bleeding concealed. The mother may be in shock if the bleeding is severe. With severe abruption FHTs may indicate distress (tachycardia, loss of beat-to-beat variability, or late decelerations) or may be absent.

Diagnosis

The diagnosis of abruptio placentae is based on the patient's history, physical examination, and special laboratory studies. Presence of any of the factors known to be associated with abruption should alert the obstetrical team to the possibility of abruption. The patient's complaints of vaginal bleeding and/or constant or severe abdominal pain always should be investigated thoroughly until serious pathology is ruled out. Analgesia/anesthesia should be withheld until the diagnosis is confirmed. Findings upon physical examination may include some or all of the following: vaginal bleeding, uterine tenderness (local or generalized), increased uterine tone, maternal shock, fetal distress, or lack of FHTs. Specific diagnosis is made by ultrasound examination excluding placenta previa and demonstrating a retroplacental clot. With marginal separation of the placenta or revealed hemorrhage, a retroplacental clot may not be evident, and the diagnosis is presumptive, based on history, physical examination, and clinical course. If a sonogram is unavailable, presumptive diagnosis also may be based on the absence of placenta previa on double set-up examination (see p. 354). The diagnosis usually can be confirmed by placental inspection after delivery.

Maternal and Fetal Outcome

With current obstetrical management, the maternal mortality is less than 1% overall in cases of abruptio placentae. Maternal mortality is as high as 10% if the abruption is undetected until it is severe enough to cause fetal death (2, p 193).

Disseminated intravascular coagulation occurs in up to 30% of mothers who experience an abruption. Petechiae, excessive vaginal bleeding, or bleeding from puncture wounds, gums, the gastrointestinal tract, or urinary tract may result. See Chapter 8 for further information on consumptive coagulopathies.

Other potential maternal sequelae include maternal shock, renal failure secondary to hypovolemia, amniotic fluid embolism, uterine rup-

ture, Couvelaire uterus (severe uterine apoplexy), postpartum endometritis, and pituitary necrosis (Sheehan's syndrome). The incidence of postpartum hemorrhage is doubled after abruptio placentae, but if coagulopathy occurs, the incidence may be as much as eight times greater than in the general population. Fortunately, postpartum hemorrhage usually responds to oxytocin and correction of the coagulopathy so that hysterectomy rarely is needed. (2, p 204).

Perinatal mortality is much greater than maternal mortality. It has been reported to range from 20–80% (1, p 111). Perinatal mortality depends to a great extent on how much of the circulation has been disrupted by separation; if over half of the placenta has separated before birth, fetal death usually will result. Fetal bleeding may occur if the chorionic villi are torn. Since half of cases of abruption occur before 36 weeks' gestation (2, p 193), the baby may be delivered prematurely with all the sequelae of prematurity. If a term infant survives the insult of the abruption, however, there is little increase in morbidity (2, p 193).

Medical Management

When a patient presents with vaginal bleeding, the first step is diagnosis. It is especially important to rule out placenta previa. *No vaginal or rectal examination is done until placenta previa is ruled out* (Table 31.1).

Once the diagnosis of abruption is made, the patient is admitted to the hospital and placed on bed rest. Vital signs are checked frequently, and an intravenous line is started with a 16- or 18-gauge catheter. Blood is drawn for type and cross-match of at least two to four units of fresh whole blood. Studies to evaluate blood loss and clotting status as well as to provide a baseline for comparison later include hematocrit (HCT), complete blood count, platelet count, fibrinogen, fibrinogen-fibrin degradation products, thrombin, prothrombin, partial thromboplastin time, Lee White clotting time, serum fibrinolysin, anticoagulant factor, and electrolytes. FHTs are electronically monitored, preferably internally. The fundal height is marked on the abdomen as a baseline for change. (Rising fundal height indicates concealed hemorrhage.) A central venous pressure (CVP) line is started, especially if there are signs or symptoms of shock since monitoring the CVP gives a better indication of blood volume than pulse or blood pressure.

With abruptio placentae there is no room for expectant management. The mode of delivery depends upon maternal and fetal status. Cesarean section is chosen if any of the following occur: fetal

Table 31.1.

CAMPARISON OF ABRUPTIO PLACENTAE AND PLACENTA PREVIA

ABRUPTIO PLACENTAE	PLACENTA PREVIA
Bleeding usually is accompanied by pain.	Bleeding usually is painless.
Blood usually is dark.	Blood usually is bright red.
The first episode of bleeding usually is profuse and usually continues until delivery.	The first episode of bleeding usually is scant at onset. The patient may have several "warning" hemorrhages.
The patient usually is in labor when bleeding begins.	The patient usually is not in labor when bleeding begins.
Signs of shock may be out of proportion to visible bleeding.	Signs of shock and visible blood loss are compatible.
Uterus is firm, tender, tetanically contracted.	Uterus is soft and nontender.
The fetus is hard to palpate. Fetal heart tones may be irregular or absent.	The fetus is easily palpable. Fetal heart tones usually are present.
The patient may have toxemia or hypertension (although the blood pressure may be low from blood loss).	The patient usually does not show evidence of toxemia.
The patient may have proteinuria or anuria.	The urine usually is within normal limits.
A clotting defect may be present.	Clotting usually is normal.
The placenta cannot be felt on double set-up examination.	The placenta can be felt on double set-up examination.
Sonogram shows a normally implanted placenta, perhaps with a retroplacental clot.	Sonogram shows the placenta implanted in the lower uterine segment.

distress, increasing uterine resting tone, severe hemorrhage, coagulopathy, or poor labor progress (2, p 202). Vaginal delivery is anticipated if the fetus is alive and in no distress or is dead and the mother's condition allows it.

Fortunately, labor often proceeds rapidly in cases of abruptio placentae. If vaginal delivery is chosen as the route of choice, all preparations should be made for emergency cesarean section in case circumstances change. Efforts are directed toward correcting hypovolemia and coagulopathy. Strict intake and output (I and O) are monitored. Coagulation studies are performed every 2–3 hours or as needed. Rapid infusion of D$_5$RL (Ringer's lactate solution) and whole blood may be required. An attempt is made to keep the HCT at 30% or more and urinary output at 30 cc/hour or more. Coagulopathy may be corrected by the administration of whole blood, fresh frozen plasma, and cryoprecipitate. (Fibrinogen may be substituted if cryoprecipitate is unavailable.)

The fetus should be monitored continuously by internal electronic fetal monitoring and fetal blood gas sampling when indicated. Amniotomy should be performed as soon as possible because it may help decrease bleeding into the uterus, may decrease the amount of thromboplastin released into the circulation, may speed labor, and will allow for the placement of internal fetal electrode and intrauterine pressure catheter. Oxytocin may be used to speed labor if necessary. Oxygen may be administered to the mother by mask.

At the time of delivery, careful hemostasis must be achieved. Episiotomy is avoided if possible. Postpartum hemorrhage is managed as usual (see Chapter 42). A pediatrician should be present for neonatal resuscitation.

During the postpartum period, coagulation problems usually resolve quickly. Anemia and electrolyte imbalances are corrected. I and O are monitored to guide and evaluate fluid volume replacement. The perineum and vagina or cesarean section incision should be monitored for the presence of hematoma.

NURSING MANAGEMENT

Nursing care specific for patients with abruptio placentae:

☐ Carefully assess women at risk for the signs and symptoms of abruptio placentae including increased risk of abruptio with crack use. (It is common street "knowledge" that crack will help start labor or make labor easier.)

☐ Provide information to the patient and her family about abruptio placentae, including etiology, treatment, expected course for both mother and baby. Provide realistic reassurance as appropriate.

☐ Provide information about every procedure before it is done, including reasons for it, and expected benefits.

NURSING MANAGEMENT

- [ ] Admit the patient and place her on bedrest, preferably in a side-lying position to maximize uteroplacental circulation.
- [ ] Check vital signs frequently, at least every 15 minutes, until the patient is stable. Observe for signs and symptoms of shock, including cool, clammy skin, thirst, and anxiety.
- [ ] Observe for vaginal bleeding (may or may not be present) and mark height of uterine fundus in order to evaluate increase in height as evidence of continuing hemorrhage.
- [ ] AVOID VAGINAL/RECTAL EXAMINATIONS UNTIL PLACENTA PREVIA HAS BEEN RULED OUT.
- [ ] Assess uterus for contractions, resting tone between contractions, tenderness, change in size, rigidity, and pain.
- [ ] Encourage patient to verbalize changes in sensations and pain level.
- [ ] If vaginal delivery is planned, assist with amniotomy and oxytocin augmentation of labor as necessary.
- [ ] Prepare for emergency cesarean section even if vaginal delivery is anticipated: alert operating room personnel including anesthesiologist and pediatrician, perform abdominal shave and prep, insert Foley catheter, ensure that at least two units of blood are ready for transfusion, and be sure operative consent has been signed.

- [ ] Observe the patient frequently for signs and symptoms of bleeding disorders, including petechiae, bleeding gums, or bleeding from other locations in the body.
- [ ] At delivery, assist with newborn resuscitation. After delivery, assess uterine tone and the amount of lochia carefully. Check sites of incision and/or laceration carefully for bleeding or hematoma formation.
- [ ] Allow the mother and her family ample opportunity to express their feelings about neonatal outcome and the loss of the birth experience they had hoped for.

Nursing diagnoses most frequently associated with *abruptio placentae* (see Section V):
- [ ] Anxiety/fear.
- [ ] Grieving related to potential/actual loss of infant or birth of an imperfect child.
- [ ] Anticipatory grieving related to actual/perceived threat to self.
- [ ] Pain.
- [ ] Knowledge deficit regarding etiology, disease process, treatment, and outcome.
- [ ] Altered fetal cardiac and cerebral tissue perfusion.
- [ ] Altered maternal tissue perfusion.
- [ ] Fluid volume deficit.

PLACENTA PREVIA

Definition

Placenta previa is an abnormally implanted placenta, placed totally or partially in the lower seg-

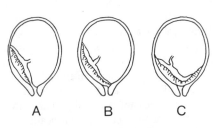

Figure 31.3. The three classifications of placenta previa. *A,* Low lying. *B,* Partial. *C,* Total. (From Buckley KA, Kulb NW (eds): In *Handbook of Maternal Newborn Nursing.* New York, John Wiley & Sons, 1983, p 420. Copyright © 1983. Reprinted by permission of Delmar, Inc.)

ment of the uterus rather than in the corpus. When the cervix begins to efface and dilate, the placenta separates, allowing bleeding from the open blood vessels.

Again, there are systems for classifying the severity or degree of placenta previa (Fig. 31.3):

1. Complete (also called *total* or *central*): The internal os is covered completely by the placenta.
2. Incomplete: The internal os is not covered completely by the placenta. Incomplete previa is further divided into:
   a. Partial: A portion of the cervical os is covered by the placenta.
   b. Marginal: The edge of the placenta extends to the edge of the cervical os (1, p 107).

Note that this system of classification depends upon the degree of dilatation of the cervix. For example, a marginal previa at the onset of labor would become a partial previa as the cervix dilates. Similarly, a complete previa at the onset of labor could become a partial previa as the cervix dilates.

An alternative system of classification is based on a projection of what the circumstances will be at full dilatation:

Type I: The placenta is low lying, with the inferior margin extending into the lower uterine segment but not reaching the cervical os.

Type II: The placental border reaches the edge of the internal os at full dilatation.

Type III: The placenta partially covers the os when the cervix is dilated fully.

Type IV: The placenta covers the os completely when the cervix is dilated fully (2, p 181).

The incidence of placenta previa depends to a great extent on gestational age. In the second trimester as many as 45% of placentas appear to be implanted in the lower uterine segment, but in the third trimester, with development and elongation of the lower uterine segment, the site of implantation appears to move up and away from the cervical os. By term, the incidence of placenta previa is 0.5–1.0%. Even when the previa appears to be complete in the second trimester, only 1 in 12 will be previa at term (4).

Placenta previa occurs more often in multiparae (80% of cases are in multiparae), although there is disagreement about whether age or parity is the more important factor (1, p 107; 2, p 183; 4, p 219). It tends to recur; the incidence in women with a history of previa is 12 times that of the general population. Also, it is more common after a history of abortion, cesarean section, or molar pregnancy.

Etiology

The cause of placenta previa is unknown. It is thought that when the embryo is ready to implant, if the decidua in the fundus is deficient, it will "choose" another site, finally implanting in the lower uterine segment. This theory is supported by the fact that the maternal portion of the placenta tends to be larger than normal in placenta previa, and the cord often is of a marginal or velamentous insertion, suggesting that the placenta was growing toward more favorable decidua.

Interestingly, the factors that predispose to placenta previa might contribute to damage and scarring in the endometrium: endometritis after a previous pregnancy, uterine scars, tumors altering the internal contours of the uterus, close pregnancy spacing, and multiparity. A large placenta,

such as in multiple gestation or erythroblastosis fetalis, also may predispose to placenta previa.

Signs and Symptoms

The classic sign of placenta previa is painless vaginal bleeding, usually not occurring before the third trimester. Sometimes previa will be suspected because of fetal oblique or transverse lie, occurring because the low-lying placenta prevents fixation of a fetal pole in the inlet of the pelvis. Occasionally, previa is diagnosed during an ultrasound examination being done for other reasons.

In 80–90% of cases, however, bleeding occurs. Its onset is without warning and often without precipitating events. Sometimes it occurs during sleep. The bleeding is bright red. The first episode often is scant and, fortunately, rarely fatal unless accompanied by an "ill-advised vaginal or rectal exam" (2, p 183). The uterus is nontender with normal resting tone. Recurrence of bleeding is unpredictable.

Patients with more severe forms of previa tend to have an earlier onset of bleeding. Shock may occur in up to 25% of patients, more commonly in those with the more severe types of previa.

In the past there were several methods for determining the location of the placenta, but ultrasound now is the method of choice. In the third trimester of pregnancy, ultrasound is 97% accurate in diagnosing placenta previa (2, p 189). There are no known risks. Pre- and postvoiding sonograms may be required to determine the relationship of the placenta to the cervix. If the placental edge is at least 6 cm from the cervical os, the diagnosis of placenta previa can be ruled out (4, p 219). If previa is diagnosed early in the third trimester, repeat sonograms should be done to determine whether the condition still exists as the lower uterine segment develops.

A double set-up examination, although less popular since the advent of sonography, still may be required in some cases to make a final diagnosis. A double set-up always is done in an operating room with full preparations made either for vaginal or cesarean delivery. Preparations include abdominal shave and preparation; Foley catheter; patent intravenous line; at least two units of blood type- and cross-matched and ready; signed operative consent; instruments set up; surgical assistants scrubbed; and presence of anesthesiologist and pediatrician. The double set-up begins with a speculum examination to rule out vaginal causes of bleeding, such as cervicitis or ruptured vaginal varices. An examining finger then is passed through the cervix to palpate for the placenta. If the placenta is encountered and catastrophic bleeding ensues, the baby is delivered immediately by cesarean section. Otherwise, there is no emergency, and observation and/or labor may be allowed until vaginal delivery occurs or the circumstances change, necessitating cesarean section.

Maternal and Fetal Outcome

Maternal prognosis with placenta previa is good. The mortality is less than 1%, and morbidity is about 20%. Most women with placenta previa will have at least one significant hemorrhage, and up to 25% will go into shock (2, p 183). Because previa may result from poor endometrial vascularization, the placenta is likely to be larger than average and may have a succenturiate lobe. Postpartum hemorrhage may result and may be exacerbated by the less efficient muscular contraction of the lower uterine segment. Cervical and uterine lacerations also are more common after vaginal delivery of patients with placenta previa. Poor endometrium may contribute to placenta accreta.

Fetal mortality in cases of placenta previa is approximately 20%, primarily from prematurity, hypoxia in utero, and developmental anomalies (2, p 192). There is no relationship between perinatal outcome and the number of bleeding episodes, but there may be a relationship to the amount of blood lost. Certainly, the outcome depends to a great extent on the severity of the placenta previa. After delivery the baby has a higher risk of death than other infants of the same birth weight and gestational age because of developmental anomalies and lingering effects of hypoxia. After the first month of life, there is no further impact on the baby's ability to survive (2, p 193).

Medical Management

The immediate management of placenta previa depends upon the severity of hemorrhage and fetal maturity. If the bleeding is not severe and the baby is less than 36 weeks' gestation, the patient is admitted to the hospital and placed on strict bed rest. An intravenous line is started with a 16- or 18-gauge catheter, and at least two units of type- and cross-matched blood are made available. Blood is drawn for HCT, complete blood count, and clotting studies. If the HCT drops below 30% or the hemoglobin below 10 gm/dl, a blood transfusion is given. Pelvic examinations are contraindicated absolutely (except in a double set-up when committed to delivery). If the uterus is contracting, tocolysis may be attempted. The management is conservative unless there is evidence of fetal demise or fetal distress, advanced labor, or uncontrollable hemorrhage.

The woman is placed on strict bed rest for at least 72 hours. If bleeding stops soon after admission, she may be allowed to ambulate after 72 hours. Continuous hospitalization until delivery is the rule, but if the woman is discharged to her home near the hospital, she must have immediate transportation available to return to the hospital if bleeding recurs, and she should have someone with her at all times. Blood is kept matched and ready in the hospital. The patient is cautioned strictly against douching or coitus and is advised to stop smoking and to maintain good nutrition.

Amniocentesis may be done weekly until fetal maturity is documented. At that point, with central previa, cesarean section is indicated since the risks to mother and baby are less than the risks of another bleeding episode. With marginal previa and no bleeding, the pregnancy may be followed until term and delivered vaginally if the placenta migrates upward from the os. Sometimes, pressure from the descending fetal head will tamponade bleeding and allow vaginal delivery with a marginal previa, but active bleeding still requires cesarean section. If vaginal delivery is attempted, the mother should be given oxygen by mask throughout the labor. Oxytocin may be used if necessary.

It is important to perform serial sonograms to determine whether the placenta has "moved away" from the cervical os and also to document that the baby is growing well, since intrauterine growth retardation may occur whenever there is interference with placental circulation.

When a patient is admitted at term with central placenta previa, there is no place for conservative management. Cesarean section is done. Only if the placenta is marginal should vaginal delivery be considered.

Similarly, if the patient presents with severe hemorrhage, regardless of gestational age, cesarean section is required. Again, an intravenous line is begun with a 16- or 18-gauge angiocatheter; baseline HCT, complete blood count, and clotting studies are drawn; and at least two units of blood are type- and cross-matched. A CVP line is started to monitor fluid volume. Preparations are made for immediate cesarean section. A pediatrician should be present at delivery to manage neonatal resuscitation.

After delivery, the danger of clotting disorders diminishes rapidly. Fluid volume replacement is guided by the CVP, and blood replacement by the hemoglobin and HCT.

NURSING MANAGEMENT

Nursing care specific for patients with placenta previa:

☐ *Never* perform a vaginal or rectal examination on a bleeding maternity patient until the cause of bleeding is diagnosed.

☐ Provide information to the patient and her family about placenta previa, including etiology, treatment, and expected outcome for both mother and baby; provide realistic reassurance as appropriate.

☐ Provide information about every procedure before it is done, including reasons for it and expected benefits.

☐ Admit the patient to the hospital, and place her on bedrest; advise her that she will receive nothing by mouth until stable.

☐ Check vital signs frequently, at least every 15 minutes, until the patient is stable; observe for signs and symptoms of shock, including cool clammy skin, thirst, and anxiety.

☐ Observe for and assess blood loss frequently, at least every 15 minutes until stable; weigh pads for a more accurate assessment of blood loss.

☐ Place or assist in placing the patient on the external fetal monitor; be continually alert for signs of fetal distress.

☐ If conservative management is planned, explain the need for strict bedrest for 72 hours, and help the patient comply; be prompt in bringing the bedpan, set up her tray when oral intake is allowed, provide or encourage her family to provide diversional activities.

☐ When ambulation is allowed, be sure the patient understands the limits on her activities.

☐ Continue to monitor the patient's blood loss and vital signs, and the baby's heart tones; be prepared at any time for emergency intervention.

☐ If the mother is to be discharged undelivered, provide teaching and counseling about: the need for a constant companion and ready access to transportation to the hospital; avoidance of douching or coitus; good nutrition; cessation of smoking; and limits on physical activity and to return to hospital immediately if any bleeding occurs.

☐ Prepare for cesarean section if indicated: alert operating room personnel including anesthesiologist and pediatrician.

☐ Assist with monitoring blood volume and clotting status: observe for signs and symptoms of bleeding disorders, monitor central venous pressure as necessary, assist with serial hematocrits and clotting studies.

☐ At delivery, assist with newborn resuscitation; continue to monitor blood volume and clotting status after delivery.

☐ Allow the mother and her family ample opportunity to express their feelings about neonatal outcome and the loss of the birth experience they had hoped for.

Nursing diagnoses most frequently associated with *placenta previa* (see Section V):

☐ Anxiety/fear.

☐ Grieving related to potential/actual loss of infant or birth of an imperfect child.

☐ Anticipatory grieving related to actual/preceived threat to self.

☐ Knowledge deficit regarding etiology, disease process, and outcome.

☐ Altered fetal cardiac and cerebral tissue perfusion.

☐ Altered maternal tissue perfusion.

☐ Fluid volume deficit.

VASA PREVIA

Definition

Vasa previa is a rare circumstance that may occur with a velamentous insertion of the umbilical cord. A velamentous insertion, which occurs in approximately 1% of singleton term pregnancies, is the condition in which the vessels of the cord separate at a distance away from the margin of the placenta, reaching the placenta surrounded only by a fold of amnion. Vasa previa occurs when some or all of these umbilical vessels cross the internal os, presenting ahead of the fetus (5) (Fig. 31.4).

Etiology

The cause of vasa previa is unknown. It is postulated that it may occur when, at the time of implantation, the inner cell mass of the zygote implants away from the endometrium, causing the cord and the placenta to lie at opposite poles. This position may allow the fetal vessels to course through the membranes on the way to the placenta (5).

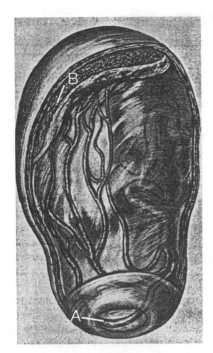

Figure 31.4. Velamentous insertion of cord with vasa previa. **A**, vasa previa; **B**, placenta.

Signs and Symptoms

Occasionally, upon careful vaginal examination, the vessels will be felt in the membranes overlying the presenting part. More commonly, however, the first sign of vasa previa is vaginal bleeding with concomitant fetal distress, occurring after the membranes have ruptured. Vasa previa should be considered in any case of vaginal bleeding with fetal distress.

Diagnosis

When fetal vessels are palpated in membranes before they are ruptured, compressing them against the presenting part will cause changes in fetal heart rate patterns. Amnioscopy will confirm the diagnosis. When vasa previa is suspected because of fetal distress and vaginal bleeding, the blood should be tested to determine whether it is of fetal origin. If so, the diagnosis is fairly certain and can be confirmed after delivery by tracing the course of the umbilical vessels to the placenta.

Maternal and Fetal Outcome

Vasa previa presents no danger to the mother because her circulation is not involved. Danger to the baby is considerable since exsanguination may occur quickly after rupture of the vessels. Blood volume in the fetus is approximately 85 ml/kg, so very little can be lost before hypovolemia, shock, and death occur.

Medical Management

If the diagnosis is made before delivery and the baby is alive, cesarean section is required whether the vessels are ruptured yet or not. The only exception is when vaginal delivery is imminent and will occur as quickly as a cesarean can be done (2, p 214). If the baby is dead, vaginal delivery should be allowed since the mother is not in any danger and cesarean section would be of no benefit.

NURSING MANAGEMENT

Nursing care specific for the patient with vasa previa:

☐ For all patients, be alert to the possibility of vasa previa when performing vaginal examinations, especially if a thickened or tubular area, with or without pulsations, is palpated in the membranes.

☐ Provide information to the patient and her family about vasa previa, if diagnosed, including etiology, treatment, and expected course for both mother and baby. Provide realistic reassurance as appropriate; if there is no time prior to surgery for this step, be sure to return to the mother and family after delivery to ensure their understanding; provide information about every procedure before it is done, including reasons for it and expected benefits.

☐ If the baby is alive, prepare for emergency cesarean section: alert operating room personnel including anesthesiologist and pediatrician, perform abdominal shave and prep, insert Foley catheter, ensure that two units of blood are being type- and cross-matched for the mother and ensure that a unit of type O-packed cells is available for transfusion to the baby.

☐ At delivery, assist with newborn resuscitation.

☐ If the baby is not alive, support the mother and family both physically and emotionally throughout the labor and delivery. Prepare them in advance for the appearance of the baby. Allow them to see, touch, and hold the baby after delivery if they desire.

NURSING MANAGEMENT

☐ Allow the mother and her family ample opportunity to express their feelings about neonatal outcome and the loss of the birth experience they had hoped for. If the baby did not survive, support them in their grieving, providing anticipatory guidance, follow-up visits or telephone calls, and appropriate referrals.

Nursing diagnoses most frequently associated with *vasa previa* (see Section V):
☐ Grieving related to potential/actual loss of infant or birth of an imperfect child.
☐ Knowledge deficit regarding etiology, disease process, treatment, and expected outcome.
☐ Altered fetal cardiac and cerebral perfusion.

PLACENTA ACCRETA

Definition

Placenta accreta is a rare condition in which all or part of the placenta is unusually adherent to the myometrium. The normal fibrinoid plane of cleavage in the spongy layer of the decidua (Nitabuch's layer) is absent or defective, allowing the placental villi to grow down through the endometrium to the myometrium. *Placenta increta* occurs when the villi invade the myometrium. *Placenta percreta* occurs when the villi grow through the uterine muscle to the serosa layer (Fig. 31.5).

Placenta accreta is said to be complete or total when all the placenta is involved, incomplete or partial when some cotyledons are involved, and focal when only one cotyledon is involved.

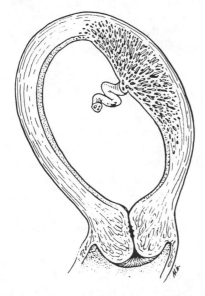

Placenta increta

Figure 31.5. Placenta increta. Reprinted with permission from Caplan RM (ed). *Principles of Obstetrics.* Baltimore, Williams & Wilkins, 1982, p 225.

The incidence of placenta accreta varies considerably in the literature, ranging from 1 in 540 to 1 in 70,000 deliveries. The average incidence is one in 7000 deliveries (5, p 884).

Etiology

The etiology is thought to be a paucity or absence of decidua, causing a defective or totally absent layer of cleavage normally found in the spongy layer of the decidua (6). Predisposing factors are those that would be likely to contribute to faulty decidual formation: implantation over a previous cesarean section scar or other surgical scar in the uterine cavity; previous curretage; prior history of endometritis or other endometrial trauma; or high parity. Placenta previa, which also may result from faulty endometrium, precedes one-third of the cases of placenta accreta (5, p 884).

Signs and Symptoms

Ordinarily, there are no signs or symptoms of placenta accreta until after delivery. The signs and symptoms depend upon site, depth of penetration and number of cotyledons involved.

If the accreta is partial, some cotyledons may separate from the uterine wall, leaving open bleeding vessels. The uterus is unable to contract because of the adherent placenta still within the uterine cavity, and the result may be profuse hemorrhage.

If the accreta is total, there is no bleeding until, when the placenta has not separated, attempts are made to remove it. Tears in the placenta or partial removal again will cause profuse hemorrhage.

Diagnosis

Normally, it is thought that the placenta is not separating because of uterine atony. The diagnosis of accreta is made when attempts at manual removal of the placenta reveal the pathological adherence.

Maternal and Fetal Outcome

The baby is not affected by placenta accreta, although it may be affected by associated conditions, such as placenta previa or rupture of a uterine scar.

The mother is affected by the hemorrhage, which may be profuse. Shock and even death may occur, although with adequate treatment, including blood and fluid replacement, mortality is rare. Occasionally, traction on the umbilical cord in the attempt to remove the placenta may lead to uterine inversion (5, p 586). Uterine perforation during attempts to remove the placenta and subsequent infection also may occur.

Medical Management

Management begins with immediate blood replacement. Manual removal of the placenta should be done only if it can be completed gently. Otherwise, hysterectomy is required. In one study attempts at "conservative" treatment (i.e., manually removing as much of the placenta as possible, followed by packing the uterus) resulted in maternal mortality four times as often as when the treatment was hysterectomy (5, p 586).

NURSING MANAGEMENT

Nursing care specific for the patient with placenta accreta:

☐ Provide information to the patient and her family about placenta accreta as time permits, including etiology, treatment, expected course for the mother; provide realistic reassurance, as appropriate.

☐ Ensure that a patent intravenous line is in place with a 16- or 18-gauge catheter, or start one to ensure blood may be replaced, as needed.

☐ Send blood specimen for type and cross-match for at least 2 units of blood.

☐ Assist with manual removal of the placenta, if it is indicated: alert anesthesiologist, provide sterile long glove for obstetrician, prepare oxytoxics for administration when called for, administer prophylactic antibiotics as ordered.

☐ Prepare for emergency hysterectomy if necessary: alert operating room personnel.

☐ After hysterectomy, support patient in grief over loss of future childbearing.

Nursing diagnoses most frequently associated with placenta accreta (see Section V):

☐ Anticipatory grieving related to actual/perceived threat to self.

☐ Knowledge deficit regarding etiology, disease process, treatment, and expected outcome.

☐ Altered maternal tissue perfusion.

☐ Fluid volume deficit.

NEOPLASTIC TROPHOBLASTIC DISEASE

Definition

The neoplastic trophoblastic diseases are a set of complications of pregnancy characterized by abnormal proliferation of the trophoblast.

Hydatidiform mole, the most common one, is a benign neoplasm that has the potential to develop into a malignancy. It is characterized by degeneration and cystic proliferation of the chorionic villi, particularly of avascular villous stroma. With a complete mole there is no fetus or amnion. With a partial mole the process is focal, and there may be a fetus or an amniotic sac present (35, p 559). Ninety-four percent of the time there is no fetus (7). The incidence varies considerably, occurring only in 1 in 2000 pregnancies in the West, 1 in 125 in Taiwan, and as often as 1 in 75 in some Eastern countries (5, p 561; 7).

Invasive mole, also called chorioadenoma destruens, essentially is the same as hydatidiform mole except that the proliferating neoplastic villi invade and penetrate the myometrium and/or metastasize to other organs. Generally, histologically, there is a well-preserved villous pattern. Although metastases occur with invasive mole, they are not as common as with choriocarcinoma.

Choriocarcinoma, also called chorioepithelioma, is a rare malignant disease occurring after some type of pregnancy. In the West, 50% of cases of choriocarcinoma are preceded by a mole, 25% by an abortion, and 25% by a normal pregnancy (7), although it may also occur after an ectopic pregnancy. Why the chorionic epithelium becomes malignant is unknown. Choriocarcinoma is characterized by a dark red or purple friable tumor, with no identifiable villous pattern. It grows rapidly, invading both muscle and blood vessels. Metastases are borne by blood and occur frequently, especially to the vagina, vulva, and lungs but also to the kidneys, ovaries, or other organs (5, p 568).

Because hydatidiform mole is the most common neoplastic trophoblastic disease and because it commonly precedes the others, emphasis in this section is on hydatidiform mole. (see Chapter 21).

Etiology

Mole usually occurs very early in pregnancy, certainly before the 12th week (8). The circulation in the villi never becomes established. Why this occurs is unknown. Because the incidence is much greater in Eastern countries than in Eastern people who have migrated to Western countries, it has been postulated that inadequate protein ingestion may be a cause or a contributing factor (8, p 527). Mole tends to recur in subsequent pregnancies. Age is a factor. The incidence in mothers over 45 years old is 10 times greater than 20–40 year olds (5, p 561). The karyotype of molar pregnancies is 46,XX, all of paternal origin. Either one spermatozoan duplicates itself, thus having a diploid number of chromosomes, and impregnates an ovum that is missing its nucleus, or two sperm fertilize one such ovum concurrently. Interestingly, there usually is a triploid karyotype in cases of partial mole (5, p 559).

Signs and Symptoms

The signs and symptoms of hydatidiform mole vary greatly. Usually, the early stage is like normal pregnancy, with all the symptoms of early pregnancy. In 89% of cases (5, p 561) some bleeding occurs, usually beginning by the 12th week, although in some cases it may not occur for as long as 6 months (9). The bleeding often is dark brown rather than bright red. It may occur as spotting or very heavy bleeding, and it may occur off and on for weeks or months, or it may occur just before the mole is aborted spontaneously. The uterus often is large for dates and of a soft, "doughy" consistency. It may, however, be small for dates. The ovaries may be enlarged and tender because of multiple lutein cysts that often accompany hydatidiform mole. No fetal heart tones or fetal activity can be detected except in the very rare occurrence of a normal "twin" with a molar pregnancy.

Occasionally, the first sign of a mole is the expulsion of vessicles characteristic of hydatidiform mole. These vessicles are clear and grape-like in that they often hang in clusters from thin pedicles.

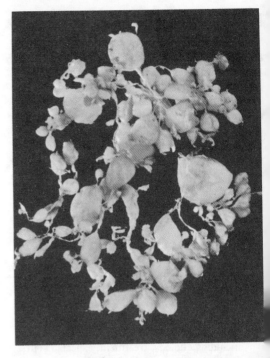

Figure 31.6. Molar villi with typical grape-like vessicles. (From Tuchmann-Duplessis H, David G, Haegel P: *Illustrated Human Embryology: Volume I, Embryogenesis.* New York, Springer-Verlag, 1972, p 85.)

The size of the vessicles may vary from a few millimeters to a few centimeters in diameter (Fig. 31.6).

Conditions often associated with mole may first make one suspicious of the diagnosis. Constant or frequent bleeding may cause anemia. Severe nausea and vomiting are associated with mole with hyperemesis gravidarum in as many as 30% of cases (9). Preeclampsia occurring before 24 weeks gestation normally is very rare, but with mole it may occur in as many as 50% of cases that pass 20 weeks' gestation (8). Hyperthyroidism occurs in only 2% of patients with mole (5, pp 562–563), but the majority have high thyroxine levels. Rarely pulmonary embolus may occur as a result of trophoblastic tissue escaping from the uterus via the venous system.

Diagnosis

The diagnosis of hydatidiform mole sometimes is made obvious by the expulsion of the characteristic grape-like vessicles. Often, however, the signs and symptoms are less obvious and other techniques are required to make the diagnosis. The differential diagnoses include normal pregnancy, a error in dates, uterine myomas, polyhydramnios, or multiple gestation (5, p 563).

Ultrasound is now the technique of choice for definitive diagnosis. It will show a characteristic "snow storm" pattern within the uterus, with no fetus or gestational sac visible.

Serial quantitative human chorionic gonadotrophin (HCG) levels may be used to assist in the diagnosis. Because HCG levels are extremely high with mole, abnormally high levels or levels that continue to rise later than 100 days after the last menstrual period suggest mole. It is imperative to compare the HCG levels to the normal curve for pregnancy, remembering that multiple gestation also causes elevated levels. It is also important to remember that no single value can distinguish normal from abnormal pregnancy (5, p 564).

The diagnosis of invasive mole can be made only when remote metastases are identified or if, after hysterectomy, the uterus is available for histologic examination.

Maternal Outcome

The ultimate prognosis for the woman with a neoplastic trophoblastic disease is quite good with appropriate medical care. During or immediately after a molar pregnancy, the associated complications must be treated: hyperemesis gravidarum, preeclampsia, hyperthyroidism, anemia, hemorrhage, uterine perforation, or infection. Immediate maternal mortality is negligible.

The overriding concern is that 5–15% of cases of hydatidiform mole develop malignant sequelae. Sometimes it is years before the choriocarcinoma develops. Fortunately, choriocarcinoma is the first gynecological malignancy to be treated successfully with chemotherapy, and it has the best remission and survival rates of any gynecological malignancy (7, p 231).

The primary site of choriocarcinoma is the uterus. Metastases are borne by blood and may occur in the lung, brain, liver, kidneys, vagina, fallopian tubes, ovaries, pancreas, or other sites. The prognosis with brain or liver metastases is worse than with other sites. The disease progresses rapidly if left untreated, often causing death in less than 1 year. However, with available chemotherapy the cure rate is 90–100% (5, p 569). Once the malignancy is cured, there is no residual adverse effect of either the disease or the chemotherapy on subsequent pregnancy outcome.

Medical Management

Once hydatidiform mole is diagnosed, there are two phases to its management: the evacuation of the mole and careful follow-up for diagnosis and treatment of any malignant changes.

The evacuation of the mole should be undertaken as soon as the woman is medically stable. Hysterectomy is the procedure of choice if the woman does not want any more children. Otherwise, however, the mole is evacuated by suction, followed by gentle sharp curettage. Evacuation by oxytocin, prostaglandins, or saline is not recommended since they may allow too much blood loss.

When the mole is to be evacuated, the patient is admitted to the hospital. An intravenous line is started with a 16- or 18-gauge angiocatheter. Two to four units of blood are type and cross matched. General anesthesia is used during the procedure. The cervix is dilated, and the uterine contents are suctioned out gently. An infusion of oxytocin is given during the entire procedure both to reduce bleeding and to reduce chances of perforating the uterus. After thorough suctioning, sharp curettage is performed. Specimens are sent to pathology to confirm the diagnosis and to detect the presence of malignant tissue. Complications of the evacuation may include hemorrhage, uterine perforation, and infection (5, p 566).

Whether to give chemotherapy prophylactically (i.e., before evacuating the mole) is controversial. However, since this may increase morbidity at the time of evacuation and since subsequent surveillance must be equally thorough and treatment is effective once malignancy is found, many experts do not recommend it.

After evacuation a baseline chest x-ray is recommended. It can be used for comparison later to establish the diagnosis of metastases. HCG values are used to detect the presence of persistent trophoblastic tissue. Usually, any trophoblastic tissue remaining will regress spontaneously. Thus, HCG levels should fall progressively. No chemotherapy is required as long as values decrease continually. Table 31.2 gives the protocol for following women after hydatidiform mole.

Chemotherapy is required in women who have evidence of metastatic disease or in those whose HCG titers either plateau or rise. Contraception is crucial during the follow-up period to avoid rises in HCG levels due to pregnancy, which would prevent evaluation of persistent trophoblastic tissue. Oral contraceptives or barrier methods may be used.

Chemotherapy for those who wish to preserve fertility is with a single agent—methotrexate or actinomycin (10). Only one course of treatment is given as long as subsequent HCG levels fall and no new sites of tumors develop. If a second course of treatment is required, the dose is not increased if

Table 31.2.

PROTOCOLS FOR FOLLOW-UP CARE AFTER HYDATIDIFORM MOLE[a]

1. Withhold chemotherapy as long as HCG levels continue to decrease and there is no evidence of metastasis.
2. Perform serum HCG titers weekly until normal for 3 weeks and then monthly for 6 months.
3. Begin chemotherapy if any of the following occur:
   a. HCG levels rise.
   b. HCG levels plateau on 2 consecutive weeks.
   c. There is evidence of metastasis.
4. Provide a reliable method of contraception, either oral contraceptives or a barrier method.

If no chemotherapy is required, discontinue follow-up and allow pregnancy 6 months after HCG levels reach normal (i.e., not detectable).

If chemotherapy is required:
1. Resume performing weekly HCG levels until normal for 3 weeks and then monthly for 12 months.
2. Withhold subsequent therapy as long as HCG levels continue to decrease.
3. Resume chemotherapy if any of the following occur:
   a. HCG levels rise.
   b. HCG levels plateau on 2 consecutive weeks.
   c. There is evidence of metastasis.
4. Change chemotherapeutic agent if HCG level plateaus after 2 consecutive courses or if values rise during or immediately after a course of treatment.
5. Discontinue follow-up and allow pregnancy after HCG values have been normal (i.e., not detectable) for 12 consecutive months.

[a]Adapted from Pritchard JA, MacDonald PC: *Williams Obstetrics*, ed 16. New York, Appleton-Century-Crofts (now Appleton & Lange), 1980, p 568.

the response to the first dose was adequate. Multiple-agent therapy is reserved for those rare cases that are resistant.

Choriocarcinoma occurring after an abortion or normal pregnancy may present with subinvolution, asymmetrical uterine enlargement, theca lutein cysts, irregular vaginal bleeding, or infection accompanied by acute pelvic pain, fever, or purulent vaginal discharge. Occasionally, the invasive tumor may cause intraperitoneal hemorrhage or severe vaginal bleeding. Sonogram, laparotomy, and/or curettage may aid in making the diagnosis. HCG levels will be elevated. Again, treatment either with methotrexate or actinomycin is extremely effective, with a cure rate of 90–100% (5, p 569).

NURSING MANAGEMENT

Nursing care specific for patients with
hydatidiform mole:
- [ ] Acknowledge and support the need for the patient and significant others to grieve the loss of this pregnancy.
- [ ] Assist with evacuation of the mole.
- [ ] Explain the rationale for frequent blood tests for HCG levels and encourage consistent compliance with follow-up regimen.
- [ ] Administer chemotherapy, as ordered, observing the patient carefully for adverse effects and alerting her to specific side effects (e.g., gastritis, anorexia, alopecia).
- [ ] Provide contraceptive counseling, as needed, emphasizing the importance of consistent and reliable use of the method chosen.
- [ ] Reassure patient/family about the favorable prognosis after neoplastic trophoblastic disease.
- [ ] Reassure that a favorable outcome can be expected in subsequent pregnancies.

Nursing diagnoses most frequently associated
with *hydatidiform mole* (see Section V):
- [ ] Grieving related to potential/actual loss of infant or birth of an imperfect child.
- [ ] Anticipatory grieving related to actual/perceived threat to self.
- [ ] Knowledge deficit regarding etiology, disease process, treatment, and outcome.
- [ ] Knowledge deficit regarding medication regimen.
- [ ] Anxiety/fear.

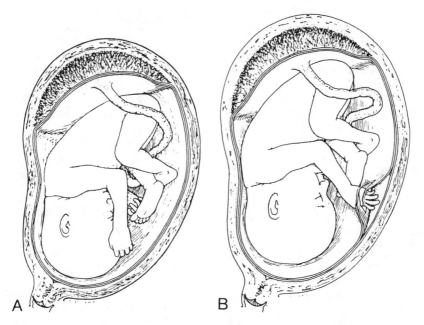

Figure 31.7. A, Intrauterine pregnancy prior to tear in amnion. **B,** Fingers entrapped in amnion bands. (From Turner BS: Amniotic band syndrome. *JOGN* July/Aug:299, 1985.)

AMNIOTIC BAND SYNDROME

Amniotic band syndrome results from a tear in the amnion, while the chorion remains intact. Strands of variable size then may wrap around the fetus, or fetal parts may protrude through the opening in the amnion, resulting in a wide variety of fetal malformations (Fig. 31.7). The reported incidence is quite variable, ranging from 1:1234 to 1:15,000 (11), perhaps because of variable accuracy in diagnosis.

The etiology of the disorder is unknown, although it occurs more often following significant abdominal trauma and in patients who conceived within 1 month after discontinuing oral contraceptives.

The signs and symptoms depend upon when in gestation the amniotic tear occurs; how long, thick, and wide the bands are; what fetal parts become entrapped in the bands; and how tightly wrapped the bands are. The bands tend to wrap around extremities at the point of least circumference. Therefore, areas between joints are more vulnerable than the joints themselves. Bands may become progressively tighter because of fetal movements as well as fetal growth. Among the possible anomalies are pseudosyndactyly; amputation of extremities or digits; club foot; craniofacial deformities that may result from pressure on the head or from a firmly attached band that the fetus has swallowed; anencephaly; and fetal death. Death may result from severe constriction of the fetus or from constriction of the umbilical cord.

Diagnosis sometimes is obvious when the baby is born with a band wrapped around a point of constriction. Careful evaluation of any fetal defects, including those thought to result from other causes, as well as careful scrutiny of the placenta and membranes for evidence of amniotic bands will improve the accuracy of diagnosis. The diagnosis may be suspected prenatally if ultrasound examination reveals deformities characteristic of the syndrome.

There are no maternal sequelae, and there are no reports of the syndrome recurring in subsequent pregnancies. Effects on the fetus vary from mild to severe, depending upon the size and tightness of the band, where it is located, and the point in gestation when it occurred.

There is no medical management during the pregnancy. Neonatal management must be based upon the individual clinical presentation.

NURSING MANAGEMENT

Nursing care specific for the patient with amniotic band syndrome:

☐ Explain the cause of the band to the patient.

☐ Allow the patient and her family ample time to express their feelings regarding the anomaly.

☐ Emphasize the normal infant features and role model maternal caretaking behaviors.

☐ Refer to parenting support groups and ongoing public health nursing home assessment.

Nursing diagnoses most frequently associated with *amniotic band syndrome* (see Section V):

☐ Grieving related to potential/actual loss of infant or birth of an imperfect child.

☐ Potential altered parenting.

REFERENCES

1. Buchheit K, Price J: Obstetrical hemorrhage emergency care. In Perez RH (ed): *Protocols for Perinatal Nursing Practice*. St. Louis, Mosby, 1981, p 109.
2. Cavanagh D, Woods RE: Hemorrhage in late pregnancy. In Cavanagh D, Woods RE, O'Connor TCF: (eds): *Obstetric Emergencies*, ed 2. Hagerstown, MD, Harper and Row, 1978, p 194.
3. Butnarescu GF, Tillotson DM: *Maternity Nursing: Theory to Practice*. New York, John Wiley and Sons, 1983, p 487.
4. Gottesfeld KR: Placenta previa. In Queenan JT, Hobbins JC (eds): *Protocols for High Risk Pregnancies*. Oradell, NJ, Medical Economics Books, 1982, p 218.
5. Pritchard JA, MacDonald PC; *Williams Obstetrics*, ed 16. New York, Appleton-Century-Crofts, 1980, p 574.
6. O'Connor TCF, Cavanagh D: Postpartum emergencies. In Cavanagh D, Woods RE, O'Connor TCF: *Obstetric Emergencies*, ed 2. Hagerstown, MD, 1978, p 299.
7. Kramer EE, Dawood MY: Pathophysiology of placental development. In Caplan RM (ed): *Principles of Obstetrics*. Baltimore, Williams & Wilkins, 1982, p 231.
8. Hawkins JW, Higgins LP: *Maternity and Gynecological Nursing: Women's Health Care*. Philadelphia, JB Lippincott, 1981, p 238.
9. Miller MA, Brooten DA: *The Childbearing Family: A Nursing Perspective*, ed 2. Boston, Little, Brown, and Co., 1983, p 517.
10. Berkowitz R, Goldstein DP, Bernstein MR: Current management of nonmetastatic gestational trophoblastic tumors. *Contemp OB-GYN* 23:139–160, 1984.
11. Turner BS: Amniotic band syndrome. *JOGN* July/Aug:298–301, 1985.

Chapter 32
Postdates Pregnancy
Angela Portale, R.N., M.S., Nancy W. Kulb, C.N.M., M.S.

DEFINITION

A human gestational period completed within 38 weeks to 42 weeks' gestation is a term pregnancy. When the gestational period continues beyond 42 weeks or 294 days from the first day of the last menstrual period (LMP), it is considered prolonged. This situation has been reported to occur in from 7–12% of all pregnancies (1). Some of these prolonged pregnancies may be the result of inaccurate dating of the LMP or failure to account for a long menstrual cycle (more than 14 days between LMP and conception).

Although the terms prolonged, postterm, and postdate pregnancy are defined differently by different authors, usually they all refer specifically to gestational age. Postmaturity (or dismaturity) is a diagnosis made after birth, based on the appearance of the infant and the placenta. This problem is caused by uteroplacental insufficiency. Most prolonged pregnancies do not result in a "postmature infant," and not all dismature infants are the result of a prolonged pregnancy. It is estimated, however, that in 10–20% of prolonged pregnancies the baby also is postmature. The incidence of postmaturity increases with advancing gestational age.

Pathophysiology of Postmaturity Syndrome

Because of its limited functional life span, the placenta is the key organ in the pathogenesis of postmaturity. Reaching its peak of function between 36–38 weeks' gestation, the natural aging process continues with the formation of fibrinoid material on the surface of its chorionic villi. The villi are finger-like projections from the fetal side of the placenta into the intervillous space. It is here that the maternal-fetal exchange of metabolic and gaseous materials takes place. As the fibrinoid material on the chorionic villi increases, the available placental surface area where maternal-fetal exchange can take place decreases. This increases the risk of fetal compromise. Prior to 42 weeks the fetal effects of placental aging usually are insignificant. However, after this point in gestation, the rapidity of placental aging inhibits the fetus's ability to meet its oxygenation and nutritional needs.

Another significant physiological aspect of prolonged pregnancy is amniotic fluid volume. Within a normal pregnancy amniotic fluid reaches its peak of 1000–1200 ml at 38 weeks. It decreases rapidly as pregnancy progresses.

ETIOLOGY

Although perinatal research has provided clues, there is no clear understanding why some pregnancies are prolonged abnormally. There is reason to believe, however, that there may be some anatomic or biochemical abnormality in the fetus or amnion that, along with failure of other multiple back-up mechanisms, prevents the normal initiation of labor. (See Chapter 38 for a discussion of the initiation of labor.)

Prolonged pregnancy is more common with certain fetal abnormalities: fetal adrenal hypoplasia, anencephaly, extrauterine pregnancy, and placental sulfatase deficiency. Maternal factors associated with an increased incidence of postterm pregnancy—therefore leading to postmaturity—are:

1. Maternal age: increased incidence in mothers less than 25 years old, and increased in mothers more than 35 years old. There also is a higher incidence of postmaturity in this older group, especially rapid in the presence of maternal hypertension.
2. History of prolonged pregnancies in the past.
3. Medical conditions that can cause placental aging: hypertension, diabetes mellitus, collagen-vascular diseases.
4. High levels of maternal anxiety.
5. Parity greater than four.
6. Use of oral contraceptives until the LMP (i.e., the LMP was withdrawal bleeding following oral contraceptive use the previous month).
7. First trimester bleeding (i.e., threatened abortion).
8. Carriers of group B hemolytic streptococcus.
9. Use of labor-inhibiting drugs (e.g., high doses of steroids, aspirin).

SIGNS AND SYMPTOMS

The obvious sign of prolonged pregnancy is gestational age greater than 42 weeks. If careful dating of the pregnancy has been done throughout (i.e., determination of LMP, date of conception, uterine size in early pregnancy, uterine growth pattern, date of quickening, date fetal heart tones are first heard with a fetoscope, and evaluation of any sonograms that were done), this sign will be obvious. The difficult question is whether the prolonged gestation is having (or will have) an adverse effect on the fetus.

Signs and symptoms of fetal jeopardy resulting from prolonged pregnancy include:

1. Decreasing amniotic fluid volume, thought to result from placental insufficiency.
2. Decreasing uterine size, because of decreased subcutaneous fat and muscle mass of the baby and decreased amniotic fluid volume.
3. Maternal weight loss (more than 3 pounds in the last weeks of pregnancy).
4. Meconium-stained amniotic fluid.
5. Decreased fetal movement.

DIAGNOSIS

Again, with careful dating of the pregnancy, the diagnosis of prolonged pregnancy is obvious. The diagnosis of fetal postmaturity is much more difficult. Many parameters of fetal assessment have been studied for their value in making that diagnosis, with conflicting results.

The nonstress test (NST) (see Chapter 6) frequently is used to assess fetal well-being. Since NSTs are known to have a high false-positive rate (27.4%) (2), nonreactive NSTs are followed by the more sensitive contraction stress test (CST) to increase accuracy of the assessment of fetal well-being. However, the NST false-negative rate has been reported to range from 0.6%–8% (2, 3). For this reason some practitioners prefer to use the CST rather than the NST. Nipple stimulation has been demonstrated to be an effective method of performing the CST (1, pp 227–228).

Ultrasound evaluation has become an increasingly important method of assessing the postdates pregnancy. It can be used early in pregnancy to establish gestational age, but in the third trimester it is of little use for dating the pregnancy. It can be used, however, to estimate placental maturity (see Chapter 6). Grade 0 or 1 placentas are not seen with postmature fetuses. Ultrasound also can be used to estimate amniotic fluid volume (AFV). AFV less than 200 ml is associated with a high rate (81%) of placental insufficiency (4). Decreased AFV repeatedly has been demonstrated to be associated with poor outcome: fetal distress, especially cord compression; intrauterine growth retardation (IUGR); and thick meconium staining. Ultrasonography is the basis for the biophysical profile (see Chapter 6), which has been shown to be quite accurate in assessing fetal well-being.

MATERNAL AND FETAL OUTCOME

Some babies in postdates pregnancies continue to grow, suggesting that the placenta is functioning quite well. These babies are not free of adverse effects, however. Continued fetal growth may result in macrosomia, with fetopelvic disproportion, dysfunctional labor, and a higher incidence of operative delivery.

Other fetuses suffer from placental insufficiency. These babies may not only stop growing but actually may lose subcutaneous fat and muscle. Because of the loss of vernix caseosa, these babies may have desquamation of the epidermis. At birth they exhibit the typical appearance of the postmature baby (Table 32.1). Babies with compromised placental function may exhibit a similar appearance at an earlier gestational age (5).

Table 32.1.
APPEARANCE OF THE POSTMATURE INFANT

1. Limbs appear long and thin.
2. Skin is parchment-like or macerated.
3. Vernix and lanugo are absent.
4. The skull is quite hard.
5. The baby appears very alert.
6. Skin, umbilical cord, and membranes may be discolored—brownish green or yellow.

Oligohydramnios is common with placental insufficiency and may contribute to fetal distress by allowing increased cord compression. Hypoxia, asphyxia, acidosis, and polycythemia can result from placental insufficiency and/or cord compression.

With hypoxia, and perhaps also because of the maturing parasympathetic reflex activity of the postdates fetus, meconium staining is not uncommon. With oligohydramnios the meconium often is thick, with increased danger from intrauterine meconium aspiration (see Chapter 39).

When compared to term infants, there is an increase in perinatal mortality after 42 weeks' gestation. This rate doubles by 43 weeks and becomes four to six times higher at 44 weeks. It accounts for 15% of all perinatal mortality and is second to prematurity as a cause of fetal and neonatal mortality (6). Thirty-five percent of these deaths occur before the onset of labor (7). Perinatal death usually is the result of placental insufficiency, cord compression, or meconium aspiration. During the neonatal period, hypoglycemia is a risk.

Risks for the mother include the risk of dysfunctional labor, induction or augmentation of labor, and operative delivery for fetal distress or fetopelvic disproportion.

In addition, the mother may experience physical and psychological stress. The discomforts of the late third trimester continue and may increase with continued fetal growth. The mother may have feelings of inadequacy and lack of control, feeling that the pregnancy will never end. The patient and her family may express concern regarding the potential thwarting of their planned birth experience, and they may have fear regarding the well-being of the mother and baby. Increased fetal testing can contribute to this fear. Anxiety, with its increase in circulating catecholamines, may be a cause of prolonged gestation. The anxiety caused by prolonged pregnancy actually may contribute to delayed onset of labor, thus setting up a continuing cycle.

MEDICAL MANAGEMENT

Management begins with careful pregnancy dating at the first prenatal visit and throughout the pregnancy so that there is no confusion about gestational age at term.

Management of pregnancy after 41 weeks is not clear-cut. Studies are controversial and conflicting, with the result that each practitioner and institution may manage the pregnancy somewhat differently. Guidelines for management are presented here.

Beginning at 41 weeks, some assessment of fetal well-being is begun. Usually, an NST is done, followed by a CST if the NST is nonreactive. The NST is repeated weekly or twice weekly. Some clinicians prefer to start with a CST, either by oxytocin infusion or nipple stimulation. Some practitioners may ask the patient to do daily fetal movement counts (see Chapter 6). Some may attempt amnioscopy—to check color of amniotic fluid—if the cervix is dilated sufficiently. If resources are available, or if there is any question regarding fetal status, a biophysical profile may be done. Fetal jeopardy requires intervention. Induction of labor with careful fetal monitoring usually is the chosen method of delivery unless overt fetal distress is evident.

At or slightly beyond 42 weeks' gestation, some clinicians choose to induce labor, regardless of cervical readiness for labor. The benefits of this approach have not been documented clearly (1), although it seems a reasonable approach given the increase in fetal morbidity and mortality after 42 weeks. Problems with induction at 42 weeks include (5):

1. The imprecision with which gestational age often is known.
2. The inability to identify which fetuses will or will not get into difficulty with continued pregnancy—and most do fairly well.
3. Labor induction is not always successful.
4. Induction leads to a higher rate of cesarean section, with increased maternal morbidity in this and subsequent pregnancies.

Some practitioners induce only if the cervix is favorable. If the cervix is not favorable, induction fails or the practitioner prefers to await spontaneous labor, intensive fetal surveillance is continued, with fetal testing at least twice weekly. Biophysical profiles, if not begun at 41 weeks, should be begun at 42 weeks. Again, fetal jeopardy requires intervention regardless of cervical readiness for labor. Because of the risks of extremely prolonged gestation, most clinicians do not allow the pregnancy to continue past 44 weeks if they are certain of the gestational age.

Before labor begins the postdates patient should be given emotional support, educated about comfort measures for the discomforts of late pregnancy, and given anticipatory guidance about assessment and treatment procedures. She should be advised to come to the hospital as soon as labor begins, since even the stress of early labor may be hazardous for the postterm baby.

Continuous electronic fetal monitoring throughout labor is indicated for the postdates pregnancy. Internal electronic fetal monitoring has the advantage of allowing the patient to remain on her left side to promote optimum uterine blood flow while providing accurate information on beat-to-beat variability and contraction intensity. However, whether artificial rupture of membranes is warranted to allow internal monitoring is controversial. It will result in less intrauterine fluid volume, with increased potential for cord compression, and thus may contribute to fetal distress. Whenever membranes rupture, the fluid should be observed for meconium staining. Fetal scalp blood sampling (see Chapter 39) should be done if there is meconium staining or a fetal heart rate abnormality.

Labor progress is monitored carefully because of the potential for dysfunctional labor. Oxytocin may be used as necessary for induction or augmentation of labor as long as fetal status is monitored carefully. Cesarean section is used as required for fetopelvic disproportion or fetal distress.

The neonatal resuscitation team should be present at the delivery. If meconium is present, the nose and pharynx should be suctioned prior to delivery of the shoulders. Immediately after birth the cord should be clamped to prevent polycythemia, and the bronchial tree should be suctioned under laryngoscopic visualization to prevent meconium aspiration.

NURSING MANAGEMENT

Nursing care specific for a patient with a postdates pregnancy:

☐ For all patients establish the gestational age as soon as possible: take a thorough history, do an accurate physical examination, and evaluate results of ultrasound done early in pregnancy (if necessary) (see Chapter 6).

☐ Educate the postdates patient regarding:
- — Assessment techniques (e.g., fetal movement counts, NST, CST, biophysical profile, amnioscopy); include risks, benefits, frequency of tests, and how results will be used in management;
- — Signs/symptoms of spontaneous labor and the importance of reporting to the hospital as soon as they occur;
- — Relief measures for discomforts of late pregnancy (e.g., urinary frequency, lower abdominal pressure, shortness of breath, varicose veins);
- — Induction (if indicated) (see Chapter 37); and
- — Observe for complications during labor, especially fetal distress and abnormal labor progress (e.g., use continuous electronic fetal monitoring; observe for meconium staining; assist with fetal blood gas sampling).

☐ Be prepared for emergency cesarean section and/or neonatal resuscitation.

Nursing diagnoses most frequently associated with postdates pregnancy (see Section V):

☐ Grieving related to potential/actual loss of infant or birth of an imperfect child.

☐ Knowledge deficit regarding etiology, disease process, treatment, and outcome.

☐ Altered fetal cardiac and cerebral perfusion.

☐ Anxiety/fear.

REFERENCES

1. Nichols CW: Postdate pregnancy: Part I. A Literature review. *J Nurse-Midwifery* 30:222–239, 1985.
2. Thornton YS, Yeh S, Petrie RH: Antepartum fetal heart rate testing and the post-term gestation. *J Perinatal Med* 10:196–202, 1982.
3. Miyazaki FS, Miyazaki BA: False reactive nonstress tests in postterm pregnancies. *Am J Obstet Gynecol* 140:269–276, 1981.
4. Beisher NA, Brown JB, Smith MA: Amniocentesis in prolonged pregnancy. *Am J Obstet Gynecol* 103:496–503, 1969.

5. Pritchard JA, MacDonald PC, Gant NF: *Williams Obstetrics*, ed 17. Norwalk, CT, Appleton-Century-Crofts, 1985, p 762.

6. Clifford SH: Postmaturity with placental dysfunction. *J Pediatr* 44:1–13, 1954.

7. Vorherr H: Placental insufficiency in relation to postterm pregnancy and fetal postmaturity. *Am J Obstet Gynecol* 123:67–103, 1975.

Chapter 33
Special Pregnancies
Nancy W. Kulb, C.N.M., M.S., Dale Bierschenk Scorza, C.N.M., M.P.H., and Nancy Campau, C.N.M., M.S.

INTRODUCTION

There are special circumstances in some pregnancies that may affect the course and outcome of pregnancy profoundly. Some are obstetrical complications in themselves, while others may predispose toward complications. They may present unique challenges to the obstetrical team because of the psychosocial issues they involve. This chapter discusses some of the most common of these special circumstances: adolescence, advanced maternal age, multiple gestation, pregnancy in the diethylstilbestrol (DES)-exposed woman, and pregnancy after infertility.

ADOLESCENCE

Introduction

It is estimated that 11 million of the 21 million teenagers in the United States are sexually active (1). A study by the Centers for Disease Control indicated that most teenagers begin sexual activity before they begin to use contraception—often as much as 1 year before (2). It is not surprising, then, that approximately one million adolescents get pregnant each year (3). It is estimated that one-half of all nonmarital adolescent pregnancies occur in the first 6 months after initiating sexual activity, and 20% of those within the first month (4).

The reason for the high incidence of teenage pregnancy is multifactorial. The mean age of menarche has decreased from an estimated 15 in 1933 to 11.6 in 1964 (5). Thus, adolescents increasingly may be physically mature before they are psychologically mature. Although contraceptive clinics are widely

available to teenagers, teenagers may not take advantage of their services for a variety of reasons:

1. They may be embarrassed to go or to admit that they are sexually active.
2. They may fear their parents will find out.
3. They may fear adverse effects of the contraception.
4. They actually may desire pregnancy.

Teenagers may overtly or covertly desire pregnancy for proof of their femininity/masculinity, for someone to love (or to love them), or to prove their love for their partner. They may not be reality oriented, thinking pregnancy cannot happen to them, or it cannot happen the first time.

Of course, all pregnant adolescents are not irresponsible. Many, especially in the 17–19 year age group, may be married with a planned pregnancy. It may be an attainment of a life goal for them to bear children.

Pregnant adolescents have many special needs specific to their age. They have a higher basal metabolic rate than older women. Therefore, they require more calories than adults of the same height and weight. Their needs for protein and calcium also are increased because of the growth of muscle and bone. At the same time, they may be very concerned about watching their figures or eating like their peers. Adolescent girls frequently have been found to be inadequately nourished—especially deficient in iron and vitamins A and C—overweight, underweight, or anemic (6). Nutrition counseling is very important, but it must include recognition of peer group practices and inclusion of the person in the household who buys and prepares food if it is not the adolescent herself (see Chapter 26).

It has been postulated that the pelvic basin and birth canal reach full maturity later than stature—about 2–3 years after menarche. It may be that pelvic adequacy depends more on time since menarche than on chronological age. However, conflicting data exist concerning the rate of labor dystocia because of pelvic inadequacy among teenagers. Some studies show no increase in cesarean section or midforceps delivery rates over the general population (5, p 87).

There is a high rate of drug and alcohol abuse among teenagers. Substance abuse may be an additional factor complicating adolescent pregnancy and may require sensitive counseling (see Chapter 19).

Suicide among teenagers is on the rise in the United States. The fear or depression that may be caused by pregnancy may be so great as to make the teenager feel that death is the best way out. The health care team therefore must be alert to the clues that a teenager is contemplating suicide and help her to get the support and assistance she needs at that critical time. Hot lines and special programs are available in many communities to help the teen who is finding it difficult to cope with life. The health care team should be aware of such programs and make referrals to them when appropriate.

Although adolescent pregnancy is not confined to any group of teens, more often than not, pregnant adolescents are of lower socioeconomic status, if only for the reason that they have not had time to finish their education and become established in a career. In many cases they are unmarried. Sometimes they are living at home with their parents, but with the coming of a child, they have a need to establish a residence on their own. All of these factors impact on adolescent pregnancy.

The following section gives information on developmental aspects of adolescence.

Developmental Aspects of Adolescence

Adolescence is a bridge between childhood and maturity. It is a time of biologic and psychosocial integration. Individual adolescents are at various points in this maturation process, and the degree of maturity is only very roughly correlated with chronological age.

Austin (7) listed four developmental tasks the adolescent must achieve:

1. Demonstration of adult behavior.
2. Management of interpersonal trust in relationships with other people.
3. Mastery of sexual impulses in a socially acceptable way.
4. Incorporation of cultural values.

Much of the psychosocial development of the adolescent centers around sexual identity and body image. Adolescents are at various stages in their emotional readiness to deal with sexuality, contraception, pregnancy, and parenthood.

Peer groups are important to the adolescent. Through relationships with others, adolescents seek to establish their own identity. Often adolescents have one best friend—a person with whom they can have an intimate give-and-take relationship.

Adolescents often are characterized as rebellious and often times do not communicate well with authority figures. They are constantly testing their limits in an effort to find out what they really are. This occurs in the health care setting as well as at home and at school.

Adolescents often are idealistic, refusing to compromise even in the face of reality. They sometimes have difficulty dealing with the discrepancy between what ought to be and what is. Fairness is very important to them.

As the adolescent matures, he or she becomes increasingly independent and responsible for her own decisions. Early in adolescence, parents and authority figures make the major decisions for the "child." But, with increasing maturity, the adolescent takes on more responsibility, although it may be very inconsistent—one moment relying on her parents and the next relying on herself. With continued growth, the adolescent reaches the point where he or she makes decisions alone and accepts the consequences.

The health care giver must identify the stage of psychosocial as well as biological development of the adolescent in order to provide optimum care. This often requires altering one's usual "style" (e.g., from authoritarian to nonauthoritarian) to communicate effectively with the patient.

Maternal and Fetal Outcome

Many pregnant adolescents are very healthy and can anticipate a normal pregnancy, labor, and delivery. In 18–19 year olds, the clinical course is much like that of a mature adult (6, p 249). High complication rates have been reported in adolescents, particularly younger ones, but it is debatable whether most of these are due primarily to socioeconomic factors rather than to age. With good obstetrical care, some studies have showed even lower complication rates in adolescents than in the general population (5, p 90).

The rate of pregnancy-induced hypertension (PIH) has been reported to range from 9–34% in adolescents (8). Many studies, however, show only a modest increase in PIH, primarily among gravidas less than 15 years old. The PIH, when it does occur, is no more severe in them than in older patients (5, p 84).

Some studies show an increased rate of anemia and a possible increase in trophoblastic disease among adolescents. There is no increase in hyperemesis gravidarum (5, p 84). Some studies show an increase in cesarean section rates, whereas others do not.

Rochat, in 1981 (9), reported an incidence of maternal mortality twice as great in patients less than 15 years old than in 16–34 year olds.

Most studies show an increased incidence of low birth weight in adolescent pregnancy. This finding, however, is not universal. Again, it is postulated that the incidence may be related more to nutritional and socioeconomic status of the adolescent than to age.

Medical Management

Management of adolescent pregnancy should begin with prevention for those patients who do not desire pregnancy. Accurate education regarding sexuality and contraception must be readily available for teenagers. Family planning services that are readily accessible and confidential must be made available. Family planning services provided in high schools have proven to decrease the incidence of teen pregnancy.

Counseling and education services should include anatomy and physiology of reproduction, signs and symptoms of pregnancy, how and where to get pregnancy tests, and the importance of early prenatal care. One effective method of conveying information to pregnant teenagers is through peer counselors or peer groups. Teens often are more responsive to and trusting of their peers than authority figures, making it easier to convey information. Peer groups that are effective can help patients change irresponsible behavior and develop realistic plans for dealing with their problems (10).

Many adolescents react with shock and denial when confronted with pregnancy. Because of this reaction or because they are afraid or embarrassed to admit they are active sexually, they may register for prenatal care very late.

Adolescents who register for care early should be counseled appropriately regarding the option of abortion. Currently, approximately one-third opt for elective abortion (3, p 277). Idealistic teens may elect to continue the pregnancy because that is what a "good mother" would do, but they may not be realistic about the demands of pregnancy amd motherhood and the impact on their education and social relationships.

Prenatal visits may be scheduled for the adolescent more frequently than normal (e.g., every 2 weeks in the first two trimesters and weekly in the third trimester). Screening for venereal disease should be a routine procedure. Periodic checks of hemoglobin/hematocrit will allow early diagnosis and treatment of anemia as well as monitoring progress toward resolving it. Screening for PIH is an important part of prenatal visits. It must be remembered that a diastolic pressure of 80–85 mm Hg may indicate hypertension in a teenager. Fundal growth should be monitored closely. Suspicion of intrauterine growth retardation requires sonographic confirmation as well as evaluation and treatment or counseling for etiologic factors (e.g., smoking, drug abuse, poor nutritional status). Teenagers should be taught the danger signs of pregnancy, including signs and symptoms of preterm labor, and how to report them.

Special programs for prenatal care for adolescents have demonstrated repeatedly that optimum medical care coupled with emotional support will result in good outcomes for pregnant teens and their babies. Several teen pregnancy programs (3, 8, 11) have nurse-midwives as the primary care providers. Because midwifery emphasizes individualized education, patient participation in care, a nonauthoritarian approach, and continuity of care, nurse-midwives have been successful in improving compliance with treatment modalities and achieving good outcomes. Table 33.1 reports selected complication rates for 738 teens seen in one such adolescent prenatal clinic. The team in these adolescent clinics has included an obstetrician consultant, nutritionists, and social workers. Sometimes psychiatrists have been included to help the teens deal with depression or fear resulting from pregnancy and impending parenthood as well as the underlying factors that may have precipitated the pregnancy.

Nutrition counseling, as discussed above, is extremely important in the prevention of low birth weight, anemia, and other pregnancy complications. Referral to the Supplemental Food Program for Women, Infants, and Children (WIC) or other food assistance programs should be made as necessary. Routine vitamin and iron supplementation may be necessary in view of the common nutritional practices of teenagers.

Social workers provide much-needed assistance with financial and housing problems. They may help the teenager plan for dealing with the stress the pregnancy places on her family if she is living at home. They also may spend a great deal of time with an adolescent discussing preparations for

Table 33.1.
RATE OF SELECTED COMPLICATIONS IN SPECIAL PRENATAL PROGRAM FOR ADOLESCENTS,
LESS THAN 18 YEARS OLD (MEDICAL UNIVERSITY OF SOUTH CAROLINA, 1974–1978)[a]

COMPLICATION	RATE IN SPECIAL PROGRAM (N = 738)	RATE IN MATCHED CONTROL GROUP[b] (N = 2014)
Low birth weight (total)	9.1%	12.7%
Low birth weight (<15 years old)	8.8%	21.0%
Preeclampsia	11.2%	——
Premature rupture of membranes	9.0%	——
Meconium staining	10.0%	——
Fetal distress (abnormal fetal heart tone pattern)	3.0%	——
Cesarean section	12.3%	——
Perinatal mortality rate	10.8/1000	22.1/1000

[a]From Piechnik SL, Corbett MA: Reducing low birth weight among socioeconomically high-risk adolescent pregnancies. *Nurse-Midwifery*. 30:88–98, 1985.
[b]Matched for age, race, socioeconomic status, perinatal risk; living in same state.

the baby, the mother's life goals (e.g., education, career, marriage), and how the patient plans to incorporate her baby into her goals.

Counseling regarding smoking, drug and alcohol abuse, sexuality, personal hygiene, and contraception is an important part of prenatal care of the adolescent. Preparation for childbirth classes should be considered an integral part of the care. Some adolescent clinics schedule classes just before or after clinic hours to make it easy for the adolescent to attend.

The majority of pregnant adolescents, especially younger ones, are having their first baby. They may not be prepared physically or emotionally for the demands of parenthood. A certain amount of information and literature can be given to the teen prior to delivery. A number of adolescent pregnancy programs have found it beneficial to continue contact through family planning care or parenting groups and classes to assist adolescents

during the first 1–3 years of parenting. Federal funding has continued to support such longitudinal case management.

The cost of providing such intensive care to the adolescent may seem, at first, to be unrealistic. However, the documented outcomes of such programs demonstrate that they can reduce dramatically the incidence of complications in teenagers. When comparing the cost of the program to the cost of treatment of low birth weight babies (and other complications), it is evident that prevention is very cost effective (11).

During labor, the teenager needs continuous emotional support. Analgesia should be used, when necessary, when comfort measures are not sufficient. Maternal-infant bonding should be promoted and observed. Any problems with maternal-infant attachment should be noted and appropriate intervention initiated.

NURSING MANAGEMENT

Nursing care specific for a patient experiencing teenage pregnancy:

☐ Educate teenagers, preconceptionally if possible, regarding sexuality, contraception, pregnancy, and parenthood. Stress importance of early diagnosis of pregnancy and early prenatal care.

☐ Provide effective counseling for pregnant adolescents:
— Use open, honest manner to inspire trust;
— Recognize readiness to learn specific information;
— Adapt counseling to developmental stage of adolescent;

— Include significant other(s), as appropriate, recognizing that it may require great sensitivity to determine appropriate degree of involvement of patient's mother, boyfriend, or others; and
— Consider influence of peer group.

☐ Encourage maturational growth by:
— Exploring with the patient her life goals (e.g., education, career, marriage) and how the baby will fit in, and
— Encouraging the patient to make responsible decisions.

☐ Explain the importance of frequent prenatal visits; if possible, allow the patient to see the same provider at each visit to enhance rapport.

NURSING MANAGEMENT

☐ Educate the patient at the appropriate time in pregnancy regarding:
- Options (e.g., therapeutic abortion, giving the baby up for adoption);
- Impact of smoking, alcohol, and drugs on successful pregnancies,
- Nutrition:
  * Extra nutritional needs (e.g., protein, calories, iron, calcium) of pregnant adolescents and food sources, and
  * iron and vitamin supplements, with an explanation of their importance and how to take them;
- Signs/symptoms of preterm labor and how to report them;
- Preparation for childbirth (or refer to classes specifically for adolescents); and
- Sexuality, hygiene, infant feeding, parenting, and postpartum contraception.

☐ Provide appropriate referrals:
- Visiting nurse service prenatally to monitor patient's health status and readiness for the baby and postpartum to assess adjustment to parenthood;
- Social worker;
- Nutritionist and/or WIC; and
- Psychologist.

☐ Screen for common complications of adolescent pregnancy:

- Iron or folic acid deficiency (see Chapter 8).
- Intrauterine growth retardation (see Chapter 27).
- Preterm labor (see Chapter 28).
- PIH (see Chapter 13);
- Sexually transmitted diseases (see Chapter 22); and
- Fetopelvic disproportion (see Chapter 35).

☐ Provide a continuing presence during labor; assist with breathing/relaxation techniques and comfort measures.

☐ If possible, provide a telephone number or initiate contact periodically after hospital discharge to encourage patient to ask questions or express concerns.

Nursing diagnoses most frequently associated with *teenage pregnancy* (see Section V):
☐ Disturbance in body image, self-esteem.
☐ Ineffective individual coping.
☐ Ineffective family coping: compromised.
☐ Potential altered parenting.
☐ Anxiety/fear.
☐ Knowledge deficit regarding pregnancy, process of labor and delivery, concerns of the postpartum period, parenting.
☐ Altered nutrition: less than body requirements.

ADVANCED MATERNAL AGE

Introduction

The commonly accepted definition of advanced maternal age is pregnancy with an expected date of confinement (EDC) after the patient's 35th birthday. Some studies of pregnancy outcome in the older woman, however, use 30 or 40 as the definition of advanced maternal age.

The largest increase in fertility rates in recent years has been in women 30–35 years old. The 35–40 year olds also have had a significant increase in pregnancies. There are several sociological trends that have contributed to this change. Many women have postponed childbearing (and sometimes marriage) until their education is complete and their careers are established. Many have reached their early thirties and realized that their "biological time clock" is running out (i.e., they must have children soon or face the possibility of never having any). Some have been working and waiting for greater economic security before bearing children. Others have remarried and are ready to begin a "second family" when they reach their thirties.

Thus, many women over 35 are very happy to be pregnant and look forward eagerly to motherhood. There are others, however, who did not plan their pregnancies. Older multiparas may have thought they had finished childbearing and raising small children. These women may view pregnancy as disruptive to their lives. They may perceive that other pregnant women are younger, their contemporaries are not caring for small children, and therefore there is no one with whom to share their feelings. These women need extra support during their pregnancies if they elect to continue the pregnancy.

Maternal and Fetal Outcome

Maternal and fetal outcome commonly have been reported to be less favorable in the woman over 35 than in younger age groups. What is not always clear is how much of the difference is due to medical complications of pregnancy and how much is due to age alone. There is much misinformation regarding risks in these patients. The levels of risk vary with time, locale, and income class. Many older patients seek prenatal care early and have the socioeconomic advantage of better education and income class.

The incidence of infertility is greater in women over 35 than in younger women. The age-related causes include premature menopause, endometriosis, leiomyomas, medical illness, and psychological factors (12). Age may just allow more time for medical illness, such as pelvic inflammatory disease, hypertension, and diabetes, to occur or accumulate.

The currently available sensitive tests of pregnancy indicate that spontaneous abortion occurs in one-half to three-quarters of fertilized ova in women over 35. Half of the spontaneous abortions for which older women seek care are due to chromosomal abnormalities, but older women also have a greater incidence of spontaneous abortion in chromosomally normal conceptions (12, p 69–70).

The incidence of chromosomal anomalies also is increased in fetuses that are carried to viability. Table 33.2 lists the incidence of trisomy 21 (Down's syndrome) by age. Trisomy 21, of course, is not the only anomaly that can occur. Table 33.3 gives the incidence of all clinically significant cytogenetic anomalies by age. The role of the male factor in genetic abnormalities is not yet clear. Older women often are married to older men. Whether part of the increased incidence of genetic anomalies is related to age of the father is under investigation.

Congenital anomalies are not limited to those of chromosomal etiology. Older women may also have a greater incidence of anomalous offspring because of problems with the intrauterine environment or accumulation of environmental teratogens (12, p 70).

The risk of perinatal mortality is increased in patients over 35. The Collaborative Perinatal Project, 1959–1966, showed a perinatal mortality rate of 25:1000 in 17–19 year olds compared to 69:1000 in women over 39. This increase in perinatal mortality was independent of parity. Half of the increase was thought to be due to preexisting medical

Table 33.2.
INCIDENCE OF DOWN'S SYNDROME BY MATERNAL AGE[a]

MATERNAL AGE	INCIDENCE
Less than 35	1/600
37	1/100
40	1/50
44	1/20

[a]From Hogan LR: Pregnant again—at 41. *MCN* 4:175, 1979.

Table 33.3.
RATE OF CLINICALLY SIGNIFICANT CYTOGENETIC ABNORMALITIES BY MATERNAL AGE[a]

MATERNAL AGE	RATE OF CYTOGENETIC ABNORMALITIES
<30	2/1000
30	2.6/1000
35	5.6/1000
40	15.8/1000
45	53.7/1000

[a]From Hook EB: Rates of chromosome abnormalities at different maternal ages. *Obstet Gynecol* 58:282, 1981.

problems and half to uteroplacental underperfusion (e.g., abruption, large placental infarcts, placental growth retardation). Ninety-two percent of the increased perinatal mortality in older patients was due to stillbirths (12, p 70). Kajanoja and Widholm report a stillbirth rate of 23:1000 in women over 35 compared to 8:1000 in controls. Causes included prematurity, dismaturity, and congenital anomalies (13).

Morrison reported that older primigravidas had a 14% rate of premature deliveries and an 11% rate of intrauterine growth retardation (14). Some other researchers have confirmed the increased incidence of prematurity, but others have not.

Maternal mortality is higher in the older gravida than the younger one. Most of the increased risk is thought to be related to concurrent medical problems, such as hypertension, underlying renal, vascular, cardiac, or malignant disease, or obstetrical hemorrhage. Risk increases with age and parity. A 1982 study suggests that the maternal death rate in women over 35 dropped to 50% of that in 1974–1978. Possible explanations include a decrease in the overall maternal death rate, a greater proportion of older women in relatively high socioeconomic classes, and an increase of 35- to 39-year old gravidas who are not grand multiparas (15).

Many clinicians and researchers report prolonged labor in older women, up to 25% longer in nulliparas over 30. Proposed etiologies for the prolonged labor include cervical rigidity, decreased elasticity of the soft tissue of the vagina, immobility of pelvic joints, and uterine dysfunction because of aging of the myometrium (16–18).

As already stated, older women have the attendant risks of any accompanying medical disease—especially hypertension, diabetes mellitus, and cardiovascular disease. Primigravidas over 35 are more likely to have preeclampsia, uterine myomas, oxytocin induction, and cesarean section. All of these conditions and procedures, of course, carry their own risks for mother and baby. The reader is referred to the appropriate chapter of the text for more detailed information on each.

There is, unequivocally, an increased risk both for mother and baby when the mother is older. However, it is not clear whether age alone is a factor or whether the increased incidence is due solely to associated complications. Certainly, if the patient has no medical illnesses, age alone is not a reason to deter pregnancy. Careful medical management, nursing case management, and genetic screening can do much to decrease the risks for mother and baby.

Medical Management

Management of the gravida over 35 essentially is the same as for other pregnant women. The primary difference is in the necessity to offer genetic counseling and screening. Because of the increased risk of genetic abnormalities, the woman should be given the options of amniocentesis or chorionic villi sampling (see Chapter 6) and therapeutic abortion if an anomaly is found.

Associated medical/obstetrical problems, of course, require proper diagnosis and treatment to minimize adverse sequelae.

Since many older gravidas have delayed childbearing, each may see her baby as a "premium baby." Of course, in the eyes of the medical team, all babies are equally important. These women may need suggestions on books to read on pregnancy and childbearing as well as extra counseling and anticipatory guidance during the prenatal period and referral to preparation for childbirth classes. During pregnancy, older gravidas may need counseling regarding life-style changes and reorientation of career goals required by parenting. After delivery, these women need some anticipatory guidance regarding future reproductive potential prior to menopause and appropriate contraception.

NURSING MANAGEMENT

Nursing care specific for a patient with
advanced maternal age **(over 35 years):**

☐ Counsel the older woman preconceptionally, if possible, regarding her risk status based on her current health and medical history.

☐ Screen for signs/symptoms of medical illness and/or obstetric complications in the older gravida:

— Genetic defects (see Chapter 25);

— Diabetes mellitus (see Chapter 10);

— Hypertension (see Chapter 13);

— Preterm labor (see Chapter 28);

— Intrauterine growth retardation (see Chapter 27); and

— Dystocia of labor (see Chapter 34).

☐ Provide emotional support and sensitive care for the older woman with an unplanned pregnancy.

☐ Encourage preparation for childbirth and parenting:

— Refer to preparation for childbirth classes;

— Teach relaxation techniques/comfort measures for dealing with a labor that may be prolonged;

— Provide books, films, and so on about pregnancy, labor, delivery, and parenting; and

— Assist patient and partner to develop realistic plan for coping with baby and career.

☐ Counsel patient regarding future reproductive potential and contraception: provide sterilization counseling as needed.

Nursing diagnoses most frequently associated with *advanced maternal age* (see Section V):

☐ Disturbance in body image, self-esteem.

☐ Ineffective individual coping.

☐ Anxiety/fear.

☐ Knowledge deficit regarding pregnancy, process of labor and delivery, concerns of the postpartum period, parenting.

MULTIPLE GESTATION

Definition

Multiple gestation is the simultaneous presence of two or more fetuses in the uterus. There are two types: fraternal—dizygotic gestations resulting from the fertilization of two or more ova in one ovulatory cycle—and identical—monozygotic siblings resulting from a single fertilized ovum that divides into two or more similar structures that then develop into separate individuals.

The incidence of monozygotic twins is 1 in 250 births and does not seem to be affected by race, age, parity, heredity, or fertility medications (19).

Dizygotic twinning, however, is influenced by race, heredity, maternal age, parity, and, especially, ovulation-inducing medications. The incidence increases with maternal age up to about 40 and parity up to 7. Oriental women have the lowest incidence of multiple birth (about 1:155), followed by white women (1:100). The highest incidence is in black women (1:79). The overall incidence of multiple birth is approximately 1:85; however, the incidence increases to about 1:9 with the use of fertility drugs. The incidence of multiple gestation after gonadotropin therapy is 20–40%, with up to 11 fetuses at one time reported (none survived). After clomiphene therapy, the incidence is much lower, approximately 7.5% (19, p 506).

The early use of ultrasound to detect the occurrence of multifetal pregnancy has shown that the incidence of conception of multiple fetuses may be twice as high as the incidence of delivery of multiple fetuses. Thus, half of multiple gestations may be lost due to blighted ovum, missed abortion, or fetal death (19).

Etiology

The etiology of monozygotic twinning is unknown, but it occurs when a single fertilized ovum divides to form two individuals. If division occurs within the first 72 hours following conception, two amnions and two chorions with two distinct placentas or a fused placenta result. Division between the 4th and 8th days results in a single chorion with two amnions and a common placenta. Division after the 8th day results in only one amnion and chorion, and if cleavage is incomplete, conjoined twins may result (19, pp 503–504). Dizygotic twinning is a result of multiple ova being released and fertilized in one ovulatory cycle.

Signs and Symptoms

Family history of multiple gestation or a history of taking fertility drugs should alert the practitioner to the possibility of multiple gestation. The mother's symptoms may include excessive fetal movement, excessive weight gain, and exaggeration of the common discomforts of pregnancy (e.g., nausea, edema, fatigue).

The most common sign of multiple gestation is the discrepancy between uterine size and gestational age by menstrual history and previous examinations. The discrepancy is most striking in the middle trimester of pregnancy. The differential diagnoses for the large fundal height for dates include an error in dating the pregnancy, erroneous measurement of fundal growth, uterine fibroids, polyhydramnios, and macrosomia.

Another sign is the palpation of more than one fetus; however, usually this is not possible before the third trimester and is very difficult in obese women. The detection of two fetal heart rates distinct from one another by more than 10 beats per minute at the same time and distinct from the maternal rate also can be a sign. Finally, when the fetal head is palpated on vaginal examination and feels too small to be compatible with the estimated fetal weight, multiple gestation is suspected.

Diagnosis

Recent studies have reported accurate antepartum diagnosis of multiple gestation in 93% of cases. However, without careful evaluation of the patient's family history, pregnancy history, uterine growth, and appropriate use of sonogram, the rate of diagnosis prior to labor may slip to 50% (19, p 510).

Sonogram provides the definitive diagnosis of multiple gestation. As early as the 6th week of gestation separate sacs can be seen. Beginning around the 14th week, diagnosis is made by visualizing two or more fetal heads. However, the diagnosis often is difficult, and only careful scanning can assure accuracy. The accuracy of diagnosis decreases with an increased number of fetuses since their position may make it difficult to see all of them.

Maternal and Fetal Outcome

The physiological and psychological stress of pregnancy is increased for the mother with a multiple gestation. Minor disorders associated with pregnancy often are exaggerated. There is increased nausea and vomiting. Constipation and indigestion may be more severe. Sleeping problems are common. Abdominal discomfort as well as lower back

Table 33.4.

COMPLICATIONS OF PREGNANCY
ASSOCIATED WITH MULTIPLE GESTATION[a]

1. Abortion
2. Increased perinatal mortality
3. Low birth weight
   a. Prematurity
   b. Intrauterine growth retardation
4. Congenital anomalies
5. Fetus-to-fetus hemorrhage
   a. Hypovolemia and anemia
   b. Hypervolemia, hyperviscosity, and polycythemia
6. PIH or aggravated hypertension
7. Maternal anemia
   a. Acute hemorrhage
   b. Iron or folic acid deficiency
8. Placental accidents
   a. Abruptio placentae
   b. Placenta previa
9. Postpartum hemorrhage (atony)
10. Cord accidents
    a. Prolapse
    b. Entwinement
    c. Vasa previa
11. Polyhydramnios
12. Labor dysfunction
    a. Preterm labor
    b. Labor dystocia
    c. Abnormal fetal presentation

[a]Adapted from Pritchard JA, MacDonald PC, Gant NF: *Williams Obstetrics*, ed 17. Norwalk, CT, Appleton-Century-Crofts (now Appleton & Lange), 1985, p 503.

pain is more pronounced with the more distended and heavy uterus. Increased edema and problematic varicose veins result form mechanical blockage, leading to decreased venous return.

Other medical and obstetrical problems also increase in cases of multiple gestation (Table 33.4). Spontaneous abortion occurs more frequently and with it the risk of excessive blood loss. An increased incidence of hyperemesis gravidarum may lead to depletion of the mother's nutritional stores. Anemia may result from poor intake of nutrients, especially iron and protein, but also may result from increased demand. There are increased fetal demands for blood proportional to the number of fetuses and increased maternal demands because of greater expansion of maternal blood volume. Women pregnant with multiple fetuses have greater requirements for calories and protein as well as other nutrients (see Chapter 26) and may have a more difficult time consuming them because of the pressure imposed by a large uterus. Maternal renal function may be become impaired seriously as a consequence of obstructive uropathy, especially when polyhydramnios occurs, a frequent occurrence in multiple gestation. PIH also is more common and the onset of hypertension usually is

earlier and the course more severe (20). Early termination of pregnancy may be necessary if the preeclampsia cannot be controlled.

Other associated maternal complications include placental accidents and labor dysfunction. Both of these may require operative delivery. The incidence of postpartum hemorrhage is increased owing to atony from overdistention of the uterus.

Perinatal morbidity and mortality in multiple gestation are increased for the fetus and newborn to a certain extent because of the increased incidence of medical complications for the mother but largely because of the frequent occurrence of prematurity. Spontaneous rupture of the membranes and/or the onset of labor prior to term is very common, and preterm delivery is the norm rather than the exception (19, p 514). In addition, competition for nutrients, crowding, and twin-to-twin transfusion (in monochorionic twinning) may result in intrauterine growth retardation for one or more fetuses, or the spontaneous death of one fetus. Perinatal mortality has been estimated at four times the rate for all fetuses (21).

The cesarean section rate is increased with multiple gestation for many reasons. One predisposing factor is the increase in malpresentation; the most common malpresentation is with the second fetus in the breech position or in a transverse lie. Malpresentation alone is not an indication for cesarean section in the infant weighing more than 1000 g. It may increase fetal morbidity, however, and may be one of the factors increasing the rate of cesarean birth. Prolapse of the umbilical cord increases with multiple gestation because of associated polyhydramnios, prematurity, and/or malpresentation.

Medical Management

Management begins with an awareness of the signs and symptoms of multiple gestation and prompt diagnosis. It then requires meticulous monitoring throughout the prenatal, intrapartal, and postpartal course. The overriding concerns in the management of multiple gestation include (22):

1. Control of nausea and vomiting.
2. Frequent screening for signs and symptoms of toxemia.
3. Prevention of premature labor.
4. Supplementation of iron and folic acid stores.
5. Evaluation of fetal well-being and growth through ultrasonography.
6. Careful conduct of labor and delivery.
7. Diagnosis and treatment of postpartum hemorrhage.

The goals for maternal care are individualized. The mother's physiology will be stressed enormously in its effort to provide the optimum intrauterine environment, and the demands on lifestyle change may be great. However, if the mother's health already is compromised with cardiac disease, renal disease, or another life-threatening condition, a careful assessment must be made of the effect of the pregnancy. The mother must be informed fully of all risks. Termination of pregnancy may be an option.

The provision of an optimum intrauterine enviroment is related directly to fetal nourishment. Dietary calorie and protein intake as well as vitamin and mineral consumption must be increased to meet the needs of multiple fetuses as well as increased maternal demands. Agnes Higgins of the Montreal Diet Dispensary recommends an extra 25 g protein and 500 calories per day for each fetus to support necessary growth (23). Encouragement to maintain strict adherence to intake of prenatal vitamins, iron, and folic acid is important. Increased maternal rest, especially in the left lateral recumbent position, will increase uterine blood flow and nutrients available to the fetus while at the same time preventing excessive edema and perhaps preterm labor.

Biweekly or weekly prenatal visits to determine fetal growth and maternal well-being are advisable, with frequent assessment of maternal hemoglobin levels.

Following the diagnostic sonogram, the growth of the fetuses should be followed by serial scans. The biparietal diameters should be no smaller than those of singletons up to 33 weeks' gestation, and the difference between fetuses optimally is no more than 3 mm. Fetal weight can be monitored with abdominal circumference measurement. Widely discrepant growth may indicate intrauterine growth retardation of the smaller baby and may require early delivery.

Weekly or biweekly evaluation of effacement and dilatation of the cervix beginning at 24–26 weeks' gestation can help to predict preterm labor or diagnose it early. The patient should be taught the subtle signs and symptoms of preterm labor (see Chapter 28). At the earliest sign of preterm labor, the patient should be admitted to the hospital, placed on bed rest, hydrated, monitored, and given tocolytic drugs as indicated.

The patient also should be hospitalized for any indication of medical complications (e.g., hypertension, severe anemia, any indication of poor fetal growth, poor maternal weight gain, or a home environment that is not conducive to sufficient rest and adequate nourishment. Associated complications of pregnancy require vigorous treatment.

Although the major concern in multiple gestation is preterm labor, at term during labor a dysfunctional contraction pattern also may occur, with or without rupture of membranes. Intravenous oxytocin can be used to augment or induce labor in pregnancies with multiple gestation when all the appropriate safeguards are used. This practice is controversial however. Cesarean section is the choice of some practitioners (19, p 520).

A sonogram or x-ray during labor may be required to determine the position of each baby. An intravenous infusion should be in place during labor because of the potential for operative delivery and hemorrhage. Electronic fetal monitoring should be used for each baby if possible. The presenting fetus can be monitored internally if the membranes are ruptured. The other one(s) can be monitored externally if the position is such that fetal heart tones are accessible. Often, with triplets or higher order multiple gestations, it is not possible to get all fetal heart rates monitored. Each fetus requires a separate monitor, of course.

Analgesia/anesthesia for labor and delivery must be selected according to the status of mother and babies. Prematurity or fetal distress may contraindicate use of narcotics during labor.

When vaginal delivery is imminent, a large delivery room should be prepared, with a complete set of equipment for each baby and a neonatal resuscitation team for each baby. An anesthesiologist should be present in case rapid induction of general anesthesia is required.

Delivery of the first infant proceeds as usual. After delivery of the first infant, careful assessment of the second infant's position and lie is essential. The fetal heart is monitored and labor is allowed to resume. Real-time sonography in the delivery room can be useful in assessing the exact position of the second fetus. With cephalic or breech presentation, the presenting part can be guided into the pelvis, the membranes ruptured, and delivery effected with maternal pushing. If labor does not resume, intravenous oxytocin is started, because the optimum time for delivery of the second baby is between 3 and 15 minutes after the delivery of the first baby. If the second baby is in the transverse or oblique position, internal podalic version is done with the patient under general anesthesia, and the baby is delivered by total breech extraction. As soon as the third stage of labor is completed and the patient is inspected for any lacerations that can be repaired along with the episiotomy, anesthesia is discontinued. Uterotonic agents are administered because of the possibility of hemorrhage resulting from uterine overdistention and a large placental site. Careful monitoring of postpartum bleeding is important in vaginal as well as cesarean birth, and the liberal use of uterotonic agents is the rule.

Cesarean section accounts for about half of the deliveries in multiple gestation. The greater incidence of severe maternal hypertension and extreme prematurity and/or malpresentation accounts for the majority of cesarean sections. The incidence is much higher with three or more fetuses since all of the potential complications of twin delivery are intensified. All of the usual indications for cesarean section also may occur in multiple gestation.

NURSING MANAGEMENT

Nursing care specific for a patient with
multiple gestation:

☐ Be aware of predisposing factors for multiple gestation (e.g., use of fertility drugs, family history of multiple gestation).

☐ Be alert to signs/symptoms of multiple gestation (e.g., exaggeration of the common discomforts of pregnancy, such as nausea, fatigue, edema, rapid weight gain; patient's report of excessive fetal movement; progressing discrepancy between fundal growth and dates).

☐ Assist in simultaneous counts of fetal heart rates heard in separate quadrants of the mother's abdomen.

☐ Educate patient regarding:
   — Sonograms for diagnosis and serial sonograms to monitor fetal growth and position.
   — Importance of frequent prenatal visits.
   — Nutritional requirements:
      * 25 g protein and 500 calories per day for each additional fetus;
      * Expected extra weight gain to account for weight of each fetus, placenta, and amniotic fluid sac; and
      * Vitamin and iron supplements.
   — Left lateral bed rest to enhance uteroplacental blood flow and minimize risk of preterm labor.
   — Comfort measures for the discomforts of pregnancy.
   — Proper use of maternity support hose.
   — Importance of avoiding practices that may contribute to intrauterine growth retardation (e.g., smoking, alcohol, drug use).
   — Signs/symptoms of preterm labor and how to report them.

☐ Provide emotional support to patient/family who may be overwhelmed by the diagnosis; assist the family in making realistic plans for the care of the babies.

☐ Screen for complications common in multiple gestation:
   — Hyperemesis gravidarum (see Chapter 11);
   — PIH (see Chapter 13);
   — Anemia (see Chapter 8);
   — Preterm labor (see Chapter 28);
   — Labor dystocia (see Chapter 34); and
   — Fetal distress (see Chapter 39).

☐ Provide appropriate referrals;
   — Visiting nurse service prenatally to assist in monitoring maternal/fetal status and to assess preparation for babies and postpartum to assist adjustment to parenting; and
   — Mothers of twins groups.

☐ Assist with sonogram or x-ray during labor, if required, to diagnose fetal positions.

☐ Monitor each fetus, if possible, by using external fetal monitors or a combination of internal and external modalities.

☐ Ensure that a patent intravenous infusion is in place.

☐ Provide nursing support and comfort measures during labor since analgesia/anesthesia may be contraindicated.

☐ Prepare for emergency cesarean section.

☐ Prepare for delivery:
   — Alert anesthesiologist and pediatric team to attend delivery, and
   — Ensure that there is a complete set of equipment (including identification papers, cord clamps, infant warmers, resuscitation equipment) and a neonatal resuscitation team for each baby.

☐ Note time of delivery of first baby; be prepared to start an oxytocin infusion if contractions do not resume spontaneously within a few minutes.

NURSING MANAGEMENT

☐ After delivery, monitor uterine consistency and bleeding; observe for excessive fatigue.

☐ Assist with the initiation of breastfeeding for mothers who desire to do so.

Nursing diagnoses most frequently associated with *multiple gestation* (see Section V):

☐ Grieving related to potential/actual loss of infant or birth of an imperfect child.

☐ Disturbance in body image, self-esteem.

☐ Ineffective individual coping.

☐ Ineffective family coping: compromised.

☐ Potential altered parenting.

☐ Anxiety/fear.

☐ Knowledge deficit regarding etiology, disease process, treatment, and outcome.

☐ Altered nutrition: less than body requirements.

☐ Altered fetal cardiac and cerebral tissue perfusion.

PREGNANCY IN THE DIETHYLSTILBESTROL-EXPOSED WOMAN

Introduction

DES is a synthetic, nonsteroidal estrogen that was developed in the 1930s. It is one of the most potent synthetic estrogens currently on the market. The use of DES was recommended in 1946 as a therapeutic agent to prevent spontaneous abortions; infertility; and complications of pregnancy, such as toxemia, prematurity, and intrauterine death (24, 25).

From 1948–1971 it is estimated that between four and six million women and their offspring were exposed to DES (25). DES therapy frequently began at the time that pregnancy was confirmed and continued until fetal viability or about the 35th week of pregnancy.

An increase in the reported incidence of vaginal clear cell adenocarcinoma in DES offspring spurred the research by Herbst and coworkers in 1971 (26) that demonstrated a statistically significant association between DES exposure in utero and adenocarcinoma. Other studies followed, associating DES exposure with squamous dysplasia and metaplasia (25, 27–29), infertility, vaginal and cervical abnormalities (30), uterine malformations and cervical incompetence (31, 32), and menstrual dysfunction (33). Structural abnormalities of the cervix and vagina that have been widely reported include a cervical hood or collar, cervical hypoplasia, and endocervical pseudopolyps. Almost two-thirds of women exposed to DES in utero have some uterine abnormalities on hysterosalpingography, even though laparoscopy findings are normal (34–36). These abnormalities may include T-shaped uterus, intrauterine synechia, or shaggy endometrium. Table 33.5 lists the effects of DES exposure on sons and daughters.

In a recent review of the literature on the subject of DES exposure in utero (37), it was con-

Table 33.5.
ADVERSE EFFECTS OF IN UTERO EXPOSURE TO DES[a]

Effects on daughters
  Anatomic abnormalities
    Lower müllerian tract
      Adenosis and clear cell adenocarcinoma
      Cervicovaginal structural abnormalities
        Collars, hoods, septa, and cockscombs
        Cervical mucus effects
        Cervical incompetence
    Upper müllerian tract
      Uterine structural abnormalities
      Fallopian tube structural abnormalities
  Reproductive abnormalities
    Menstrual dysfunction
    Reproduction dysfunction
      Infertility
      Adverse pregnancy outcome
        Spontaneous abortion
        Ectopic pregnancy
        Premature delivery
        Perinatal death
Effects on sons
  Anatomic abnormalities
    Hypoplastic testes
    Cryptorchidism
    Capsular induration
    Microphallus
  Reproductive dysfunction
    Altered semen analysis
    Altered fertility potential

[a]From Stillman RJ: In utero exposure to diethylstilbestrol: adverse effects on the reproductive tract and reproductive performance in male and female offspring. *Am J Obstet Gynecol* 142:905, 1982.

cluded that although the incidence of clear cell adenocarcinoma of the vagina is increased in DES-exposed women, it is not as great an increase as once thought. Vaginal epithelial changes appear to progress toward normal epithelium as the woman ages (38). The overall cancer incidence in a population exposed to DES in utero studied by Hadjimichael et al. was not different from that of the general population. He found that cancer developed somewhat more fre-

Table 33.6.

REPRODUCTIVE PERFORMANCE IN DES-EXPOSED AND NONEXPOSED WOMEN[a]

	DES-EXPOSED WOMEN	NONEXPOSED WOMEN
Spontaneous abortion	24%	12%
Preterm delivery	16%	5%
Live births	67% of all pregnancies	87% of all pregnancies
Fertility (at least one surviving infant)	80%	95%

[a]From U.S. Dept of Health, Education and Welfare: *Health Effects of the Pregnancy Use of Diethylstilbestrol. Physician Advisory, Rx 1948-1971.* Government Printing Office, Washington, DC, 1978.

quently in the exposed women; however, it was not found to be statistically significant (39).

Maternal and Fetal Outcome

Poor reproductive performance of DES-exposed females has been reported (40). There is an increased incidence of infertility and pregnancy loss (see Table 33.6). One study concluded:

One out of every twenty-four exposed parous women will have at least one ectopic pregnancy, and one out of every thirty pregnancies in exposed women will be ectopic (41).

The population that is being studied for DES-related sequelae is still young—the oldest being less than 45. More time and studies need to be devoted to this area before final conclusions and recommendations can be reached.

Medical Management

As with any patient, treatment should be individualized depending upon symptomatology. Along with routine screening and laboratory work, special consideration should be given to the DES-exposed female who is pregnant.

Prior to conception the woman exposed to DES should be counseled regarding her potential reproductive performance based on her own clinical presentation (e.g., uterine abnormalities), if possible. Women with previous second trimester losses may benefit from a laparoscopy or hysterosalpingography prior to pregnancy for an evaluation of possible uterine or tubal abnormalities.

Once the patient is pregnant, she should be taught the signs and symptoms of spontaneous abortion and ectopic pregnancy (see Chapter 24). A careful pelvic examination and early sonogram can be used to identify ectopic pregnancy before it becomes an emergency.

Women with a history of cervical incompetence or those who have documented cervical change in the second trimester may benefit from cerclage. Thus, weekly or biweekly cervical examinations may be appropriate, beginning in the second trimester.

Since DES-exposed women are at high risk for preterm labor, they should be taught the signs and symptoms of it. Weekly cervical examinations beginning at 24–26 weeks also can contribute to early diagnosis of preterm labor. Tocolytic agents may be used as necessary.

Routine Pap smears should be a part of prenatal care and may be performed more often in the DES-exposed woman. Referral for colposcopy can be made for evaluation of abnormal results, as necessary.

There is no evidence that DES exposure affects the course of labor and delivery. Therefore, the intrapartum course should be managed as usual, with cesarean section reserved for obstetric indications.

The expected postpartum course is not altered in the DES-exposed patient. She should be counseled appropriately regarding methods of contraception; for example, the intrauterine device (if available) also is associated with an increased incidence of ectopic pregnancy and therefore should be discouraged. Low dose combination birth control pills may be used, but the patient should be followed closely for adverse side effects and breast masses.

The patient should be reminded of the importance of frequent (annual or semiannual) pap smears, with colposcopic evaluation if abnormalities occur.

NURSING MANAGEMENT

Nursing care specific for a patient with DES exposure:

☐ Counsel the patient preconceptionally, if possible, regarding the risks of pregnancy. Encourage her to seek early diagnosis of pregnancy and early prenatal care.

☐ Educate the patient/family regarding:
— Importance of frequent prenatal visits;

NURSING MANAGEMENT

- Rationale for frequent pelvic examinations;
- Signs/symptoms of complications associated with DES exposure and how to report them:
  * Ectopic pregnancy (see Chapter 24);
  * Spontaneous abortion (see Chapter 24);
  * Incompetent cervix (see Chapter 24); and
  * Preterm labor (see Chapter 28).
- After adverse pregnancy outcome, assist with diagnostic procedures (e.g., hysterosalpingogram, laparoscopy) to determine and/or treat cause.

Nursing diagnoses most frequently associated with *DES exposure* (see Section V):
- Grieving related to potential/actual loss of infant or birth of an imperfect child.
- Anticipatory grieving related to actual/perceived threat to self.
- Disturbance in body image/self-esteem.
- Knowledge deficit regarding etiology, disease process, treatment, and outcome.
- Anxiety/fear.

PREGNANCY AFTER INFERTILITY

Infertility has been an increasing obstetric/gynecologic complication in recent years. It is defined as the inability to achieve a pregnancy after approximately a year of regular, unprotected coitus two to three times a week. Table 33.7 lists the causes of male and female infertility.

The diagnostic workup of the infertile couple may be extensive and time-consuming. Therefore, in the patient over 30, the evaluation may begin before a full year of attempting pregnancy. A full discussion of the infertility evaluation and treatment is beyond the scope of this book; Table 33.8 lists steps in the diagnostic workup. Depending upon the findings, treatment modalities may be instituted when an abnormality is found; the order of tests may be altered and some eliminated. It is evident that many couples have undergone a very time-consuming, expensive, and sometimes painful process, with invasion of their sexual privacy, before finally achieving pregnancy.

Table 33.7.
GENERAL CAUSES OF INFERTILITY[a]

MALE	FEMALE
Abnormal seminal fluid–cervical mucus interaction	Congenital uterine/vaginal anomalies
Immunologic	Endometriosis
Infectious	Hormonal disorders
Disturbed insemination	Adrenal
Anatomic anomalies	Ovarian
Genital surgery	Pituitary
Hernia repair	Thyroid
Prostatectomy	Immunologic disorders
Sexual dysfunction	Pelvic infections
Spinal cord injuries	Contraception related
Venereal disease	IUDs
Disturbed spermatogenesis	Steroids
Chronic illness	Postsurgical
Exposures	Appendectomy
Chemicals	Colon surgery
Heat	Diagnostic tests
Radiation	Pelvic surgery
Genetic disorders	Pregnancy related
Genital injuries	Abortion
Hormonal disorders	Cesarean section
Varicocele	Vaginal delivery
Viral infections	Sexual dysfunction

[a]From Behrman SJ, Kistner R: *Progress in Infertility*. Boston, Little, Brown, & Co., 1975, pp 207–221.

Table 33.8.
DIAGNOSIS OF INFERTILITY[a]

1. History
   a. Female
      Menstrual history
      Obstetric history
      Contraceptive history
      Abdominal pelvic surgery
      Pelvic infection (pelvic inflammatory disease,
         puerperal sepsis)
   b. Male
      Undescended testicles
      Inguinal hernia
      Testicular injury
      Mumps orchitis
      Occupational/environmental hazards
   c. Both
      Acute or chronic illness
      Drug therapy or use
      Family history
      Pubertal development
      Age
      Duration of infertility
      Frequency of coitus
      Sexual dysfunction
      Previous marriage
      Previous venereal disease
      Occcupation
2. Physical examination (both)
   Genitalia: development, hair distribution
   Secondary sexual characteristics
   Somatic anomalies
3. Special diagnostic tests
   a. Female
      Basal body temperature
      Hysterosalpingography
      Hysteroscopy
      Postcoital test
      Timed endometrial biopsy
      Selected hormone levels
      Laparoscopy
   b. Male
      Semen analysis
      Postcoital test
      Selected hormone levels

[a]Adapted from Grimes EM: For infertile couples—a holistic approach. *Contemp OB/GYN* 23:179–196, 1984.

It is no wonder, then, that the parents view the pregnancy as very special and very important.

Some remain overconcerned throughout the pregnancy; for example, they may be very anxious until fetal heart tones are heard and then switch to a preoccupation with how fast or slow it is (42). Others may be bewildered when they experience many of the same anxieties, fears, and even ambivalence that other couples experience. They need the continuing support of the entire medical team as they experience the normal joys and anxieties of pregnancy.

Some couples have gone to great lengths to pursue pregnancy. Some may have had to go into debt, change their life-style, or perhaps change a job or quit working during the process. Some may have "blamed" the other partner for the inability to achieve pregnancy, and occasionally these feelings may persist after conception.

The maternal and fetal outcome depends largely on the cause of the infertility problem and any concurrent medical/obstetrical risk factors. Usually, a normal pregnancy, labor, and delivery can be anticipated once conception and implantation have occurred. Of course, ectopic pregnancy, spontaneous abortion, or preterm labor may occur if abnormalities of the reproductive tract are present. Couples who experience pregnancy loss will need continuing support as they go through the grief process.

The use of fertility drugs increases the risk of multiple gestation. The couple should be made aware of that possibility before initiating fertility drugs. The obstetrical team should carefully observe for any signs or symptoms of multiple gestation. A sonogram done early in the second trimester, specifically to look for multiple gestation, might be warranted.

The couple should be counseled regarding their future reproductive potential—specifically, whether infertility should be expected to recur and whether contraception is recommended until future childbearing is desired.

NURSING MANAGEMENT

Nursing care specific for a patient *after* infertility:

☐ Provide education/support for the patient/family:
   — Teach common emotional and physiological changes of pregnancy;
   — Discuss common discomforts of pregnancy and prevention/relief measures;
   — Refer for preparation for childbirth classes; provide books, films, and so on to reinforce learning;
   — Refer for financial or psychological support as necessary; and
   — Encourage the patient/family to express feelings or concerns regarding pregnancy, observing for exaggerated anxiety.

NURSING MANAGEMENT

☐ Screen for complications of pregnancy, particularly multiple gestation in the patient who took fertility drugs.

☐ Provide accurate information regarding the individual patient's reproductive potential and appropriate methods of contraception.

Nursing diagnoses most frequently associated with *pregnancy after infertility* (see Section V):

☐ Disturbance in body image, self-esteem.

☐ Knowledge deficit regarding etiology, disease process, treatment, and outcome.

☐ Ineffective individual coping.

☐ Ineffective family coping: compromised.

☐ Anxiety/fear.

REFERENCES

1. Sanfilippo JS: Meeting the unique needs of teenage patients. *Contemp OB/GYN* 21:177–192, 1983.

2. Hale M: Better care for adolescents. *Contemp OB/GYN* 21:150–175, 1983.

3. Brucker MC, Muellner M: Nurse-midwifery care of adolescents. *Nurse-Midwifery* 30:277–279, 1985.

4. Bearman DL: Quotation in Hale M: Better care for adolescents. *Contemp OB/GYN* 21:161, 1983.

5. Sherline DM: When the mother is a child herself. *Contemp OB/GYN* 24:83–90, 1984.

6. Butnarescu GF, Tillotson DM: *Maternity Nursing Today: Theory to Practice*. New York, John Wiley and Sons, 1983, pp 133–147.

7. Austin SH: Cognitive and psychosocial development of adolescence. In Schuster CS, Ashburn SS (eds): *The Process of Human Development: A Holistic Approach*. Boston, Little, Brown, and Co., 1980, p 481–498.

8. Piechnik SL, Corbett MA: Reducing low birth weight among socioeconomically high-risk adolescent pregnancies. *Nurse-Midwifery* 30:88–98, 1985.

9. Rochat RW: Maternal mortality in the United States of America. *WHO Stat Quart* 34:2, 1981.

10. Sewall KS: Peer-group reality therapy for the pregnant adolescent. *MCN* 8:67–69, 1983.

11. Leppert PC, Namerow PB: Costs averted by providing comprehensive prenatal care to teenagers. *Nurse-Midwifery* 30:285–289, 1985.

12. Dorfman SF: Age as a factor in pregnancy. *Contemp OB/GYN* 27:64–77, 1986.

13. Kajanoja P, Widholm A: Pregnancy and delivery in women aged 40 and over. *Obstet Gynecol* 51:47–51, 1978.

14. Morrison I: The elderly primigravida. *Am J Obstet Gynecol* 121:465–470, 1975.

15. News from the Literature. *Contemp OB/GYN* 27:264, 1986.

16. Pritchard JA, Hellman LM: *Williams Obstetrics*. New York: Appleton-Century-Crofts, 1971.

17. Donald I: *Practical Obstetrical Problems*. London, Lloyd-Luke, 1969.

18. Halfar MM: Frequency of labor dysfunction in nulliparas over the age of thirty. *Nurse-Midwifery* 30:333–339, 1985.

19. Pritchard JA, MacDonald PC, Gant NF: *Williams Obstetrics*, ed 17. Norwalk, CT: Appleton-Century-Crofts, 1985, p 504.

20. Varney H: *Nurse-Midwifery*. New York, Blackwell Scientific Publications, 1980, p 325.

21. Naeye RL, Tafari N, Judge D, Marboe CC: Twins: causes of perinatal death in 12 United States cities and one African city. *Am J Obstet Gynecol* 31:267, 1978.

22. Buckley KA: Antepartum deviations. In Buckley KA, Kulb NW (eds): *Handbook of Maternal-Newborn Nursing*. New York, John Wiley & Sons, 1983, p 389.

23. Higgins AC: Nutritional status and the outcome of pregnancy. *J Can Diet Assoc* 37:17–34, 1976.

24. Smith OW, Smith GV, Hurowitz D: Increased excretion of pregnanediol in pregnancy from diethylstilbestrol with special reference to the problem of late pregnancy accidents. *Am J Obstet Gynecol* 51:411, 1946.

25. U.S. Department of Health, Education, and Welfare: *Health Effects of the Pregnancy Use of Diethylstilbestrol. Physician Advisory, Rx 1948–1971*. Government Printing Office, Washington, DC, 1978.

26. Herbst AL, Ulfelder H, Poskouzer DC: Adenocarcinoma of the vagina. Association of maternal stilbestrol therapy with tumor appearance in young women. *N Engl J Med* 284:878–881, 1971.

27. Ulfelder H: The stilbestrol disorders in historical perspective. *Cancer* 45:3008–3011, 1980.

28. Robboy SJ, et al.: Pathological findings in young women enrolled in the National Cooperative Diethylstilbestrol Adenosis (DESAD) Project. *Obstet Gynecol* 53:309–317, 1979.

29. Herbst AL, et al.: Prenatal exposure to stilbestrol. A prospective comparison of exposed female offspring with unexposed controls. *N Engl J Med* 292:334–339, 1975.

30. Pomerance W: Post-stilbestrol secondary syndrome. *Obstet Gynecol* 42:12, 1973.

31. Kaufman RH, Adam E: Genital tract anomalies associated with in utero exposure to diethylstilbestrol. *Isr J Med Sci* 14:353, 1978.

32. Singer MS, Hochman M: Incompetent cervix in a hormone exposed offspring. *Obstet Gynecol* 51:625, 1978.

33. Bibbo M, Gill WB, Azizi F, Blough R, Fang VS, Rosenfield R, Schumacher GF, Sleper KM, Sinek M, Wred GL: Follow-up study of male and female offspring of D.E.S. exposed mothers. *Obstet Gynecol* 49:1, 1977.
34. Kaufman RH, Binder GL, Gray PM, et al.: upper genital tract changes associated with exposure in utero to diethylstilbestrol. *Am J Obstet Gynecol* 128:51, 1977.
35. Pillsbury SG Jr: Reproductive significance of changes in the endometrial cavity associated with exposure in utero to diethylstilbestrol. *Am J Obstet Gynecol* 137:178, 1980.
36. Rosenfeld DL, Bronson RA; Reproductive problems in the D.E.S. exposed female. *Obstet Gynecol* 55:453, 1980.
37. Glaze GM: Diethylstilbestrol exposure in utero: review of the literature. *J Am Osteopath Assoc* 83:435, 1984.
38. Antoncoli DA, Burke L, Friedman EA: Natural history of diethylstilbestrol associated genital tract lesions. Cervical ectopy and cervical vaginal hood. *Am J Obstet Gynecol* 137:847–853, 1980.
39. Hadjimichael OC, Meigs JW, Falcier FW, Thompon WD, Flannery JT: Cancer risk among women exposed to exogenous estrogens during pregnancy. *J Natl Cancer Inst* 73:831, 1984.
40. Kaufman RH, et al: Upper genital tract changes and pregnancy outcome in offspring exposed in utero to D.E.S. *Am J Obstet Gynecol* 141:1019–1028, 1981.
41. Sandberg EC, Riffle NL, Higdon JV: Pregnancy outcome in women exposed to diethylstilbestrol in utero. *Am J Obstet Gynecol* 140:194, 1981.
42. Grimes EM: For infertile couples—a holistic approach. *Contemp OB/GYN* 23:179–196, 1984.

Section III:
Deviations of
the Intrapartum
Period

Chapter 34
Dystocias of Labor
Suzanne M. Smith, C.N.M., M.S., M.P.H.

INTRODUCTION

Normal labor is characterized by progress in cervical effacement and dilatation and descent of the fetus (Table 34.1 and Fig. 34.1). Dystocia, or difficult labor, is characterized by no progress or abnormally slow progress in labor (Figs. 34.2 and 34.3). The causes of dystocia can be thought of as problems with the powers (uterine contractions and maternal expulsive efforts), the passenger (the fetus), the passageway (the birth canal), or a combination of the three. This chapter discusses hypertonic and hypotonic uterine dysfunction. Chapter 35 discusses fetopelvic disproportion.

HYPERTONIC LABOR

Definition

Hypertonic uterine dysfunction, or incoordinate uterine dysfunction, is abnormal labor characterized by an elevated tonus of the uterus, by a distortion of the normal pressure gradient pattern of contractions, or by both. When it occurs spontaneously, it is usually during the latent phase of labor and results in a prolonged latent phase with failure to establish active, progressive labor. It is a relatively rare condition. Hypertonicity may occur as a result of overstimulation of the uterus during oxytocin induction or augmentation. See Chapter 37 for a discussion of prevention and treatment of oxytocin-induced hypertonicity.

Etiology

Fetopelvic disproportion or fetal malposition may be the cause of uterine dysfunction, but quite often the cause is unknown. Hypertonic labor oc-

curs more often in nulliparas and may be related to maternal anxiety.

Signs and Symptoms

Hypertonic labor is characterized by pain that seems to be greater than would be expected based upon objective assessment of the intensity of the contractions. Contractions are frequent and irregular in intensity. Often, the normal pressure gradient pattern of the uterus is disrupted, with areas of hypertonicity throughout the uterus or, more commonly, with the midsection contracting more strongly than the fundus. Sometimes, even when the pressure gradient pattern is normal, the uterus does not relax well between contractions. There may be coupling of contractions, with two contractions occurring close together without proper relaxation between them, or contractions may develop double peaks of intensity. (It should be noted that spontaneous coupling of contractions occasionally occurs during normal labor and requires no intervention if progress is being made and the fetus is in no distress.) Because of the disproportionate amount of pain, the patient may become anxious and/or exhausted. Lack of progress in dilatation, effacement, and descent results from the inefficiency of the hypertonic contractions.

Diagnosis

The diagnosis of hypertonic labor is based upon the following:

1. The observation of frequent, excessively painful uterine contractions and/or incomplete uterine relaxation between contractions during the latent phase of labor.

Table 34.1.

PARAMETERS FOR NORMAL PROGRESS IN LABOR[a]

PHASE	NULLIPARA	MULTIPARA
Latent phase	Less than 20 hours	Less than 14 hours
Active phase	<6, average 4	<4, average 2
Phase of maximum slope	At least 1.2 cm/hour	At least 1.5 cm/hour
Second stage	Less than 2 hours	Less than 1 hour

[a]Adapted from Buckley K, Kulb NW. *Handbook of Maternal-Newborn Nursing.* New York, John Wiley & Sons, 1983, pp 235–237.

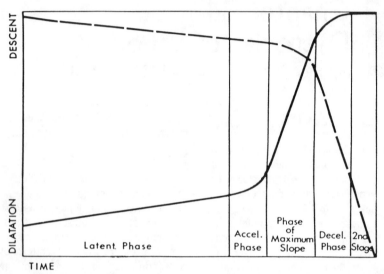

Figure 34.1. Cervical dilatation and descent patterns in the labor of nulliparas. The time period from the onset of the acceleration phase to the end of the deceleration phase is known as the active phase. (From Friedman EA: In Caplan RM, Sweeney WJ: (eds): *Advances in Obstetrics and Gynecology.* Baltimore, Williams & Wilkins, 1978, p 247.)

2. The lack of progress in dilatation, effacement, and fetal descent.

Although the diagnosis of hypertonic labor may be facilitated by the use of internal electronic fetal monitoring to document tonus and contraction pressures, artificial rupture of membranes may not be warranted for the purpose of initiating internal monitoring. One of the possible treatment regimens is to sedate the mother, which would be contraindicated with ruptured membranes (see below, Medical Management).

Maternal and Fetal Outcome

If hypertonic labor is diagnosed and treated appropriately, maternal and fetal sequelae should be minimal. If the labor is prolonged, the mother may become exhausted, and there is an increased risk of infection and postpartum hemorrhage. If the labor is obstructed but allowed to continue, the normal physiological retraction ring can become excessive, developing into a pathological retraction ring, with the potential for uterine rupture.

Because of the elevated intrauterine pressure, blood flow to and oxygen perfusion of the placenta may be impaired, causing uteroplacental insufficiency. The fetus may experience late decelerations and severe fetal distress.

Medical Management

Cesarean section is warranted if the fetus is in distress or if fetopelvic disproportion is strongly suspected. Otherwise, if the membranes are intact, an attempt is made to interrupt the discoordinate contraction pattern. Usually, this is done by administering morphine or meperidine (Demerol) in a sufficient

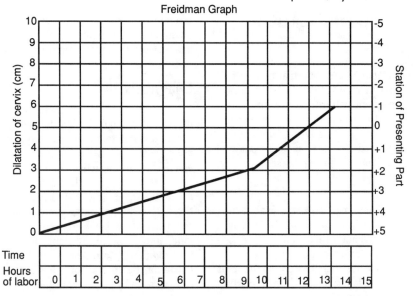

Figure 34.2. Friedman graph. Example of a graph illustrating a protraction disorder (primigravida).

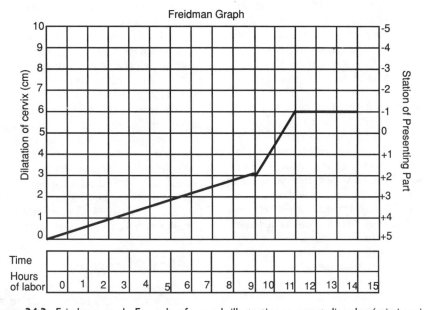

Figure 34.3. Friedman graph. Example of a graph illustrating an arrest disorder (primigravida).

dose to relieve pain and allow the patient to sleep for several hours. Narcotics are preferred over other drugs that could be used for sedation because of the ready availability of narcotic antagonists such as Narcan and Nalline. If the treatment is successful, when the patient awakes, the uterus will resume a normal labor pattern. Tocolytic agents have been used successfully in other countries to arrest hypertonic labor (1).

Administration of oxytocin rarely, if ever, is indicated to treat hypertonic labor. If it is used at all, it is only after rest has proved unsuccessful. Oxytocin is used for a short time only in the attempt to establish a normal labor pattern. Close monitoring of both intrauterine pressure and fetal heart rate is mandatory if oxytocin is used in the presence of hypertonic labor. If a normal labor pattern cannot be established or if fetal distress occurs, delivery by cesarean section is necessary.

HYPOTONIC LABOR

Definition

Hypotonic labor is the abnormal pattern that results from uterine contractions that have a normal pressure gradient pattern but are insufficient in intensity or frequency to result in cervical change or fetal descent. This type of uterine dysfunction usually occurs during the active phase of the first stage of labor or during the second stage.

Etiology

There are many maternal and fetal factors known to cause or contribute to hypotonic labor. However, in an individual case it is often not possible to determine the specific etiology.

Any factor that obstructs descent of the fetus may cause hypotonic labor: fetopelvic disproportion (e.g., from a large fetus or a contracted maternal pelvis—see Chapter 35), fetal anomalies (e.g., hydrocephaly), fetal malpresentation or position (see Chapter 36), or abnormalities of the soft tissue of the birth canal (e.g., tumors). The development of hypotonic labor in this case seems to be protective against the futility of continued strong contractions that may result eventually in uterine rupture.

Many maternal factors may cause or contribute to hypotonic labor. The muscle contractions of normal labor require adequate calories and electrolytes. Electrolyte imbalance, dehydration, and nutritional deprivation may all contribute to ineffective uterine contractions. The role of maternal anxiety is less clear, but it may be that catecholamines released during a "fight or flight" response divert blood flow away from the uterus and result in poor uterine action.

Excessive analgesia or regional anesthesia, particularly if administered before active labor is well established, may cause hypotonic labor for a time. A normal labor pattern usually resumes when the anesthesia or analgesia wears off. Amnionitis may cause hypotonic labor (or it may result from the prolonged labor caused by the hypotonic contractions). Overdistention of the uterus, as with multiple gestation or polyhydramnios, also may cause hypotonic uterine dysfunction.

Signs and Symptoms

Hypotonic labor is characterized by abnormally slow progress in cervical effacement and dilatation and fetal descent. The contractions are mild and may be infrequent. Since hypotonic labor usually occurs after the onset of active labor, the contractions become progressively milder, less frequent, and less painful. The patient feels quite well and may use the break from painful contractions to rest or sleep.

Diagnosis

The diagnosis of hypotonic labor is made only during active labor. It must be clear that the slow progress is due to a problem with active labor and *not* to a normal latent phase. Cervical dilatation and descent in the active phase may be abnormally slow (protracted—less than 1.2 cm/hour dilatation for nulliparas or less than 1.5 cm/hour for multiparas), or they may stop completely (arrest). This abnormally slow labor progress is accompanied by mild, infrequent contractions. Internal electronic fetal monitoring can be used to document the intensity of the contractions, but the diagnosis also can be made by palpation of the uterus.

Maternal and Fetal Outcome

Although the mother may feel well during hypotonic uterine dysfunction, the potential sequelae are not benign. The labor may be prolonged, with the potential for maternal exhaustion, intrauterine infection (especially if the membranes are ruptured), and postpartum hemorrhage. The incidence of cesarean section is increased.

The fetus usually does well initially during hypotonic labor since the contractions usually are not strong enough to threaten uteroplacental blood flow. However, the malpresentation, malposition, and/or fetopelvic disproportion that often cause hypotonic labor may in themselves threaten fetal well-being (see Chapters 35 and 36). Because of the potential for prolonged labor, the fetus is at risk for intrauterine infection, especially if the membranes are ruptured.

Medical Management

Medical management begins with prevention of hypotonic labor. All laboring patients should be given intravenous fluids or oral fluids and perhaps easily digestible foods to maintain their hydration, electrolyte balance, and energy for the work of labor.

Since a full bladder may interfere with effective uterine contractions, and occasionally a full bladder or rectum may impede fetal descent, attention must be paid to elimination status. The laboring patient should be encouraged to empty her bladder frequently. Catheterization should be performed if necessary to ensure that the bladder is empty. An enema should be given if it seems possible that a full rectum could obstruct fetal descent.

Ambulation or an upright position may enhance labor. Gravity may aid descent of the fetal presenting part. This will encourage pressure of the presenting part or the amniotic sac against the cervix, thus enhancing their function as a dilating wedge. Mechanical stretching of the cervix resulting from the increased pressure will stimulate the Ferguson reflex, which enhances uterine activity. The exact physiologic mechanism of the Ferguson reflex is not clear. It once was thought that stretching the cervix stimulated the release of oxytocin from the pituitary gland, but this has not been proven. It may be that it stimulates local production and release of prostaglandin $F_2\alpha$ (1, p 308).

Uterine contractions have been shown to be of greater intensity and of greater effectiveness in producing cervical dilatation in the lateral recumbent position as opposed to the supine position. The lateral position or squatting may increase pelvic diameters slightly and thus allow delivery of a larger infant than could be delivered in the lithotomy position.

Position changes also may be useful in helping a fetus in a posterior or transverse position to rotate to the more favorable occiput anterior position. The hands and knees position or laying on the same side as the fetal small parts may help facilitate rotation to the anterior position.

Since an excessive dose or early administration of analgesia or anesthesia may inhibit uterine contractions, the judicious use of analgesia/anesthesia may prevent hypotonic labor. Patient education and emotional support by the patient's family and friends and the staff may help allay maternal anxiety and thus prevent hypotonic labor.

Once the diagnosis of hypotonic labor has been made, the first step is to try to determine the cause. Fetopelvic disproportion often is the cause (see Chapter 35). Except in rare cases, however, fetopelvic disproportion cannot be diagnosed without a trial of labor (i.e., documentation of lack of progress in labor in the presence of adequate uterine contractions). Therefore, an adequate labor pattern must be reestablished, if possible. Cesarean section is indicated whenever there is fetopelvic disproportion, fetal distress, inability to reestablish a normal contraction pattern, failure to progress over a 2- to 3-hour period in the presence of adequate contractions, or fetal or maternal abnormalities that prevent delivery (e.g., fetal hydrocephaly or maternal soft tissue tumors obstructing the birth canal).

If there is no obvious mechanical cause of the dystocia and the fetus is in good condition, the goal of management is to reestablish a normal labor pattern. All of the measures cited above may be used to try to enhance the effectiveness of the contractions before more intervening steps are taken.

Several additional steps may be taken to try to reestablish normal labor. An enema may be given both to evacuate the bowel and to try to stimulate labor, although the effectiveness of the latter is controversial. It is postulated that irritation of the bowel causes irritation and stimulation of the nearby uterus.

Amniotomy may be performed in an attempt to stimulate labor. The manipulation of the cervix or the change in pressure on the cervix may stimulate the release of prostaglandins. If the amniotic sac has been an ineffective dilating wedge, amniotomy may allow the presenting part of the fetus to descend and exert more effective mechanical pressure on the cervix. Clinical research has not documented the effectiveness of amniotomy in shortening labor except in multiparas in the latent phase of labor. Many practitioners, however, report that amniotomy often seems to improve the labor pattern. Some practitioners employ it as an intermediate step since amniotomy is necessary for the institution of internal electronic fetal monitoring, which should be used if oxytocin augmentation is to be started.

Nipple stimulation has been used as a method of endogenous oxytocin augmentation. A sample protocol is as follows. The patient is given a rough-textured cloth, such as a towel, and is instructed to rub one nipple for 30 seconds. If no increase in the contraction pattern develops over the next 4–5 minutes, she is instructed to rub the nipple again, this time for 1 minute. If no increase in the contraction pattern develops after another 4–5 minutes, she is instructed to rub the other side for 1 minute. If an improved contraction pattern is not seen after several attempts, nipple stimulation is discontinued.

There is some evidence that nipple stimulation can cause hypertonic contractions, so it should be used only when electronic fetal monitoring, preferably internal monitoring, can be employed and only when an attendant can time it carefully.

The final treatment for improving labor quality is oxytocin (Pitocin) augmentation. Chapter 37 discusses in depth the indications, protocols, and precautions for oxytocin augmentation.

Again, cesarean section or forceps delivery may be necessary if contractions sufficient to effect spontaneous delivery cannot be achieved or if fetal distress ensues.

NURSING MANAGEMENT

Nursing care specific for a patient with *dystocia of labor:*

☐ For all patients
— Screen for abnormal labor patterns:
* Evaluate contraction pattern, clinically or by electronic fetal monitoring, noting frequency, intensity, and duration of contractions, and time between contractions; and
* Evaluate progress in cervical dilation and effacement and descent of the presenting part; compare to normal parameters of labor (see Fig. 35.1 and Table 35.1).
— Enhance normal progress in labor:
* Ensure adequate nutrition/hydration by oral or intravenous route;
* Encourage ambulation; encourage position changes (avoiding dorsal recumbent) if patient is confined to bed;
* Ensure that bowel and bladder are empty; encourage patient to empty bladder at least every 2 hours; catheterize if necessary; administer enema if necessary; and
* Encourage relaxation (e.g., by use of comfort measures, breathing/relaxation techniques, presence of support person).

☐ For patients experiencing *labor dystocia*:
— Be alert to signs/symptoms of sequelae of prolonged labor dystocia (e.g., maternal exhaustion, intrauterine infection, development of pathological retraction ring).
— Be prepared for cesarean section, forceps delivery, neonatal resuscitation, and/or postpartum hemorrhage.

☐ For patients with *hypertonic labor,* administer narcotics for sedation, as necessary; monitor effectiveness; have narcotic antagonist available.

☐ For patients with *hypotonic labor*:
— Assist with amniotomy, as necessary; note color, amount, odor of amniotic fluid; note fetal heart rate before and after amniotomy.
— Teach patient/partner how to perform nipple stimulation; monitor effectiveness, fetal status.
— Administer oxytocin augmentation of labor as required (see Chapter 37).

Nursing diagnoses most frequently associated with *dystocia* **(see Section V):**

☐ Knowledge deficit regarding etiology, disease process, treatment, and outcome.
☐ Altered fetal cardiac and cerebral tissue perfusion.
☐ Pain.
☐ Anxiety/fear.
☐ Knowledge deficit regarding pregnancy, process of labor and delivery, concerns of the postpartum period, parenting.

REFERENCE

1. Pritchard JA, MacDonald PC, Gant NF: *Williams Obstetrics,* ed 17. Norwalk, CT, Appleton-Century-Crofts, 1985, p 647.

Chapter 35
Cephalopelvic Disproportion
Suzanne M. Smith, C.N.M., M.S., M.P.H.

INTRODUCTION

The pelvis consists of four bones: the two innominate bones made up of the ileum, the ischium, and the pubis; the sacrum; and the coccyx. Together they form the curved passageway through which the fetus must pass during labor. The inclination of the pelvis, when the woman is upright, is 60°. The axis of the birth canal, called the curve of Carus, is the direction the baby must move as it passes through the pelvis (i.e., down and backward to the level of the ischial spines, and then down and forward (Fig. 35.1).

The pelvic architecture is not identical in all humans. There are significant differences between male and female pelves, not considered here. However, there also are differences in size and shape of the female pelvis, which vary from woman to woman. Historically, many researchers and practitioners have attempted to identify and classify pelvic differences.

In 1933 Caldwell and Moloy (1) classified the female pelvis into four pure types according to the shape of the inlet and the morphology of the mid and lower pelvis. Not all women possess a pelvis of pure type. In many cases the inlet shape may be identified, followed by a description of the mid and/or lower pelvic morphology. In still other mixed types, two classifications may be hyphenated, with the first term referring to the shape of the posterior segment and the second term referring to the shape of the anterior segment.

The four pure types of Caldwell and Moloy are:

1. Gynecoid (typical female)
2. Android (similar to male configuration)
3. Anthropoid (upright or ape-like)
4. Platypelloid (flat)

See Table 35.1 and Fig. 35.2 for comparison of the four pelvic types.

Clinical Evaluation of the Pelvis

In many institutions the nurse performs vaginal examinations during labor. In such cases, attention should be directed not only to effacement and dilatation of the cervix, status of the amniotic membranes, and station of the presenting part but also to clinical

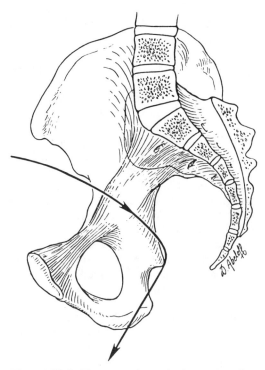

Figure 35.1. The axis of the birth canal is illustrated. The axis turns forward at the level of the ischial spine. (Used with permission from Caplan RM (ed): *Principles of Obstetrics.* Baltimore, Williams & Wilkins, 1982, p 86.)

Table 35.1.

PELVIC TYPES

CHARACTERISTIC	GYNECOID	ANDROID	ANTHROPOID	PLATYPELLOID
Shape of inlet	Round or slightly oval	Wedge or heart shaped	Long, narrow anteroposterior oval	Long, transverse oval
Retropubic angle (anterior segment) (forepelvis)	Well rounded, wide	Angulated, narrowed	Well rounded, long, narrow, deep	Rounded or slightly flattened; very wide, shallow
Posterior segment	Well rounded, roomy	Flat, wide, sacral promontory protrudes	Long, narrow, deep	Flat, very wide, shallow
Inclination curvature of sacrum	Average, concave	Inclined forward, flat	Average—backward sacrum is long (may have six vertebrae) and narrow	Average sacrum may be shallow or hollow
Sidewalls	Straight, parallel	Converging	Straight or converging	Straight or may converge slightly
Sacrosciatic notch	Medium width	Narrow, high arch	Shallow, very wide	Narrow
Ischial spines	Not prominent	Prominent	Variable	Variable
Bispinous diameter	Wide	Narrow	Less than average	Very wide
Bituberous diameter	Adequate	Reduced	Adequate	Very wide
Subpubic arch	Wide, ≥90° "Norman arch"	Narrow, wedge-shaped 70° "Gothic arch"	Normal or slightly narrow	Very wide
Bone structure overall	Medium delicate	Medium heavy	Average delicate	Medium delicate
Prognosis for delivery	Good	Poor	Good	Poor; often requires cesarean section for CPD

evaluation of the pelvis. The procedure and findings of clinical pelvimetry are presented here.

After completion of routine bimanual pelvic examination, the bony pelvis is evaluated and its dimensions estimated. Performance of clinical pelvimetry generally causes some discomfort to the mother; thus, measures to aid her in relaxation are beneficial. Perhaps the most useful comfort measure is communication. Explanation of what is being done, why, and the findings will greatly facilitate the mother's cooperation with the examination. Likewise, avoidance of obvious causes of discomfort, such as examination during uterine contractions or excessively long examinations, will aid in evaluation of the pelvis. The mother should be prevented from feeling that she is "failing" the examination.

A consistent, organized, and thorough method of pelvic evaluation will permit the examiner to obtain comprehensive information that can be evaluated for specific dimensions as well as determination of pelvic type.

Before beginning the examination, the patient's bladder should be empty, and she should be in the lithotomy position.

The procedure, findings, and illustration of clinical pelvimetry are found in Table 35.2 and Figure 35.3A-E. The most important pelvic measurements that can be determined clinically are found in Table 35.3. A knowledge of the average diameters of the pelvis is necessary for comparison with the clinical pelvimetry findings in order to evaluate normalcy or deviations from normal. Average pelvic dimensions are listed in Table 35.4 (see also Fig. 35.4A and B).

DEFINITION

Fetopelvic disproportion is the inability of the fetus to pass through the maternal pelvis. However, since the majority of fetuses present as cephalic, cephalopelvic disproportion (CPD) is the term commonly used.

Successful vaginal delivery depends upon the relationship of the powers (uterine contractions and maternal expulsive efforts), the passageway (the maternal pelvis), and the passenger (the fetus). Disproportion may occur when there is a problem with any of the three.

Disproportion may be absolute or relative. Absolute CPD exists when the fetus cannot be delivered safely through the pelvis. Cesarean section is required. Relative CPD exists when other factors

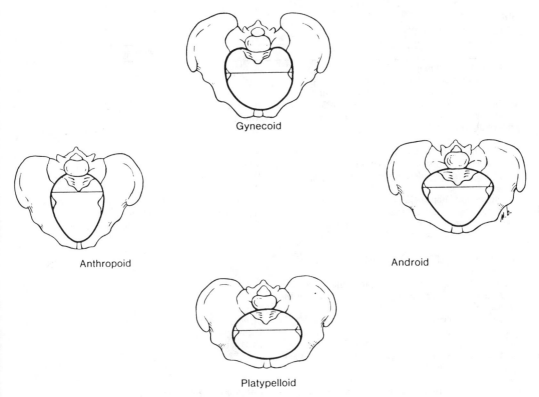

Gynecoid

Anthropoid

Android

Platypelloid

Figure 35.2. The four "pure" types of pelves. (Used with permission from Caplan RM (ed). *Principles of Obstetrics.* Baltimore, Williams & Wilkins, 1982, p 245.)

contribute to the problem. With appropriate treatment, labor complicated by relative CPD may result in vaginal delivery.

ETIOLOGY

As is evident by the definition, CPD is caused primarily by the difference between the size of the fetus and that of the maternal pelvis. Relative CPD may be caused by fetal factors such as an unfavorable fetal position or presentation, incomplete flexion of the fetal head, large baby, relative inability of the fetal head to mold, and fetal anomalies. Factors that affect the passageway are the size and shape of the bony pelvis and soft tissue resistance. The shape of the bony pelvis may be disadvantageous by genetic design or may be altered by musculoskeletal problems, such as rickets or scoliosis (see Chapter 14). The size of the pelvis *may* be small in young teenagers who reached menarche within the past 2–3 years (2). Soft tissue abnormalities such as a rigid cervix, vaginal septum, uterine fibromyomas, and ovarian cysts may impede delivery. Finally, factors related to the powers are inefficient uterine contractions (see Chapter 34) or

poor maternal expulsive efforts from exhaustion, regional anesthesia, or ineffective pushing techniques.

SIGNS AND SYMPTOMS

CPD commonly is indicated by abnormalities in labor. There may be delay or arrest of cervical dilatation during the first stage of labor. Failure or cessation of descent of the fetus through the pelvis also may occur either during the first or second stage (see Chapter 34).

DIAGNOSIS

Clinical estimation of pelvic type and size is particularly beneficial to alert the practitioner to the possibility of CPD. Clinical pelvimetry should be evaluated initially during the antepartum course and repeated during labor. Estimation of fetal weight as well as determination of presentation, position, and station within the pelvis also should be done during labor.

If the pelvis is estimated to be borderline or contracted in size; if the fetus appears unusually

Table 35.2.
CLINICAL PELVIMETRY

PROCEDURE	FINDINGS[a]
Evaluation of the symphysis pubis	
Care is taken not to exert undue pressure on the sensitive anterior structures (urethra and clitoris).	
○Estimation of overall bone structure. Gentle palpation of the symphysis between the vaginal fingers internally and the thumb externally.	*Average* Thin Thick
○Determination of retropubic angle and shape of the forepelvis. Side-to-side movement of the vaginal fingers against the internal surface of the symphysis.	*Average (gently rounded)* Wide (flattened) Narrow (sharply angled)
○Evaluation of subpubic arch (angle). Position the fingers along the undersurface of the symphysis and separate them until the descending rami are felt.	*Average (approximately 90° angle or 2 fingerbreadths)* Wide (greater than 2½ fingerbreadths) Narrow (tight placement of 2 fingerbreadths; unable to separate fingers)
Evaluation of the pelvic sidewalls and ischial spines/bispinous diameter	
Maintain the vaginal fingers as near to the pelvic brim as possible while moving along to the right side of the pelvis.	
○Splay of the sidewalls. Place the thumb of the examining hand on the ischial tuberosity externally and draw the vaginal fingers downward, maintaining contact along the ramus of the ischium, to the inner aspect of the tuberosity.	*Straight (parallel)* Convergent Divergent
○Palpation of the ischial spine. Maintain the thumb in contact with the tuberosity after the vaginal fingers are drawn down to the inside. Direct the vaginal fingers backward and upward at a 45° angle for approximately one-third to one-half the distance traveled along the sidewall. If the ischial spine is not readily appreciated by this maneuver, release the thumb's position. Move the fingers backward and upward until contact is lost with the bony pelvis. The fingers should now be in the greater sciatic notch, and the sacro-spinous ligament may be located at its base. The ligament will feel like a tautly stretched rubberband. By palpating along the ligament forward, the ischial spine will be the point of contact with bone since the ligament inserts onto the spine. The length of the ligament and thus the width of the sacrosciatic notch also is evaluated in this way.	*Not prominent (blunt or flat)* *Average/palpable (readily identified)* Prominent (sharp or encroaching) *Average = 2–2½ fingerbreadths (3–4 cm)*
○Evaluation of the opposite (left) sidewall and ischial spine. The examining hand is pronated and the maneuvers are repeated on the left side of the pelvis.	
○Estimation of the bispinous diameter. After both ischial spines have been located, the fingers should be swept across the pelvis, touching each spine. Alternatively, one finger may be placed on one of the spines and the fingers separated until the other spine is reached. This is only possible, however, in the case of a very narrow bispinous diameter.	Cannot be measured clinically, but impression can be obtained. *Average bispinous diameter is 10.5 cm* Generally recorded as adequate or reduced by impression
Evaluation of the sacrum and coccyx.	
○The examing fingers should be swept both side to side and up and down the sacrum to determine both lateral and longitudinal curves.	Sacrum: *Concave (gently curved)* Hollow (curvature accentuated, J shaped) Flat (minimal curve)
○The relationship of the coccyx to the sacrum and the mobility of the coccyx are evaluated by moving the	*Average (curves smoothly with the sacrum)* Forward inclination (protrudes into pelvis, relative to

Table 35.2.

(Continued)

PROCEDURE	FINDINGS[a]
fingers downward until the coccyx is reached. Gentle pressure and release of the coccyx should provide the sensation of slight movement.	sacrum) Backward inclination (curves away behind direction of sacral curve) Coccyx: *Mobile* Fixed
Estimation of diagonal conjugate 　Evaluation of the diagonal conjugate is the most uncomfortable portion of clinical pelvimetry determination and thus is performed as the final intravaginal maneuver. Pressure should be exerted against the perineum, not against the anterior surfaces throughout the maneuver. The examining fingers are "walked" upwards along the sacrum as far as possible. When it is not possible to move higher in the pelvis or when the sacral promontory has been reached, the examining hand is raised so that the area between the index finger and the thumb rests along the undersurface of the symphysis pubis. This maneuver is facilitated if the examiner's leg on the same side of the body (ipsilateral) is rested upon a small step stool or the base of the examining table. The elbow of the examining arm should then be placed on the knee to align the elbow, forearm, wrist, hand, and fingers in a straight line. This provides the maximum reach with minimum patient discomfort. (The examiner should measure the distance from the tip of the longer finger to the junction of the thumb and forefinger in centimeters.)	If the sacral promontory is reached, the exact diagonal conjugate is measured. If the promontory is not reached, the diagonal conjugate is recorded as "greater than" the examiner's known measured distance. *Average diagonal conjugate = 12.5 cm*
Estimation of the bituberous diameter ○After removing the examining fingers from the vagina but before removing the glove, a fist is made and placed against the perineum, touching the inner surface of one tuberosity. The other tuberosity then is identified, and estimation of the total distance is made. (The examiner should measure the width of the clenched fist along the knuckles in centimeters).	If the examiner's fist fits or is smaller than the distance between the tuberosities, the exact bituberous diameter is recorded. If not, "greater than" the examiner's known measurement is recorded. *Average bituberous diameter = 11.0 cm*

[a]Normal findings are in italics.

large; or if malposition, malpresentation, or high presenting station is determined, careful observation of the labor pattern is warranted. Electronic fetal monitoring may be used to document the contraction pattern, and a graph of cervical dilatation and station versus time may be used to document labor progress (see Chapter 34, Fig. 34.2).

Confirmation of CPD may be made in several ways. Current practice most often utilizes a trial of labor when suspicion of CPD exists based on assessment of maternal or fetal factors. A trial of labor requires good contractions over a period of 2–3 hours. If spontaneous contractions are not adequate, oxytocin augmentation usually is undertaken if there is not absolute proof of CPD in order to maximize the uterine forces. Failure to progress after 2–3 hours of adequate contractions strongly suggests CPD.

In some cases, or at some institutions, ultrasonographic evaluation of the fetus or x-ray pelvimetry of the maternal pelvis may be employed. However, both technologies have limited usefulness in predicting the outcome of labor. Although the maternal pelvis may be measured accurately, it is not possible to assess the dynamic changes of fetal head molding, the effect of a change in fetal position, or the influence of maternal position on the pelvic diameters. Additionally, radiation exposure of the fetus is known to increase the risk of subsequently developing leukemia. Thus, the benefits of x-ray versus clinical pelvimetry are regarded as doubtful by some practitioners. It is progress in labor that determines both management and outcome rather than absolute measurements.

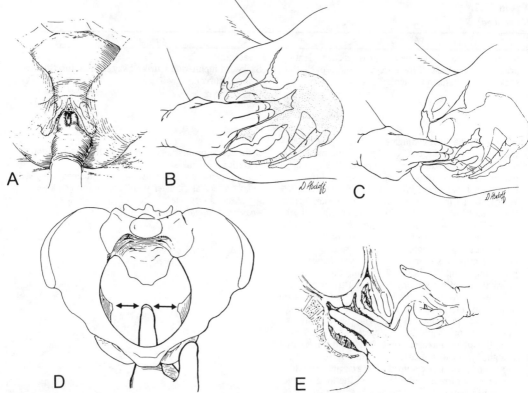

Figure 35.3. A, Estimation of contour of suprapubic angle. (From Wilson JR: *Management of Obstetric Difficulties,* ed 6. St. Louis, Mosby, 1961.) **B,** Palpating the pelvic sidewall. **C,** Palpating the ischial spine. (From Caplan RM (ed). *Principles of Obstetrics.* Baltimore, Williams & Wilkins, 1982, p 248.) **D,** Estimation of bispinous diameter. (From Moloy HC: *Evaluation of the Pelvis in Obstetrics.* Philadelphia, WB Saunders, 1951.) **E,** Estimation of diagonal conjugate diameter. (From Willson JR: *Management of Obstetric Difficulties,* ed 6. St. Louis, Mosby, 1961.)

MATERNAL AND FETAL OUTCOME

If CPD is diagnosed and treated properly, the outcome for both mother and baby can be expected to be good, although there is an increased likelihood of operative delivery. Continued labor in the presence of CPD may lead to abnormal thinning of the lower uterine segment, the development of the pathologic retraction ring of Bandl, and possibly uterine rupture. The mother's bladder may be damaged by the pressure of the presenting part. Pelvic lacerations may result from instrumental delivery. Postpartum hemorrhage or uterine infection may

Table 35.3.
OBSTETRICALLY SIGNIFICANT PELVIC MEASUREMENTS

PELVIC MEASUREMENT	NORMAL FINDINGS
1. Obstetric conjugate	11.0 cm
2. Diagonal conjugate (Note: Diagonal conjugate minus 1.5 cm approximates obstetric conjugate)	12.5 cm
3. Transverse diameter of the plane of least pelvic dimensions (bispinous)	10.5 cm
4. Transverse diameter of the outlet (bituberous)	11.0 cm
5. Subpubic angle	90° (2 fingerbreadths)
6. Curve and length of the sacrum	Concave, average curvature
7. Sacrospinous ligament (width of the sacrosciatic notch)	2–2½ fingerbreadths

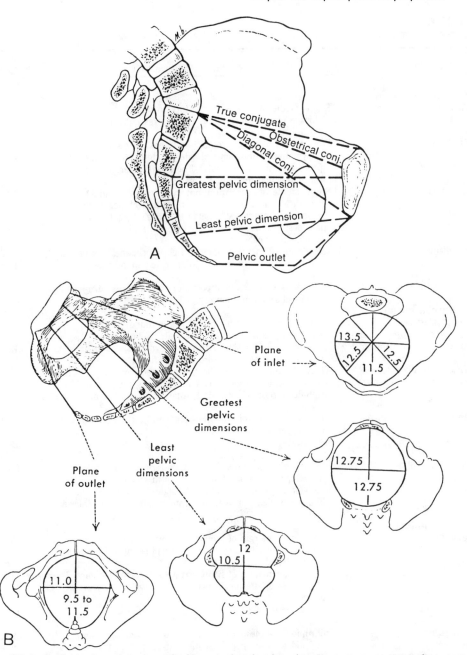

Figure 35.4. A, Sagittal section through the articulated pelvis showing anteroposterior diameters and major planes. (From Caplan RM (ed). *Principles of Obstetrics.* Baltimore, Williams & Wilkins, 1982, p 86.) **B,** Diameters in centimeters of various planes of pelvis. (From Danforth DN (ed). *Obstetrics and Gynecology,* ed. 3. Hagerstown, MD, Harper & Row, 1977, p 478.)

occur if labor is prolonged. Ultimately, maternal death may occur.

Fetal outcome may include fetal distress, intracranial hemorrhage, skull fracture, neurologic damage, or perinatal death.

MEDICAL MANAGEMENT

Initial management is directed toward recognizing and/or confirming the diagnosis of

Table 35.4.
PELVIC DIAMETERS

PLANE/DIAMETER	DESCRIPTION/SIGNIFICANCE	AVERAGE MEASUREMENT
Inlet		
Anteroposterior diameters		
Anatomic conjugate (true conjugate)	From middle of sacral promontory to middle of superior surface of symphysis pubis (pubic crest). No obstetric significance.	11.5 cm
Obstetric conjugate	From middle of sacral promontory to posterior superior margin of symphysis pubis (approximately 1 cm below pubic crest; protrudes into pelvic cavity). The anteroposterior diameter through which the fetus passes.	11.0 cm
Diagonal conjugate	From middle of sacral promontory to subpubic angle. Significant because it can be measured clinically and the obstetric conjugate estimated by subtracting 1.5 cm.	12.5 cm
Transverse diameter	The widest distance between the iliopectineal lines (linea terminalis or pelvic brim).	13.5 cm
Oblique diameters	Left: From left sacroiliac joint to right iliopectineal eminence.	12.5 cm
	Right: From right sacroiliac joint to left iliopectineal eminence.	12.5 cm
Posterior sagittal	From intersection of anteroposterior and transverse diameters to middle of sacral promontory.	4.5 cm
Midpelvis (pelvic cavity)		
Plane of greatest pelvic dimensions	The roomiest plane of the pelvis, nearly round. Obstetric significance is minimal because of its spaciousness.	
Anteroposterior diameter	From midpoint of posterior surface of symphysis pubis to junction of second and third sacral vertebrae.	12.75 cm
Transverse diameter	Widest distance between the lateral aspects of the midpelvis.	12.75 cm
Plane of least pelvic dimensions	The smallest, least roomy plane of the pelvis, thus the most significant obstetrically. Most instances of arrest of progress occur at this level.	
Anteroposterior diameter	From lower border of symphysis pubis to junction of fourth and fifth sacral vertebrae.	12.0 cm
Transverse diameter (bispinous)	Between the ischial spines.	10.5 cm
Posterior sagittal	From the intersection of the anteroposterior and transverse diameter to junction of fourth and fifth sacral vertebrae.	4.5–5.0 cm
Outlet	An angulated plane made of two triangle-shaped planes with the bituberous diameter as their common base and most inferior part.	
Anteroposterior diameters		
Anatomic	From inferior margin of symphysis pubis to tip of coccyx. Not significant because a mobile coccyx will be pushed out of the way by the advancing fetus.	9.5 cm
Obstetric	From inferior margin of symphysis pubis to sacroiliac joint. The actual anteroposterior diameter through which the fetus passes.	11.5 cm
Transverse diameter (bituberous)	Between the inner surfaces of ischial tuberosities.	11.0 cm
Posterior sagittal	From middle of bituberous diameter to sacrococcygeal joint.	9.0 cm
Anterior sagittal	From middle of bituberous diameter to subpubic angle.	6.0 cm

CPD. The process begins, as mentioned above, during the antepartum course. Clinical examination of the pelvis commonly is performed during the initial antepartum examination. Fetal size, engagement, presentation, and position are estimated in late pregnancy and during labor. Reevaluation of clinical pelvimetry and comparison of pelvic capacity with the dimensions of the presenting part are made early in labor. Except in rare instances of absolute disproportion, a trial of labor is indicated. Final estimation of disproportion by x-ray pelvimetry to compare pelvic and fetal dimensions may or may not be performed.

In cases of relative CPD, management may be directed toward relieving factors that contribute to CPD. Fetal position may be improved by having the mother change position (e.g., lying on the same side as fetal small parts or assuming a hands and knees position to facilitate rotation of the baby into an anterior position). A squatting position may increase the anteroposterior diameter of the outlet as much as 0.5–2.0 cm (3). Maternal pushing efforts can be facilitated by avoidance of regional anesthesia and by proper instruction and support during the second stage of labor. The efficiency of uterine forces may be enhanced by adequate nutrition and hydration; an empty bladder; ambulation or an upright position; patient education and support to minimize anxiety; and perhaps by an enema, amniotomy, or nipple stimulation.

In most cases careful oxytocin stimulation of labor will be attempted while monitoring both maternal and fetal well-being (see Chapter 37). Cesarean section without adequate trial of labor is appropriate only in those instances in which the risks to the mother or fetus are excessive.

Instrumental delivery with forceps or vacuum extractor may be employed for delivery. Cesarean section is the ultimate treatment when CPD has been demonstrated.

NURSING MANAGEMENT

Nursing care specific for a patient with cephalopelvic disproportion:

☐ Enhance normal progress in labor by:
— Ensuring that the patient maintains adequate hydration and nutrition, either orally or intravenously;
— Encouraging ambulation if appropriate, or frequent position changes (avoiding the dorsal recumbent position) if the patient is in bed;
— Ensuring that bladder and bowel are empty, encourage the patient to empty her bladder at least every 2 hours, catheterize her if necessary, administer an enema if necessary; and
— Encouraging the patient to relax by the presence and support of her significant other, and by use of breathing and relaxation techniques, comfort measures, and patient education.

☐ Enhance fetal descent in the second stage by:
— Teaching proper pushing techniques; and
— Encouraging a position that will maximize pelvic diameters and utilize the force of gravity, e.g., squatting, pushing on the toilet, sitting upright.

☐ Administer oxytocin as ordered (see Chapter 37).

☐ Be alert to signs/symptoms of sequelae of prolonged CPD (e.g., pathological retraction ring, uterine rupture [see Chapter 41], intrauterine infection [see Chapter 30]).

☐ Be prepared for cesarean section, forceps delivery, neonatal resuscitation, and postpartum hemorrhage.

Nursing diagnoses most frequently associated with cephalopelvic disproportion (see Section V):

☐ Disturbance in body image, self-esteem.

☐ Knowledge deficit regarding etiology, disease process, treatment, and outcome.

☐ Altered fetal cardiac and cerebral tissue perfusion.

☐ Pain.

☐ Anxiety/fear.

☐ Impaired skin integrity.

☐ Altered nutrition: less than body requirements.

REFERENCES

1. Caldwell WE, Moloy HC: Anatomical variations in the female pelvis. *Am J Obstet Gynecol* 26:479, 1933.

2. Sherline DM: When the mother is a child herself. *Contemp OB/GYN* 24:83–90, 1984.

3. Roberts J: Alternative positions for childbirth. *J Nurse-Midwifery* 25:13–19, 1980.

Chapter 36
Abnormal Fetal Presentation
Suzanne M. Smith, C.N.M., M.S., M.P.H.

INTRODUCTION

Presentation refers to the part of the fetus that lies over the pelvic inlet, becomes engaged, and can be felt through the cervix during vaginal examination (1). The most frequent presentation (96%) is cephalic, with the occiput the most dependent part. Other less frequent presentations include breech and shoulder.

In order to describe presentation in terms of abdominal and vaginal findings, the following terminology is used (2):

1. Lie—relationship of the long axis of the fetus to the long axis of the mother (e.g., longitudinal, transverse, or oblique).
2. Attitude—relationship of the fetal parts to one another (e.g., flexed or extended).
3. Denominator—an arbitrarily chosen point on the presenting part of the fetus used to describe position. Each presentation has its own denominator.
4. Position—relationship of the denominator to the right or left anterior, transverse, or posterior portion of the maternal pelvis (e.g., left occiput posterior [LOP]).

COMPOUND PRESENTATION

Definition

Compound presentation is the prolapse or concurrent presentation of an extremity with the presenting part. Most often, a fetal hand or arm presents alongside or before the vertex. An arm or hand presents approximately one out of every 700 deliveries

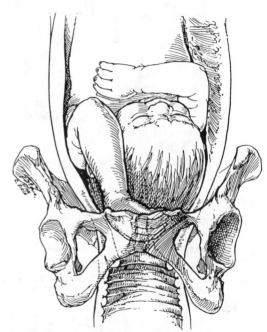

Figure 36.1. Compound presentation. The right hand is lying in front of the vertex. With further labor the hand and arm may retract from the birth canal and the head descend normally. (From Cunningham FG, MacDonald PC, Gant NF: *Williams Obstetrics*, ed 18. Norwalk, CT, Appleton-Lange, 1988, p 365.)

(2, p 659) (Fig. 36.1). Less frequently, an arm may prolapse alongside a breech presentation, and, even more rarely, a leg may present alongside the vertex.

Etiology

No specific cause has been identified for compound presentations. However, any factors that predispose to a loose-fitting presenting part are contributory. For example, an extremely large maternal pelvis may predispose toward compound presentation simply because it is too roomy. However, compound presentation most often occurs in small or premature babies when the presenting part is not big enough to fill the pelvis or in cases where the presenting part has not entered the pelvis prior to labor.

Signs and Symptoms

Signs and symptoms are similar to those of fetopelvic disproportion. In such cases the progress of labor may be impeded, since the compound presentation may interfere with the pressure of the presenting part on the cervix. The contractions may become less frequent and less intense, cervical dilatation will cease or occur very slowly, and little descent occurs.

The mother occasionally may report movement of the extremity in the pelvis or lower uterine segment.

Diagnosis

The compound presentation, particularly that of a hand alongside the vertex, often is not identified before delivery. In a normal spontaneous vaginal delivery, the hand may deliver with the vertex.

At other times the prolapsed extremity will be palpated during vaginal examination in labor. Rarely, compound presentation will be diagnosed by x-ray or ultrasonogram performed for another indication.

Maternal and Fetal Outcome

In most cases the presence of a compound presentation has no effect on the mother or the course of labor. Generally, as labor progresses, the presenting part will descend further into the pelvis and deliver before the extremity. In some cases, as mentioned above, the extremity may deliver with the presenting part. The increased diameter of the compound presentation may necessitate an episiotomy or cause a more extensive vaginal laceration. As stated before, delay in descent or cervical dilation may be the first clinical appearance of compound presentation. If no progress has been made, cesarean section with all its attendant risks may be necessary.

Fetal risks vary. A compound occiput and hand usually present very little, if any, sequelae to the fetus. However, any compound presentation does carry with it the risk of umbilical cord prolapse, because the compounding part prevents the presenting part from filling the pelvic inlet completely. Hypoxia and, finally, anoxia can result from compression of the umbilical cord. In addition, there is increased risk of fracture or nerve damage to the extremity during delivery.

Medical Management

In situations where labor progress is slow or arrest of labor has occurred, particularly if the compound presentation has not been diagnosed, the management discussed in Chapter 34 regarding dystocia of labor would be utilized. When the situation is suspected or diagnosed, vaginal examination should be done gently in order to avoid dislodging the presenting parts and causing cord prolapse. The fetus should be monitored continuously and the tracing evaluated for signs and symptoms of distress that may result from occult cord compression.

Oxytocin may be used to stimulate or augment labor as needed. If the labor progresses normally, a vaginal delivery can be anticipated. A large episiotomy usually is performed to allow the larger presenting diameter to deliver without excessive trauma to maternal tissue.

If the vertex delivers with the arm or hand alongside, the extremity is grasped and guided gently and smoothly across the face to complete its delivery in the normal range of motion.

Forceps delivery may be indicated to hasten abnormally slow labor progress during the second stage. As in all forceps applications, it is critical that a careful and thorough vaginal examination be performed to identify the specific position of the fetus and to avoid the risk of trauma to the extremity caused by faulty application of the forceps (see Chapter 40).

Finally, cesarean section may be warranted because of failure of the labor to progress even with oxytocin or other methods of labor stimulation.

Cord prolapse and/or fetal distress are other indicators for emergency cesarean section.

ABNORMAL CEPHALIC PRESENTATIONS

Definition

The normal cephalic presentation is termed vertex. The attitude is well flexed, with the chin touching the chest. Any presentation other than a well-flexed vertex is abnormal. There are three abnormal cephalic presentations that occur as the degree of extension increases (Fig. 36.2).

1. Military: The fetal head is neither flexed nor extended. The attitude is called "military" because the head is the same degree of flexion/ extension as a soldier standing at attention. The denominator continues to be the occiput.

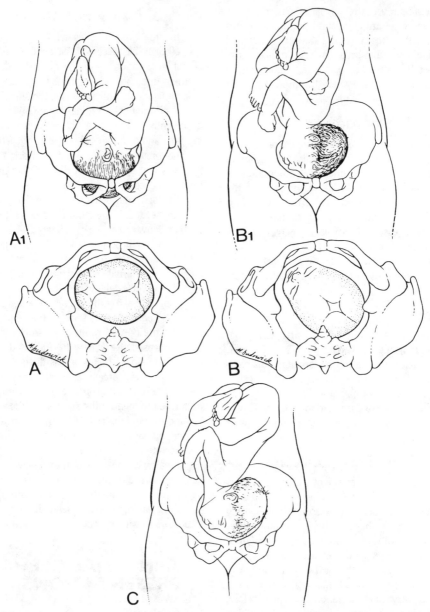

Figure 36.2. A, Longitudinal lie, cephalic presentation, left occiput transverse position. The fetal sagittal suture is in a transverse position. **B**, Brow presentation. On vaginal examination, the anterior fontanelle and brow are palpable; the posterior fontanelle is not. **C**, Extended attitude, face presentation. (From Caplan RM (ed). *Principles of Obstetrics*. Baltimore, Williams & Wilkins, 1982, pp 121, 264.)

2. Brow: The fetal head is extended partially so that the brow or forehead of the fetus presents to the pelvis. The denominator is the forehead (frontum).
3. Face: The fetal head is completely extended (hyperextended). In a face presentation, the occiput (back of the head) touches the back. The denominator is the chin (mentum).

Etiology

Generally, cephalic malpresentations result from a poor fit between the passenger and the passageway (the fetus is too large or the maternal pelvis is too small). Changes in attitude occur as the presenting part attempts to negotiate the birth canal.

Cephalic malpresentation may be caused by maternal or fetal factors. Maternal factors include alteration in the abdominal musculature, the pelvis, the uterus, or the placenta. Lax abdominal musculature allows the fetus excessive mobility and may prohibit proper alignment of the occiput over the birth canal. Pelvic malformations that decrease the size or the symmetry alter the pelvic diameters. Hip fracture, pelvic fracture, and rickets may decrease pelvic size and distort pelvic symmetry. Uterine fibroids and neoplasms also may encroach into the birth canal and decrease the diameter of the birth canal. Placenta previa interferes with the presenting part's ability to enter the birth canal.

Any congenital anomaly resulting in an abnormal fetal biparietal diameter is a causative factor. Thus, hydrocephaly or anencephaly often are associated with cephalic malpresentation and must be considered in the differential diagnosis. Fetal tumors of the neck or thyroid also are implicated. Polyhydramnios may allow the fetus to assume an abnormal presentation due to excessive mobility.

Signs and Symptoms

Labor may be prolonged or dysfunctional because of the less than optimum fit of the fetal presenting part within the lower uterine segment and pelvis. As in any such labor, careful assessment to identify a cause of dysfunction must be performed. There also may be findings associated with the predisposing factors (e.g., polyhydramnios, pelvic contracture, and uterine fibroid).

Diagnosis

Vaginal examination, combined with abdominal palpation, is the principal means of diagnosing an abnormal cephalic presentation. Table 36.1 details the technique used to perform abdominal examination. In the normal vertex presentation, the cephalic prominence on abdominal palpation is the forehead and will be on the side opposite the fetal back. On vaginal examination, the triangular-shaped posterior fortanel, sagittal suture, parietal bones, occipital bone, and part of the lambdoidal suture are palpable. The anterior fontanel and coronal and frontal sutures may not be palpable except through a well-dilated cervix and will be at a higher level in the pelvis.

Abdominal and vaginal findings diagnostic of military, brow, and face presentation are listed below (3):

1. Military: Abdominal palpation reveals essentially the same findings as in the normal vertex presentation. However, since the head is neither flexed nor extended, a cephalic prominence will not be identified. On vaginal examination, both anterior and posterior fontanels are palpable and will be at the same level within the pelvis. The position at time of diagnosis is most often transverse (left occiput transverse or right occiput transverse). In most cases the military presentation will flex to vertex during labor. Occasionally, however, further extension may occur either to a brow or a face presentation. Thus, this presentation rarely is seen at delivery.

2. Brow: The presenting part is the fetal forehead, between the orbital ridges and the bregma (anterior fontanel). On abdominal palpation, the occiput is the cephalic prominence and thus will be palpated on the same side as the fetal back. On vaginal examination, the anterior fontanelle and the frontal and coronal sutures will be palpable, but the sagittal suture generally will be out of reach. If the orbital ridges are identifiable, the diagnosis of brow presentation is confirmed. The brow may feel similar to the vertex on examination, and both molding and edema may obscure the differences further.

3. Face: The presenting part is the fetal face, between the orbital ridges and the chin. On abdominal palpation, the occiput is the cephalic prominence and thus will be palpated on the same side as the fetal back. Vaginal examination findings often are uncertain and may be confused with a breech. The face is soft and irregular rather than round, hard, and with the identifiable suture lines and fontanels of the vertex. However, identification of specific facial features (mouth, nose, and eyes) confirm the diagnosis. In some cases, particularly when labor progresses normally, the diagnosis may not be made until the face is visible at the introitus.

Following is a comparison of the diameters of the fetal head passing through the maternal pelvis:

Presentation	Diameter	Measurement
Vertex	Suboccipito-bregmatic	9.50 cm
Military	Occipitofrontal	11.75 cm
Brow	Occipitomental	13.50 cm
Face	Trachelobregmatic/submentobregmatic	9.50 cm

Table 36.1.
LEOPOLD'S MANEUVERS[a]

	PROCEDURE	FINDINGS	SIGNIFICANCE
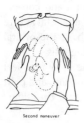First maneuver	**Step 1** Facing the woman's head, place the palmar surfaces of both hands over the fundus and palpate gently for the consistency, shape, size, and mobility of the fetal part in the fundus. Is it round, hard, smooth, and ballotable (as in a vertex) or softer, irregular in contour, and not ballotable (as in a breech)?	1.1 Fetal part feels round and hard, is readily movable, and can be ballotted between the thumb and a finger of one hand. 1.2 Fetal part feels irregular, larger/bulkier, and less firm than a head. It cannot be well delineated, readily moved, or ballotted. 1.3 Neither of the above is felt in the fundus.	1.1 Indicative of the fetal head. The mobility is a result of the head's being able to move independently of the trunk. The lie is longitudinal. 1.2 Indicative of the fetal breech, which cannot move independently of the trunk. The lie is longitudinal. 1.3 Indicative of a transverse lie.
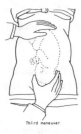Second maneuver	**Step 2** Continue to face the woman's head. Slide hands down from the top of the uterus over both sides equidistant from the midline. Stabilize the uterus with one examining hand and gently—but with deep pressure and rotary movement—palpate the other side for smoothness, resistance, convexity, and/or knobby, irregular masses. Repeat this procedure for examination of the other side of the uterus.	2.1 A firm, convex, continuously smooth, and resistant mass extends from the breech to the neck. 2.2 Small, knobby, irregular masses. May move when pressed on or may kick or hit the examiner's hand. 2.3 (See 1.1 and 1.2 above.) The head or breech is palpated on either side instead of in the fundus or at the symphysis pubis.	2.1 Indicative of the fetal back. The location of the back on the left or right side of the woman's abdomen indicates the position in a longitudinal lie. 2.2 Indicative of the fetal small parts (e.g., hands, feet, knees, and elbows). They should be on the opposite side of the woman than the fetal back. 2.3 Indicative of a transverse lie.
Third maneuver	**Step 3** The *Pawlick grip* confirms fetal lie and presentation. Continue to face the woman's head. It is essential that she have her knees slightly bent in order to avoid discomfort during this maneuver and the next. Grasp the presenting part between the fingers and the thumb of the right hand and grasp the part in the fundus with the other hand. It will be necessary to gently but firmly press into the abdomen in order to feel the presenting part below and between the fingers and thumb. As in the first step, palpate for size, shape, consistency, and mobility of the fetal part in the upper and lower pole of the uterus. Compare simultaneously what is in the two poles.	3.1 If the presenting part is the head, it will feel round and hard. It may not be readily movable if it is engaged. If the head is above the pelvic brim, it is readily movable and ballotable as described for the first maneuver. 3.2 Presenting fetal part feels irregular, larger/bulkier, and less firm than a head. 3.3 Neither of the above is palpated.	3.1 Confirmation of longitudinal lie and cephalic presentation. 3.2 Confirmation of longitudinal lie and breech presentation. 3.3 Confirmation of transverse lie.

Table 36.1.
(Continued)

	PROCEDURE	FINDINGS	SIGNIFICANCE
 Fourth maneuver	**Step 4** This step will be used to determine the descent of the presenting part. Face the woman's feet. Place two hands gently on either side of the lower abdomen just below the level of the umbilicus and lower the fingers slowly on each side of the symphysis pubis. Note the contour, size, and mobility of the presenting part.	4.1 The examining hands converge around the presenting part with the fingertips touching in the abdominal midline. If the presenting part is the head, it will be readily movable. If the presenting part is the breech, it will move along with the trunk of the fetus. 4.2 The examining hands diverge from the presenting part and the abdominal midline. There is no mobility of the presenting part. 4.3 There is complete absence of any presenting part.	4.1 Indicative of unengaged presenting part floating at or above the pelvic inlet as determined by being at or above the symphysis pubis. 4.2 Indicative of either dipping or engaged presenting part. Dipping occurs when the presenting part has entered the pelvic inlet but has not yet descended to the point of engagement. 4.3 Indicative of a transverse lie.
	Step 5 Finally, share the findings with the woman and offer to help her feel and identify various fetal parts.		

a Adapted from Buckley K, Kulb NW: *Handbook of Maternal-Newborn Nursing.* New York, John Wiley & Sons, 1983, p 10.

Maternal and Fetal Outcome

All abnormal cephalic presentations predispose to prolonged or dysfunctional labor. The problems associated with such labor (i.e., intrauterine infection, postpartum hemorrhage, and maternal exhaustion) therefore may occur.

Since military attitude most often flexes to vertex presentation, there is generally a normal maternal/fetal outcome.

In a brow presentation, since the presenting diameters of the fetus are much larger than normal, normal labor progress and delivery often do not occur. Cesarean section may become necessary for persistent brow presentation. If vaginal delivery occurs, the mother often suffers extensive perineal, vaginal, or rectal lacerations as a result of the larger diameters. The extensive molding of the fetal skull may increase the risk of brain damage and fetal mortality. However, because a brow presentation may flex to a vertex or extend to a face presentation during labor, trial of labor with careful monitoring of maternal and fetal well-being is appropriate.

In a face presentation labor generally takes longer since the face dilates the cervix poorly. The mother generally experiences greater discomfort during labor and, as with delivery of a brow presentation, may receive more extensive lacerations. The fetus usually does well unless significant trauma occurs during delivery, although the baby's face generally becomes quite edematous, bruised, and misshapen as a result of the pressure from the maternal soft tissues. However, facial edema and bruising will resolve spontaneously within a few days. Edema of the larnyx, however, may lead to respiratory difficulty. Mentum posterior positions are the most traumatic and cannot be delivered vaginally (Fig. 36.3).

Medical Management

In cases of abnormal cephalic presentation, careful observation of labor progress and monitoring of maternal and fetal well-being are critical to optimum outcomes. In brow presentation labor may be stimulated or augmented with oxytocin. With good labor a brow presentation usually will convert to a vertex. However, if the diagnosis of face presentation is made and labor progress is poor, the treatment of choice is cesarean section to prevent trauma to the fetal head, larynx, and spine. Labor stimulation probably would result in poor fetal outcome. If arrest of descent in face presenta-

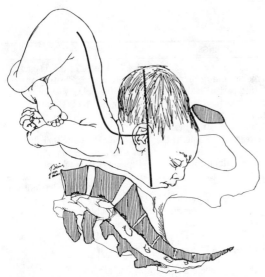

Figure 36.3. Face presentation. The occiput is on the longer end of the head lever. The chin is directly posterior. Vaginal delivery is impossible unless the chin rotates anteriorly. (Used with permission from Cunningham FG, MacDonald PC, Gant NF: *Williams' Obstetrics*, ed. 18. Norwalk, CT, Appleton-Lange, 1988, p 358.)

tion occurs deep in the pelvis, forceps delivery may be performed.

BREECH PRESENTATIONS

Definition

A breech presentation is a longitudinal lie of the fetus in which the head is in the fundus of the uterus and the fetal pelvis is in the lower segment (Fig. 36.4.). The fetal sacrum is the denominator. There are four types of breech presentation:

1. Frank breech: The buttocks present with the hips flexed and the knees extended. The thighs and lower legs are in front of the abdomen and chest.
2. Complete breech: The buttocks and feet present with both the hips and the knees flexed.
3. Single or double footling breech: The leg(s) present(s) with both hip and knee extended.
4. Single or double kneeling breech: The knee(s) present(s) with the hip extended and the knee flexed.

An alternative classification of breeches is frank, complete, and incomplete. Both the footling and the kneeling breech are termed incomplete.

Etiology

In many instances the cause of the breech presentation is not known. However, prematurity is the most common cause of breech presentation since the relationship between fetal size and intrauterine volume allows the fetus freedom of movement to assume any position. Other fetal factors include hydrocephalus, large baby, multiple gestation, polyhydramnios, and fetopelvic disproportion. It is thought that in these cases the smaller presenting bitrochanter diameter somehow is selected naturally over the larger biparietal diameter. Maternal factors include multiparity; uterine abnormalities such as septum, bicornua, or fibroids; and pelvic contracture. Placental factors include placenta previa and fundal or cornual implantation.

Signs and Symptoms

The mother may report signs and symptoms of fetal movement or kicking in the lower abdominal quadrants or directly on the urinary bladder. Increased discomfort under the ribs, heartburn, and/or dyspnea because of increased pressure of the larger, harder head also may be reported. The fetal heart tones generally are most distinct above the level of the umbilicus.

Diagnosis

Careful abdominal palpation will identify most cases of breech presentation. The hard, round, ballotable head is located in the upper pole of the uterus, with the larger, irregular, and nonballotable breech in the lower pole. Most breech presentations do not engage prior to the onset of labor. Vaginal examination should identify or confirm the breech presentation. There are no sutures or fontanels; rather, the presenting part generally is soft and irregular. If the sacrum is palpated, it will feel hard and may be identified incorrectly as a face or brow presentation. Palpation of the ischial tuberosities with the anus on line between them is diagnostic of a breech presentation. After the membranes have ruptured, the anus may be differentiated from the mouth by its failure to suck on the examining finger. Further, meconium may be present after palpating the anus. Sometimes, one or both feet are palpated and must be differentiated from a hand.

Diagnosis

When a breech presentation is suspected or known, an ultrasonogram or single x-ray film should be obtained to confirm the diagnosis and position of the fetus and the attitude of the fetal head.

Maternal and Fetal Outcome

The type of delivery is a major factor in the maternal/fetal outcome. Cesarean section principally increases maternal risk, whereas vaginal delivery carries risk for the fetus.

In a vaginal breech delivery a generous episiotomy most likely will be performed. Soft tissue lacerations of both the vagina and the cervix may occur either spontaneously or as a result of forceps application or other manipulations. In the case of a cesarean delivery, it may be necessary to make a classical or T-shaped uterine incision in order to conduct the delivery. These incisions are more likely to rupture in subsequent labors. (Both incisions are discussed in Chapter 40.)

Postpartum hemorrhage and/or infection may occur if labor is prolonged or significant manipulation is required.

Fetal outcome is poorer than in vertex presentations. In some cases, however, the probable cause of the breech presentation also is the cause of the poor outcome (e.g., congenital malformations or prematurity). Fetal asphyxia may be caused by difficult or prolonged labor, prolapse of the umbilical cord, compression of the umbilical cord between the fetus and maternal pelvis during vaginal delivery, or amniotic fluid or meconium aspiration. Injuries that may occur as a result of vaginal delivery include skull fracture; intracranial hemorrhage, tentorial tears, or other lacerations; fractures of the femur, humerus, clavicle, or neck; spinal cord trauma; organ damage of kidneys, adrenal glands, liver, or spleen; paralysis of the cervical and/or brachial plexus; and injury to the pharynx.

Medical Management

When a breech presentation has been diagnosed late in the third trimester, attempts to aid in conversion to a cephalic presentation may be warranted. The most noninterventive means of encouraging the breech to convert to cephalic presentation is maternal positioning. The mother is asked to assume a position in which her pelvis is higher than her shoulders. While she is in this position, the fetal head is lower than the breech, and the breech is lifted out of the pelvis and has a chance to turn naturally. The mother may be in knee-chest position, resting on her shoulders and forearms, or she may lie supine with several pillows beneath her hips or on an inverted slantboard. A slantboard may be improvised by resting the end of an ironing board upon a chair seat. The knee-chest position often is preferable since it avoids the risk of supine hypotension syndrome or aortic/vena caval compression by the uterus. The position should be assumed two or three times each day for 10–20 minutes at a time. Some mothers massage their fetus upwards along the back, across the head, and downwards along the chest toward the pelvis while

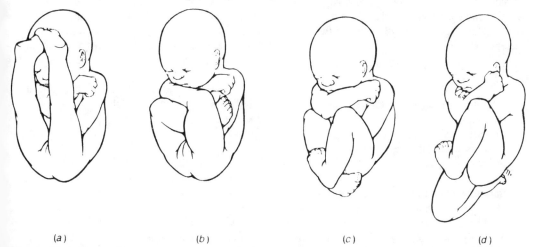

(a)	(b)	(c)	(d)

Figure 36.4. Types of breech presentations. **A,** Frank breech. **B,** Complete breech. **C,** Incomplete (foot below buttocks). **D,** Incomplete (knee below buttocks). (From Butnarescu JF, et al: *Maternity Nursing, Theory to Practice.* New York, John Wiley & Sons, 1983, p 515.)

in the tilted position. Once the breech has turned, the exercise should be stopped.

External version, or manipulation to turn the fetus, may be attempted. Cephalic version is the turning of a fetus to cephalic presentation. Some physicians will attempt external cephalic version if the fetus remains in breech presentation several weeks before term. The following conditions must be present:

1. The presenting part is not engaged.
2. Uterine irritability should be minimal.
3. Amount of amniotic fluid is adequate.
4. Fetal heart tones must be monitored continuously.

Sonography often is used to rule out fetal anomalies or placenta previa. Anesthesia should not be used in order to prevent use of excessive force. Some clinicians use tocolytics to relax the uterus before version is attempted. The version technique involves grasping both fetal poles, one in each hand, and moving the fetal head gently toward the inlet while the breech is moved away. Dangers in the procedure include cord prolapse and placental abruption. Thus, the technique always should be undertaken where it is possible to perform emergency cesarean section—never on an outpatient basis. For women who are Rh negative, many recommend immunoprophylaxis before the version is attempted. If fetal distress does occur during the attempted version, the procedure is stopped immediately and the fetus gently returned to the original position.

A decision to deliver a breech presentation vaginally should be made only after a comprehensive evaluation of maternal and fetal status. The following factors increase the risk of poor outcome for both mother and fetus:

1. Advanced maternal age
2. History of infertility
3. Intrauterine growth retardation
4. Postdates pregnancy
5. Preeclampsia
6. Diabetes and/or uterine myomas or neoplasms
7. Nulliparity

Radiography or ultrasonography of the pelvis should be done in order to (1, p 240):

1. Assess the size and shape of the maternal pelvis. A pelvis inadequate to attempt vaginal breech delivery is characterized by the following:

a. Interspinous diameter less than 9.0 cm;
b. Forward jutting of the sacrum; and
c. Narrow subpubic arch.
2. Confirm the presentation.
3. Diagnose the type of breech presentation.
4. Diagnose congenital anomalies.
5. Rule out hyperextension of the head.

If a trial of labor is allowable, the course of labor should be evaluated. Deviations from expected progress should indicate the need to reevaluate the route of delivery rather than the need for oxytocin stimulation. Oxytocin stimulation is not recommended because failure to progress may be due to fetopelvic disproportion. The fetus should be monitored electronically continuously in order to diagnose fetal distress quickly.

The presence of meconium in the amniotic fluid of a breech baby does not necessarily indicate fetal distress. Meconium may be passed as a mechanical response of the fetal intestines to compression by the uterine contractions and/or pressure of the maternal pelvis. Artificial rupture of the membranes is avoided because of the danger of cord prolapse as well as cord accident. If membranes rupture spontaneously, the laboring woman must be confined to bed in the Fowler's or semi-Fowler's position in order to facilitate the breech filling the pelvis completely—aided by gravity. Thus, cord prolapse will be prevented. If the pelvis is contracted, anomalies are present, the head is hyperextended, or placenta previa is evident, cesarean section is mandated. Of particular importance in the decision to deliver a breech vaginally is the attitude of the fetal head because of the high rate of fetal mortality and morbidity associated with this presentation. A fetus with a completely hyperextended head has been clinically described as a "star gazing fetus," and star gazing is an absolute indicator for cesarean section in order to save the fetus from trauma.

If the initial radiography is favorable, a trial of labor may be considered. A standardized obstetric tool has been developed to evaluate this decision further. Scores of 3 or less are associated with:

1. Prolonged labor
2. High incidence of fetal morbidity
3. High rate of cesarean sections

A score of 3 or less indicates the need for cesarean section without a trial of labor (Table 36.2).

When the cervix becomes fully dilated, the laboring woman is moved from the labor room to the

Table 36.2.
BREECH SCORE[a]

	0 POINTS	1 POINT	2 POINTS
Parity	Primigravida	Multipara	
Gestational age	39 weeks or more	38 weeks	37 weeks or less
Estimated fetal weight	>8 pounds	7–8 pounds	<7 pounds
	>3630 g	3176–3630 g	<3176 g
Previous breech >2500 g	None	1	2 or more
Cervical dilatation on admission by vaginal examination	2 cm or less	3 cm	4 cm or more
Station on admission	−3 or higher	−2	−1 or lower

[a]*Note*: A score of 3 or less is associated with a high incidence of fetal/newborn morbidity and should be considered an indication for Cesarean section.

Table 36.3.
MECHANISM OF LABOR: BREECH PRESENTATION

In breech presentations there are three successive mechanisms of labor for the three successively larger segments of the fetus—the buttocks and legs, the shoulders and arms, and the head.

Descent occurs throughout labor for each segment.

THE BUTTOCKS AND LEGS

Engagement and *descent* occur in one of the oblique diameters of the pelvis. Engagement is achieved when the bitrochanteric diameter has passed through the inlet of the pelvis; the sacrum of the fetus should be approximately at 0 station.

Internal rotation. Since the anterior hip generally descends more rapidly than the posterior, internal rotation occurs when it meets the resistance of the pelvic floor. The anterior hip rotates forward 45 degrees toward the pubic arch, bringing the bitrochanteric diameter into the anteroposterior diameter of the pelvic outlet.

Lateral flexion (birth of the buttocks). The anterior hip impinges under the pubic arch as the posterior hip continues to descend along the sacrum to the perineum. Lateral flexion at the waist increases, and the posterior hip is born over the perineum. The body then straightens and the anterior hip slips below the symphysis and delivers. The legs and feet generally deliver spontaneously.

Restitution occurs as the buttocks untwist 45 degrees to align with the engaging shoulders.

External rotation occurs as the buttocks rotate another 45 degrees in response to internal rotation of the shoulders.

THE SHOULDERS AND ARMS

Engagement occurs with the bisacromial diameter passing through the pelvic inlet in one of the oblique diameters of the pelvis.

Internal rotation occurs as the anterior shoulder strikes the pelvic sidewall and rotates 45 degrees to the anteroposterior diameter of the pelvis.

Lateral flexion (birth of the shoulders). The anterior shoulder impinges under the pubic arch, and the posterior shoulder and arm are born over the perineum. Then the anterior shoulder and arm deliver under the symphysis.

THE HEAD

Engagement. The head enters the pelvis when the shoulders are at the pelvic outlet. The head normally is well flexed, with the chin touching the chest. It enters the pelvis in one of the oblique diameters.

Internal rotation. The occiput strikes the pelvic sidewalls and rotates 45 degrees to bring the occiput into the anteroposterior diameter of the pelvis, with the nape of the neck under the pubic arch.

Flexion (birth of the head). The nape of the neck pivots under the symphysis, and the chin, mouth, nose, forehead, bregma (brow), and occiput are born over the perineum by flexion.

delivery room. Every effort should be made to maximize her expulsive efforts. The patient should continue to be positioned in a semi-Fowler's position, and she should be instructed in the bearing down technique.

There are three types of vaginal breech delivery (1, p 53). In spontaneous delivery the fetus delivers completely by the normal mechanisms of labor without assistance, other than support of the body, by the attendant. Mechanisms of labor are de-scribed in Table 36.3 and shown in Figure 36.5. The assisted breech delivery or partial breech extraction is conducted by the attendant after spontaneous delivery to the level of the umbilicus or above. The use of Piper forceps to the after-coming head thus is classified as an assisted breech delivery. Breech extraction is the complete delivery of the breech by the attendant and also may include the use of Piper forceps. Figure 36.6 details breech extraction.

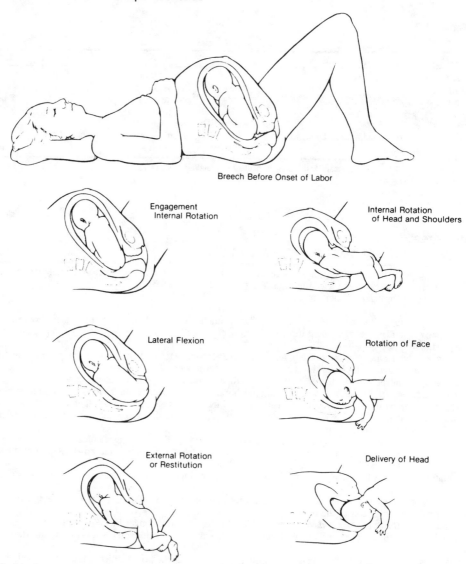

Breech Before Onset of Labor

Engagement
Internal Rotation

Internal Rotation
of Head and Shoulders

Lateral Flexion

Rotation of Face

External Rotation
or Restitution

Delivery of Head

Figure 36.5. Mechanisms of labor: breech presentation. (From Butnarescu JF, et al: *Maternity Nursing, Theory to Practice.* New York, John Wiley & Sons, 1983, p 516.)

In nearly all cases of breech delivery, a generous episiotomy also provides sufficient room to conduct maneuvers or apply forceps to aid the delivery if necessary. Most breech deliveries are best assisted if a second skilled attendant also is present and scrubbed to aid the delivery if necessary.

Although oxytocin induction or augmentation is not recommended for labor of a breech presentation, some practitioners use oxytocin augmentation once vaginal delivery has begun to maintain the strength and frequency of contractions and to avoid delay in delivery. As the umbilicus is born, a loop of cord should be drawn down gently to prevent trac-

tion and resultant hemorrhage or trauma. Delivery may occur slowly until the umbilicus has been delivered. After that, delivery must be completed in 5 minutes in order to avoid fetal hypoxia from cord compression. The baby is covered with a warm towel and the body is supported.

Once the shoulders are born, the head will have descended from the fundal portion of the uterus into the lower segment, the cervix, or the upper vaginal canal. Thus, fetal descent can be aided no longer by the expulsive efforts of the uterus. This is the time for the second attendant to apply suprapubic pressure. Suprapubic pressure

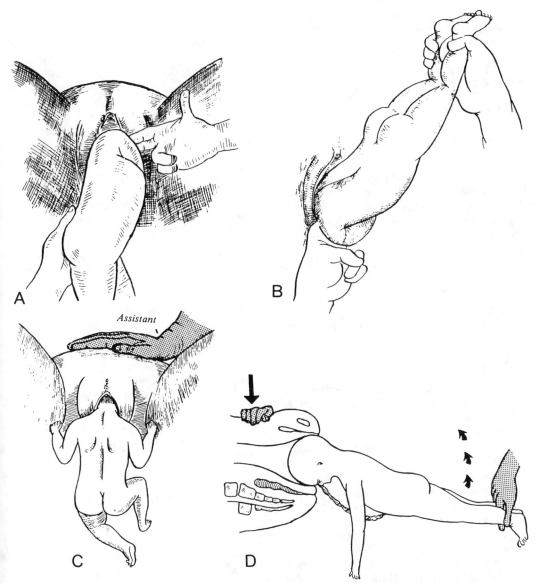

Figure 36.6. Breech. **A**, Right arm is delivered. **B**, Posterior arm is delivered by hooking left index finger over baby's shoulder while trunk is elevated with right hand. (Redrawn from Eastman: *Williams Obstetrics*, ed 11. New York, Appleton-Century-Crofts, 1956.) **C**, Delivery of after-coming head by Burn's maneuver. Baby's body is allowed to hang downward while fundal pressure is applied by assistant. **D**, After slight initial downward traction, child's body is swung upward in an arc. Suprapubic pressure is maintained throughout by an assistant to minimize neck traction. (From Cavanaugh D, Woods RE, O'Connor TCF: *Obstetric Emergencies*, ed. 2. Hagerstown, MD, Harper & Row, 1978, pp 231, 232, 235, 236.)

will continue fetal descent and maintain flexion of the head.

Another benefit of suprapubic pressure is that a well-flexed head will fill the birth canal and prevent the fetal arms from slipping up around the head. The enlarged diameter of this compound presentation impedes delivery and may pose grave risks to mother and infant.

As the face is born, the nares and face should be suctioned. Since the infant will be able to breathe, delivery of the rest of the head may occur more slowly. The pediatrician should be present to resuscitate the newborn and to evaluate the baby for evidence of trauma.

SHOULDER PRESENTATION (TRANSVERSE LIE)

Definition

When the long axis of the fetus is perpendicular or at right angles to the long axis of the mother, the term "transverse lie" is used. In this case the shoulder commonly presents over the pelvic inlet, and the scapula or acromion is the denominator. Transverse lie occurs in 0.4% of singleton deliveries (2, p 664).

Less frequently, the fetus may present obliquely, with either the head or the breech in one of the iliac fossae. This also may be termed a transverse lie. This presentation generally is transitory and converts either to cephalic or breech presentation prior to or at the beginning of labor.

Etiology

Transverse lie most often occurs as a result of a contracted or obstructed pelvic inlet. Transverse lie occurs during pregnancy when the intrauterine volume still is large enough to allow the small fetus great mobility (i.e., generally, prior to 32–34 weeks' gestation). Polyhydramnios also increases intrauterine volume, thus contributing to transverse lie. An abnormal intrauterine cavity because of fibroids, especially of the lower uterine segment, a uterine septum, or bicornuate uterus predisposes to transverse lie. Poor maternal abdominal musculature will permit the uterus to fall forward and the fetus to lie transversely. Fetal factors include anomalies or fetal demise, which permit increased flexibility. Transverse lie may occur in multiple gestation when the second or subsequent fetus occupies available space transversely. Pelvic contraction or fetopelvic disproportion also may lead to transverse lie. Finally, factors include placental abnormalities such as placenta previa.

Signs and Symptoms

The mother generally reports fetal movement in both flanks and does not complain of either pelvic pressure or upper abdomen or chest compression as would be anticipated with a longitudinal lie. There also may be signs and symptoms of associated conditions, such as polyhydramnios or multiple gestation.

Diagnosis

Abdominal palpation reveals the uterus to be shorter in length as measured from symphysis pubis to uterine fundus and wider in breadth than anticipated. Palpation of the fetus reveals the head and breech on opposite sides of the abdomen, with nothing occupying the fundus or lower pole of the uterus. The back and small parts may be located either inferiorly or superiorly, anteriorly or posteriorly.

Pelvic examination reveals no presenting part in the pelvis except in cases in which an arm or the umbilical cord has prolapsed.

In most cases, either ultrasonogram or x-ray is obtained to confirm the diagnosis and to identify the exact position of the fetus.

Maternal and Fetal Outcome

Unless recognized and managed properly, the outcome for both mother and fetus will be tragic. Continued labor with a transverse lie will result in impaction of the fetus in the pelvic brim and will lead eventually to formation of a pathologic retraction ring and uterine rupture as the myometrium attempts to expel the fetus (Fig. 36.7). Both the mother and fetus in such a case likely will die.

The possible causes of the transverse lie increase the risks to mother and fetus. Prematurity, fetal anomalies, and multiple gestation all increase the possibility of perinatal morbidity and mortality. Intrauterine manipulations for either vaginal or cesarean delivery may cause trauma or fetal distress. The possibility of prolapsed cord also increases the risks to the fetus. Placenta previa increases the risk of hemorrhage to the mother and hypoxia to the fetus. Risk of maternal sepsis is high if membranes have ruptured and the arm prolapses into the vagina because the arm acts as a conduit for vaginal flora to enter the uterus. The required surgical delivery carries an increased risk of infection and bleeding, as well as anesthetic complications.

Medical Management

Current practice requires the cesarean delivery of a viable fetus in transverse lie at the onset of labor. In rare instances external version to a vertex or breech presentation may be attempted prior to labor or in very early labor, particularly in a grand multipara. The second twin may be delivered vaginally by an internal podalic version and breech extraction.

In the case of a dead fetus, labor and vaginal delivery may be attempted as long as there is no evidence of pelvic obstruction or increased risk of maternal sequelae.

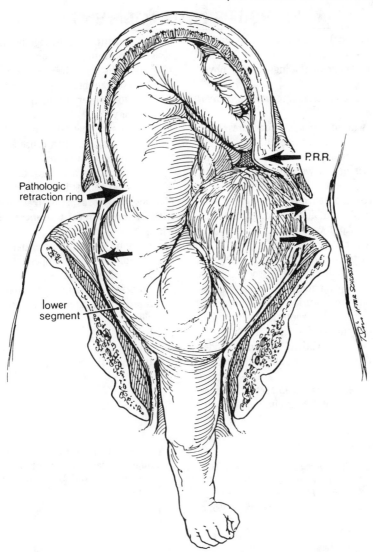

Pathologic
retraction ring

P.R.R.

lower
segment

Figure 36.7. Neglected shoulder presentation. A thick muscular band to form a pathologic retraction ring has developed just above the very thin lower uterine segment. The force generated during a uterine contraction is directed centripetally at and above the level of the pathologic retraction ring. This serves to further stretch and possibly to rupture the very thin lower segment below the retraction ring. *P.R.R.*, pathologic retraction ring. (From Cunningham FG, MacDonald PC, Gant NF: *Williams' Obstetrics,* ed.18, Norwalk, CT, Appleton-Lange, 1988, p 363.)

As mentioned above, failure to diagnose the transverse lie, mismanagement in labor, or maternal delay in presenting to the hospital may require heroic efforts to save mother and/or fetus.

NURSING MANAGEMENT

Nursing care specific for a patient with an abnormal fetal presentation:

☐ For *all patients* screen for abnormal fetal presentation:

— Perform careful abdominal palpation on all patients in labor;

— Carefully palpate presenting part (including sutures and fontanelles with cephalic

NURSING MANAGEMENT

presentations) when performing vaginal examinations; and

— Report abnormal findings to the physician.

☐ For the patient experiencing *abnormal fetal presentation*:

— Assist with diagnostic procedures (e.g., sonogram, x-ray) as needed.

— Avoid rupturing membranes if presenting part does not fit well in maternal pelvis; confine patient to bed if membranes are ruptured spontaneously to prevent prolapse of the umbilical cord. Place folded blanket or pillow under right hip to prevent vena caval occlusion.

— Be alert to signs/symptoms of other maternal/fetal abnormalities associated with abnormal presentations (e.g., polyhydramnios, prematurity, placenta previa).

— Ensure that pelvic room is maximized:

  * Give enema if ordered, and
  * Encourage patient to empty bladder at least every 2 hours; catheterize if necessary.

— Be prepared for cesarean section, forceps delivery, neonatal resuscitation, or post-partum hemorrhage because of extensive lacerations or atony.

— Assist in delivery as necessary (e.g., apply suprapubic pressure to maintain flexion for delivery of the head in a breech delivery).

— Assess neonate for evidence of birth trauma; explain cause and transitory nature of unusual features (e.g., facial edema in face presentation, unusual position of legs in breech presentation).

Nursing diagnoses most frequently associated with *abnormal fetal presentation* (see Section V):

☐ Grieving related to potential/actual loss of infant or birth of an imperfect child

☐ Knowledge deficit regarding etiology, disease process, treatment, and outcome.

☐ Altered fetal cardiac and cerebral tissue perfusion.

☐ Pain.

☐ Anxiety/fear.

☐ Impaired skin integrity.

REFERENCES

1. Oxorn H, Foote WR: *Human Labor and Birth*, ed 5. Norwalk, CT, Appleton-Century-Crofts, 1985, p 53.
2. Pritchard JA, MacDonald PC: *Williams Obstetrics*, ed 17. Norwalk, CT, Appleton-Century-Crofts, 1985, p 666.
3. Smith SM: Intrapartum deviations. In Buckley K, Kulb NW (eds): *Handbook of Maternal-Newborn Nursing*. New York, John Wiley and Sons, 1983, p 415.

Chapter 37
Oxytocin Induction/
Augmentation of Labor

Nancy W. Kulb, C.N.M., M.S.

INTRODUCTION

Physiology of Labor

The onset of labor (see Chapter 28) is difficult to distinguish from the end of the "prelabor" period. Labor usually is said to begin with the onset of regular, coordinated uterine contractions that lead to the progressive effacement and dilatation of the cervix. Often, the point at which true labor begins is determined in retrospect or roughly estimated at best.

Labor is a continuous, slowly accelerating process that normally begins weeks before term. Braxton Hicks contractions may be noted as early as 24 weeks' gestation. In the third trimester they may occur as frequently as every 10 minutes and may reach an intrauterine pressure of 40–60 mm Hg (1). But contractions alone are not sufficient to produce the biochemical changes in the uterus and cervix that are prerequisite to labor.

At about 30 weeks' gestation, mechanical changes in the cervix begin to occur: the cervix moves anteriorly to the center of the birth canal from its former posterior position, it softens, and it may begin to efface. These changes can be induced by prostaglandins and are independent of uterine contractions, which usually are irregular in frequency and intensity at this point. Meanwhile, the myometrium of the uterus begins to "ripen," forming the gap junctions that are required to conduct electrical impulses throughout the uterus, thus allowing uterine contractions to be coordinated.

The normal resting tone of the uterus is 5–12 mm Hg. Blood flow through the uterus is unimpeded at this pressure. Contraction pressure of at least 25 mm Hg is required to produce progress in labor (1, p 117). Contraction strength tends to increase as labor progresses, often reaching an intensity of 60–70 mm Hg by the end of the first stage of labor.

There is a reciprocal relationship between contraction frequency and pressure. During a uterine contraction with a pressure of 30–70 mm Hg, the blood flow through the spiral arteries in the myometrium is stopped. Because blood flow is arrested, the available oxygen is used up quickly, and anaerobic metabolism is necessary until the contraction resolves. Metabolites of the anaerobic process accumulate in the myometrial tissue. An adequate period of relaxation between contractions is crucial to restore oxygen and nutrients and to remove metabolites, or the subsequent contraction will be weak. Although frequency of contractions is important, it is adequate contraction pressure that is necessary to effect labor progress.

Each contraction also affects oxygenation of the fetus. Initially, myometrial pressure compresses veins that drain the intervillous space (IVS) in the placenta. Blood flow continues through the arteries, resulting in an expansion in the size of the IVS. As contraction pressure continues to increase, the blood flow through the arteries also is halted. Fetal circulation continues, but stored oxygen is extracted from the maternal blood in the IVS. The fetus undergoes a mild, transient hypoxia, leading to some anaerobic metabolism. The result of this anaerobic metabolism is a slow decline in pH. Recovery of oxygenation normally occurs between contractions, but if contractions are too frequent, recovery does not occur, and the fetus becomes increasingly hypoxic and acidotic.

Many factors normally affect contraction frequency and pressure. The supine position decreases uterine blood flow, with the result that contractions are more frequent but weaker than in the more favorable lateral position. Standing increases efficiency of contractions because of the additional 20–30 mm Hg pressure on the cervix from the effect of gravity. Anxiety results in the release of epinephrine, which increases blood pressure and inhibits uterine blood flow, resulting in decreased efficiency of contractions and decreased fetal oxygenation. Narcotics not only may relieve the ill effects of anxiety but also may stimulate the coordination and efficiency of uterine contractions (2).

Oxytocin

Role in Normal Labor

The exact role of oxytocin in the initiation and maintenance of normal labor is not completely clear. Whereas prostaglandins can be used to initiate labor at any stage of pregnancy, the uterus is unresponsive to oxytocin until near term. Even then, the response varies widely from woman to woman.

Oxytocin is a hormone synthesized in the neural cell bodies in the supraoptical and paraventricular nuclei in the hypothalamus. It is transported down neural tracts to nerve terminals in the posterior pituitary, where it is stored until it is secreted into the circulation. Oxytocin is secreted in response to vaginal distention, cervical distention or pressure, or nipple stimulation. It circulates as a free peptide until it binds to cell membrane receptors on the target tissue—namely, myometrial cells of the uterus and the myoepithelial cells of the breasts (3).

The number of myometrial receptor cells in the uterus increases rapidly near term, peaking early in the first stage of labor. The serum concentration of oxytocin reaches a peak in the second stage. Its exact mechanism of action is not known, but it may act by increasing free intracellular calcium in the target tissue, thus enhancing muscle contraction (3, p 140).

Pharmacology

The commercially available preparations of the hormone are Pitocin and Syntocinon. Both are available in vials of 10 USP units for parenteral use only. (Oxytocin is not effective when given by mouth.) Approximately 500 USP units is the equivalent of 1 mg of oxytocin. The circulatory halflife of oxytocin is very short—approximately 3–5 minutes, although uterine effects may persist as long as 20–30 minutes. Oxytocin is rendered ineffective by the enzyme oxytocinase. After intravenous infusion of the drug at a given rate for a period of 20–30 minutes, equilibrium is achieved (i.e., the plasma level plateaus) as the rate of destruction balances the rate of administration.

The uterine response to oxytocin administered exogenously during labor is triphasic (1, p 120):

1. Uterine activity increases as the dose increases.
2. A stable phase is reached in which uterine activity remains constant in spite of increases in dosage. Eventually, if dosage continues to be increased, an increase in frequency with a decrease in intensity will result.
3. Baseline tone increases and may result in hyperstimulation.

Ergonovine and methylergonovine (commercially available as Ergotrate and Methergine) are the other commonly used oxytoxic-like drugs. They are very similar in their actions. Both may be administered intravenously, intramuscularly, or by mouth. Both are very powerful stimulants of uterine contractions, with an effect that lasts for hours. The pregnant uterus is very sensitive to these drugs. Although the powerful, prolonged uterine contractions they cause are very beneficial in the treatment of postpartum hemorrhage, they are extremely dangerous to both mother and fetus prior to delivery and therefore are contraindicated absolutely prior to delivery.

Adverse Effects

Oxytocin, when used properly, is a safe drug. However, with improper use, serious sequelae may occur. Rapid injection of 5 USP units (0.5 ml) intravenously may result in severe tetanic contractions that last several minutes. It also may result in marked maternal hypotension, followed by an increase in cardiac output. These effects may be quite dangerous if the patient already is hypovolemic, if she has cardiac disease that limits cardiac output, or if she has right-to-left shunts. Therefore, oxytocin should not be given by rapid intravenous injection but instead by intramuscular injection or dilute, continuous intravenous injection (4).

Even with a physiologic dose of oxytocin in intravenous solution, the patient may initially experience a mild decrease in blood pressure. After a prolonged period, she may experience a rise in blood pressure—up to 30% above baseline. Stroke volume and cardiac output also may increase (2, p 25).

Oxytocin in doses as low as 20 mU/minute exerts an antidiuretic effect because of the reabsorption of free water and decreased urinary output. Large doses of oxytocin (20–40 mU/minute) can result in water intoxication, particularly if it is given in large volumes of electrolyte-free dextrose solution. The hypoosmotic, hyponatremic state can result in convulsions, coma, and even death. Neonatal convulsions also have been reported. Therefore, it is recommended that oxytocin be administered only in balanced salt solution. If high doses of oxytocin are required, it is preferable to increase the concentration rather than increase the rate of flow of a dilute solution. The antidiuretic effect is reversible within a few minutes after stopping an intravenous infusion. Intramuscular injection is not so likely to cause water intoxication because it is not administered in an aqueous solution (4, p 346).

An association has been found between neonatal jaundice and oxytocin infusion; it is dose related. It is postulated that oxytocin causes a decrease in erythrocyte flexibility, causing erythrocytes to become lodged in capillaries, and eventually they are destroyed (1, p 119).

Other adverse effects of oxytocin generally are the result of improper (usually too vigorous) administration. Fetal distress may result from hypertonic uterine contractions. Placental abruption, cervical laceration, and amniotic fluid embolus also may result from overstimulation. Uterine rupture may occur and may result in maternal and/or fetal death. If fetal maturity is not properly documented prior to induction, iatrogenic prematurity may occur.

Oxytocin is administered for three major reasons: induction of labor, augmentation of labor, and prevention or treatment of postpartum hemorrhage. (See Chapter 42 for a discussion of postpartum use.) This chapter focuses on the intrapartum use of oxytocin.

AUGMENTATION AND INDUCTION OF LABOR

Induction of labor is the artificial initiation of labor. Augmentation of labor is the stimulation of already established labor.

Many methods for initiating labor other than oxytocin administration have been tried. For example, sexual intercourse, because of the prostaglandins in semen and the prostaglandins that may be released by pressure on the cervix, has been used popularly (but not documented to be effective). Stripping membranes, which may cause local prostaglandin release because of manipulation of the cervix, has been used. Nipple stimulation, by stimulating the release of endogenous oxytocin, has been demonstrated to be effective in 70% of mul-

tiparas (5). Amniotomy has been tried, but in the presence of an unripe cervix, the effectiveness is low, and the rate of chorioamnionitis is high. "Ripening" the cervix prior to induction has been attempted with laminaria (seaweed), but vaginal administration of prostaglandin gel has been found to be far more effective. Labor often occurs within 48 hours after prostaglandin gel is used. However, it is not yet approved by the United States Food and Drug Administration (FDA).

Alternative methods of augmenting labor have included the following: ambulation to increase pressure on the cervix from gravity; enemas to cause irritation of the bowel and, hopefully, the nearby uterus; nipple stimulation; and amniotomy. Some practitioners avoid amniotomy to stimulate or induce labor, stating that the fluid acts as a cushion for the fetal head and umbilical cord, equalizing the pressure of each contraction over the baby's body and thus reducing fetal heart rate abnormalities and formation of caput succedaneum.

Contraindications

The most common (and very effective) means of inducing or augmenting labor is with administration of exogenous oxytocin. Table 37.1 lists the absolute and relative contraindications for administration of oxytocin for induction or augmentation of labor.

Indications

Indications for labor induction include those cases in which prolonging the pregnancy is more dangerous for mother and/or fetus than delivery but in which emergency delivery by cesarean section is not required. Table 37.2 lists some common indications for induction, but the list is not exhaustive. In each case the expert clinical judgment of the physician must be used to determine that induction is indicated and the optimal time to initiate it.

When termination of the pregnancy is indicated, the urgency may determine whether immediate cesarean section is necessary or whether induction may be tried. The Bishop score (see Table 37.3) has been used to predict the success of induction. A score greater than or equal to 6 carries with it a high probability of success, whereas a score of 3 or less indicates that induction may be lengthy or unsuccessful. As mentioned above, in other countries a prostaglandin gel applied vaginally has been used successfully to ripen the cervix prior to induction (increasing the Bishop score) and sometimes is effective in inducing labor.

Table 37.1.

CONTRAINDICATIONS TO INDUCTION OR AUGMENTATION OF LABOR WITH OXYTOCIN

Absolute Contraindications
1. Evidence of mechanical obstruction to delivery (e.g., cephalopelvic disproportion)
2. Fetal distress (e.g., abnormal fetal heart rate tracing, thick meconium)
3. Patient refusal
4. Inability to document medical indication for it (i.e., elective procedure)
5. Hypertonic uterine activity
6. Placenta previa

Relative Contraindications
1. Abnormal fetal presentation or position
2. Uterine overdistention (e.g., polyhydramnios, multiple gestation, macrosomic fetus)
3. High parity (more than 5)
4. Previous uterine scar
5. Fetal immaturity
6. Unripe cervix

Table 37.2.

COMMON INDICATIONS FOR INDUCTION OF LABOR

Diabetes mellitus (class B or greater)
Pregnancy-induced hypertension
Chronic maternal hypertension
Intrauterine growth retardation
Positive contraction stress test
Postmaturity (42 + weeks' gestation)
Premature rupture of membranes (at or near term)
Chorioamnionitis
Cyanotic maternal cardiac disease
Rh isoimmunization
Fetal demise

Augmentation is indicated only when true labor has been established (i.e., there is documentation of progressive dilatation and effacement of the cervix, with dilatation of at least 3 cm), and there is subsequent hypotonic uterine dysfunction. Augmentation is not appropriate for prodromal or normal latent phase labor, and it is not appropriate unless labor progress truly is abnormal. Finally, it is not appropriate unless the abnormal labor progress is due to hypotonic uterine contractions and *not* absolute fetopelvic disproportion or some other cause. If these criteria are met, augmentation of labor will decrease the risk of maternal exhaustion, intrapartum or postpartum infection, operative

Table 37.3.

BISHOP SCORE[a]

FACTOR	0	1	2	3
Dilatation (cm)	Closed	1–2	3–4	≥5
Effacement (%)	0–30	40–50	60–70	≥80
Station	−3	−2	−1/0	+1/+2
Consistency	Firm	Medium	Soft	—
Cervical position	Posterior	Midposition	Anterior	—

[a]Adapted from Bishop EH: Pelvic scoring for elective induction. *Obstetrics and Gynecology*, 1964, p. 267.

delivery, or fetal distress or death from uterine dysfunction.

Protocols for Administering Oxytocin during Labor

During labor, the intravenous route is used for administering oxytocin, for with the intramuscular route, the rate of absorption cannot be controlled, and the drug cannot be stopped immediately when necessary. The drug is administered in a dilute balanced electrolyte solution. It is mandatory that both fetal heart rate and contraction pattern be monitored continuously, preferably electronically. Internal monitoring has the distinct and important advantages of measuring actual intrauterine pressure and showing fetal heart rate variability accurately. It can be instituted, however, only when the membranes are ruptured, so it may not be possible when amniotomy is contraindicated or early in an induction that may require more than 1 day.

Before initiating an oxytocin infusion, the baseline fetal heart rate and uterine contraction pattern should be determined, preferably by electronic fetal monitoring. This practice will ensure that there is no evidence of fetal distress and that there is not already adequate uterine activity.

A constant infusion pump (IVAC, IMED, Harvard pump) should be used to ensure accurate, constant administration of the drug. The oxytocin infusion should be inserted ("piggybacked") into a well-functioning main intravenous line as near the intravenous insertion site as possible. If the oxytocin infusion must be stopped for any reason, there will not be a large amount of oxytocin remaining in the line going to the patient.

In general, a higher dose of oxytocin is required for induction of labor than for augmentation. This probably is because the gap junctions and oxytocin receptor sites have been developed fully in

Table 37.4.

NURSING PROTOCOLS FOR ADMINISTRATION OF OXYTOCIN FOR INDUCTION/
AUGMENTATION

1. Document indication for oxytocin induction or augmentation and vaginal examination findings. Be certain the physician has documented fetal maturity, presentation of fetus, and indication for induction/augmentation.
2. Explain to the patient and her significant other(s) the indication(s) and procedures to be used. Include an explanation of the equipment to be used (electronic fetal monitor, constant infusion pump).
3. Apply fetal monitor and obtain the baseline fetal heart rate and uterine activity over a 15- to 20-minute period.
4. Prepare the intravenous solution as ordered. Usually 10 USP units of Pitocin are added to 1000 cc D₅RL or other balanced electrolyte solution. Label the intravenous bottle appropriately, including the amount of oxytocin in the solution, the date, time, patient's name, and the name of the nurse who prepared the solution.
5. Prepare the constant infusion pump according to the specific instructions for that pump. Insert the oxytocin line, with the flow turned off, into the mainline intravenous infusion, as close to the patient as possible.
6. Begin the infusion, as ordered, at 0.5–1 mU/minute. Increase the dose as ordered, until adequate uterine activity is achieved (i.e., contractions occur every 3–4 minutes with a duration of 50–60 seconds and an intensity of ≥60 mm Hg. Suggested protocols for changing the dose follow:
   a. Increase oxytocin 2 mU/minute every 20 minutes until adequate labor is achieved or a dose of 20 mU/minute is reached. Consult with the physician and obtain an order to increase the dose beyond 20 mU/minute. Do not increase the dose above 20 mU/minute faster than 4 mU/minute in 20 minutes. Once an adequate labor pattern is established and dilatation is at least 6–8 cm, decrease the dose by 2–4 mU/minute every 10–20 minutes to maintain adequate labor but avoid hyperstimulation (2, p 28).
   b. Increase the dose 2 mU/minute every 15 minutes. When uterine activity stops increasing over a 30-minute period, the stable phase has been reached. Decrease the dose to one-half that at which the stable phase was entered. If uterine activity again increases, decrease the dose by half again (1, p 120).
   c. For induction: Begin at 1 mU/minute and double the dose every 30–45 minutes until an adequate, stable contraction pattern has been established or a dose of 32 mU/minute is reached. For augmentation: Begin at 1 mU/minute and increase by 1 mU/minute every 30–45 minutes until adequate labor is established or a dose of 4 mU/minute is reached. Maintain the dose at 4 mU/minute for 2 hours and then increase by 1 mU/minute every 30–45 minutes if necessary (3, pp 145, 150).
   d. Increase the dose gradually, reaching a maximum dose of 10 mU/minute for augmentation and 30–40 mU/minute for induction (4, p 644).
7. Encourage the patient to remain in the left lateral position.
8. Document on the patient's chart and the fetal monitor strip each oxytocin dosage change and time; maternal vital signs with each change in dose; all procedures, vaginal examinations, position changes, etc.; and all consultations with the physician. Document on the chart fetal heart rate and uterine contraction pattern with each change in oxytocin dose or at least every 30 minutes.
9. Decrease the dose and consult with the physician if uterine activity decreases with increasing dosage of oxytocin. Overdosage may have occurred.
10. Terminate the oxytocin infusion if any of the following occur: precipitous labor, hyperstimulation, unusual vaginal bleeding, or fetal distress. Consult with the physician.
11. If fetal distress occurs, discontinue the oxytocin infusion, notify the physician, turn the patient to the left side, administer oxygen at 6–8 liters/minute, increase the rate of flow of the mainline intravenous line, and observe for imminent delivery (see Chapter 39).
12. If hyperstimulation occurs, discontinue the oxytocin, notify the physician, and turn the patient to her left side. Wait at least 15 minutes before restarting oxytocin, and begin it at a dose no greater than that being used 30 minutes before the hyperstimulation occurred.

the uterus that began labor spontaneously. Also endogenous oxytocin levels may be higher.

Table 37.4 gives a suggested protocol for preparation and administration of the oxytocin infusion. The specific setting to deliver a particular dose of oxytocin will vary with the particular constant infusion pump. In order to ensure correct dosage, it is suggested that each institution have detailed written instructions for preparing the intravenous infusion and the settings that are required to deliver given dosages for each type of constant infusion pump. This is especially important in institutions that use more than one type of pump.

The patient should never be left alone while the oxytocin infusion is in progress. A physician or nurse trained to manage the oxytocin infusion should be present to decide whether and when it is appropriate to increase or decrease the dose and to respond immediately if hyperstimulation or fetal distress occur.

The goal with oxytocin administration is to use the minimum dose necessary to get the required uterine response. The frequency, duration, and intensity of contractions should not be greater than in normal labor. Oxytocin acts quickly and effectively—it should not be needed for more than a few hours (except in the case of induction with an unripe cervix). If no progress in cervical dilatation has been made after 3–4 hours with adequate uterine activity, the cause is presumed to be absolute dystocia requiring delivery by cesarean section. When the stable phase of uterine activity has been reached, it is often possible to decrease the dose and yet maintain the same uterine activity. Efforts to force a faster than normal rate of dilatation are likely to end in hyperstimulation and/or fetal distress.

Hyperstimulation is said to occur clinically when contractions last longer than 90 seconds, frequency is greater than every 2–3 minutes, or resting tone between contractions is greater than 15 mm Hg. When hyperstimulation does occur, the first action is to stop the oxytocin infusion. Oxygen should be given to the patient if there is evidence of fetal distress, and the patient should be turned to the left lateral position to enhance uteroplacental blood flow. Unless absolutely necessary, vaginal examination should be avoided, since dilating the cervix or vagina may stimulate the release of endoge-

nous oxytocin. Since the half-life of oxytocin is short—3–5 minutes—the recovery should be rapid. The oxytocin should not be restarted for at least 15 minutes, and it should be started at a dose equal to or less than that 30 minutes prior to the episode of hyperstimulation (3, p 148).

If after 12 hours of steady administration of oxytocin for induction there is no active labor, the infusion should be stopped and the patient allowed to rest overnight. Often, this will allow the uterine contractile mechanisms to mature more fully. The induction can be resumed the next morning, starting the entire procedure from the beginning (see Protocols).

When oxytocin is used properly for labor induction or augmentation, it is quite safe—indeed, far less hazardous than the conditions for which it is indicated. But it must be used by properly trained personnel, with well-functioning equipment and with an understanding of its actions, respect for its power, and careful observation for any untoward effects.

NURSING MANAGEMENT

Nursing care specific for a patient with oxytocin induction/augmentation of labor:

☐ Encourage all laboring women to enhance the forces of labor through ambulation, frequent voiding, maintaining nutrition/hydration status, and by squatting during the second stage, if possible.

☐ Administer oxytocin according to protocol—NEVER leave the bedside of the patient receiving oxytocin.

☐ Be alert for complications of oxytocin administration (e.g., hyperstimulation, water intoxication, fetal distress) as well as sequelae of the

complication requiring induction/augmentation.

Nursing diagnoses most frequently associated with oxytocin induction/augmentation of labor (see Section V):

☐ Grieving related to potential/actual loss of infant or birth of an imperfect child.

☐ Altered fetal cardiac and cerebral tissue perfusion.

☐ Pain.

☐ Knowledge deficit regarding medication regimen.

☐ Anxiety/fear.

REFERENCES

1. Steer PJ: Bettering control of oxytocin infusions. *Contemp OB/GYN* 19:117–141, 1982.
2. Marshall C: The art of induction/augmentation of labor. *JOGNN* Jan/Feb: 22–28, 1985.
3. Ross MG, Hayashi R: How can we use oxytocin more effectively. *Contemp OB/GYN* 24:139–152, 1984.
4. Pritchard JA, MacDonald PC, Gant NF: *Williams Obstetrics*, ed 17. Norwalk, CT, Appleton-Century-Crofts, 1985, pp 345–346.
5. Jhirad A, Vago T: Induction of labor by breast stimulation. *Obstet Gynecol* 41:374, 1973.

Chapter 38
Analgesia/Anesthesia during Pregnancy and Labor
Hilda Pedersen, M.D.

INTRODUCTION

More women with complicated pregnancies are coming to our delivery suites every year. The implications for anesthetic management during parturition are numerous. In addition, it has been estimated that as many as 1.6% of all pregnant women undergo surgery (and, therefore, anesthesia) unrelated to parturition at some time during gestation (1). An awareness of the physiological changes of normal pregnancy as they relate to anesthesia is an essential part of the approach to the problems and management of the critically ill obstetric patient.

PHYSIOLOGICAL CHANGES IN NORMAL PREGNANCY

Although major alterations occur in nearly every organ system during pregnancy, the discussion in this chapter is limited to the changes of greatest interest to the anesthesiologist—namely, those involving hemodynamics, the respiratory system, acid-base balance, and the gastrointestinal tract.

Hemodynamic Changes

Cardiac output begins to rise during the eighth week of pregnancy, initially through an increase in the stroke volume, and reaches its peak of 30–50% above normal at 30–34 weeks. Alterations in cardiac output in the remaining 6–10 weeks are a subject of controversy. Older studies, performed in the supine position, indicated that by the 38th to 40th week the cardiac output declines to the non-pregnant level (2). It was postulated subsequently that the low cardiac output seen in the supine position was due to compression of the inferior vena cava by the enlarged uterus since, when measured in the lateral decubitus, cardiac output during the last few weeks of pregnancy was no lower than that seen in the second trimester (3). Yet another study indicates that there is a decline in maternal cardiac output after the 32nd week of pregnancy whether the woman is in the sitting, lateral, or supine position (4). The greatest reduction occurs when the mother is supine; the cardiac output measured in this position was less than in the nonpregnant state, as determined at 6–8 weeks postpartum.

Vena caval compression can begin to develop during the second trimester and becomes maximal at 36–38 weeks. It may decrease thereafter, with the descent of the fetal head into the pelvis. It has been known since 1953 to account for the "supine hypotensive syndrome," characterized by arterial hypotension, tachycardia, pallor, and faintness. This occurs in approximately 10% of pregnant women at term who are placed in the supine position (5). More recently, a radiographic study revealed that complete obstruction of the inferior vena cava occurs in approximately 90% of pregnant women at term, when lying supine (3). Venous blood from the lower part of the body reaches the heart through the superior vena cava after diversion via the intervertebral venous plexus and the azygous vein. The engorgement of the intervertebral plexus reduces the size of the epidural and subarachnoid spaces, consequently diminishing the drug requirement for regional anesthesia.

425

As already mentioned, reduced cardiac output is another result of vena caval occlusion. Most women manage to maintain normal or near normal brachial arterial pressure by increasing the peripheral resistance. The compensatory response seems to involve the uteroplacental vasculature, with harmful effects on the fetus (6).

In the supine position the lower aorta also may be compressed, as was demonstrated by aortography in 1968. (7). This phenomenon affects primarily the renal and uteroplacental blood flows.

Thus, the supine position should be avoided during the second and third trimesters of pregnancy, even in the absence of maternal arterial hypotension.

Heart rate increases throughout pregnancy, reaching an average of 92–95 beats per minute at term. Arterial blood pressure decreases slightly because the decrease in peripheral resistance exceeds the increase in cardiac output. Changes in the electrocardiogram are attributable to the shift in the position of the heart (left axis deviation) resulting from the upward displacement of the diaphragm by the gravid uterus. There also is an increased tendency toward premature contractions, sinus tachycardia, and paroxysmal supraventricular tachycardia (8).

Respiratory System Changes

Anatomical Changes

Capillary engorgement throughout the respiratory tract occurs in the majority of pregnant women (9). Swelling in the area of the nasopharynx makes nose breathing difficult for some women and increases the risk of bleeding following nasotracheal intubation. The level of the diaphragm rises by a maximum of approximately 4 cm, but diaphragmatic breathing remains unimpeded (10). As a matter of fact, breathing in pregnancy is more diaphragmatic than costal. The upward shift of the diaphragm is counterbalanced by an increase in the anteroposterior and transverse diameters of the thoracic cage and by flaring of the ribs. These changes result in important modifications of lung volumes during pregnancy.

Lung Volumes and Dynamics

Lung volumes undergo progressive changes beginning in the fifth month of pregnancy. There is a decrease in expiratory reserve volume, residual volume, and functional residual capacity (11). At term, functional residual capacity is approximately 1350 ml or 20% less than that in the nonpregnant state. There is a concomitant increase in inspiratory capacity and inspiratory reserve volume so that total lung capacity remains unchanged.

The closing volume of the lung is the pulmonary gas volume below which bronchiolar airways close off, trapping gas in pulmonary alveoli. These rapidly become atelectatic and augment the pulmonary shunt. Closing volumes in young, nonpregnant women are well below expiratory reserve volume. Measurements made during pregnancy have yielded contradictory results. In one study the closing volume exceeded the expiratory reserve volume in 30% of subjects lying supine (12), but none of the pregnant women showed this phenomenon in a more recent investigation (13).

Lung compliance also is unchanged, but total pulmonary resistance is diminished, primarily because of progesterone-induced relaxation of bronchiolar smooth muscle, resulting in decreased airway resistance (14).

Ventilation

Ventilation increases early in pregnancy, approaching maximum in the second or third month (15). At term, tidal volume is increased by 40% and respiratory rate by 15%, with a net minute ventilation of approximatley 50% above the nonpregnant level. Since dead space does not change significantly, alveolar ventilation at term is approximately 70% above that in the nonpregnant state. (See Chapter 16.)

Acid-Base Balance Changes

Basal oxygen consumption increases during pregnancy but is offset by hyperventilation, so there is an increase in maternal PaO_2 to a mean of 106 torr and a decrease in the mean $PaCO_2$ to 32 torr. At the same time, the plasma buffer base decreases from average of 47 mEq/liter to 42 mEq/liter, and the pH remains practically unchanged. All these changes occur early in pregnancy.

Increased alveolar ventilation along with decreased functional residual capacity (FRC) enhances maternal uptake and elimination of inhalation anesthetics. On the other hand, decreased FRC and increased metabolic rate predispose the mother towards hypoxemia, even during a brief period of airway obstruction or the apnea of intubation.

Gastrointestinal Tract Changes

During the course of pregnancy, the stomach and intestines gradually are pushed upward by the enlarging uterus. Eventually, the stomach assumes a horizontal position, with the pylorus displaced upward and posteriorly, thus slowing the evacuation of gastric contents. It has been noted that gastric retention of a watery meal is prolonged from the 34th week onward (16). Pain, anxiety, and administration of narcotics and belladonna alkaloids may delay gastric emptying further. Near term, there is an increase in intragastric pressure, particularly in the lithotomy and Trendelenburg positions. In most women this is exceeded by the rise in the opening pressure of the gastroesophageal sphincter (17) so that in most unanesthetized patients, the risk of regurgitation is not enhanced by pregnancy. Women with heartburn appear to be an exception. In this group the sphincter tone has been found to be greatly reduced. The administration of general anesthesia and of muscle relaxants obviously enhances the risk of regurgitation in all pregnant patients by producing relaxation of the sphincter.

Placental Transfer

The ease with which most pharmacologic agents administered to the pregnant patient cross the placenta is now fully appreciated, and improved methods of detection and assay of drugs and metabolites have improved our knowledge of the tissue distribution, metabolism, and excretion of drugs in the patient, fetus, and newborn infant. The unique anatomic and physiologic characteristics of the placental and fetal circulations play a significant role in placental transport.

Physiochemical Properties

A prime factor in placental transfer of drugs is their degree of ionization. Organic substances are transferred mainly in the undissociated or nonionized form, whereas ions penetrate only with difficulty. Fat solubility determines the rate of transfer of these nonionized molecules; drugs that are highly fat soluble pass across the membrane rapidly. Molecular weight also is important. Assuming adequate lipid solubility, most nonionized drugs of molecular weights under 600 cross the cell boundaries with ease, whereas those with weights exceeding 1000 cannot cross. The concentration gradient between maternal and fetal blood, along with the surface area available for transfer and the thickness of the membrane, also determines the rate of diffusion.

Anatomic and Hemodynamic Factors

Among maternal factors influencing placental transport is uterine blood flow, which increases throughout pregnancy to reach an average value at term of 500–700 ml/minute (approximately 10% of resting cardiac output). About 80% of this flow reaches the placenta; the remaining 20% perfuses the uterine muscle. However, complications that may occur during the antepartum period, such as maternal arterial hypotension caused by hemor-

rhage, spinal or epidural anesthesia, or vena caval compression, may reduce uteroplacental blood flow and decrease drug delivery to the fetus. Further, uterine contractions may impose an intermittent obstruction to placental perfusion and drug transfer.

Drug uptake in fetal tissues depends both upon the tissue/blood partition coefficient of a given drug and upon the extent of tissue perfusion. Most of the umbilical vein blood perfuses the fetal liver and enters the vena cava through the hepatic vein, while a small fraction is shunted through the ductus venosus directly into the inferior vena cava. Consequently, a greater proportion of any drug carried by the umbilical vein blood is strained through the liver before gaining access to other fetal tissues.

Furthermore, a progressive dilution occurs during transit to the arterial side of the circulation as blood within the umbilical vein becomes admixed with venous blood from the gastrointestinal tract, the lower extremities, the head and upper extremities, and the lungs. This unique pattern of fetal circulation delays equilibration between fetal blood and fetal tissues, as manifested by the persistence of a drug concentration gradient between umbilical vein and artery.

Anesthetized patients in uncomplicated term deliveries usually give birth to vigorous infants, which indicates that there is a delay in drug uptake by fetal brain tissue. This delay can be explained in part by the interposition of the fetal blood compartment between maternal blood and fetal brain. The persistent gradient between umbilical vein and artery concentrations, as well as uptake by the fetal liver, has been demonstrated for a variety of anesthetics, including thiopental (Pentothal) and nitrous oxide. With use of thiopental, the rapid fall in maternal plasma concentrations following intravenous injection ensures that fetal exposure to high maternal blood levels will be very short. The placental transfer of any drug given intravenously can be hindered if injection is carried out at the beginning of a uterine contraction, which temporarily diminishes or perhaps arrests perfusion of the intervillous space.

Inhalation agents also cross the placenta readily, although analgesic concentrations do not produce significant neonatal depression, even when administered continuously for prolonged periods. Low Apgar scores correlate with prolonged induction-to-delivery time, however, when anesthetic concentrations are used. For example, concentrations of 70% will depress the fetus within approximately 10 minutes.

Formerly, it was believed that muscle relaxants, commonly used for "balanced" anesthesia during cesarean section, could not cross the placenta in significant amounts because of their high degree of ionization and low lipid solubility. Recently developed sensitive and specific radioimmunoassay techniques show measurable, albeit low, concentrations of D-tubocurare in blood specimens taken from the umbilical vessels at delivery, even following use of recommended doses. Pancuronium bromide (Pavulon) has been detected in the neonatal urine. Similarly, studies on rhesus monkeys have shown placental transmission of succinylcholine to be more rapid and extensive than believed previously. And, as recently reported, succinylcholine given to a patient with atypical serum cholinesterase can cause neonatal flaccidity and apnea in atypical homozygous infants. Succinylcholine does not seem to affect a heterozygous infant seriously.

The growing use of regional anesthesia for relief of pain in labor and delivery has led to increased concern about the effects of local anesthetics on the fetus and neonate. All amides have been found to cross the placenta within 1–3 minutes of injection. Mepivacaine (Carbocaine) reaches peak concentrations in maternal blood within 25–40 minutes following a single epidural injection; peak concentrations in fetal blood occur within 30–45 minutes. Since blood levels in both mother and fetus fall slowly, repeated injections may result in maternal and fetal drug accumulation. Absorption of local anesthetics from the paracervical area appears to be more rapid than from the epidural space, probably because of the higher vascularity of paracervical tissues; the result is occasional fetal overdosage. Serial determinations of fetal and maternal blood concentrations of lidocaine following paracervical block reveal mean maternal and fetal drug concentrations at maximal values within 9–10 minutes. This rapid rate of absorption may be decreased by depositing the drug at a depth no greater than 2–3 mm below the mucosal surface. With this technique maternal blood levels tend to rise more slowly (i.e., for 20 minutes).

Rapidly metabolized or long-acting drugs should reduce the problems of maternal and fetal toxicity. Unlike most clinically used amides, which are metabolized slowly by hepatic microsomal enzymes, chloroprocaine (Nesacaine) is an ester that is hydrolyzed rapidly by plasma pseudocholinesterase. It has an in vitro half-life of 21 seconds in maternal blood and of 43 seconds in fetal blood. Compared to lidocaine and mepivacaine, long-acting agents such as bupivacaine (Marcaine) and etido-caine (Duranest) have the advantage of requiring less frequent injection, thus lessening the risk of accumulation in both mother and fetus.

Indirect Effects

The adequacy of the uteroplacental circulation, so vital to the well-being of the fetus, is easily affected by drugs and anesthetic procedures.

Placental blood flow is directly proportional to the net perfusion pressure across the intervillous space and inversely proportional to the resistance of the spiral arterioles supplying the intervillous space, as well as the resistance imparted to the blood vessels by the myometrial tension. Thus, any anesthetic procedure or agent that would tend to decrease the perfusion pressure and/or increase vascular resistance may result in a placental hypoperfusion and fetal asphyxia.

Perfusion pressure across the intervillous space may be diminished consequent to maternal systemic hypotension, which, in turn, may be due to the use of epidural or spinal anesthesia, to aortocaval compression in the supine position, or to hemorrhage. It has been proposed that, in normal circumstances, the placental vasculature is dilated maximally so that the perfusion is the major determinant of uterine blood flow (18). However, with general anesthetics, such as halothane, a small drop in maternal blood pressure may even be associated with an increase in uterine blood flow because of uterine muscle relaxation and a decrease in uterine vascular resistance (19).

Conversely, increased uterine activity may result in reduced placental perfusion. Thus, the use of alpha-adrenergic drugs, such as methoxamine, to correct maternal hypotension (20) and anesthetics, such as ketamine (in doses above 1 mg/kg), may produce increased uterine tone sufficient to endanger the fetus (21).

Hyperventilation of the mother, if severe, also may reduce uterine blood flow. Originally, this was attributed to hypocapnia or respiratory alkalosis. More recently, a study performed in pregnant sheep has established that placental hypoperfusion results from the mechanical effect of hyperventilation since it could not be corrected by restoring $PaCO_2$ to normal or above normal levels (22).

Finally, it has been shown in experimental animals that epinephrine and norepinephrine infusion results in a decrease in uterine blood flow and deterioration in fetal condition (23). Administration of local anesthetic solutions containing epinephrine or maternal pain and apprehension may similarly affect the fetus.

CLINICAL
APPLICATIONS

As a result of the special experience gained by anesthesiologists in recent years in the intraoperative and intensive care management of critical illness, their help can be an invaluable part of the care of the complicated pregnant patient and should be sought early. Evaluation of the medical history, current problems, and past anesthetic experiences are important, as well as a review of all medications the patient has received recently or is receiving. Many drugs used by anesthesiologists may interact with current medications, and physiological parameters can be assessed fully only in relation to preexisting pharmacologic modifications. Possible difficulties with airway management or endotracheal intubation should be considered before the necessity for these procedures arises.

Of particular importance is the preparation of the mother for any special monitoring or anesthetic techniques that may be considered essential for the control of *her* status at the time of labor and delivery. *Fetal* monitoring during labor has become a standard practice, but the value of central venous, arterial, or pulmonary artery pressure monitoring or the benefits of controlled regional anesthesia in certain situations may have to be explained carefully. The anesthetic procedures involved in cesarean section also should fully be discussed in advance, either when planned electively or to allay the anxiety that may occur if an emergency intervention should prove necessary. It is generally agreed that only emergency nonobstetric surgery should be performed during pregnancy.

Based on our knowledge of the anesthetic hazards particularly related to pregnancy, the following guidelines for analgesia/anesthesia seem indicated:

1. Apprehension should be allayed as much as possible by personal reassurance and adequate premedication. Belladonna alkloids may be used.
2. Pain should be relieved whenever possible.
3. Administration of an antacid, 15–30 ml, approximately 1 hour prior to induction of anesthesia usually will raise the pH of gastric juice above the critical level of 2.5. Clear antacids produce fewer sequelae when aspirated.
4. Beginning in the second trimester, mothers should not be transported or placed on the op-

erating table in the supine position. The lateral decubitus position or left uterine displacement will minimize the risk of vena caval compression.
5. Hypotension related to spinal or epidural anesthesia should be prevented as much as possible by rapid intravenous infusion of at least 1 liter of a crystalloid solution prior to induction of anesthesia. Should maternal blood pressure fall despite this pretreatment, a beta-adrenergic vasopressor, such as ephedrine, should be promptly administered intravenously.
6. General anethesia should be preceded by careful denitrogenation to avoid maternal and fetal hypoxemia during induction and intubation.
7. The risk of aspiration should be minimized by application of cricoid pressure and rapid endotracheal intubation with a cuffed tube.
8. To reduce fetal hazard, particularly during the first trimester, it appears preferable to choose drugs with a history of safe usage over many years. These would include thiopental, morphine, merperidine, succinylcholine, curare, and low concentrations of nitrous oxide. However, ketamine, 0.5–0.75 mg/kg, might be preferable to thiopental as an induction agent in the face of severe hypovolemia. In these low doses, ketamine should have practically no effect on uterine tone. Halothane offers the specific advantage of relaxing the uterus when this is required during delivery or for procedures such as cervical cerclage (Shirodkar procedure).
9. In order to avoid maternal hyperventilation, one should monitor arterial blood gases or end-expiratory PCO_2.
10. It is also advisable to monitor the fetal heart rate continuously throughout surgery and anesthesia provided that placement of the transducer does not encroach upon the surgical field (24). Using the directional Doppler apparatus, this monitoring is technically feasible from the 16th week of pregnancy. Uterine tone also may be monitored with an external tocodynamometer if the uterus has grown enough to reach the umbilicus or above.
11. Special procedures, such as hypothermia and induced hypotension, might be desirable to facilitate surgery. Successful fetal outcome following both procedures for intracranial operations (25, 26) has been reported.

NURSING MANAGEMENT

Nursing care specific for the pregnant patient receiving *analgesia/anesthesia*:

☐ Educate the patient regarding analgesia/anesthesia, including procedure, risks, benefits, expected outcome.

☐ Assess maternal and fetal vital signs before analgesia/anesthesia is given; continue to monitor after it is given.

☐ Assess bladder and encourage frequent voiding since patient may be unaware of bladder pressure.

☐ Encourage left lateral position to promote uterine perfusion

For the patient having *general anesthesia*:

☐ Assess for factors that increase anesthetic risk:
  — Use of alcohol, medications, street drugs, cigarettes;
  — Poor nutritional status (e.g., anemia);
  — Fluid/electrolyte imbalance; and
  — History of recent food/fluid intake.

☐ Encourage use of relaxation techniques prior to induction to promote fetal oxygenation.

For the patient receiving *narcotic analgesia*:

☐ Administer the intravenous narcotic properly:
  — Begin injecting narcotic at the beginning of a contraction to minimize fetal absorption; and
  — Give slowly (approximately 2 minutes) to prevent dizziness, and nausea/vomiting.

☐ Monitor effectiveness (maximum effect on both mother and fetus will occur rapidly after intravenous administration and will decrease in 1–2 hours); after intramuscular injection effects will occur more slowly and clear more slowly.

☐ Observe for untoward maternal/fetal effects (e.g., decreased fetal beat-to-beat variability); keep patient on bed rest with side rails up to prevent falling; keep emesis basin by the bed.

☐ Alert patient at the onset of a contraction so she may begin a psychoprophylactic breathing pattern rather than be awakened by a contraction at its peak.

For the patient receiving *epidural anesthesia*:

☐ Have equipment and personnel readily available in case of emergency (e.g., respiratory or cardiac arrest).

☐ Administer rapid infusion of intravenous fluids prior to administration of epidural to prevent hypotension.

☐ Assist patient to maintain correct position for insertion of epidural catheter: sitting or lying with lower back curved outward, shoulders forward, chin on chest.

☐ Assess for hypotension after epidural is given: take blood pressure every 5 minutes until stable and then every 15 minutes.

☐ Assess for fetal distress via electronic fetal monitoring.

☐ Prepare for delivery:
  — Assist patient with pushing in second stage by telling her *when* as well as *how* to *push*, and assist her into proper position for pushing;
  — Alert anesthesia team of imminent delivery so delivery dose can be given;
  — Allow extra time for transfer to delivery room since patient will need help moving to delivery table; and
  — Do not discharge the patient from the recovery area until the epidural catheter is removed and the patient has recovered full sensory and motor ability.

For the patient receiving *spinal anesthesia*:

☐ Have equipment and personnel readily available in case of emergency (e.g., respiratory or cardiac arrest).

☐ Administer rapid infusion of intravenous fluids prior to administration of spinal anesthesia.

☐ Assist patient to assume correct position after transfer to delivery room: sitting during administration (to facilitate downward flow of anesthetic solution by gravity) with lower back curved outward, shoulders forward, and chin on chest; assist to lying position at proper time.

☐ Assess for hypotension after spinal is given: take blood pressure every 5 minutes until stable, and then every 15 minutes.

☐ Teach patient to remain flat in bed for 12 hours after delivery to avoid spinal headache syndrome.

☐ Do not discharge the patient from the delivery area until she has recovered full sensory and motor ability.

Nursing diagnoses most frequently associated with *analgesia/anesthesia* (see Section V):

☐ Altered maternal tissue perfusion.
☐ Altered fetal cardiac and cerebral tissue perfusion.
☐ Pain.
☐ Anxiety/fear.
☐ Altered patterns of urinary elimination.
☐ Knowledge deficit regarding analgesia and anesthesia.

REFERENCES

1. Shnider SM, Webster GM: Maternal and fetal hazards of surgery during pregnancy. *Am J Obstet Gynecol* 92:891–900, 1965.
2. Bonica JJ: Basic considerations: obstetric analgesia-anaesthesia, recent advances and current status. In Bonica JJ. (ed): *Clinics in Obstetrics and Gynaecology*. London, WB Saunders, 1975, vol 2, pp 469–497.
3. Kerr MG, Scott DB, Samuel E: Studies of the inferior vena cava in late pregnancy. *Br Med J* 1:532–533, 1964.
4. Ueland K, Novy MJ, Peterson EN, Metcalfe J: Maternal cardiovascular dynamics. IV. The influence of gestational age on the maternal cardiovascular response to posture and exercise. *Am J Obstet Gynecol* 104:856–864, 1969.
5. Howard BK, Goodson JH, Mengert WF: Supine hypotensive syndrome of late pregnancy. *Obstet Gynecol* 1:371–377, 1953.
6. Humphrey MC, Chang A, Wood EC, Morgan S, Hownslow D: A decrease in fetal pH during the second stage of labour when conducted in the dorsal position. *J Obstet Gynaecol Br Commonw* 81: 600–602, 1974.
7. Bieniarz J, Crottogini JJ, Curuchet E, Romero-Salinas G, Yoshida T. Poseiro JJ, Caldeyro-Barcia R: Aortocaval compression by the uterus in late human pregnancy. II. An angiographic study. *Am J Obstet Gynecol* 100:203–217, 1968.
8. Mendelson CL: Disorders of the heartbeat during pregnancy. *Am J Obstet Gynecol* 72:1268–1301, 1956.
9. Bonica JJ: *Principles and Practice of Obstetric Analgesia and Anesthesia*. Philadelphia, FA Davis, 1967, p 21.
10. McGinty AP: The comparative effects of pregnancy and phrenic nerve interruption on the diaphragm and their relation to pulmonary tuberculosis. *Am J Obstet Gynecol* 35:237–248, 1938.
11. Cugell DW, Frank NR, Gaensler A, Badger TL: Pulmonary function in pregnancy. I. Serial observations in normal women. *Am Rev Tuberc* 67:568–597, 1953.
12. Bevan DR, Holdcroft A, Loh L, MacGregor WG, O'Sullivan JC, Sykes MK: Closing volume and pregnancy. *Br Med J* 1:13–15, 1974.

13. Baldwin GR, Doraswamy SM, Whelton JA, MacDonnell KF: New lung functions and pregnancy. *Am J Obstet Gynecol* 127:235–239, 1977.
14. Gee JBL, Packer BS, Millen JE, Robin ED: Pulmonary mechanics during pregnancy. *J Clin Invest* 46:945–952, 1967.
15. Anderseon GJ, James GB, Mathers NP, Smith EL, Walker J: The maternal oxygen tension and acid-base status during pregnancy. *J Obstet Gynaecol Br Commonw* 76:16-19, 1969.
16. Davison JS, Davison MC, Hay DM: Gastric emptying time in late pregnancy and labour. *J Obstet Gynaecol Br Commonw* 77:37–41, 1970.
17. Lind FJ, Smith AM, McIver DK, Coopland AT, Crispin JS: Heartburn in pregnancy—a manometric study. *Can Med Assoc J* 98:571–574, 1968.
18. Greiss FC Jr: Pressure-flow relationship in the gravid uterine vascular bed. *Am J Obstet Gynecol* 96:41–47, 1966.
19. Palahniuk RJ, Shnider SM: Maternal and fetal cardiovascular and acid-base changes during halothane and isoflurane anesthesia in the pregnant ewe. *Anesthesiology* 41:462–472, 1974.
20. Vasicka A, Hutchinson H, Eng J, Allen CR: Spinal and epidural anesthesia, fetal and uterine response to acute hypo- and hypertension. *Am J Obstet Gynecol* 90:800–810, 1964.
21. Galloon S: Ketamine for obstetric delivery. *Anesthesiology* 44:522–524, 1976.
22. Levinson G. Shnider SM, de Lorimier AA, Steffenson JL: Effects of maternal hyperventilation on uterine blood flow and fetal oxygenation and acid-base status. *Anesthesiology* 40:340–344, 1974.
23. Rosenfeld CR, Baron MD, Meschia G: Effects of epinephrine on distribution of blood flow in the pregnant ewe. *Am J Obstet Gynecol* 124:156–163, 1976.
24. Katz JD, Hook R, Barash PG: Fetal heart rate monitoring in the pregnant patient under surgery. *Am J Obstet Gynecol* 125:267–269, 1976.
25. Hehre FW: Hypothermia for operations during pregnancy. *Anesth Analg (Cleve)* 44:424–428, 1965.
26. Donchin Y, Amirav B. Sahar A, Yarkoni S: Sodium nitroprusside for aneurysm surgery in pregnancy: report of a case. *Br J Anaesth* 50:849–851, 1978.

Chapter 39
Recognition of Fetal Distress
Kathleen Buckley, C.N.M., M.S.N.

UTEROPLACENTAL PHYSIOLOGY

Assessing fetal well-being during labor through use of fetal monitoring requires first and foremost that the nurse has a basic understanding of uteroplacental physiology. Since the placenta is the organ for fetal oxygen/carbon dioxide (O_2/CO_2) exchange, most severe abnormal variations in fetal heart rate can be traced back to a malfunction of the placenta (1). Compromised maternal blood flow to the placenta and/or constricted fetal blood vessels produce hypoxia. This condition is known as placental insufficiency.

On the other hand, a properly functioning placenta with adequate maternal blood flow into the placenta ensures that the fetus will be well oxygenated and supplied with necessary electrolytes and nutrients.

The placenta is a fetal organ composed of extensively branching, closely packed fetal villi. The maternal blood flow circulates only in the intervillous space (IVS) (see Chapter 31). Three protective layers of fetal tissue separate fetal blood capillaries from maternal blood in the IVS. The fetal capillary is surrounded by a layer of endothelial cells, which is embedded in a cushion of connective tissue and, finally, wrapped in a layer of trophoblast cells (1). Therefore, fetal and maternal bloods do *not* mix.

Water, electrolytes, carbon dioxide, and oxygen are exchanged between maternal and fetal blood through the process of passive diffusion. Passive diffusion is defined as the movement of substances from an area of higher concentration to an area of lower concentration. Almost any substance dissolved in maternal or fetal blood crosses the placenta through passive diffusion, depending on the concentration gradient. The IVS has an oxygen ten-

sion averaging 40–50 mm Hg. The fetal villi have an O_2 tension of only about 35 mm Hg, causing O_2 to diffuse from the higher maternal gradient into the lower fetal gradient (1).

The effects of inadequate placental respiratory gas exchange (placental insufficiency) depend on the degree of inadequacy and the rate of onset. Chronic insufficiency results in fetal intrauterine growth retardation (see Chapter 27). Insufficiency that occurs rapidly gives the fetal system little time to compensate, and fetal death may ensue. Examples of rapidly occurring insufficiency include abruptio placentae, fetal cord accidents, and sudden onset of maternal hypertension or hypotension.

THE AUTONOMIC NERVOUS SYSTEM AND FETAL HEART RATE

The fetal autonomic nervous system plays an important part in modulating the fetal heart rate (FHR). Increases or decreases in FHR are related directly to cardiac output, which is the second important factor that affects fetal oxygenation (2).

The fetal heart has its own intrinsic pacemaker in the sinoatrial (SA) node. The two branches of the autonomic nervous system—parasympathetic and sympathetic—cause changes in the heart's inherent rate. Pressure and oxygen sensors located in the aorta and carotid sinus activate the autonomic nervous system.

The parasympathetic nervous system primarily is the vagus nerve (cranial nerve X), which originates in the medulla oblongata. Fibers supply the SA and also the atrioventricular (AV) node. Stimulation of the vagus nerve results in a *decrease* in FHR. For example, pressure on the fetal head during uterine contractions or during vaginal examination may stimulate the vagus nerve and decrease the FHR. Conversely, a substance such as atropine, which counteracts vagal nerve-ending secretions, increases the FHR.

Sympathetic nerves (SN) are distributed widely throughout the muscle of the heart. They are a reserve system to improve the pumping action of the heart during intermittent stressful situations. Stimulation of SN will release norepinephrine and increase FHR, and blood pressure. A decrease in O_2 or an increase in CO_2 triggers the sympathetic nervous system. When blood pressure rises, stretch receptors called baroreceptors, found in the arch of the aorta and in the carotid sinus, send impulses via the vagus nerve to the heart to slow it down.

Peripheral chemoreceptors also are found in the arch of the aorta and in the carotid sinus. Central chemoreceptors are found in the medulla oblongata. Increase of CO_2 or decrease in O_2 results in tachycardia and increase in blood pressure. An increase in blood pressure then may cause the baroreceptors to fire and decrease FHR.

In the adult heart the amount of blood pumped per minute (stroke volume) is inversely proportional to the heart rate. As the heart rate decreases, the stroke volume increases. This mechanism (Frank-Starling mechanism) helps to maintain a constant level of tissue perfusion (2).

In the fetus that mechanism is not well developed. When the FHR decreases, the stroke volume does *not* increase. Therefore, the fetus can only increase cardiac output and, hence, oxygen perfusion by increasing the heart rate. A poorly oxygenated fetus first will manifest tachycardia and increased blood pressure—an attempt to increase oxygen supply to fetal cells. A severely asphyxiated fetus will manifest bradycardia. This is a reflex reaction activated by the autonomic nervous system baroreceptors in response to elevated blood pressure. The fetus with a slow heart rate is severely jeopardized because the only fetal mechanism for increasing oxygen flow is tachycardia, and that has failed (3).

TYPES OF FETAL HEART RATE CHANGES

FHR data are divided into two main categories: baseline rate and periodic change. Baseline FHR is defined as the rate pattern in the absence of or in between contractions. Periodic FHR change is defined as modulation of the FHR occurring with uterine contractions.

FACTORS AFFECTING THE BASELINE FETAL HEART RATE

The average baseline FHR at term is 140 beats per minute (BPM). Variations of 20 BPM above or below these values are within normal limits. Thus, the normal range is 120–160 BPM (4).

Variations in baseline FHR are tachycardia, bradycardia, and variability (Fig. 39.1). These three changes are produced in response to stimulation by the autonomic nervous system or by oxygen deprivation, which depresses the action of the myocardium directly.

Tachycardia

Fetal tachycardia is defined as a rise in the baseline heart rate to greater than 160 BPM. The most common cause is maternal fever. During labor, dehydration from vomiting or inadequate oral or intravenous intake is a frequent cause of temperature elevation (4).

Other etiologies of fetal tachycardia include the following (5):

1. Fetal hypoxia (an early, compensated sign)
2. Fetal infection
3. Fetal movement or stimulation
4. Fetal cardiac arrhythmias
5. Maternal anxiety
6. Maternal hyperthyroidism

Certain drugs that block the parasympathetic nervous system, such as scopolamine or atropine, produce tachycardia. Other drugs such as isoxsuprine or ritodrine, mimic the cardiac stimulation of epinephrine and also produce tachycardia (6).

Bradycardia

Fetal bradycardia is a decrease in baseline FHR to less than 110 BPM. Bradycardia always is a sign of severe, decompensated anoxia (4, p 617).

The etiology of bradycardia includes the following (5, p 232):

1. Acute oxygen deprivation from placental abruption, cord prolapse, or uterine rupture
2. Chronic oxygen deprivation resulting in intrauterine growth retardation
3. Tetanic uterine contractions (often seen with oxytocin hyperstimulation)

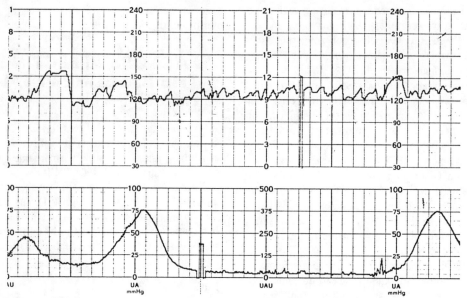

Figure 39.1. Normal tracing. Baseline FHR = 130 BPM, with short-term beat-to-beat variability of 3–5 BPM and good cyclicity. There are accelerations with movement and contractions. Uterine activity is excellent, with contractions of 75 mm Hg and low baseline tone. (Used with permission from Caplan RM (ed): *Principles of Obstetrics.* Baltimore, Williams & Wilkins, 1982, p 270.)

4. Vagal stimulation because of pressure on the fetal head—common during vigorous vaginal examination and application of fetal scalp electrode
5. Congenital fetal heart block (seen in systemic lupus erythematosus)
6. Maternal hypertension or hypotension
7. Maternal hypothermia

Sympathetic agents such as propranolol slow the heart rate. Anesthetic agents used for epidural or spinal anesthesia also slow the FHR indirectly by producing maternal hypotension. Agents used for pudendal anesthesia or paracervical block may slow the heart rate directly if they are inadvertently injected into the fetal blood system (6, p 44).

Variability

Irregular, random oscillations between 110–160 BPM in the fetal baseline pattern are termed variability. Variability reflects the maturation of the autonomic nervous system (4, p 619). Therefore, a term, healthy fetus will evidence more baseline variability than a preterm infant. Average short-term variability is between 6–10 BPM. Suppressed variability is associated with the following (4, p 619):

1. Chronic hypoxia
2. Prematurity
3. Fetal cardiac arrhythmias

4. Fetal sleep periods (short term—lasting approximately 20 minutes)

Tranquilizers, narcotics, barbiturates, or anesthetics can decrease short-term variability. Depressed variability because of drugs does not necessarily indicate fetal hypoxia. A healthy fetus will regain a normal baseline pattern as the drug is metabolized. However, injudicious drug administration to a compromised fetus may be the deciding factor in producing profound distress (7).

FETAL HEART RATE CHANGE ASSOCIATED WITH UTERINE CONTRACTIONS

Beginning in 1959, Hon first described the relationship between uterine contractions and FHR changes. Using animal models, he found consistent patterns between FHR decelerations and uterine activity. In South America Caldeyro-Barcia, working independently, at the same time documented similar findings (8, 9).

In 1967 the American College of Obstetricians and Gynecologists developed a standard terminology to clinically describe decelerations of the FHR

Table 39.1.
PERIODIC FETAL HEART RATE CHANGES[a]

EARLY DECELERATION

DEFINITION

Early deceleration is a transitory decrease in FHR caused by compressions of fetal head. Compression of fetal head stimulates vagus nerve to decrease heart rate. Early deceleration is not considered a sign of fetal distress.

ETIOLOGY

1. Sterile vaginal examination
2. During second stage of labor with pushing efforts
3. During application of scalp electrode
4. In cephalopelvic disproportion
5. In vertex presentations
6. Imminent delivery (vertex crowning)

DIAGNOSIS OF EARLY DECELERATION

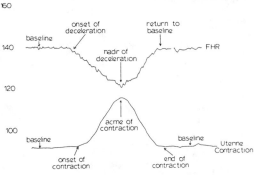

Early deceleration.

1. Uniform shape of deceleration on fetal monitor strip
2. Begins at beginning of contraction and ends with end of contraction
3. Depth of deceleration is related to intensity of contraction
4. Deceleration rarely goes below 110 beats/minute

VARIABLE DECELERATION

DEFINITION

Variable decelerations consist of transitory decreases in FHR caused by compression of umbilical cord. Variable decelerations are not associated with poor fetal outcome if baseline heart rate remains stable and variability is not decreased.

ETILOGY

1. Prolapse of cord
2. Nuchal cord (cord around the neck)
3. Cord occlusion (true knot)

DIAGNOSIS OF VARIABLE DECELERATION

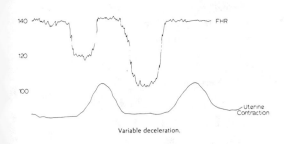

Variable deceleration.

1. Variable shape (often V or U shaped) of deceleration on fetal monitor strip
2. Variable onset: may begin at any time in relation to contraction
3. Heart rate may fall below 90 beats/minute; variable decelerations below 60 beats/minute are severe
4. Variable duration (greater than 40–60 seconds = prolonged deceleration)
5. Occur more frequently in active labor
6. Severe decelerations constitute a presumptive diagnosis of cord prolapse

LATE DECELERATION

DEFINITION

Late deceleration is a transitory decease in FHR caused by uteroplacental insufficiency; uteroplacental insufficiency means that there is decreased blood flow and oxygen to the fetus. *All late decelerations are ominous.*

ETIOLOGY

1. Hematological disorders: anemia, sickle cell disease, Rh isoimmunization
2. Bleeding disorders: abruptio placentae, placenta previa
3. Hypertensive disorders
4. Placental dysfunction: infarcts, postmaturity
5. Diabetes
6. Maternal hypotension
7. Uterine hyperstimulation and tetanic contractions

Table 39.1.
(Continued)

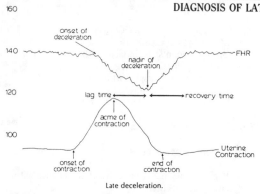

DIAGNOSIS OF LATE DECELERATION

Late deceleration.

1. Uniform shape of deceleration on fetal monitor strip
2. Begins after onset of contraction and ends after contraction completed
3. Often begins with peak of contraction
4. Depth of deceleration related to intensity of contraction
5. Depth of deceleration unrelated to degree of fetal hypoxia (i.e., drop in FHR of 5–10 points may connote *severe* hypoxia)

*aAdapted from Vestal K, McKensie C: *High Risk Perinatal Nursing.* Philadelphia, WB Saunders, 1983, pp 232–234.

occurring with contractions. These are detailed below (see Table 39.1):

1. Early decelerations—The onset, peak, and recovery coincide with the occurrence of the uterine contraction. It is designated *early* because the onset of the deceleration occurs early in the contracting phase of the uterus. The etiology is the compression of the fetal head during contractions, mediated by the vagus nerve. The shape of the deceleration reflects the shape of the contraction (uniform). The usual range of this type of deceleration is 140–100 BPM. It carries no association with fetal morbidity or mortality.

2. Late decelerations—The peak of the FHR deceleration occurs after the peak of the uterine contraction. The shape of the deceleration is uniform. The etiology is placental insufficiency, resulting in fetal hypoxia. This, in turn, interferes with the ability of the fetal myocardium to maintain FHR. It is frequently seen in high risk pregnancy, uterine hyperactivity, and/or maternal hypotension and occurs in 4–8% of all labors. This ominous pattern associated with asphyxiated newborns may be insidious because it is usually found in the normal FHR range.

3. Variable decelerations—These decelerations show variable shape as well as occur at variable times in relation to contractions. The etiology is transient compression of the umbilical cord. These decelerations change fetal status only if they are frequent, profound, and prolonged. In most cases change in maternal position (turning to right or left side) can cause complete

reversal of these decelerations. The range of variable decelerations is 140–60 BPM.

INTERMITTENT EVALUATION OF FETAL STATUS

This method involves the use of the fetoscope or doptone to count fetal heart tones and palpation of uterine contractions. Several studies have documented the safety and effectiveness of intermittent FHR monitoring (10, 11) for the low risk gravida. The World Health Organization has urged the adoption of an international standard that supports use of intermittent monitoring for normal labor and birth. However, since this text deals with the high risk gravida, the reader is referred to other nursing texts for further details regarding assessment techniques.

CONTINUOUS EVALUATION OF FETAL STATUS

Two types of electronic fetal monitoring—external monitoring system (EMS) and internal monitoring system (IMS)—provide for a continuous data read-out of both the FHR and the uterine contraction pattern. Each method has its place along a continuum of normal to high risk perinatal assessment. Women who fall into high risk categories must be monitored continuously during labor. Use of continuous monitoring is an invaluable aid to the obstetrical health care team in developing a management plan for the compromised, hypoxic fetus (see Table 39.2).

Table 39.2.
CRITERIA FOR ELECTRONIC MONITORING[a]

PRENATAL FACTORS	INTRAPARTUM FACTORS
Toxemia	Falling estriol levels
Maternal weight of <45.4 kg (<100 pounds) or >90.7 kg (>200 pounds), or a weight gain of <7.7 kg (<17 pounds).	No prenatal care
	Gestational age <37 or >42 weeks or small for gestational age
Rh-sensitized pregnancy	Toxemia
Maternal age <17 or >35 years	Hydramnios or oligohydramnios
Drug or alcohol abuse	Premature rupture of membranes of >12 hours
Anemia	Failure to progress in labor
Metabolic disease (diabetes, thyroid condition, etc.)	Use of medication (magnesium sulfate, oxytocin, narcotics, etc.)
Cardiac disease	Meconium staining
Renal disease	FHR abnormalities
Chronic hypertension	Abnormal presentation or lie
Maternal obstetric history (previous stillbirth, neonatal death, premature infant, previous cesarean section, etc.)	Grand multiparity
Seizure disorder	
Suspicious or positive NST or OCT	

[a]Adapted from Hobel C: Prenatal and intrapartum high risk screening. *Am J Obstet Gynecol* Sept: 1-9, 1973.

External Monitoring System

The most common method of obtaining an external recording of the FHR is with an ultrasound transducer containing a transmitting and receiving crystal that picks up the motion of the fetal heart valves (12, p 374–375). This is mounted in a capsule and held firmly in place on the maternal abdomen with an elastic strap. A conductive jelly should be applied to the transducer in order to improve sound transmission through the abdomen. A strain gauge transducer is used to monitor uterine contractions externally. It is placed over the uterine fundus and held in place with a second elastic strap. The heart rate sounds and uterine contractions are translated into electrical impulses that are reproduced on a strip chart on a fetal monitor.

Both heart rate and uterine transducers may pick up extraneous sounds or movement. Fetal movement, maternal bowel sounds, and maternal coughing or vomiting should not be confused with the true reading.

External FHR tracings cannot accurately assess FHR variability. Moreover, external uterine contraction monitoring does not quantify the relative strength of uterine contractions.

EMS is thought to be a noninvasive technique. However, in order to obtain an accurate fetal heart tracing, the laboring woman's movements usually must be restricted. It should be noted that positioning the woman flat in bed in order to obtain a "better" tracing will cause iatrogenic fetal hypoxia because of portocaval occlusion and maternal hypotension. Such mismanagement of technology should not occur.

Although the laboring woman will need to be in bed with this method of monitoring, she should be positioned on her side—never flat on her back. If the dorsal recumbent position must be used, a bedroll should be placed under the right hip in order to keep the weight of the uterus off the vena cava.

Internal Fetal Monitoring

While internal fetal monitoring is the most reliable means of monitoring the FHR, it is also the most invasive. It is used when labor has begun, membranes are ruptured, and the cervix is dilated enough to allow application of the monitoring equipment (12, p 374–375).

A stainless steel spiral electrode is inserted just under the skin of the presenting part of the fetus. A special safety lock prevents penetration of the skin by more than 2 mm. These electrode signals are recorded on the strip chart on the fetal monitor. Beat-to-beat variability may be assessed accurately by this method.

A fluid-filled strain gauge catheter placed in the uterine cavity transmits the pressure of a uterine contraction to a transducer. This transducer converts the pressure into millimeters of mercury. Unlike the EMS, IMS gives a precise evaluation of contraction strength measured in millimeters of mercury (7, p 171).

The laboring woman wearing the IMS can move easily from side to side in bed, sit with her legs over the side of the bed, or even move to a nearby chair. A variety of positions for second-stage pushing (i.e., squatting in bed, left lateral) are possible and will not dislodge the IMS.

Table 39.3.
CLASSIFICATION OF FETAL HEART RATE PATTERNS[a]

CLASSIFICATION	BASELINE FEATURES	PERIODIC FEATURES
Reassuring	Stable rate	No change
	Average variability	Uniform accelerations
		Early decelerations
Suspicious	Decreased variability	Absent deceleration
	Tachycardia	Absent deceleration
	Bradycardia	Absent deceleration
Threatening	Stable rate	Late decelerations
	Average variability	Variable decelerations
Ominous	Absent variability	Late decelerations
	Tachycardia	Variable decelerations
	Bradycardia	Variable decelerations

[a]Reprinted with permission from Cohen W, Friedman E: *Management of Labor*. Baltimore; University Park Press, 1983, p 182.

The most frequently reported fetal complication of IMS is scalp abscess at the site where the FHR electrode was attached (7, p 179). Currently, there is some concern regarding increased transmission or inoculation of the AIDS virus via the scalp electrode. The incidence of infection increases if multiple attempts at placement are involved. Because of this, many institutions have developed policies requiring the following:

1. Application of a bacteriostatic solution to the electrode placement site immediately after delivery.
2. Documentation of IMS in the nursery record in order to alert nursery staff to assess the scalp for presence of infection.

Puncture of the fetal umbilical vessels by the uterine strain gauge catheter has been reported (7, p 179). The most common maternal complication of IMS is postpartum infection. Both the fetal scalp electrode and the strain gauge catheter act as conduits for vaginal flora to enter the uterus (7, p 179). Women who are monitored internally and have cesarean sections have the highest overall rate of uterine infection. In diminishing order of frequency of infection are those who have a cesarean section and are not monitored; those with a vaginal delivery who are monitored; and those with a vaginal delivery who are unmonitored.

FETAL SCALP BLOOD SAMPLING

Clinical studies have shown a strong correlation between a normal FHR tracing via continuous electronic monitoring and good fetal outcome as measured by Apgar scores of 7 or above at 5 minutes. In fact, the correlation is on the order of 99% (4, p 634).

However, the converse is *not true*. An abnormal FHR tracing is not always associated with poor outcome. The false-positive rate is as high as 50%.

This discrepancy has led to the development of a further assessment technique—fetal scalp blood sampling (FSBS). A small amount of blood is taken directly from the fetal scalp and measured for pH. A pH of 7.25–7.35 indicates a well-oxygenated fetus and correlates with a good outcome. Values of 7.20 or lower are always suggestive of significant hypoxia. A pH of 7.20–7.24 is equivocal and must be repeated frequently as labor progresses (7, p 175).

Physiologically, pH is a reliable indicator of fetal oxygen status because of the following (7, p 175):

1. Poor placental functioning produces a carbon dioxide debt that causes a modest fall in pH, producing a *respiratory acidosis*.
2. Because of oxygen deprivation, fetal aerobic pathways of metabolism cannot function, and anaerobic metabolism of glucose (the major fetal metabolite) results in build-up of organic acids, causing a *metabolic acidosis*.

Timing of the sample in relation to the uterine contraction pattern is important. A pH determination obtained directly *before* a contraction gives the best indication of fetal reserve and ability to recover from the previous contraction. Conversely, samples taken immediately after a contraction or a deceleration will be abnormal. However, this acidosis usually is respiratory (not metabolic) and resolves quickly; therefore, it is an unreliable measure of the true fetal pH (7, p 175).

Fetal complications arising from FSBS include scalp infection and cellulitis at the site of the sampling incision. Although rare, significant fetal hemorrhage has been associated with the procedure even though subsequent newborn coagulation profiles were defined as normal (13). FSBS should

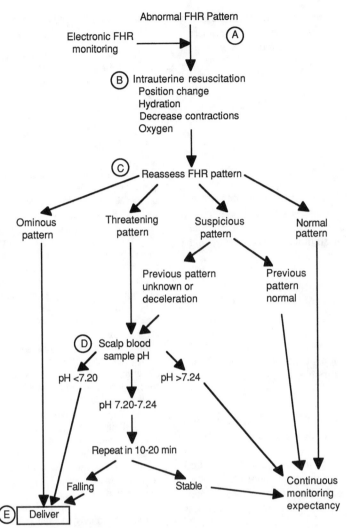

Figure 39.2. Schema for management of fetal distress in labor. (Adapted with permission from Friedman E: *Obstetrical Decision Making.* St. Louis, Mosby, 1982, p 139.)

be used cautiously in those fetuses diagnosed with coagulation defects or with coagulation deficits owing to maternal conditions or ingestion of drugs (i.e., salicylates).

Maternal complications include cervical hemorrhage or laceration because of manipulation during the procedure.

MANAGEMENT OF LABOR

Management of labor can be planned safely even for the most compromised fetus by using continuous monitoring and FSBS. FHR patterns should be evaluated and classified as reassuring, suspicious, threatening, or ominous (Table 39.3) (7).

Suspicious signs—tachycardia, bradycardia, or decreased variability—should be assessed to eliminate correctable causes such as maternal dehydration or portocaval hypotension. Analgesia and regional anesthesia hold the risk of synergistic compromise and should be withheld unless the tracing becomes reassuring. Oxytoxics may be used, but only after fetal oxygenation is documented as adequate by FSBS.

Recurrent variable or late decelerations constitute a threatening pattern. Emergency delivery should be considered if the quality of the baseline characteristics declines or if the FSBS decreases.

Ominous FHR patterns in the presence of low fetal pH should prompt immediate cesarean section, because these patterns almost always signify severe fetal asphyxia.

Figure 39.2 provides a schematic plan for management of labor based on baseline and periodic FHR changes.

Charting

Guidelines for charting nursing notes on the continuous monitor graph vary from institution to institution. However, all procedures performed should be written legibly on the monitor print-out graph as well as in the nurse's notes. The graph is a legal document and remains with the mother's chart. Examples of significant information to be written on the graph include:

1. Application of monitor—time and type (EMS or IMS) and name of caregiver who applied it.
2. Maternal vital signs—recorded with onset of fetal tachycardia, bradycardia, or severe variables.
3. Maternal position—time and position change (i.e., left or right side, in chair).
4. Vaginal examination—time performed and results.
5. Rupture of membranes—whether spontaneous or artificial, time, and character of amniotic fluid.
6. Medications (narcotics, oxytocin, MgSO$_4$, etc.) —time, type, amount, and route.
7. Physician evaluation of graph—document time and name of physician who evaluates tracing.

Response to Continuous Fetal Monitoring

Research has documented a consistent pattern of emotional response to fetal monitoring. In general, women with previous poor obstetric outcome and/or with the potential for poor outcome with a current pregnancy are reassured by use of continuous fetal monitoring and welcome its use. On the other hand, obstetrically normal women may perceive its use as dehumanizing or as an interference in the normal birth process.

Perhaps the most important research finding to date has documented the patient's need for continuous nursing presence throughout the entire course of electronic monitoring (14).

The National Institute of Child Health and Human Development has recommended guidelines for using continuous monitoring in order to promote family-centered care regardless of the method of fetal assessment employed during labor.

Standards for Use of Electronic Fetal Monitoring

1. Electronic fetal monitoring or any other technology should never be a substitute for clinical judgment. Electronic fetal monitoring is only one parameter of fetal assessment.

2. Proper use of both intermittent auscultation and continuous electronic fetal monitoring in both high and low risk patients should at the outset include a discussion with the patient of her wishes, concerns, and questions concerning benefits, limitations, and risks of fetal monitoring. Women should have the opportunity to discuss the use of all forms of monitoring during the course of prenatal care and again upon admission to the labor suite.

The use of all forms of monitoring should be accompanied by supportive and knowledgeable personnel who are attentive to the patient's expectations regarding the conduct of her labor. Hospital personnel should be cognizant of the potential impact of electronic fetal monitoring upon family-centered childbirth.

3. Periodic auscultation of the FHR (for 30 seconds every 15 minutes in the first stage of labor and every 5 minutes during the second stage, immediately following a contraction) is an acceptable method of assessing fetal condition for women at low risk of intrapartum fetal distress. Interpretation of auscultated FHR data should include an understanding of the relationship of FHR changes to uterine contractions.

Although the Task Force on Antenatal Care finds that the weight of present evidence does not show a benefit of electronic fetal monitoring in low risk patients, it recognizes that under certain circumstances, mothers or physicians may choose to use electronic fetal monitoring in low risk patients.

4. The use of electronic fetal monitoring should be considered strongly in high risk patients. Some of the high risk situations may include: (1) low birth weight, prematurity, postmaturity, and intrauterine growth retardation; (2) medical complications of pregnancy; (3) meconium staining of the amniotic fluid; (4) intrapartum obstetrical complications; (5) use of oxytocin in labor; and (6) the presence of abnormal auscultatory findings.

The medical record should reflect careful consideration of the benefits and risks to each individual, including a discussion of the indications for electronic fetal monitoring.

5. Since unexpected risk factors may arise during labor in patients without prior evidence of risk, all hospitals and birthing centers providing maternity care should have the necessary trained staff and equipment to assess carefully the status of each fetus in labor and to take appropriate action.

6. To ensure that electronic fetal monitoring is used appropriately, the medical profession and others should encourage, through their various educational modalities, a thorough understanding of the principles and procedures of intrapartum FHR assessment by all personnel responsible for the care of pregnant

women. Special attention should be given to the benefits, limitations, and risks of each mode of assessment. Acquisition of expertise in the use of continuous FHR and intrauterine pressure data requires the opportunity for supervised practical training in the interpretation of monitor tracings, use of FSBS, and the integration of such data into the clinical setting.

7. The use of fetal scalp blood pH determination is encouraged strongly as an adjunct to electronic FHR monitoring.

8. Attention to the known potential hazards of electronic fetal monitoring should accompany its use. Placement of the fetal scalp electrode and intrauterine pressure catheter should be performed with attention to aseptic and atraumatic technique. Prolonged supine position of the mother should be avoided, and maternal mobility should not be limited unnecessarily.

9. Hospital personnel should be cognizant of the potential impact of electronic fetal monitoring upon family-centered childbirth. Family-centered care and indicated intrapartum fetal monitoring are not mutually exclusive. Maternity services should be encouraged to integrate concepts of family-centered care with care of women who are monitored electronically. (Adapted from National Institute for Child Health and Human Development: *Task Force on Antenatal Care*. United States Department of Health, Education and Welfare, 1979, pp III-159–III-164.)

NURSING MANAGEMENT

Nursing care specific for a patient experiencing *fetal distress*:

☐ Recognize signs of fetal distress and take appropriate action:
— Bradycardia (FHR under 110);
— Tachycardia (FHR above 160);
— Decreased variability; and
— Early, late, or variable decelerations.

☐ Be alert to indications for using electronic fetal monitoring: e.g., prematurity, postmaturity, meconium stained amniotic fluid, FHR abnormalities heard on auscultation, and high risk pregnancy.

☐ Explain electronic fetal monitoring to the patient and her significant other(s), including the specific indication(s), the equipment and procedure, and risks and benefits.

☐ Continue to provide the patient the nursing support she needs throughout labor, including comfort measures and providing a continuing presence.

☐ Apply the external fetal monitor when indicated:
— Position the patient in the semi-Fowler's position;
— Place the tocodynamometer over the uterine fundus;
— Locate fetal heart tones with a fetoscope; place the ultrasound transducer, with coupling gel, over the spot where fetal heart tones were heard;
— Adjust belts so they are secure, but not uncomfortable for the patient;
— Inform the patient what activities she may perform with the monitor in place; inform her when to get assistance from the nurse to move about; and

— Readjust placement of the tocodynamometer and ultrasound transducer if they become dislodged, the patient changes position, or as necessary with fetal rotation and descent during labor.

☐ When indicated, apply the fetal scalp electrode and insert intrauterine catheter, if properly trained and supervised; or assist the physician with application of internal fetal monitoring equipment:
— Turn on the monitor to let it warm up;
— Apply the fetal scalp electrode over a bony area—not over a fontanel or suture;
— Fill pressure catheter with sterile water before it is inserted to prevent introduction of air into the uterus;
— Insert pressure catheter between the cervix and fetal presenting part until the tip is approximately the level of the patient's umbilicus (i.e., when the black line on the catheter is at the introitus);
— Flush the catheter with sterile water once it is in place;
— Flush the strain gauge on the monitor, and place it about the same level as the tip of the catheter in the uterus;
— Attach the catheter and stopcock to the strain gauge; open the stopcock to air to adjust the pressure line on the monitor readout to 0. Turn the stopcock so the catheter is "on" to the strain gauge;
— Place the leg plate securely on the patient's thigh with conductive paste; Attach the wires of the fetal scalp electrode, matching the colors of the wires with the color of the terminals on the leg plate;

NURSING MANAGEMENT

— Secure the catheter and leg plate, if necessary, to the mother's thigh with tape; and

— Take the mother's temperature hourly to observe for infection.

☐ Periodically verify the accuracy of the fetal monitor tracing by auscultating the fetal heart tones and palpating the uterine contractions.

☐ Frequently evaluate the fetal monitor tracing; notify the physician of any abnormalities in contraction pattern or FHR.

☐ When early decelerations are present, continue to observe; since early decelerations in early labor *may* indicate cephalopelvic disproportion (CPD), observe for signs and symptoms of CPD (see Chapter 35); since early decelerations late in labor usually indicate fetal descent, observe for progress in descent or imminent delivery.

☐ When late decelerations or bradycardia is present:
— Notify the physician;
— Turn the patient to her left side to enhance uteroplacental blood flow;
— Start an intravenous infusion, or increase the rate of flow to ensure adequate uterine perfusion;
— If pitocin is being administered, discontinue it;
— Give oxygen by mask at 6–8 liters/minute to enhance fetal oxygenation (the effectiveness of this step is questionable, but since it carries no risk and may be beneficial, it is often tried);
— Take maternal temperature to rule out hypothermia (for bradycardia);
— Assess the patient for imminent delivery;
— Assist with fetal blood gas sampling, as needed;
— Be prepared for emergency cesarean section or forceps delivery; and
— Alert the neonatal resuscitation team to attend the delivery; be prepared to assist with resuscitation.

☐ When variable decelerations are noted:
— Notify the physician;
— Turn the patient to whatever position is found to relieve the cord compression: left side, right side, hands and knees, Trendelenberg;
— If indicated, perform vaginal examination to rule out cord prolapse (or if the decelerations are severe to try to lift the presenting part to relieve pressure on the cord);
— Observe for imminent delivery; and
— If decelerations are severe and cannot be relieved by position changes, the nursing actions for late decelerations should be employed (see above).

☐ When fetal tachycardia is present:
— Notify the physician;
— Take maternal temperature to rule out fever;
— Assess maternal hydration status; if necessary, start an intravenous infusion or increase the rate of flow to ensure adequate hydration;
— Evaluate whether medication that might increase baseline FHR (e.g., ritodrine hydrochloride, atropine) has been used; and
— Position the patient on her left side to maximize uteroplacental blood flow.

☐ When decreased baseline variability is present:
— Evaluate whether medications, especially analgesics, may be suppressing variability; if so, continue to observe, and allow time for medication to be metabolized;
— In early labor, evaluate whether the fetus is sleeping; attempt to awaken the fetus by abdominal palpation, gently moving the fetal head and buttocks back and forth; and
— If variability does not improve, utilize the nursing actions for late decelerations or bradycardia (see above).

☐ Document on the patient's chart:
— Type of monitoring instituted;
— Time monitoring began;
— Indication for monitoring;
— Any abnormalities noted on the FHR tracing;
— All nursing actions instituted in response to FHR or uterine contraction abnormalities—including notification of the physician;
— Response to treatment measures instituted; and
— All events and procedures that may affect the FHR or uterine contraction tracing: e.g., vaginal examinations, rupture of membranes, medications, maternal vital signs.

☐ Document directly on the fetal monitor strip:
— Identifying information: e.g., the number of this strip, the patient's name, age, par-

NURSING MANAGEMENT

ity, gestational age, date, time, indication for monitoring, type of monitoring, maternal vital signs, last vaginal examination findings, status of membranes, estimated fetal weight, presentation and position of fetus;

— Maternal position;

— Maternal vital signs, as they are taken (at least hourly);

— Time of vaginal examinations, and findings;

— Time of rupture of membranes, whether spontaneous or artificial, and characteristics of the fluid;

— Medications, including time, dose, and route;

— Other events, e.g., vomiting, coughing;

— Evaluation of tracing by physician, including time and physician's name;

— Time of fetal blood gas sampling, and results; and

— Measures to correct abnormalities in FHR or uterine contractions.

☐ After delivery of a baby who had a fetal scalp electrode, cleanse the puncture site with providone iodine or other acceptable solution; notify nursery personnel to observe the baby for abscess at the site.

☐ Alert the postpartum staff to observe the patient for postpartum infection.

Nursing diagnoses most frequently associated with *fetal distress* (see Section V):

☐ Grieving related to potential/actual loss of infant or birth of an imperfect child.

☐ Altered fetal cardiac and cerebral tissue perfusion.

☐ Anxiety/fear.

☐ Knowledge deficit regarding etiology, disease process, treatment, and expected outcome.

CORD PROLAPSE

Definition

Prolapse of the umbilical cord is protrusion of the cord along side of (occult) or ahead of the presenting part of the fetus (Fig. 39.3). Cord prolapse occurs in 1 out of 400 pregnancies (14).

Etiology

Risk of cord prolapse is increased in breech presentation, transverse lie, unengaged fetal presenting part, preterm labor or premature rupture of membranes, delivery of the second twin, AROM at a high station polyhydramnios. In essence, this complication occurs when the presenting part does not fill the pelvic inlet completely (15).

Signs and Symptoms/Diagnosis

Diagnosis is made when a loop of cord can be seen externally or can be palpated in the vagina or along side the presenting part. Severe recurrent variable decelerations that do not respond to maternal position change, oxygen therapy, or hydration should be considered a presumptive diagnosis of occult prolapse (15).

Maternal and Fetal Outcome

Prolapse of the umbilical cord is life-threatening for the fetus because compression of the cord by the presenting part cuts off placental circulation, thus causing anoxia.

Maternal complications may result from the emergency induction of anesthesia and/or delivery either by cesarean section or forceps. If the baby dies or is impaired neurologically, the mother will experience grief. The trauma of this frightening experience or grief over loss of a normal birth experience may be harmful psychologically.

Medical Management

Diagnosis of cord prolapse calls for immediate intervention (Fig. 39.3). The nurse or physician should place the patient in the knee-chest or Trendelenburg position and perform a vaginal examination in order to lift the presenting part off of the cord manually. The presenting part should continue to be held off of the cord without interruption until delivery is accomplished. Help should be summoned. In order to prevent chilling of any part of the cord that falls outside the vagina (which would stimulate the vagus nerve), warm towels moistened with normal saline are used to cover the cord.

The anesthesiologist and pediatrician are notified. The patient must be moved quickly to the delivery room. An intravenous line is inserted, the maternal abdomen is shaved and prepared for surgery, and oxygen is administered. Auscultation of the fetal heart should be continuous. If the heart rate returns to normal through positioning maneuvers, it is better to allow a period of 10–20 minutes for the fetus to recover from the anoxic incident in utero than to deliver a severely hypoxic infant.

Cesarean section is the routine mode of delivery in this emergency situation. However, in some instances, if the cervix is dilated fully, forceps delivery is chosen because it is the quickest route.

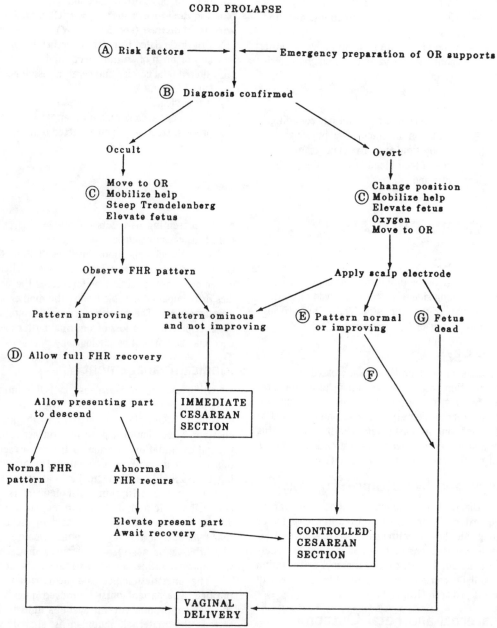

Figure 39.3. Schema for management of cord prolapse. Reprinted with permission from Friedman E: *Obstetric Decision Making.* St. Louis, Mosby, 1982, p 153.

NURSING MANAGEMENT

Nursing care specific for a patient experiencing *cord prolapse*:

☐ Perform all vaginal examinations gently, assessing not only for station, dilation, effacement and position, but also for presence of cord.

☐ Be aware of factors that predispose toward cord prolapse including:
— Breech presentation;
— Transverse lie;
— Unengaged presenting part;
— Twin gestation; and
— Polyhydramnios.

☐ Position the patient at risk for cord prolapse in semi-Fowler's position in order to use the force of gravity to encourage engagement of the presenting part; limit ambulation.

☐ Electronically monitor the patient at risk for cord prolapse continuously.

☐ Be aware that profound variable decelerations constitute a presumptive diagnosis of occult cord prolapse.

☐ When membranes spontaneously rupture or are artificially ruptured:
— Observe the perineum for presence of cord; and
— Note fetal heart rate (bradycardia when membranes rupture is presumptive sign of prolapse).

☐ Immediately after artificial or spontaneous rupture of membranes, perform vaginal examination to rule out cord prolapse.

☐ If prolapse occurs:
— Position the patient in Trendelenburg or knee-chest position;
— Perform a vaginal examination in order to push the presenting part away from the cord; *do not* remove examining hand until the infant is delivered;
— Call for help;
— Administer oxygen, as ordered;

— Monitor fetal heart rate by either EMS or IMS and call out rate to emergency team frequently; Note: It may be possible initially to count FHR by counting the cord pulsations, however, this must be done gently in order to avoid constricting the cord; over time, the examining hand becomes less able to feel the cord pulsations due to the continued pressure of the presenting part on it;

— Have staff prepare for emergency cesarean section:
* Draw blood for type and cross match;
* Start intravenous line, if not in place;
* Insert Foley catheter; and
* Shave abdomen (if time allows).

— Continuously provide patient and significant other(s) with supportive explanation of emergency procedures.

☐ In the postpartum period:
— Observe for maternal complications including anemia, signs and symptoms of infection, or hemorrhage;
— If perinatal morbidity or mortality occur, support the parents through the grief process;
— Review the course of the emergency experience with the patient and the significant other(s), emphasizing the positive effect of *their* actions during the crisis on speed of delivery and newborn outcome.

Nursing diagnoses most frequently associated with *cord prolapse* (see Section V):

☐ Grieving related to potential/actual loss of infant or birth of an imperfect child.

☐ Altered fetal cardiac and cerebral tissue perfusion.

☐ Anxiety/fear.

☐ Knowledge deficit regarding etiology, disease process, treatment, and expected outcome.

MECONIUM STAINING

Definition

Meconium is dark green, tarry material that is collected in the fetal intestine throughout the gestational period. Meconium consists of desquamated cells, digestive secretions, mucus, bile pigments, and lanugo and vernex caseosa that the fetus swallows (12, p 86). Fetal swallowing begins at 13–16 weeks' gestation, and by full term, the fetus swallows 500 ml of amniotic fluid daily, which is then reabsorbed from the gastrointestinal system. Thus, considerable meconium may accumulate in the fetal gut. The fetal bowel usually is inactive (12, p 86). However, acute or chronic fetal hypoxia may cause reflex relaxation of the anal sphincter and passage of the meconium into the amniotic fluid, which then becomes green colored or stained.

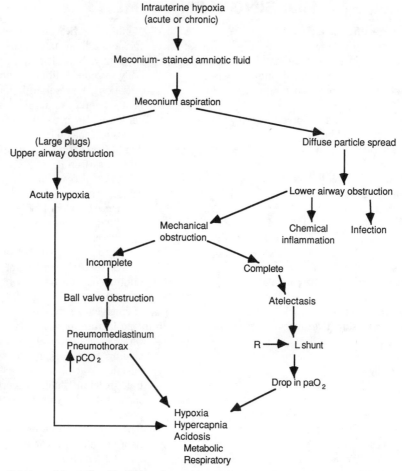

Figure 39.4. Schema of the pathophysiology of meconium aspiration. (From Cloherty J, and Stark A: *Manual of Neonatal Care*. Boston: Little, Brown & Company, 1980, p 163.)

Overall incidence of meconium staining ranges from 9–15%. Meconium staining universally is considered a sign of significant fetal distress.

Etiology

Uteroplacental insufficiency usually is the causative factor. Conditions closely associated with meconium passage include the following (3, p 163):

1. Toxemia
2. Heavy smoking
3. Chronic respiratory disease
4. Cardiovascular disease
5. Intrauterine growth retardation
6. Postmaturity

Postmaturity is considered to be a special risk category for meconium aspiration. Not only does the placental function deteriorate, producing hy-

poxia, but the fetal gut matures and, thus, is more likely to empty. The perinatal mortality rate increases up to five times from 42–44 weeks' gestation, and the most common cause of postmature perinatal death is meconium aspiration (12, p 637).

Signs and Symptoms

Meconium staining ranges from barely visible and clear to a light greenish brown to a thick, particulate "pea soup." The more thick the meconium, the greater the fetal jeopardy. Yellow meconium usually is old. It should be noted that passage of meconium in breech presentation often is due to mechanical compression and is not necessarily a sign of fetal distress.

Meconium staining most often is associated with late FHR decelerations—an ominous sign of fetal anoxia (5, p 190). Meconium staining associated with FHR tachycardia connotes an infected fetus who is compromised profoundly (16). Passage of meconium *late* in labor is an equivocal sign and may or may not be associated with fetal distress. Late meconium passage is best evaluated by IMS and FSBS (17).

Diagnosis

Diagnosis is made during labor when the membranes are ruptured. Prenatally, if the pregnancy is postterm, amnioscopy may be performed to rule out presence of meconium. This presupposes that the cervix is dilated enough to allow introduction of the amnioscope. Failure to see meconium does not necessarily mean that passage has not occurred. Many times an engaged presenting part prevents meconium from reaching the forewaters. Because amnioscopy is difficult to perform and because results are inconclusive, some clinicians may not use this procedure.

Meconium also may be discovered during amniocentesis done for some other reason (e.g., to document fetal maturity).

Maternal and Fetal Outcome

Hypoxia not only causes passage of meconium but also may cause reflex fetal gasping. If the fetus gasps and aspirates large amounts of amniotic fluid contaminated with thick meconium, severe respiratory distress, pneumonia, and death may ensue (Fig. 39.4). The perinatal mortality rate with thick meconium aspiration is 30% (7).

Aspirated meconium not only causes airway obstruction but also chemical inflammation. It is an excellent medium for bacterial growth and favors development of bacterial pneumonitis. The pathophysiology of meconium aspiration sequelae is detailed in Figure 39.4.

The newborn is not only at risk because of meconium aspiration but must recover from the acute or chronic hypoxia that caused the meconium passage.

Medical Management

During labor, when meconium staining is diagnosed, the fetus should be monitored continuously, preferably by IMS. If meconium is present, many clinicians recommend obtaining a baseline FSBS. The FSBS may be repeated at periodic intervals or if other signs of fetal distress are noted. Clear evidence of fetal hypoxia (i.e., FSBS $\leq$7.20) requires emergency cesarean section.

If the fetus has gasped in utero and aspirated meconium, it is not possible to prevent the sequelae of the insult. However, risk of initial aspiration or repeated aspiration can be minimized by removal of meconium from the nasopharynx before the infant's first breath. At birth, the obstetrician or midwife should suction the mouth and nares thoroughly after the head is delivered and before the shoulders and thorax are delivered. A DeLee suction catheter is a more effective suction apparatus for removing meconium than a bulb syringe.

Once the infant is delivered, the cord is cut and clamped immediately, and the infant is handed over to the pediatric team, who will intubate the child and suction the trachea. Positive pressure oxygenation should not be used until the trachea is suctioned thoroughly because it would force the meconium further into the bronchial tree. Use of a DeLee suction catheter will stimulate the vagus nerve and cause a drop in heart rate. Decelerations may be particularly deleterious before 1 minute of age. Suctioning should be continued only if the infant's heart rate remains above 40 beats per minute (3, p 165).

After the meconium is removed and the infant is stabilized, careful evaluation of respiratory status must be ongoing. Risk of bacterial or chemical pneumonia, atelectasis, or air-leak pneumothorax are proportional to the thickness and amount of meconium aspirated.

NURSING MANAGEMENT

Nursing care specific for a patient experiencing *meconium staining*:

☐ When membranes rupture spontaneously or are artificially ruptured, always note the color, amount, and odor of the amniotic fluid.

☐ Continuously assess the character of the amniotic fluid throughout labor.

☐ Be aware of conditions that predispose toward meconium staining including:
— Toxemia;
— Heavy smoking;
— Cardiovascular disease;
— Intrauterine growth retardation; and
— Postmaturity.

☐ If meconium is noted, notify the physician immediately.

☐ Provide the patient and her significant other(s) with information about fetal status and the rationale for intensive evaluation.

NURSING MANAGEMENT

☐ Be prepared to assist the physician to apply the IMS.

☐ Carefully assess the FHR for late decelerations, a sign of fetal hypoxia; notify the physician if they occur.

☐ Be prepared to assist the physician with FSBS as ordered.

☐ Administer oxygen, as ordered.

☐ Position patient on her left side in order to maximize placental perfusion.

☐ If FSBS falls below 7.20, prepare for emergency cesarean section.

☐ If vaginal delivery is anticipated:
  — Provide a DeLee suction catheter to the birth attendant to use after the delivery of fetal head;
  — Coach the mother to pant after the delivery of the head in order to delay delivery of the shoulders and thorax and allow complete suctioning of the nasopharanyx on the perineum; and

  — Assist the pediatrician in resuscitation efforts including visualization of the cord, suctioning, and intubation.

☐ In the postpartum period:
  — If perinatal morbidity or mortality occur, support the parents through the grief process; and
  — Review the course of the traumatic labor and birth experience with the patient and her significant other(s), emphasizing the positive effect of their cooperation on birth outcome.

Nursing diagnoses most frequently associated with *meconium staining* (see Section V):

☐ Grieving related to potential/actual loss of infant or birth of an imperfect child.

☐ Altered fetal cardiac and cerebral tissue perfusion.

☐ Anxiety/fear.

☐ Knowledge deficit regarding etiology, disease process, treatment, and expected outcome.

REFERENCES

1. Martin C, Gingerich B: Uteroplacental physiology. *JOGN* 5:18, 1976.
2. Parer JT: Physiological regulation of fetal heart rate. *JOGN* 5:27, 1976.
3. Cloherty J, Stark A: *Manual of Neonatal Care*. Boston, Little, Brown and Company, 1984, p 39.
4. Oxorn H: *Human Labor and Birth*, (ed 5.) Norwalk, CT, Appleton-Century-Crofts, 1986, p 623.
5. Vestal K, McKensie C: *High Risk Perinatal Nursing*. Philadelphia, WB Saunders, 1983, p 231.
6. Ettinger B, MaCart D: Effects of drugs on the fetal heart rate during labor. *JOGN* 5:49, 1976.
7. Cohen W, Friedman E: *Management of Labor*. Baltimore, University Park Press, 1983, p 182.
8. Hon E: *An Introduction to Fetal Heart Rate Monitoring*. Los Angeles Postgraduate Division University of Southern California School of Medicine, 1973.
9. Caldeyro-Barcia H, Alvarez H: *Segundo Congress Latino-Americano de Obstetricay Ginecologia*. Sao Paulo, Brazil, 1954.
10. Butler JM, Parer JT: Is intensive intrapartum monitoring necessary. *JOGN* 5:65, 1976.
11. Chognon L, Heldenbrand C: Nurses undertake direct and indirect fetal monitoring at a community hospital. *JOGN*:45, 1974.
12. Zeigal E, Cranley M: *Obstetric Nursing*. New York, Macmillan, 1984.
13. Chawla R, et al.: Hemorrhage after fetal scalp blood sampling. *Am J Obstet Gynecol*, 149:92, 1984.
14. Shields D: Maternal reactions to fetal monitoring. *Am J Nurs* 78: 2110, 1978.
15. Friedman E: *Obstetric Decision Making*. St. Louis, Mosby, 1982, p 152.
16. Blot P: Fetal tachycardia and meconium staining. *Int J Gynaecol Obstet*, 21: 194, 1982.
17. Meis P, Hobel C, Ureda J: Late meconium passage in labor. *Obstet Gynecol*, 59:332–335, 1982.

Chapter 40
Complications of Delivery
Suzanne M. Smith, C.N.M., M.S., M.P.H.

INTRODUCTION

The "three P's" of labor and delivery are the *powers*, the *passageway*, and the *passenger*. It is necessary to recognize the interrelationships between these factors before discussing the possible complications of delivery. The *powers* refer to uterine contractions and maternal voluntary expulsive efforts. Caldeyro-Barcia has described normal uterine contractions as having three characteristics (1): the contraction wave begins at the fundus of the uterus and progresses downward; the duration of the contraction is longest in the upper portion of the uterus and shortest in the lower uterine segment; likewise, the intensity of the uterine contraction is strongest at the top. This is known as the triple descending gradient theory. The *passageway* or birth canal refers to the bony pelvis as well as to the soft tissue, including the pelvic floor muscles and the perineum. The *passenger* is, of course, the fetus and includes consideration of size, presentation, and position.

FORCEPS DELIVERY

Definition

A forceps delivery is the vaginal delivery of a fetus accomplished through the use of obstetrical forceps. The American College of Obstetricians and Gynecologists recognizes three categories of forceps delivery:

1. Low or outlet forceps: The application of forceps to the fetal skull when the scalp is visible at the introitus, the skull has reached the pel-

vic floor, and the sagittal suture is in the anteroposterior diameter of the outlet.
2. Midforceps: The application of forceps to the fetal skull after engagement has occurred but before the criteria for low forceps are met. Furthermore, any forceps operation requiring rotation of the fetal skull to the anteroposterior diameter is classified as midforceps.
3. High forceps: The application of forceps at any time prior to engagement of the fetal head. High forceps are not justified in modern obstetric practice.

Other classifications include a subdivision of midforceps:

1. Midforceps: The application of forceps when the leading bony portion of the head is at or just below the level of the ischial spines, with the biparietal diameter below the pelvic inlet. The head nearly fills the hollow of the sacrum.
2. Low midforceps: The application of forceps when the biparietal diameter is at or below the level of the ischial spines and the leading bony portion of the head is within one fingerbreadth of the perineum between contractions. The head fills the hollow of the sacrum.

All forceps are composed of four parts; the handle, the shank, the lock, and the blade. The handle is used by the attendant to grip the forceps. The shank connects the handle and the blade. When the head is low in the pelvis, a short shank is sufficient. If the head is above the perineum, a longer shank is necessary. Finally, the lock holds the forceps together. There are three major types of locks. The English lock has a socket (shoulder and flange) located on each shank at the junction with

Table 40.1.
OBSTETRICAL FORCEPS

NAME	DESCRIPTION	PURPOSE
Classical instruments		
Elliot	Fenestrated blade with a short, round cephalic curve; overlapping shanks	Chosen for a round, unmolded head
Simpson's	Fenestrated blade with a long, tapered cephalic curve; parallel and separated shanks; English lock	General duty forceps; fits well on a long, molded head; may deliver as OP from some android or anthropoid pelves; may be used for rotation
Tucker-McLean	Elliot type forceps with a solid blade	Good general purpose forceps; may be used for rotation
Special use instruments		
Kielland's (Kjelland's)	Inner surface of fenestrated blade is beveled to decrease injury to fetal head; very slight pelvic curve with backward angle; overlapping shanks; sliding lock	Useful in rotation from transverse position; also used for OP, face, and brow presentations; gives traction in AP diameter with android and anthropoid pelves; blades may be locked even with asynclitism
Barton	Anterior blade attached to shank by hinge, flexible over an arc of 90°; other blade has a deep cephalic curve; anteriorly, no pelvic curve; transversely, a perfect pelvic curve; sliding lock; separate traction handle	Used with deep transverse arrest, posterior positions, and face presentations; allows the blades to be locked even with marked asynclitism; gives traction for descent in transverse position in a platypelloid pelvis
Piper	Fenestrated blade with small cephalic and slight pelvic curve; longer shank with downward curve results in handle being lower than the blade	Construction forms a double pelvic curve that allows application to aftercoming head in breech presentation

the handle that fits together. Articulation thus is fixed at a given point. The French lock is composed of a screw or eyebolt on the left shank that fits into a notch on the right shank. After application and positioning, the screw is tightened to lock the forceps together. A sliding lock has a lock built on the left shank only through which the right shank fits. Articulation is not fixed, and the shanks may move forward and backward independently.

The blade encloses the fetal head. Both the construction and the curvature of the blade are important. Solid blades may cause less trauma to the head, while fenestrated (open or cutout) blades grip the fetal head more firmly and are less likely to slip from position. The shape of the blade corresponds to the pelvic curve, and its angle of connection to the shank conforms roughly to the shape or axis of the maternal pelvis. The pelvic curve facilitates application to and extraction of the fetus and minimizes the risk of maternal trauma. The cephalic curve is the lateral curve of the blade that conforms to the shape of the fetal head.

There are two general types of forceps. Classical, or forceps for general use, are constructed according to the standards described above and are used in the majority of cases. Elliot and Simpson forceps are examples of classical instruments. Spe-

cial forceps have been modified in design for use in specific situations. Piper forceps are an example of a special type. Table 40.1 describes several forceps and their use.

Indications

There are a number of criteria to consider before forceps are used. The fetal head should be engaged. The fetus must present as a vertex or face with mentum anterior, except in the case of Piper forceps applied to the aftercoming head of a breech presentation. The position of the head must be known accurately for correct forceps application. The cervix must be dilated fully, with the amniotic membranes ruptured and no absolute cephalopelvic disproportion (CPD) at the midpelvis or outlet. Pelvic type and architecture must be identified. The practitioner must be knowledgeable of the advantages, disadvantages, and use of different types of forceps and skilled in the techniques of their use.

Maternal indications for the use of forceps include the need to prevent the Valsalva effect of pushing in the second stage, as in patients with heart disease, acute pulmonary edema, or cardiopulmonary disease. Maternal exhaustion, epidural anesthesia, the inability to push effectively, and uterine inertia not overcome by oxytocin stimulation may necessitate forceps for vaginal delivery. Intrapartum infection may require prompt delivery to minimize risk to both mother and fetus. Marked perineal resistance may require forceps delivery. The term *elective forceps* is used when the obstetrician chooses to use low forceps when not absolutely indicated. Elective forceps delivery may be chosen to shorten the second stage when the perineum is somewhat resistant or analgesia/anesthesia decreases the woman's voluntary expulsive efforts.

Fetal indications include malposition of the head (occiput transverse or posterior, and some face presentations). Fetal distress, including bradycardia and tachycardia in the second stage, and late passage of meconium may require forceps delivery. Failure to progress (descent or rotation) in the second stage because of relative CPD may be overcome by forceps delivery. Piper forceps may be used for the aftercoming head of a breech that does not flex and descend spontaneously. Less frequent indications may include premature separation of the placenta and prolapsed umbilical cord when delivery may be effected more quickly by forceps application than by cesarean section. In the past some obstetricians chose to deliver premature babies with forceps to prevent intracranial hemorrhage from pressure of the small, relatively soft head on the perineum. Recent evidence, however, indicates that there is no advantage to the use of forceps, and there is the potential for more neurological damage resulting from the use of forceps in these cases (2).

Maternal and Fetal Outcome

While forceps are used to optimize the outcome for both mother and fetus, there are adverse outcomes that may occur as a result of the delivery. Lacerations of the vulva, vagina, and cervix, as well as third or fourth degree extensions of the episiotomy or fracture of the coccyx, may occur as a result of the size or position of the fetus or because of poor forceps technique. Bladder injury, atony, or infection and rectal injury may be due to pressure from the fetus or to forceps trauma. Uterine rupture, hemorrhage, and postpartum infection also may occur. The most common and generally benign fetal outcomes are bruising at the site of forceps application or cephalohematoma from the pressure exerted. Facial paralysis, brachial palsy, or skull fracture may result from improperly applied forceps or excessive pressure to the fetus. Asphyxia, brain damage, intracranial hemorrhage, cord compression, or death may be a result of poor technique or a progressive result of the complication requiring the forceps delivery.

Medical Management/Technique

During forceps delivery, the patient must be in the lithotomy position, and an episiotomy is required in all but the rarest instances to minimize maternal trauma. Catheterization of the bladder is advisable to reduce the risk of injury. Pediatric attendance at the birth generally is mandatory owing to the increased risk to the fetus, not only from the indication for the procedure but also from the possible trauma of the forceps application and traction. To minimize the risks associated with the procedure, it is essential that the physician know the precise position of the fetal head and apply the blades perfectly.

Episiotomy may be performed prior to application of the forceps, but it is done more commonly after traction has brought the head low enough to distend the perineum. Traction on the forceps is best applied intermittently—with the uterine contractions—to approximate the effect of spontaneous delivery as closely as possible, except, of course, in instances when time is critical for fetal well-being. In some cases the forceps are removed prior to complete delivery of the head, and expulsion is continued spontaneously or aided by exerting forward pressure on the chin of the fetus through the perineum in front of the coccyx (the modified Ritgen maneuver) to assist the extension of the head manually.

Forceps delivery almost always requires the use of anesthesia. Pudendal block anesthesia may not be possible because of the low station of the fetal head, or it may not provide sufficient anesthesia for the procedure. Regional anesthesia generally is the most frequently used, provided that the indication for forceps delivery permits the time required for induction. General anesthesia may be necessary if the delivery must be accomplished rapidly.

Forceps are used to accomplish specific maneuvers allowing delivery of a fetus that would otherwise require cesarean section. These maneuvers result in the rotation of the fetal head from a posterior or transverse position to the anterior. The Scanzoni-Smellie maneuver requires two separate applications. The first forceps application is followed by rotation of the fetus from the occiput posterior (OP) to the occiput anterior (OA) position, and a second forceps application is needed for traction and delivery. The Kielland's forceps rotation uses a special forceps to allow a single application to a fetus in the transverse position. Both rotation to anterior and delivery then can be accomplished, although some practitioners remove the Kielland

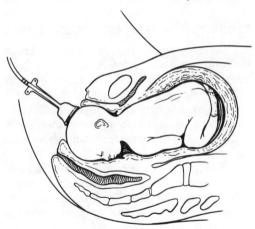

Figure 40.1. Vacuum extractor. (Courtesy of Beth Anne Willert, medical illustrator.)

forceps and apply a classical type for traction and delivery. The application of another special forceps—Pipers—to the aftercoming head of a breech permits the assisted delivery of the unflexed head.

VACUUM EXTRACTION

Definition

The vacuum extractor is a mechanical device that provides traction to the fetal head by means of suction on the fetal scalp to effect vaginal delivery (Fig. 40.1). Vacuum extraction is classified according to the same three categories as forceps delivery.

The successful use of vacuum extraction for delivery began during the mid 1950s. A metal cup was applied to the fetal head and suction applied, creating an artificial caput succedaneum. When it was applied correctly, the suction maintained the cup against the scalp, and traction was effected by means of a handle connected to the cup via a chain inside the rubber suction tubing. There is now available a soft cup that conforms better to the fetal head and with which the vacuum pressure may be increased more rapidly.

Indications

The major indications for use of the vacuum extractor are the same as those for forceps. Exceptions to these indications are face presentations and the aftercoming head of a breech. The inability to apply forceps because of uncertainty of exact fetal head position or unavailability of general or conduction anesthesia may be another indication. Finally, in some cases of fetal distress prior to full cervical dilatation, it may be appropriate to apply the vacuum extractor. The cervix must be dilated

sufficiently to allow application of the vacuum cup to the fetal scalp. There are several diameters of cups available, with the larger sizes providing better traction. Furthermore, the greater the dilatation, the shorter the procedure time.

Theoretical advantages of the vacuum extractor over forceps include the ability to apply the suction cup prior to complete cervical dilatation, the continued ability of the head to spontaneously flex and/or rotate to accommodate to the pelvis, and the lack of need for additional space in the pelvis to accommodate forceps.

Maternal and Fetal Outcome

As with forceps or other complications of delivery, there may be adverse outcomes. The mother may suffer cervical or vaginal lacerations or trauma. The vacuum pressure on the fetal scalp may cause an artificially induced caput succedaneum (chignon) or cephalohematoma. Lacerations, abrasions, or bleeding of the scalp or necrosis or ulceration at the site of application may occur. Finally, neurologic damage, intracranial hemorrhage, retinal hemorrhage, or death may be caused by poor technique or may result from the indication for the procedure.

Medical Management/Technique

Consideration of the appropriate route of delivery (vaginal or abdominal) and, if vaginal, the appropriate instrument (vacuum extractor or forceps) must be based on the specific indication and the time constraints in each situation.

For vacuum extraction, the membranes must be ruptured, with the fetus presenting as a vertex—ideally, well flexed—with no evidence of absolute CPD and with sufficient cervical dilatation for safe application of the suction cup. The cup should be positioned over the occiput or as close to it as possible. Sufficient time to develop caput must be allowed before beginning traction in order for the cup to maintain suction on the fetal head. Traction should be maintained at approximate right angles to the cup, perpendicular to the pelvic plane of the vertex, and in unison with uterine contractions and voluntary maternal expulsive efforts. Attempts to turn the cup to effect rotation of the head, rocking motions, or other maneuvers increase the risk of fetal or maternal trauma. Finally, failure to effect progress after a few attempts warrants reevaluation of the case.

Protocols for the preparation of the equipment depend on the specific type used and should be part of the procedure manual in hospitals that use the vacuum extractor. The suction cup, tubing, chain, and handle are sterile, while the remainder of the apparatus is not. Increase in the vacuum pressure must be gradual (requiring 2–10 minutes) to allow sufficient caput formation to maintain suction on the scalp. The pressure should be between 380 and 580 mm Hg for the traction and must never exceed 600 mm Hg in order to prevent fetal trauma.

NURSING MANAGEMENT

Nursing care specific for care of a patient experiencing a _complication of delivery_:

☐ Ensure patient's bladder is empty by encouraging frequent voiding in labor or by sterile catheterization if unable to void.

☐ Assist with the administration and monitoring of the anesthesia given for the delivery.

☐ Be prepared for neonatal resuscitation; alert pediatrician to attend delivery; assess neonate for evidence of injury resulting from traumatic delivery.

☐ Provide opportunity for maternal-infant contact as early as the condition of both will allow.

For the patient having an _instrumental delivery_:

☐ Know conditions requiring instrumental delivery:

— Maternal: prevention of Valsalva's effect for patients with cardiopulmonary disease; exhaustion; epidural anesthesia; inability to push.

— Fetal: fetal distress, malposition.

☐ Educate patient/partner regarding:

— Type of instrument(s) to be used;

— Rationale for their use;

— General description of procedure; and

— Expected outcomes.

☐ Provide nursing care directed to specific complication requiring use of instrumental delivery (e.g., fetal distress, prolonged second stage, cardiac disease).

☐ Prepare/gather equipment necessary for the instrumental delivery, maintaining sterile technique.

☐ Be familiar with specific equipment and protocols for use of vacuum extractor; assist with its use according to protocols.

☐ Observe for maternal complications of instrumental delivery (e.g., lacerations, infection, urine retention).

Nursing diagnoses most frequently associated with _instrumental delivery_ (see Section V):

☐ Grieving related to potential/actual loss of infant or birth of an imperfect child.

☐ Knowledge deficit regarding etiology, disease process, treatment, and outcome.

☐ Altered fetal cardiac and cerebral tissue perfusion.

☐ Pain.

☐ Anxiety/fear.

☐ Impaired skin integrity.

CESAREAN SECTION

In the United States today, the cesarean section rate ranges between 25 and 40%. In _An Evaluation of Cesarean Section in the United States_ (3) 11 factors are identified that may have contributed to the recent rise in cesarean section rates. They are, in order of significance:

1. Threat of malpractice suits
2. Routine repeat cesarean section
3. Obstetrical training focusing on intervention
4. Belief in a "superior outcome" from cesarean section
5. Changed and/or expanded indications
6. Maternal age, parity, and fertility characteristics
7. Economic factors
8. Increased use of technological procedures
9. Birth weight (estimated large or small)
10. Severe maternal medical complications
11. Herpes virus type II

Currently, more consumers and practitioners are seeking to reduce the performance of cesareans and to avoid unnecessary cesareans without increasing maternal or perinatal morbidity or mortality. Factors that may influence the course and outcome of labor and birth include the following:

1. Choice of practitioner and birth environment
2. Induced labor versus spontaneous onset
3. Early intervention in normal labor
4. Maternal position and activity
5. Electronic fetal monitoring—external or internal
6. Epidural anesthesia in labor
7. Analgesia or sedation in labor

Definition

Cesarean section is the surgical delivery of the fetus through an incision into the uterus. Actually, it requires two operative procedures: first, a laparotomy or incision into the abdomen and, second, a hysterotomy or incision into the uterus.

The subumbilical vertical incision is the quickest abdominal incision to perform, but a Pfannenstiel's incision (lower abdominal transverse incision, frequently at or below the pubic hairline) is preferred by most women for its cosmetic appearance. In addition to the appearance of the Pfannenstiel's incision, it is thought to be less likely to predispose to dehiscence or to hernia formation. The principle disadvantage is the limited exposure of the pregnant uterus and adnexae, particularly in obese women.

The abdominal skin scar direction does not always coincide with the uterine incision. There are three types of cesarean section, classified according to the incision through the uterine wall. In a classical cesarean section the uterine incision is made vertically through the contractile body of the uterus above the lower uterine segment and extended to the fundus. It is rarely performed today because of the risk of dehiscence in subsequent pregnancy or labor. The low segment vertical incision (Kronig's technique) is made through the lower uterine segment. Unless the lower segment has been lengthened by labor, the incision will involve contractile uterine wall. Therefore, it also is performed infrequently. Either vertical incision may be necessary in cases of placenta previa or anterior placental implantation, in a transverse lie, in some cases of breech presentation, or in multiple gestation. The classical incision may be used in an emergency for speed. The low segment transverse incision (Kerr's technique) is made horizontally through the lower uterine segment. It is also called the low flap transverse cesarean. This is the most frequently performed cesarean today.

There are two other incisions occasionally required by unexpected difficulty at the time of surgery. The J-shaped and T-shaped incisions are upward extensions performed after the low segment transverse incision has been found to be inadequate for delivery of the fetus or the placenta has been found implanted beneath the incision. Both types of incision should be regarded as classical incisions and indeed carry more risk of poor healing and subsequent rupture than a transverse incision alone.

Indications

Cesarean section is performed for a variety of maternal and fetal indications. Indications are considered absolute, mandating cesarean section, or relative, in which the decision is based on the specific situation. Absolute CPD, placenta previa, significant abruptio placentae, uncontrollable hemorrhage, and active genital herpes in labor (unless membranes have been ruptured longer than 6 hours) or at the time of spontaneous rupture of the membranes are absolute maternal indications. Fetal indications that mandate cesarean section include transverse lie, deep transverse arrest in which the head cannot be rotated manually or instrumentally, erythroblastosis fetalis, and most instances of prolapsed umbilical cord.

Relative maternal indications include certain maternal diseases such as severe diabetes mellitus, heart disease in which labor or vaginal delivery is not considered safe, benign or malignant neoplasms obstructing the birth canal, and invasive cervical cancer. Severe preeclampsia or eclampsia in which induction will take too much time may necessitate cesarean. Failed induction of labor or dysfunctional labor that is not corrected by other means, including oxytocin augmentation, will lead to cesarean section unless the attempted induction or augmentation can be continued or restarted later. Previous cesarean section, particularly via a classical incision, or previous uterine surgery such as a myomectomy or septal repair must be evaluated individually. A failed attempt of forceps delivery, premature rupture of membranes complicated by amnionitis, and some elderly primigravidas will require cesarean section. Finally, if the mother requires abdominal surgery for another cause such as acute appendicitis or trauma, it may be necessary to deliver the fetus at the same time, and a cesarean section would be performed.

Relative fetal indications include breech presentation, particularly kneeling, footling, or complete breech presentation; a deflexed or extended head; or a primigravid mother. Significant fetal distress, particularly if caused by uteroplacental insufficiency, may warrant a cesarean section unless delivery is imminent or the distress is corrected by other means. Finally, both prematurity and relative CPD may result in cesarean section in order to reduce the risks of vaginal delivery to the fetus, specifically intracranial hemorrhage.

Maternal and Fetal Outcome

Morbidity and mortality of both mother and fetus are higher following cesarean section than vaginal delivery. However, it must be remembered that the indication for the cesarean section rather than the procedure itself may be responsible for part of this increased risk.

Maternal complications include renal failure owing to hypotension, paralytic ileus, intestinal obstruction, hemorrhage, thrombophlebitis, and pulmonary embolism. Urinary tract infection may occur because of catheterization for the surgery. It is more common with repetitive Pfannenstiel's incisions. The rate of postoperative endometritis or wound infection after primary cesarean section is high, particularly in indigent patients and those in whom the membranes have been ruptured for longer than 6 hours. Patients undergoing primary cesarean section do not have the advantage of preparation for surgery that patients undergoing elective surgical procedures have. In addition, the cervical dilatation that occurs during labor allows vaginal flora to ascend to the operative site. Prolonged ruptured membranes, multiple vaginal examinations, and use of intrauterine monitoring equipment may contribute to the high incidence of postoperative infection. Other types of postoperative infection include pulmonary or upper respiratory infection and unexplained fever.

Anesthetic complications such as aspiration or atelectasis may follow general anesthesia, while spinal headaches or nerve pain may follow regional. Late complications of cesarean section include dehiscence of the uterine scar in subsequent pregnancies and intestinal obstruction due to adhesions. As with all surgery, death is a rare but potential result.

Some patients may have a negative psychological reaction to cesarean section. Some may feel that their femininity depends in part on their ability to conceive, carry, and deliver a child normally. The failure to deliver the baby normally may diminish self-esteem. Other patients look forward to a joyous birth experience and are disappointed bitterly when their expectations are not met. Such reactions may be short lived, but if they are not resolved, they may affect the mother's relationship with her child, or they may resurface at a later time, particularly in a subsequent pregnancy.

Fetal outcome depends primarily upon the indication for cesarean section. Anesthesia may cause a lowered Apgar score and respiratory depression at birth. The pressure on the fetal thorax that occurs during vaginal delivery is thought to contribute to drainage of fluid from the fetal lungs, and the recoil at birth is thought to contribute to the initiation of respirations. Lack of these normal events at birth may cause depression initially.

Iatrogenic prematurity and respiratory distress syndrome may occur if cesarean section is performed prior to term. Anemia may result from a fetal-placental transfusion, whereas jaundice may result from a placental-fetal transfusion. Birth trauma, including lacerations during uterine incision, also may occur. There may be abnormal or suspicious neurologic findings, a decreased sucking reflex, or changes in quiet-alert periods owing to anesthetic drugs that are cleared slowly from the neonate's system.

The importance of a time immediately following the birth for mother-infant bonding has been emphasized in recent years. The mother undergoing cesarean section, particularly under general anesthesia, may not have the opportunity for this early bonding or for early initiation of breastfeeding. Thus, there is the potential for alteration in early mother-infant interaction after cesarean.

Medical Management/Technique

Since primary cesarean section is done for emergency (i.e., unpredictable) indications, many institutions and individual practitioners treat all patients in labor as potential candidates for cesarean. In anticipation of cesarean section, patients may not be given food or fluids by mouth during labor. They may be given antacids every 4–6 hours to neutralize gastric acidity in case general anesthesia is required. A blood specimen may be sent to the laboratory for type and cross-matching to have two units of blood available if necessary. An intravenous infusion may be administered routinely. Other practitioners and institutions will institute these measures as they become necessary.

Patients for whom cesarean section is planned (e.g., those who have had a prior cesarean and are not candidates for vaginal birth) should be followed carefully during the pregnancy. Particular attention is paid to confirming the gestational age to avoid iatrogenic prematurity. Two sonograms—one as early as possible in pregnancy, and the other in the second trimester—are suggested, along with the usual historical and physical examination parameters. Elective cesarean section usually is scheduled for around 39 weeks' gestation. The patient is counseled to come to the hospital at once if labor or spontaneous rupture of membranes occurs before the date the cesarean is scheduled.

The decision regarding the type of incision, both abdominal and uterine (see above), is based on the indication for the cesarean section. The choice of regional or general anesthesia depends on the indication for cesarean, the urgency of effecting the delivery, the ability and preference of the anesthetist, and the preference of the mother. Specific information regarding obstetric anesthesia is included in Chapter 38. As a rule, however, general anesthesia is used when the fetus must be delivered rapidly or the mother chooses not to be awake for the birth. Regional anesthesia is used if the mother wishes to be awake and, in many institutions, if she has had oral intake (solid or liquid) within a specified period of time.

An indwelling urinary catheter is placed during the preparation for surgery to drain the bladder during the cesarean and is removed postoperatively.

In cases where tubal sterilization is to be performed as well as cesarean section, the surgery proceeds routinely until the uterine incision has been closed and the serosa overlying the uterus and bladder is reapproximated. At that time, each fallopian tube is identified and bilateral tubal ligation is performed.

The abdominal wall is closed in layers. The final layer—skin closure—may be done by silk mattress sutures or by surgical clips or staples that must be removed, or it may be done by absorbable subcuticular sutures. The incisional wound is covered by a sterile dressing.

Postoperative care usually includes narcotic analgesia for several days, followed by oral nonnarcotic analgesia. Vital signs, the amount of vaginal bleeding, and the status of the fundus are monitored frequently for at least 4 hours and then at least every 4 hours thereafter. The diet is progressed as the patient can tolerate it, usually beginning with clear fluids the day of surgery and progressing to a general diet by 2 days after surgery. Some physicians remove the urinary catheter almost immediately postoperatively while others maintain it for 24–48 hours. The physician's preference regarding oral intake and postoperative activity may influence the decision regarding catheter removal. Bowel sounds are monitored daily. They usually are not present the first day after surgery but are active by the third day. Ambulation with assistance should begin the day of surgery or the day after. A shower or tub bath usually is allowed the third day after surgery after removal of the dressing. The incision is inspected daily. Prophylactic antibiotics may be given, depending upon the risks imposed by the circumstances leading to cesarean and the philosophy of the physician. Other aspects of care are similar to those for normal postpartum patients.

NURSING MANAGEMENT

Nursing care specific for the patient having a cesarean section:

☐ Recognize indications for potential emergency cesarean section:
- Maternal: CPD, placenta previa, significant abruptio placentae, active herpes, obstruction of birth canal, previous uterine surgery.
- Fetal: fetal distress, malpresentation, erythroblastosis fetalis, prolapsed umbilical cord.

☐ Ensure that patient understands she has a right to a second medical opinion regarding route of delivery if urgency of situation permits.

☐ Prepare patient, staff, and equipment for cesarean section:
- Ensure that proper informed consent is obtained;
- Ensure that at least two units of blood are readily available for administration;
- Ensure that a patent intravenous line is in place;
- Perform abdominal shave and prep;
- Insert an indwelling urinary catheter, using sterile technique; and

- Alert operating room personnel, including anesthesiologist and pediatrician.

☐ Prepare partner to accompany patient to operating room if allowed by hospital policy, including role, environment, and attire.

☐ Monitor for postoperative complications:
- Circulatory collapse (e.g., shock, hypotension, dehydration);
- Respiratory problems (e.g., diminished expansion, aspiration, congestion, atelectasis);
- Hemorrhage;
- Urinary problems (e.g., infection, retention, bladder rupture); and
- Gastrointestinal problems (e.g., ileus, nausea, vomiting).

☐ Encourage the patient to request pain medication before pain becomes severe.

☐ Teach routine postoperative activities (e.g., coughing, deep breathing, ambulating).

☐ Assist with breastfeeding.

☐ Prior to hospital discharge, teach patient self-care (e.g., bathing, resumption of activity, resumption of intercourse, diet, danger signs).

☐ Educate patient regarding the indication for her cesarean, the type of scar, the need for

NURSING MANAGEMENT

postoperative follow-up, and implications for future vaginal delivery.

☐ Ensure that all cesarean section mothers leave the hospital with a 3 months' supply of vitamins and iron (if postoperative hematocrit is below 34%).

Nursing diagnoses most frequently associated with *cesarean section* (see Section V):

☐ Grieving related to potential/actual loss of infant or birth of an imperfect child.

☐ Knowledge deficit regarding etiology, disease process, treatment, and outcome.
☐ Altered maternal tissue perfusion.
☐ Altered fetal cardiac and cerebral tissue perfusion.
☐ Pain.
☐ Potential altered parenting.
☐ Anxiety/fear.
☐ Impaired tissue integrity.
☐ Disturbance in body image, self-esteem.

VAGINAL BIRTH AFTER CESAREAN/TRIAL OF LABOR

Definition

Vaginal birth after cesarean (VBAC) is self-defined. In this case, trial of labor refers to the spontaneous onset of uterine contractions that result in cervical effacement and dilatation with the expectation of vaginal delivery in a woman who has undergone a cesarean previously.

The decision to attempt labor and vaginal birth after cesarean must be based on individual circumstances. The mother, her spouse and/or others close to her, and her care giver should consider her previous and present situation in the decision making. Previous history includes the indication for the previous cesarean. Some cases, such as maternal cardiac disease, diabetes mellitus, or other chronic illness may mandate repeat cesarean. Other indications, such as placenta previa or breech presentation, may not be repeated and thus do not routinely warrant another cesarean. The number of previous cesareans, any other uterine surgery, type of uterine incision, and time since the previous surgery must be considered when evaluating the risks of complications from labor and vaginal delivery versus a repeat cesarean. Postoperative course and complications also must be evaluated since infection or other complications may increase maternal risk.

Present history to be considered in making the decision includes the course of this pregnancy, maternal and fetal well-being, duration of gestation, fetal presentation (vertex or breech), or multiple gestation. These factors must be considered when planning a VBAC since normal progress and well-being improves the outcome in any pregnancy and reduces the risks of labor and vaginal delivery.

Situational factors include the immediate availability of an operating room, anesthesia, blood bank, and pediatrician. All of these must be accessible rapidly in the event that a repeat cesarean becomes necessary.

Finally, the patient's full understanding of both VBAC and repeat cesarean is essential. It is the responsibility of the physician or other health care professional to obtain informed consent for a repeat cesarean as well as for VBAC. Objective information regarding the risks, benefits, alternatives, concomitant procedures, and anticipated effects should be provided by the professional obtaining the consent. However, it is also the responsibility of the mother and her support system to educate themselves in order to participate fully in the decision-making process.

Indications/Contraindications

Protocols for VBAC are determined by each practitioner and institution. The following is a list of generally stated *contraindications* to VBAC. There are, however, caregivers and institutions who disagree with one or more of the items included. It is necessary to evaluate each patient individually regarding:

Uterine scar other than low flap transverse.
More than one prior uterine incision.
Complications with previous cesarean section (e.g., hemorrhage or infection).
Estimated fetal weight larger than 4000 g.
Lack of immediately available operating room, anesthesia, blood bank, or pediatric care.
Need to use oxytocin for induction or augmentation of labor.

Maternal and Fetal Outcome

The occurrence of uterine rupture with VBAC is small—less than 1%. The connotation of the word "rupture" is a catastrophic, life-threatening hemorrhage and/or shock because of a tear through the uterine wall. Indeed, this is the picture of a rupture of an unscarred uterus (no previous surgery). In the majority of cases of "rupture" of a cesarean section scar, the picture is one of a window, dehiscence, or partial separation of the scar associated with little or no bleeding. The rupture actually may have occurred before the onset of labor. There is commonly little or no increase in maternal or fetal mortality or morbidity.

Symptoms of significant uterine rupture may include abdominal pain; vaginal bleeding; shock; fever; tachycardia and/or falling blood pressure; swelling of the lower uterine segment or the area of uterine incision; or a noncontracting, rigid, or board-like uterus (see Chapter 41, Injuries to the Birth Canal). A window or small dehiscence may be detected only by uterine exploration after vaginal delivery or may be seen at the time of cesarean performed for another indication.

The outcome for both mother and fetus is statistically better for vaginal birth than for routine repeat cesarean section. The specific situation will influence the outcome in each case. Various studies, using various criteria for allowing a trial of labor, report successful vaginal deliveries in 38–75% of patients (4). The possible outcomes of cesarean section, forceps delivery, and other labor or delivery complications are found in the appropriate section of the text.

Medical Management

Protocols for management should be developed by the institution and/or practitioner. In January 1985, the Committee on Obstetrics: Maternal and Fetal Medicine of the American College of Obstetricians and Gynecologists released the following guidelines for use in developing protocols (5).

Fetal heart rate and uterine activity monitoring should be utilized throughout labor in order to identify abnormalities rapidly. The use of oxytocin induction or augmentation is controversial; the indication for oxytocin may be an indication for cesarean, and it is possible that artificially strong contractions might be more likely to cause rupture of the scar. Likewise, the use of epidural anesthesia is controversial since it may mask symptoms of rupture, but it is not absolutely contraindicated. Intravenous infusion should be in place with 24-hour blood bank facilities available. A physician capable of performing cesarean delivery should be present along with professional and institutional resources with the ability to begin the surgery within 30 minutes after the time the decision has been made.

After successful vaginal delivery, uterine exploration is indicated to check the integrity of the cesarean section scar since rupture may be asymptomatic.

NURSING MANAGEMENT

Nursing care specific for the patient having a *vaginal birth after cesarean section*:

☐ Screen patient for contraindications to VBAC, evaluating the following:
- History of number of prior cesareans or other uterine surgeries, type of uterine scar(s), indication(s), complications of prior uterine surgeries;
- Fetal status (e.g., fetal distress, macrosomia, multiple gestation); and
- Labor abnormalities.

☐ Assist patient/partner in participating in making informed decision regarding optimum route of delivery; include information on risks, benefits, alternatives, concomitant procedures, and expected outcome; support their decision.

☐ Observe continually during labor for signs/symptoms of uterine rupture (e.g., abdominal pain, vaginal bleeding, tachycardia, hypotension, fetal distress).

☐ Prepare for emergency cesarean section:
- Patent intravenous line;
- Two units of blood, type and cross-matched; and
- Operating room personnel and equipment prepared.

☐ Assist with uterine exploration after delivery; explain rational for procedure; assist with relaxation techniques and/or administer analgesics as ordered.

Nursing diagnoses most frequently associated with *vaginal birth after cesarean section* (see Section V):

☐ Anxiety/fear.

☐ Knowledge deficit regarding pregnancy, process of labor and delivery, concerns of the postpartum period, parenting.

SHOULDER DYSTOCIA

Definition

Shoulder dystocia refers to difficulty encountered during delivery of the shoulders, after the birth of the head, and occurs in less than 1% of deliveries. The anterior shoulder or, rarely, both shoulders become impacted above the pelvic brim, usually in the anteroposterior (AP) diameter. True shoulder dystocia is an obstetric emergency that will result in severe fetal morbidity or even mortality if not recognized and successfully managed rapidly.

Etiology

Shoulder dystocia is more common with a large baby. There are elements in the history and physical examination that should lead the astute practitioner to anticipate the possibility of shoulder dystocia. Maternal diabetes, including gestational diabetes, may cause macrosomia and a large baby. A previous history or family history of large infants or shoulder dystocia as well as maternal obesity or excessive weight gain during the pregnancy also may indicate a large fetus. If the estimated fetal weight is above 4000 g or significantly larger than previous infants, shoulder dystocia should be anticipated. In a prolonged second stage of labor, particularly if the delivery is effected by midforceps, the incidence of shoulder dystocia is increased.

Diagnosis

Shoulder dystocia may be anticipated but cannot be diagnosed until after the head is born. The first sign is the retraction of the fetal head against the perineum after delivery. Often, restitution and/or external rotation of the head does not occur or occurs only after manual rotation by the attendant. Vaginal examination reveals that the shoulders have not entered the pelvis, and abdominal palpation will identify the anterior shoulder impinging above the symphysis pubis. Since the oblique diameters of the pelvic inlet are larger than the AP diameter (Chapter 35), the shoulders normally enter the pelvis slightly obliquely, to the side of the midline. In most cases of shoulder dystocia, the shoulders are directly AP. When downward traction on the head fails to deliver the anterior shoulder or upward traction the posterior shoulder, the diagnosis is confirmed.

Maternal and Fetal Outcome

While the major risks associated with shoulder dystocia are to the fetus, there are also negative outcomes that may occur to the mother. Perineal or vaginal lacerations and bladder trauma may occur because of the mechanical pressure from the fetus, or they may result from the manipulations performed to complete the delivery. Postpartum hemorrhage from overdistention of the uterus by the large baby or from lacerations may occur. Infection may occur owing to the lacerations and manipulations required for delivery.

The compression of the fetal neck by the pelvis impairs the circulation, hindering venous return from the head and thus trapping increasing amounts of blood in the head. Increased intracranial pressure, anoxia, intracranial hemorrhage, depressed Apgar score, and brain damage may occur as a result of the circulatory problem. Brachial plexus palsy (Erb's palsy) or fracture of the humerus, clavicle, or cervical vertebrae may result from compression by the mother's pelvis or from the delivery manipulations. Pneumothorax may result from a fractured clavicle. Ultimately, death may occur as a progressive result from any of these complications or from the failure to overcome the dystocia successfully.

Medical Management

Medical management is focused on anticipating difficulty at delivery and preparing to act quickly and competently if shoulder dystocia should occur. If shoulder dystocia is anticipated, the patient should have an empty bladder at the time of delivery (she should be catheterized if necessary). The patient also should have an intravenous infusion in place. The delivery should take place in the delivery room where equipment is available, and the pediatrician should be called to attend the delivery. Some practitioners choose to position the patient in the lithotomy position on the hard surface of the delivery table to facilitate the manipulations that might be required. Others prefer to use the labor bed for the delivery because it is easier for the patient to assume different positions that may facilitate delivery.

It is important that the patient and her support person(s) be informed of the problem and the procedures used in attempting to overcome the dystocia so that she/they may participate effectively in dealing with the emergency. There may be instances in which one or more of the management steps are performed in an order other than the one described here.

In the normal delivery steady downward traction is applied to the head after external rotation has occurred. If one or two attempts of approximately 5 seconds each have failed to produce delivery of the shoulders, an attempt may be made to deliver the posterior shoulder with upward traction. If that is unsuccessful, specific maneuvers to overcome shoulder dystocia should be employed. It should be mentioned that inexperience or poor technique may lead to identification of shoulder dystocia when it does not in reality exist or is merely a soft tissue dystocia.

Vaginal examination is performed to rule out other causes of dystocia (tight loops of nuchal cord, compound presentation of arm or hand) and to determine the position of the shoulders. If necessary, the bladder should be catheterized before further manipulations are performed in order to reduce the risk of trauma. The mother is repositioned to maximize pelvic dimensions if necessary; possible position choices include exaggerated lithotomy, left lateral, squatting, or all fours. The AP diameter may be increased by as much as 0.5–2.0 cm in these positions (6).

Since the oblique diameter of the pelvis is larger than the AP, the shoulders may be rotated manually to an oblique diameter by pressure on the scapula (back of the shoulder). Twisting of the fetal head is not effective and is likely to be traumatic. A large episiotomy may be performed or extended if additional room is needed posteriorly. Some practitioners prefer to use a mediolateral episiotomy, while others prefer a midline with 4° extension if necessary.

While an assistant applies suprapubic pressure (not fundal pressure) down toward the sacrum and in the direction of the fetal chest to disengage the anterior shoulder, traction is exerted on the fetal head directly posteriorly, not outwardly.

Fundal pressure in the attempt to overcome shoulder dystocia will fail. It will waste time and may cause injury to the fetus, or it may cause uterine rupture. There is, however, one appropriate use of fundal pressure—during the screw maneuver of Woods (see below).

If the shoulders have not been disengaged, the screw maneuver of Woods is performed to rotate the posterior shoulder 180° to the anterior. The rotation always is directed so that the *back* rotates anteriorly. An assistant should apply *fundal* pressure during this maneuver only. Fundal pressure is appropriate during this maneuver to help push the baby through the pelvis as the shoulders negotiate the widest diameters of each plane of the pelvis. The transverse diameter of the inlet is widest, so when the shoulders are transverse, fundal pressure will assist descent through the inlet. The AP diameter of the midpelvis and outlet is longer than the transverse, so as the baby is turned, with the shoulders through the inlet and now AP, pressure will aid descent through those planes. If necessary, the screw maneuver is repeated in the opposite direction. If progress is being made, the maneuver may be repeated alternately clockwise and counterclockwise until delivery is achieved.

The final two measures to effect delivery are traumatic. Extraction of the posterior arm over the perineum, across the face in the normal range of motion, may be attempted. It may result in either nerve damage or fracture of the humerus. Deliberate fracture of one or both cavicles results in reduction of the shoulder (bisacromial) diameter and delivery of the fetus.

NURSING MANAGEMENT

Nursing care specific for the patient experiencing *shoulder dystocia*:

☐ Screen for conditions predisposing to shoulder dystocia (e.g., history of shoulder dystocia, large estimated fetal weight, prolonged second stage).

☐ Never apply fundal pressure as a routine measure in a normal delivery, as this may *cause* shoulder dystocia.

☐ Prepare for management of shoulder dystocia when predisposing conditions are present:
   — Plan delivery in delivery room where equipment for neonatal resuscitation will be readily available; position patient on delivery table or labor bed according to preference of birth attendant; and

   — Have equipment (e.g., stool) ready for correct application of force if suprapubic pressure is requested.

☐ Assist with management of shoulder dystocia, as required:
   — Note time of delivery of head and be prepared to inform the attendant of elapsed time, if requested;
   — Apply suprapubic pressure down and in the direction of the fetal chest when requested;
   — Apply fundal pressure only during screw maneuver of Woods when requested;
   — Explain to the patient/partner condition, treatment, expected maternal/fetal outcomes; explain the importance of patient

NURSING MANAGEMENT

cooperation in the management (e.g., pushing, position changes); and
— Monitor the patient after delivery for excessive bleeding and assist with management of postpartum hemorrhage and/or repair of maternal lacerations.

Nursing diagnoses most frequently associated with *shoulder dystocia* (see Section V):

☐ Grieving related to potential/actual loss of infant or birth of an imperfect child.

☐ Knowledge deficit regarding etiology, disease process, treatment, and outcome.
☐ Altered fetal cardiac and cerebral tissue perfusion.
☐ Pain.
☐ Potential altered parenting.
☐ Anxiety/fear.

REFERENCES

1. Caldeyro-Barcia R, Posiero JJ: Physiology of the uterine contraction. *Clin Obstet Gynecol* 3:386, 1960.
2. Pritchard JA, MacDonald PC, Gant NF: *Williams Obstetrics*, ed 17. Norwalk, CT, Appleton-Century-Crofts, 1985, p 840.
3. Marieskind HI: *An Evaluation of Cesarean Section in the United States*. Washington, DC, U.S. Government Printing Office, Office of the Assistant Secretary for Planning and Evaluation/Health, June 1979.
4. Richart RM: Is there a scientific basis for repeat cesarean? *Contemp OB/GYN* 19:158–163, 1982.
5. Committee on Obstetrics: Maternal and Fetal Medicine: Guidelines for vaginal delivery after a previous cesarean section. *ACOG Newsletter*, February, 1985.
6. Roberts J: Alternative positions for childbirth. *J Nurse-Midwifery* 25:13–19, 1980.

Chapter 41
Injuries to the Birth Canal during Labor and Birth
Linda V. Walsh, C.N.M., M.P.H.

LACERATIONS

Lacerations of the birth canal are defined by the extent of injury and the structures involved (Table 41.1). There are common predisposing factors to all lacerations: precipitous deliveries, induction or augmentation with oxytocin, abnormal position or presentation of the fetus, large infant, rigid tissue (particularly, scarring from previous incision or laceration), poor quality tissue, and use of instrumentation (1–3). Most lacerations are minor and without short- or long-term complications. A few may result in serious morbidity such as hemorrhage, infection, scarring, and descensus of pelvic organs (3).

Labial, Clitoral, and Periurethral Lacerations

Most anterior external lacerations are associated with premature extension of the fetal head in the occiput anterior position and rapid delivery. A further contributing factor can be poor delivery technique by the birth attendant. Some authors feel that prevention is possible by the use of episiotomy. Labial lacerations usually are seen as superficial trauma to the inner surface of the labia; occasionally, there will be a tearing of the whole structure (4). Blood loss tends to be minimal. Conversely, clitoral lacerations may exhibit extensive bleeding because of the vascular network of the area. Clitoral lacerations also can be very painful because of the neurological makeup of the area. Periurethral lacerations usually are superficial lacerations in the area of the urethral meatus. Suturing is recommended if there is active bleeding (1, p 735). Some practitioners recommend repair even in the absence of bleeding in order to decrease the level of pain noted by the woman, particularly with urination. Often, even with repair, the woman may have difficulty urinating postpartum because of the resultant trauma and edema.

Perineal Lacerations

Although there may be variations in the classification of perineal lacerations, the most commonly

Table 41.1.
LACERATIONS

TYPE	STRUCTURES INVOLVED
Perineal, first degree	Skin of perineum, vaginal mucosa, posterior fourchette
Perineal, second degree	Skin, vaginal mucosa, underlying muscles and fascia
Perineal, third degree	Skin, vaginal mucosa, underlying muscles and fascia, external anal sphincter
Perineal, fourth degree	Skin, vaginal mucosa, underlying muscles and fascia, anal sphincter, rectal mucosa
Labial	Labial mucosa, underlying tissue
Clitoral	Clitoris, clitoral hood, prepuce
Periurethral	Tissue of vestibule surrounding urethral meatus
Vaginal	Vaginal mucosa, underlying muscle and fascia

Table 41.2.

FACTORS INCREASING THE RISK OF PERINEAL LACERATIONS

FACTOR	EXPLANATION
Persistent occiput posterior position	Causes overdistention of perineal body because of posterior position of the wider biparietal diameter and incomplete flexion of the fetal head
Abnormal presentation (i.e., face, breech)	May cause overdistention of perineal body and inconsistent pressure on tissues
Pelvic type/tendency exhibits a narrow pubic arch (i.e., android)	Narrowing of the anterior pelvis forces the presenting part into the posterior portion of the outlet, causing overdistention of the perineal body

used terms are described in Table 41.1. Perineal lacerations cannot always be avoided, but the skilled practitioner will use his or her expertise to decrease the extent of trauma to the tissues. Table 41.2 lists factors that increase the risk of perineal lacerations in addition to the general risk factors noted previously.

First degree lacerations may not require repair. Bleeding is minimal, and healing occurs easily because of the anatomic approximation of tissue. Second degree lacerations are repaired like episiotomies, with suturing of both deep and superficial tissues. Third and fourth degree lacerations require meticulous repair in order to assure the woman's future bowel control and prevent rectovaginal fistulas.

Vaginal Lacerations

Vaginal lacerations most often occur from extension of perineal tears from instrumentation used during delivery or by manual rotation of the fetal head. Only occasionally do they occur spontaneously (5). Isolated lacerations involving the middle or upper third of the vagina but unassociated with lacerations of the cervix or perineum are rarely observed (5). These may present as sulcus tears—second degree lacerations along one or both sides of the vaginal wall rather than extending midline. Those lacerations that extend into deep tissues may result in copious bleeding, usually readily controlled by suturing, and effective repair yields no long-term ill effects. However, because of poor visualization, repair may be difficult.

Episiotomies

Episiotomy—surgical incision of the perineum—has become a routine intervention for many practitioners. Rationales for the procedure are listed in Table 41.3. However, there is little evidence in the literature that episiotomy improves or maintains the condition of the pelvic floor and no evidence that it reduces the likelihood of cystocele or rectocele or that it improves sexual functioning after birth (6). Cogan and Edmunds state, "Most striking in the literature is the absence of clear evidence as to the advantages of the procedure." They found "no data showing a positive relationship between episiotomy and subsequent maternal or infant health in births that are not forceps delivered" (9).

Certain common interventions may, in fact, increase the need for episiotomy. Use of analgesic/anesthetic agents, particularly regional anesthesia, may inhibit the mother's expulsive efforts. Posi-

Table 41.3.

REASONS FOR EPISIOTOMY

MATERNAL	FETAL	LABOR	OTHER
Prevention of overdistention of perineum because of pelvic architecture, fetal size, position, and presentation	Shortened second stage— decrease stress of labor, fetal distress	Prevention of prolonged second stage	Practitioner preference— influenced by education, philosophy, and practice patterns
Provision of a clean, incised wound for repair	Protection of fetal head in preterm infant		
Shortened second stage— prevention of maternal exhaustion	Anticipation of shoulder dystocia		
Prevention of inevitable tears			

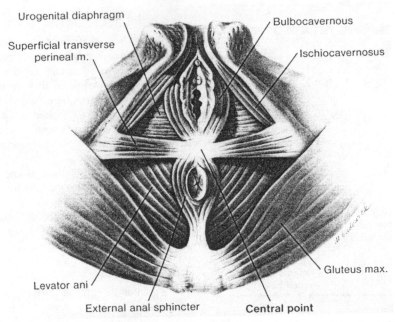

Figure 41.1. The muscles of the perineum as seen from below. (Used with permission from Caplan RM (ed): *Principles of Obstetrics.* Baltimore, Williams & Wilkins, 1982, p 91.)

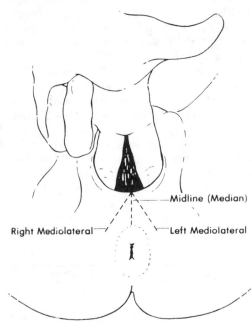

Figure 41.2. Location of midline and mediolateral episiotomies. (From Varney H: *Nurse-Midwifery* Originally Boston, Blackwell Scientific Publications, 1980, p 221. Now St. Louis, C.V. Mosby, p 618.)

tioning in the supine position may decrease uterine blood flow, leading to fetal distress and

the necessity of instrumentation to hasten delivery. Positioning in the lithotomy position may put enough tension on perineal tissue to necessitate episiotomy to prevent lacerations through rigid tissue. Changes in procedures surrounding labor and delivery may decrease the need for surgical intervention.

Midline, or median, episiotomy incises the central tendonous point of the perineum (Figs. 41.1 and 41.2). Depth of the incision determines which deep structures are involved. Most large studies concur that the midline episiotomy offers advantages over the mediolateral in terms of less blood loss, better healing, and less patient discomfort (3, p 977). Mediolateral episiotomy begins at the central tendonous point of the perineum and extends through superficial and deep muscles toward the ischial tuberosity. Advantages of this incision are that it can enlarge the vaginal outlet more than the midline, and it has less chance of extending into the anal sphincter and rectum. The chief disadvantage is that the angle of the incision causes greater trauma to the muscles and therefore results in greater blood loss and a more difficult repair.

Complications of the episiotomy include extension of the incision, breakdown of the wound, fistula formation, Bartholin's duct and inclusion cysts, endometriosis, and poor perineal tone (3, p 979).

NURSING MANAGEMENT

Nursing care specific for a patient experiencing *injuries to the birth canal*:

☐ For the patient with *lacerations and/or episisotomy*:
- Assist in prevention of lacerations:
  * Teach all patients prenatally to maintain a nutritious diet and to take vitamin and iron therapy to promote tissue integrity;
  * Teach patient/partner prenatal perineal massage;
  * Teach Kegel's exercise prenatally to enhance control of contraction/relaxation during delivery;
  * Provide childbirth education that teaches breathing/relaxation techniques to help maintain control for the birth; and
  * Position the patient for delivery with minimal stress on the perineum.
- For repair, assist in proper positioning of patient; administer analgesics as ordered.
- Observe the patient for perineal edema, apply ice to the perineum for the first 24 hours and moist heat thereafter to decrease edema and promote healing; and
- Encourage a diet high in protein and vitamin C to promote healing.

☐ Teach the patient to promote healing by:
- Wiping from front to back;
- Changing peripads every 2–3 hours;
- Using a perineal rinse after every voiding; and
- Beginning Kegel's excercises.

☐ Provide analgesics, as needed.

☐ Observe suture line for redness, swelling, bruising, pain, continued approximation of sutures, and discharge.

☐ Teach patient to delay resumption of sexual intercourse until perineum is healed and she is comfortable.

Nursing diagnoses most frequently associated with *lacerations/episiotomy* (see Section V):

☐ Disturbance in body image, self-esteem.

☐ Knowledge deficit regarding etiology, disease process, treatment, and outcome.

☐ Pain.

☐ Impaired tissue integrity.

☐ Altered patterns of urinary elimination.

☐ Altered sexuality patterns.

CERVICAL LACERATIONS

Small superficial lacerations of the cervix occur in almost all vaginal deliveries, and they rarely need repair because they do not bleed significantly and they heal spontaneously (3, p 968). Larger lacerations may be sustained with forceful, expulsive labors and with manual manipulation of the cervix. These lacerations may extend into the vaginal fornix and lower uterine segment. In severe cases the uterine vessels can become involved with resultant hemorrhage.

Cervical lacerations greater than 2 cm, should be repaired (1, p 736, 5, p 860), not only to prevent bleeding but also to prevent the possibility of incompetent cervix with subsequent pregnancies (3, p 969). Other sequelae may be leukorrhea and a feeling of pelvic pressure. Occasionally, the laceration will be extensive enough to prohibit complete visualization and repair in the delivery room. In this case laparotomy is necessary.

Rarely, avulsion (annular detachment) of the cervix occurs. This detachment is caused by excessive compression of the cervix during labor (as with an edematous anterior lip or overstimulation with oxytocin), with resultant ischemia, necrosis, and separation. Various degrees of avulsion may occur, often accompanied by portions of the upper vagina (3, p 969). Bleeding may be minimal because prolonged compression has caused the vessels to thrombose, but it may be profuse, requiring surgical intervention.

NURSING MANAGEMENT

Nursing care specific for the patient experiencing *cervical laceration*:

☐ Anticipate shock with heavy bleeding if cervical laceration is diagnosed:
- Monitor vital signs every 5 minutes until stable; and
- Ensure that blood for replacement is available.

NURSING MANAGEMENT

☐ Prepare for surgery if repair is not possible in the delivery room.

☐ Tell the patient to limit sexual activity until complete healing has occurred in 2–3 weeks.

☐ Be alert to quality of early postpartum bleeding: many times a continuous trickle of blood that does not decrease in the presence of a contracted uterus is the first sign of undiagnosed cervical laceration.

Nursing diagnoses most frequently associated with *cervical lacerations* (see Section V):

☐ Disturbance in body image, self-esteem.

☐ Knowledge deficit regarding etiology, disease process, treatment, and outcome.

☐ Fluid volume deficit.

☐ Impaired tissue integrity.

HEMATOMAS

Hematomas of the vulva and vagina are caused by the escape of blood into connective tissue beneath the skin covering the external genitalia or beneath the vaginal mucosa (5, p 915). Predisposing factors are the same as those for lacerations; in addition, there may be inadvertent damage to a vessel during local or pudendal anesthesia injection or vessel damage caused by prolonged pressure with resultant necrosis and sloughing. Usually, the hematoma will develop slowly over several hours after delivery, and the initial sign of the problem is the feeling of pressure and pain by the woman. As the hematoma enlarges, pelvic or rectal pain may become severe, and a tense, sensitive mass can be palpated. On some occasions there may be rapid development of the hematoma, with clinical signs of decreased blood pressure, increased pulse, and shock. Medical management for small hematomas can be expectant, with application of ice packs to minimize bleeding and frequent observation for an increase in size. However, with severe pain and/or significant bleeding, incision of the hematoma and ligation of the involved vessel(s) are necessary.

Broad ligament hematoma may result from dissection by blood upward from a vaginal laceration (1, p 737). More likely, the hematoma will follow undiagnosed rupture of the uterus. As the hematoma increases in size, it may extend into the retroperitoneal area or into the peritoneal cavity. Diagnosis may be difficult. As with external hematomas, pain will be present, but it may be present as general lower abdominal pain and pressure over the bladder and rectum. Eventually, a tender mass may be palpated, and the woman will exhibit signs of shock. Medical management includes replacement of blood and reexamination of the uterine cavity and upper vagina to ascertain the presence of rupture or laceration. If bleeding continues, laparotomy is indicated. When bleeding is uncontrollable, hysterectomy, bilateral ligation of the hypogastric arteries, and packing the pelvis may be necessary.

NURSING MANAGEMENT

Nursing care specific for the patient experiencing *hematomas*:

☐ Apply an ice pack to all episiotomy sites for 24 hours after birth.

☐ Observe for signs/symptoms of hematoma in all patients (e.g., pressure, pain, pelvic or rectal mass, shock).

☐ Monitor size of hematoma; observe for signs/symptoms of shock or increase in pain.

☐ Apply ice to constrict blood vessels and minimize size of hematoma if appropriate.

☐ Prepare for surgery, if required to stop bleeding.

☐ Prepare for transfusion, if appropriate.

☐ In the postpartum period, ensure a diet high in protein and vitamin C, to promote healing.

☐ Ensure that patients who have had a hematoma leave the hospital with vitamins and iron, as appropriate (hematocrit less than 34%).

Nursing diagnoses most frequently associated with *hematomas* (see Section V):

☐ Anxiety.

☐ Knowledge deficit regarding etiology, disease process, treatment, and outcome.

☐ Fluid volume deficit.

☐ Altered maternal tissue perfusion.

☐ Pain.

☐ Impaired tissue integrity.

☐ Altered patterns of urinary elimination.

RUPTURE OF THE UTERUS

Uterine rupture usually is defined in terms of complete or incomplete rupture. Complete rupture is as the name suggests—rupture through the uterine wall into the peritoneal cavity. In incomplete rupture the contents of the uterus remain covered by the visceral peritoneum (5, p 862). Estimates of the incidence vary dramatically, from 1:100 to 1:11,000, with most sources agreeing on an average of about 1:2000 births (2, p 414; 4, p 795; 5, p 862; 7). Causes include weakened scar in the uterus, placental implantation at the scar site, obstructed labor, use of oxytoxic agents, instrumentation, version in labor, and pregnancy in a rudimentary uterine horn. Exploration of the uterus after vaginal birth after cesarean section is indicated to rule out uterine rupture (see Chapter 40).

Signs and symptoms of uterine rupture include abdominal pain, possible vaginal bleeding, and shock. If the rupture occurs during labor, the woman suddenly experiences a sharp, tearing pain, followed by cessation of contractions. She may express feelings of relief. With complete rupture the uterus is able to contract effectively, and blood loss may be kept to a minimum. The contracted uterus may be felt as a firm mass to one side of the fetus. Fetal heart tones cease shortly after rupture. In incomplete rupture bleeding may be severe, and the woman can go into shock rapidly. Mortality of the fetus is estimated at 50–75% (5, p 872). The only chance of survival is immediate delivery by laparotomy. Maternal prognosis is dependent upon the availability of prompt diagnosis, efficient blood and fluid replacement, laparotomy, and antibiotic therapy. Surgical management is dependent upon the woman's condition and the degree of damage to the uterus. Hysterectomy, repair of rupture alone, and repair of rupture with sterilization are the usual choices of management.

NURSING MANAGEMENT

Nursing care specific for the patient experiencing *ruptured uterus*:

☐ Identify patients at risk for uterine rupture; monitor closely for signs/symptoms of rupture (e.g., abdominal pain, cessation of contractions, vaginal bleeding, shock, fetal distress).

☐ Prepare for immediate surgery if rupture occurs.

☐ Monitor fetal status constantly until delivered or until fetal heart tones cease.

Nursing diagnoses most frequently associated with *uterine rupture* (see Section V):

☐ Grieving related to potential/actual loss of infant or birth of an imperfect child.

☐ Anticipatory grieving related to actual/perceived threat to self.

☐ Knowledge deficit regarding etiology, disease process, treatment, and outcome.

☐ Fluid volume deficit.

☐ Altered maternal tissue perfusion.

☐ Altered fetal cardiac and cerebral tissue perfusion.

☐ Pain.

☐ Anxiety/fear.

REFERENCES

1. Danforth DN (ed): *Obstetrics and Gynecology*. Philadelphia, Harper & Row, 1982, p 735.
2. Myles MF: *Textbook for Midwives*, ed 9. London, Churchill Livingston, 1981, p 317.
3. Iffy L, Kaminetzky HA (eds): *Principles and Practice of Obstetrics and Perinatology*. New York, John Wiley and Sons, 1981, p 981.
4. Donald I: *Practical Obstetric Problems*, ed 5. London, Lloyd-Luke Ltd., 1979, p 797.
5. Pritchard JA, MacDonald PC: *Williams Obstetrics*, ed 16. New York, Appleton-Century-Crofts, 1980, p 859.
6. Cogan R, Edmunds EP: The unkindest cut? *J Nurse-Midwifery*, 23:17, 1978.
7. Cetrulo CL, Sbarra AJ: *The Problem-Oriented Medical Record for High-Risk Obstetrics*. New York, Plenum, 1984, p 386.

Section IV: Deviations of the Postpartum and Neonatal Period

Chapter 42
Abnormalities of the Third and Fourth Stages of Labor
Peggy Gallagher, C.N.M., M.S.

INTRODUCTION

The third stage of labor begins with completion of delivery of the infant and ends with expulsion of the placenta and membranes. The average duration of this stage is 5–10 minutes, but it may be considered normal for it to last up to 1 hour, unless there is excessive bleeding. It must be noted some practitioners consider 30 minutes to be the limit for a normal third stage.

During the third stage of labor, maternal blood pressure, pulse, and respirations gradually return to normal. Maternal temperature continues to be slightly elevated but below 100.4°F (37.9°C). Gastric motility and absorption begin to return to normal unless affected by drugs. Immediately after the baby is born, the placenta stops secreting both estrogen and progesterone, thereby removing any inhibitory effects these two hormones have on lactation. This allows marked increased production of prolactin by the adenohypophysis, thereby initiating milk production.

The third stage of labor may be divided into two phases: placental separation and placental expulsion. After delivery of the baby, uterine contractions resume at regular intervals. These events combine to decrease the size of the uterine cavity rapidly. This leads to a decreased area of placental attachment. The placenta initially tries to accommodate this situation by becoming thicker, but it soon buckles, thus partially or completely separating from its attachment in the spongiosa layer of the decidua. As the placenta separates, blood sinuses are torn and a hematoma—the retroplacental clot—forms between the maternal surface of the placenta and the decidua basalis. The pressure and the weight of the expanding retroplacental clot is thought to accelerate placental separation further. Bleeding is controlled by the contraction and retraction of uterine muscle fibers, which act as ligatures to compress the uterine blood vessels. The unattached placenta moves down into the lower uterine segment, exerting traction on the membranes, which then peel off the decidua.

The following are signs of placental separation:

1. There is a gush of blood from the vagina.
2. The umbilical cord appears to lengthen.
3. The uterine fundus rises as the placenta passes from the uterus into the vaginal vault.
4. The uterus becomes firm and globular.

Placental separation can be confirmed using the Brandt-Andrews maneuver once the fundus is firm. The cord is clamped at the vulva and held taut. The other hand is placed between the fundus and symphysis. Pressure is exerted down toward the spine, and toward the fundus. This elevates the uterus in the abdomen. If the cord recedes, the placenta is not separated; if the cord remains the same length or gets longer, it is separated (Fig. 42.1). Alternatively, the location of the placenta can be determined by following the umbilical cord into the vagina. The placenta will be felt in the vagina if it has separated; if not, the cord will be felt extending through the cervix.

Once the placenta has separated, it must be expelled without delay to avoid undue blood loss. The placenta is expelled by one of two mecha-

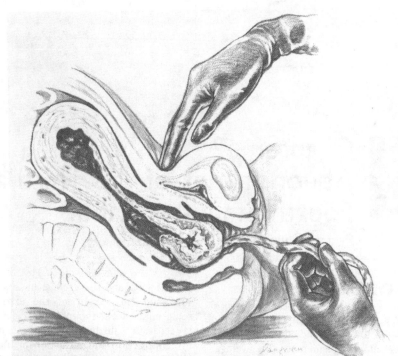

Figure 42.1. Checking for placental separation. (Reproduced by permission from Greenhill JP, Friedman EA: *Biological Principles and Modern Practice of Obstetrics.* Philadelphia, WB Saunders, 1974.)

nisms. The first method, the Schultze mechanism, occurs in about 80% of deliveries. In this method the separation of the placenta begins centrally. The retroplacental clot is formed and weighs down the central portion of the placenta, which descends first. The placenta and amniotic sac invert, and the membranes peel off the uterine wall and trail behind. Bleeding is not seen since blood is caught in the inverted sac. The placenta delivers with the smooth fetal side presenting. In the second or Duncan mechanism placental separation starts at the margin of the placenta. It descends sideways with membranes trailing behind. Blood escapes between the membrane and uterine wall and is evident before the placenta is delivered. The rough maternal side is seen first. This mechanism more frequently is followed by retained membrane fragments.

The fourth stage of labor begins following delivery of the placenta and lasts for 1 hour. Close observation of the patient is required during this time. Maternal vital signs stabilize to prelabor levels, with the exception of temperature, which may continue to be elevated slightly but below 100.4°F (37.9°C). The uterus now is situated in the

midline of the abdomen with the fundus at approximately one fingerbreadth below the umbilicus. The uterus should be firm and well contracted. Gastric motility returns to normal.

Chills are a common complaint of the patient at this time, probably owing to a release of nervous tension and/or exhaustion. The patient may experience thirst and hunger.

Trauma and pressure on the bladder during labor and delivery may cause many patients to experience urinary retention. Care must be taken to avoid bladder distention, since this could interfere with uterine contractions necessary to maintain hemostasis and could contribute to postpartum urinary tract infection.

The placenta and membranes are inspected and evaluated to determine if any placental fragments have been retained. The cervix, vagina, and perineum are inspected and repaired, and bleeding is controlled.

Third and fourth stage complications are potentially life-threatening. Maternal morbidity and mortality can be decreased greatly by meticulous management of all stages of labor and by anticipation of conditions that may lead to complications.

RETAINED PLACENTA

Definition

Retained placenta is defined as retention in the uterus of all or part of the placenta. Spontaneous detachment of the placenta occurs in 90% of patients within 5 minutes and in 95% of patients within 30 minutes of birth of the infant (1). A delay beyond 1 hour must be considered placental retention.

Etiology

Retained placenta can be divided into four categories:

1. The normally implanted placenta is separated or partially separated but retained because of absence of effective uterine contractions.
2. Entrapment prevents expulsion of a partially or completely separated placenta at the level of the physiologic retraction ring or the internal os.
3. The placenta is adherent but does not separate owing to ineffective uterine contractions.
4. The placenta is adherent and inseparable from varying degrees of placenta accreta.

Factors predisposing the patient to placental retention include:

1. History of retained placenta.
2. Prior operative procedures that increase the chance of abnormal attachment (e.g., cesarean section, myomectomy, or vigorous curettage).
3. Uterine abnormalities (e.g., subseptate or bicornuate uterus).
4. Abnormalities of placentation (e.g., low lying placenta, placenta accreta, or cornual implantation).
5. Placental abnormalities (e.g., succenturiate lobe).

In addition, inappropriate management of the patient may contribute to retained placenta. For example, improper conduct of labor leading to prolonged labor, excessive medication, or deep anesthesia may interfere with uterine contractions. Mismanagement of the third stage of labor (e.g., kneading and squeezing the uterus or administering ergot preparations prior to placental separation) or inattention to a full bladder may interfere with placental expulsion.

Diagnosis

If the placenta has not been delivered within 1 hour of birth by using controlled cord traction, retained placenta must be diagnosed by either the Brandt-Andrews maneuver or inability to palpate the placenta in the vagina. Differential diagnosis of retained placenta from constriction ring is made during an attempt at manual removal of the placenta. Placenta accreta is diagnosed during an attempt at manual removal.

Maternal Outcome

Maternal outcome depends upon the cause and treatment required to deliver the placenta. Retention of part or all of the placenta can lead to immediate or delayed postpartum hemorrhage. Manual removal carries with it an increased incidence of uterine infection. If surgery is required, the patient is exposed to the usual operative risks. If the retained placenta is due to placenta accreta and hysterectomy is required, childbearing potential obviously is lost.

Medical Management

If there is active bleeding or a delay of more than 1 hour before placental delivery, manual removal is indicated. An intravenous infusion should be started with a no. 16 or no. 18 plastic cannula. Blood should be drawn for a type- and cross-match in the event replacement therapy is warranted. Anesthesia is necessary for uterine relaxation as well as pain relief. Manual removal must be done under aseptic conditions. After removal the uterus is explored to ensure that no fragments have been missed. Oxytocin is given to ensure good uterine contractions and retraction.

If placenta accreta is diagnosed during an attempt at manual removal, attempts to complete placental separation should continue only if it can be done gently and without significant blood loss. Otherwise, the patient must be prepared for emergency hysterectomy (see Chapter 31).

INVERSION OF THE UTERUS

Definition

Inversion of the uterus occurs when the uterus turns inside out, either partially or completely. There are progressive degrees of inversion based on the anatomical position of the inverted fundus in the pelvis:

1. First degree: fundus is flattened and does not retain globular shape.
2. Incomplete or second degree: the fundus protrudes through the cervical os.
3. Complete or third degree: the fundus protrudes to the vaginal introitus.
4. Prolapsed or fourth degree: the fundus extrudes beyond the vulva.

Inversion of the uterus is rare, occurring in 1:100,000 to 1:5000 deliveries (2). Usually, it occurs immediately following delivery, but it may occur during the puerperium. This discussion focuses on acute inversion that is diagnosed during the third and fourth stages of labor.

Etiology

Factors that combine to favor uterine inversion include uterine atony, patulous or dilated cervix, fundal placement of the placenta, and fundal pressure with or without cord traction on an uncontracted uterus. In very rare instances spontaneous inversion occurs after delivery when the patient strains in an effort to expel the placenta. This increases intraabdominal pressure, thereby creating fundal pressure. However, inversion usually is a result of mismanagement of the third stage of labor. Three-fourths of the cases involve exerting cord traction prior to placental separation. Other acts of mismanagement include fundal pressure on an uncontracted uterus in an effort to expel the placenta and pulling on the placenta during manual removal.

Signs and Symptoms

Uterine inversion may present with the following signs and symptoms: sudden agonizing pelvic pain, feeling of fullness extending into the bladder, brisk vaginal bleeding, inability to palpate the fundus in the abdomen, and presence of the inverted uterus at the vaginal introitus. Shock, disproportionate to blood loss, is the outstanding sign of uterine inversion. This is probably due to traction and compression of the ovaries, fallopian tubes, and broad ligaments, leading to neurogenic shock.

Diagnosis

Diagnosis of complete uterine inversion is made simply by observation of the inverted uterus at or outside the vaginal introitus. Diagnosis of incomplete inversion is more difficult. It is suggested by a funnel-like depression instead of the fundus upon abdominal palpation. Bimanual examination is necessary to assess the degree of incomplete inversion.

Maternal Outcome

Inversion of the uterus during the third stage of labor often is followed by hemorrhage, shock, and circulatory collapse. Prompt treatment is mandatory to avoid maternal mortality.

Immediate manual replacement is indicated and, if accomplished, results are good. If this method fails, deep anesthesia is required, and manual replacement can be accomplished in about 75% of cases. The remaining 25% of cases will require immediate surgical replacement. Inversion is not likely to recur in subsequent pregnancies.

Other reported complications of inversion include infection, intestinal obstruction, paralytic ileus, anemia, embolism, and, in some cases, sterility.

Medical Management

Medical management is aimed at repositioning the uterus and treating the patient for shock. Additional assistance, including anesthesiology, is summoned immmediately. If inversion occurs after separation of the placenta and is recognized early, prior to entrapment, replacement may be accomplished simply by pushing on the fundus in the direction of the long axis of the vagina. At the same time, whole blood transfusion and intravenous fluids (Ringer's lactate) should be administered in order to counteract neurogenic and hypovolemic shock. After replacement is accomplished, oxytoxics are administered and compression of the uterus is maintained until it is well contracted.

If the placenta is attached, the inverted uterus is replaced within the vagina until intravenous fluids and blood replacements are begun. General anesthesia is needed to relax the uterus in order to replace it. The placenta is not removed until the uterus has been replaced in order to decrease the effect of hemorrhage. As soon as it is removed, anesthesia is discontinued and oxytocin begun. The fundus must be held in this position until the uterus starts to contract. Further hemorrhage can be controlled by use of bimanual compression. After uterine tone is recovered, the uterus is monitored transvaginally for evidence of recurrence.

If correction of inversion cannot be accomplished by any of the preceding methods, immediate laparotomy is mandatory. Postoperative management includes correction of fluid and electrolyte imbalance along with blood replacement. Use of broad spectrum antibiotics to prevent infection is suggested.

POSTPARTUM HEMORRHAGE

Definition

Postpartum hemorrhage is defined as blood loss in excess of 500 cc during the first 24 hours after birth of the infant. The incidence of postpartum hemorrhage ranges from 5–10% and is the leading cause of maternal death in the United States.

Etiology

The most commonly identified causes of postpartum hemorrhage include uterine atony, trauma, retention of all or part of the placenta, and bleeding from the site of the episiotomy. Other causes include preexisting blood dyscrasias (e.g., afibrinogenemia, hypofibrinogenemia) and rupture of the uterus.

Conditions that predispose to uterine atony include history of previous postpartum hemorrhage, high parity, fibroids, uterine anomalies, anemia, large fetus, multiple gestation, polyhydramnios, prolonged labor, precipitous labor, excessive analgesia or general anesthesia, placenta previa, unexpelled blood clots, and mismanagement of the third stage of labor.

Trauma can be anticipated with delivery of a large baby, operative deliveries (e.g., cesarean section and all types of forceps deliveries), vaginal delivery after cesarean section or other uterine incision, delivery through an incompletely dilated cervix, placenta previa, varices of the vagina or vulva, abnormal presentations or positions, precipitous delivery, and friability of the birth canal because of severe vaginitis or cervicitis.

Factors predisposing to retention of all or part of the placenta include the following: abnormally adherent placenta; abnormally shaped placenta (e.g., succenturiate lobe); abnormal implantation site (e.g., cornual implantation, placenta previa); and, the most common factor, mismanagement of the third stage of labor (e.g., excessive cord traction prior to placental separation or misuse of oxytoxics).

Signs and Symptoms

Signs and symptoms of postpartum hemorrhage are obvious, with heavy vaginal bleeding during the third stage of labor or within the first 24 hours postpartum, with or without hypovolemic shock.

Diagnosis

Postpartum hemorrhage from trauma is identified immediately after the second stage of labor as a continuous heavy trickle of blood from the vagina. Blood may collect in the vagina to form clots, depending on the patient's position during delivery. The uterus has good tone and usually is well contracted. Careful inspection of the perineum, vagina, cervix, and uterus is required to locate the site of bleeding.

Postpartum hemorrhage from uterine atony usually is detected after the third stage of labor as blood accumulates behind the placenta and is released as the placenta delivers. The uterus is boggy and often hard to outline as a result of uterine atony. It may be larger than normal because of the acumulation of blood within the uterine cavity. Visualization of the cervical os reveals a steady, persistent flow of blood. Bleeding in gushes may occur as the uterus is manipulated.

Maternal Outcome

Maternal conditions that determine the effect a specific blood loss will have include the patient's nonpregnant blood volume, the magnitude of pregnancy-induced hypervolemia, the degree of anemia at the time of the delivery, and the patient's general health status.

Maternal outcome depends upon the cause of bleeding, the amount lost, and the treatment required to control the hemorrhage. Maternal morbidity and mortality rates rise in direct proportion to the amount of blood loss. If hemorrhage is not checked promptly, hypovolemia and shock ensue. This may lead to renal damage, disseminated intravascular coagulation, Sheehan's syndrome, and maternal mortality. Other complications include anemia, puerperal infection, embolism, and transfusion reaction.

Medical Management

Preventive measures that can reduce the incidence of postpartum hemorrhage are screening for and treating anemia during pregnancy, ensuring that the patient is in good general health prior to labor, meticulous obstetrical management during all stages of labor, avoidance of those situations that predispose the patient to postpartum hemorrhage, close monitoring of uterine tone, and use of prophylactic oxytoxics after delivery in those patients at risk for postpartum hemorrhage.

Medical management begins with identification of patients at risk for postpartum hemorrhage. These patients should be delivered in a setting where emergency measures can be instituted immediately. They should have an intravenous infusion in place with a 16- or 18-gauge intravenous catheter prior to delivery. Two units of blood should be ready for administration. Oxytoxics should be ready to give, if necessary, after delivery.

When postpartum hemorrhage is recognized, the uterus should be palpated to determine whether it is contracted, since uterine atony is the most frequent cause of postpartum hemorrhage. If it is not contracted, the fundus is massaged and oxytoxics are given. Oxytocin causes intermittent uterine contractions, whereas ergonovine and methylergonovine cause sustained uterine contractions. However, ergonovine and methylergonovine are contraindicated for patients with hypertension. If these measures fail to control the hemorrhage, bimanual compression can be performed to achieve hemostasis by placing continuous pressure on the lower uterine segment and massaging. In very rare cases, when the hemorrhage is not controlled by these measures, aortic compression can be done in a thin woman while awaiting surgery to ligate the uterine arteries. Aortic compression is done with the fist pressing toward the spine above the level of the fundus.

If, upon palpation of the uterus, the fundus is found to be contracted, another cause for hemorrhage must be sought. The cervix, vagina, and perineum are inspected for lacerations. Any lacerations that are found are repaired. The placenta is inspected. If there is any question whether it is intact, the uterus is explored and any remaining fragments of placenta or membranes are removed.

Blood dyscrasias must be treated according to the cause.

During treatment of postpartum hemorrhage, the vital signs are monitored frequently. The following steps should be taken to prevent or control shock:

1. Provide for fluid replacement with lactated Ringer's solution.
2. Place the patient in the Trendelenburg position.
3. Provide oxygen as needed.
4. Keep the patient warm.
5. When blood is available, administer it as necessary.

If surgery is necessary, alert the anesthesiologist and the surgical team immediately.

After postpartum hemorrhage is controlled, the patient's continuing blood loss must be monitored carefully. A more accurate estimation of blood loss can be made by counting and/or weighing perineal pads. The hematocrit should be checked during the postpartum period, the frequency depending upon the severity of blood loss. It must be remembered that the normal postpartum hemodynamic changes will profoundly affect evaluation of hematocrit readings. Iron supplements and a diet high in iron, vitamin C, and protein should be prescribed.

The patient should be observed during the postpartum period for symptoms of blood loss anemia: dizziness, shortness of breath, pallor, cyanosis, rapid pulse, and hypotension. The patient is at high risk for puerperal infection and thus should be monitored frequently.

NURSING MANAGEMENT

Nursing care specific for a patient experiencing *abnormalities of the third and fourth stages of labor*:
☐ Encourage every pregnant patient to prepare for the birthing process and achieve an optimal health status, including but not limited to:
 — Eating a nutritious diet and taking iron and vitamin supplements, and
 — Reporting signs and symptoms of vaginitis and completing a full course of treatment when vaginitis is diagnosed.
☐ Intrapartum, identify patients at risk for hemorrhage and ensure that two units of whole

blood are type- and cross-matched for the patient.
☐ Ensure that a patent, large gauge intravenous line is in place, if hemorrhage occurs.
☐ Draw up oxytocic drugs and have them ready for immediate use.
☐ Postpartum, monitor maternal vital signs; height, position, and consistency of uterus; amount of lochia; presence of episiotomy redness, edema, ecchymosis, discharge, and suture approximation; and hematoma formation.
☐ Educate the patient who has had postpartum hemorrhage regarding the following:

NURSING MANAGEMENT

— Importance of maintaining a diet high in protein, iron, and vitamin C;

— Signs and symptoms of infection and where to report them (e.g, fever, malaise, abdominal pain, increased or foul-smelling lochia);

— Continuing course of iron and prenatal vitamins for at least 6 weeks postpartum; and

— To avoid dizziness or fainting, teach the patient to arise slowly from bed and to maintain adequate fluid and dietary intake.

— Assist the patient to ambulate until she is not dizzy or faint.

☐ Support the patient who has had postpartum hemorrhage by:

— Assisting the fatigued mother in early interactions with her baby;

— Helping the family to coordinate the mother's first weeks at home to minimize homemaking responsibilities.

— Ensuring the patient is given a 3-month supply of iron and vitamins (if Hct is below 34%).

Nursing diagnoses most frequently associated with *abnormalities of the third and fourth stages of labor* (see Section V):

☐ Anticipatory grieving related to actual/perceived threat to self.

☐ Knowledge deficit regarding etiology, disease process, treatment, and outcome.

☐ Fluid volume deficit.

☐ Altered maternal tissue perfusion.

☐ Potential altered parenting.

☐ Anxiety/fear.

☐ Potential for infection.

REFERENCES

1. Benson RC: *Current Obstetric and Gynecologic Diagnosis and Treatment*, ed 3. Los Altos, CA, Lange Medical Publications, 1980, p 694.

2. Oxorn H, Foote WR: *Human Labor and Birth.* ed 4, East Norwalk, CT, Appleton-Century-Crofts, 1980, p 435.

Chapter 43
Abnormalities of the
Postpartum Period
Kathleen Buckley, C.N.M., M.S.N.

INTRODUCTION

The postpartum period is a time of dramatic psychological and physiological growth and change. The maternal reproductive system returns to its nonpregnant state (Table 43.1). The mother, infant, and significant others begin the process of bonding and family integration (Table 43.2).

Maternal abnormalities of the postpartum period not only interfere with the normal physiological involutional changes, but concurrent pain/stress may also delay or inhibit the important family growth. It is one of nursing's most important challenges to continue to support mothering and family bonding in the face of chronic or acute illness. This chapter discusses the common maternal complications of the postpartum period.

PUERPERAL INFECTION

Definition

Puerperal infection is defined as infection of the genital tract after delivery through the first 6 weeks postpartum. Puerperal morbidity is defined as "a temperature of 38.0° C (100.4° F) or higher, the temperature to occur on any 2 of the first 10 days postpartum, exclusive of the first 24 hours, and to be taken by mouth by a standard technique at least four times daily" (1). While not life-threatening in itself, infection may lead to serious conditions such as thrombophlebitis, pulmonary embolism, hemorrhage, which, in turn, may result in maternal death. Incidence of puerperal infection is 5% (2).

Etiology

The normal birth process opens many portals of entry to invading microorganisms, including (3):

1. Episiotomy incision
2. Clitoral, periurethral, labial, or perineal lacerations
3. Vaginal lacerations
4. Cervical lacerations
5. Site of placental attachment
6. Trauma to the bladder.

Infections of the Perineum, Vulva, and Vagina

These infections are common. Signs and symptoms include localized pain, dysuria, low grade fever, edema, episiotomy edges reddened or inflamed, and episiotomy dehiscence.

Diagnosis is made by visual inspection of the infected wound and by culture. Although painful, these infections rarely cause permanent harm to the mother. However, the pain may interfere with her ability to care for her infant, and to rest and recover from the birth. Conservative treatment consists of moist heat (e.g., sitz bath) four times a day for 20 minutes (2, p 874). Others recommend that any infected area be incised and drained immediately (1, p 727). If the episiotomy has dehisced, the wound is allowed to heal naturally. Perineal reconstructive surgery may be required at a later date. If systemic infection is evidenced by fever, appropriate systemic antibiotics should be ordered. Analgesics may be used, if pain is severe.

Table 43.1.

ANATOMY AND PHYSIOLOGY OF THE PUERPERIUM[a]

A. Uterus
   1. Size and position after delivery
      a) Fundus hard, globular, and contracted, usually felt at umbilicus if bladder is not distended
      b) Usual weight 1000 grams
   2. The first 2 days after delivery the uterus remains stationary, then descends into pelvic cavity approximately one centimeter a day. By the tenth day, fundus usually cannot be palpated.
   3. At the end of puerperium weight of uterus is usually 40 to 60 grams.
   4. Process of involution is accomplished by
      a) Autolysis of protein of uterine lining; waste products are excreted in urine causing albuminuria
      b) Two layers of decidua are involved in involution
         (1) one is cast off as lochia
         (2) underlying layer becomes endometrial lining; entire endometrium restored by third week
      c) Placental site—completely regenerated within 6 weeks
      d) Large uterine blood vessels become smaller
      e) Well-contracted uterus clamps down on maternal blood vessels and controls hemorrhage
      f) Uterus is a very tactile organ immediately after delivery and responds to massage by contracting
      g) Involution occurs more rapidly in primipara or breastfeeding mother because of increased muscle tone in primipara and release of oxytocin during breastfeeding
      h) Factors delaying involution
         1) Muliparity
         2) Conditions causing overdistention of uterus
            a) Polyhydramnios
            b) Large-sized baby
         3) Infection
         4) Retained placenta or membranes
         5) Hormonal deficiencies
B. Cervix
   1. Immediately after delivery cervix is soft, flabby and partly open
   2. After 1 week, muscle begins to regenerate and internal os closed
   3. Small lacerations may heal spontaneously
   4. External os remains somewhat wider than in the nonparous woman
C. Lochia—contains blood from placental site, decidua, cervical secretions, epithelial cells, and bacteria
   1. Lochia rubra—1–4 days; bright red; if persists longer than 2 weeks, may indicate retained placenta or membranes
   2. Lochia serosa—4–10 days; pinkish brown in color
   3. Lochia alba—beginning about day 10, persisting 1–2 weeks;
   4. Should not be excessive, scant (during rubra), or foul smelling
   5. Blood clots may be passed immediately after delivery
D. Perineum
   1. Vaginal distention decreases
   2. Lacerations, tears, sutures, swellings gradually heal within 3 weeks
E. Abdominal wall
   1. Soft and tone poor
   2. Striae fade to silvery white, but always remain
   3. Diastasis of the recti muscle (separation of abdominal muscle) may occur due to loss of muscle tone
F. Urinary tract
   1. Ureteral dilation disappears in 2 weeks
   2. Increased output (diuresis) 2nd to 5th day due to excretion of extracellular fluid
   3. Urine may contain increased amounts of acetone (CHO breakdown), nitrogen, and albumin (protein autolysis of uterus), and lactose from production of mammary glands
G. Breasts
   1. Soft immediately after delivery
   2. Prior to delivery high levels of estrogen and progesterone secreted by placenta inhibit anterior pituitary. After delivery of placenta, inhibition is removed, and lactogenic hormone (prolactin) is secreted, which stimulates production of milk
   3. 2 days postpartum, engorgement of breasts may occur
      a) Caused by venous and lymphatic secretion stasis, not by milk production, which does occur simultaneously
      b) In most severe type, breasts are swollen, hard, red, and painful
H. Blood
   1. Decrease in volume after blood loss in delivery
   2. Hemodilution of blood (hydremia) is decreased in first week postpartum through excretion by kidneys and from skin
   3. Moderate anemia may occur due to blood loss
   4. Leukocytosis occurs during labor and immediately afterwards

Table 43.1.

(Continued)

    5. Fibrinogen levels are elevated
    6. Immediately after delivery, pulse rate slows
I. Weight loss
    1. Usually 10-11 lbs immediately after delivery, 5 more lbs the following week
    2. Loss of weight due to
        a) Delivery of baby and placenta
        b) Hydremia reduction
        c) Excretion of retained fluid
        d) Uterine involution
J. Skin
    1. Mask of pregnancy gradually fades
    2. Linea nigra fades
    3. Striae fade but remain silvery white
    4. Primary areola remain darkened
K. Hormonal
    1. Nonlactating woman
        a) Ovulation within 3-6 weeks
        b) Menstruation within 5-8 weeks
    2. Lactating woman
        a) Return of menstrual cycle varies; may be delayed until weaning
        b) Because of variation, breastfeeding is not a reliable form of contraception

[a]Adapted from Friesner A, Raff B. *Maternity Nursing*, Medical Examination Publishing Company, 1977, pp 137-139.

Table 43.2.

FACTORS INFLUENCING ADJUSTMENT TO MATERNAL ROLE[a]

I.   FACTORS
A. New sense of responsibility may be influenced by
    1. Maturity of new parents
    2. Fear of failure to measure up to ideal parent role
    3. Lack of knowledge of newborn
    4. Financial worries
    5. Marital relationships
B. Attention diverted from mother to baby
C. Development of maternal instinct may be delayed
    1. Analgesia and anesthesia, which preclude experiencing the birth process
    2. Immediate separation of mother and child may be a factor in this delay
    3. In an out-of-wedlock mother guilt, shame, and feelings of hostility toward child may be present and may have an influence on the maternal-child relationship
II. STAGES IN ADJUSTMENT TO NEW ROLE
A. After the first hour after delivery, there is a need for sleep which if interrupted, causes the patient sleep hunger (after childbirth, mother may be so exhilarated, she may not be aware of her own exhaustion)
B. Classification of phase of puerperal restoration according to Reva Rubin[b]
    1. Taking-in phase
        a) Lasts 2–3 days
        b) Mother passive and dependent
        c) Expresses own needs rather that baby's
            (1) In order for mother to meet baby's needs, her own needs must be met
            (2) Needs physical care and attention to her emotional needs
        d) Verbalizes reactions to delivery so that experience can be integrated
        e) Symbiotic relationship ends and child should be recognized as an individual
    2. Taking-hold phase
        a) 3rd to 10th day
        b) The mother strives for independence and autonomy—she wants to care for herself and her child
        c) Initiates action
        d) Strong anxiety element
            1) Unsure of mothering role
            2) Unsure of ability to care for child physically
        e) Develop maternal responsibilities and feelings
        f) Mother may experience rapid and frequent mood swings; she may have ambivalent feelings about the baby
        g) Curious and interested in care of baby
        h) Stage of maximum readiness for new learning

Table 43.2.

(Continued)

C. Establishment of new role
    1. The birth of the baby may be viewed as a developmental crisis
        a) Roles are reassigned
        b) New responsibilities added
        c) Values reoriented
        d) Needs are met in new ways
    2. New parents may not have been adequately prepared for new difficulties in adjustment
        a) Mother's relationship to husband changes
        b) Father may feel isolation, economic pressure, dissatisfaction with paternal role
        c) Mother may feel fatigued, may have decrease in satisfaction due to confinement in home, loss of social contacts, burden of additional household duties, and guilt about not being a "better mother"
D. Maternal-child interaction
    1. Immediately after delivery, the mother may not have grasped the reality of the birth
    2. The mother will react to the infant according to her perception of its needs; this perception will be based on the child's
        a) Sex
        b) Activity level
        c) Appearance
        d) Size
    3. The first interaction between mother and infant is one of exploration and examination
    4. Initial behavior is usually concerned with ability to function in mothering role; a primipara in her first contact may show signs of tension
        a) Flushed face
        b) Excessive perspiration
        c) Body rigid
        d) May be anxious for baby to be taken away
    5. Maternal cues which indicate acceptance and claiming of infant as her own
        a) Assigns cultural values regarding sex
        b) Identifies resemblance of baby to family members
        c) Calls baby by name
        d) Touching and fondling child
E. Paternal-child interaction
    1. May exhibit fear and anxiety about handling baby
    2. May show positive reaction similar to mother
III. POSTPARTAL BLUES
A. Timing and severity of symptoms vary with the individual; usually occurs within a few days of delivery.
B. Manifestations
    1. Loss of energy
    2. Crying
    3. Anxiety and fear
    4. Insomnia
    5. Concerned about her body
    6. Misinterpretation of actions and words of others, primarily her husband
    7. Extreme control; insists everything is okay
C. Theories of etiology
    1. Stress of labor and birth
    2. Hormonal changes
        a) Absence of placental hormones
        b) Lactation begins
    3. Immaturity
    4. Family, social, and economic problems
    5. Lack of sleep
D. Mother may verbalize
    1. A sensation of feeling unprotected
    2. A feeling of emptiness; removal of baby from uterus may be compared to amputation

---

[a]Adapted from Freisner A. and Raff. B. *Maternity Nursing*, Medical Examination Publishing Company, 1977 pp 140-142.
[b]Rubin R. Puerperal change. *Nursing Outlook* 9:753-755, 1961.

Table 43.3.
LOCHIAL CONTENTS[a]

COLOR	DURATION	CONTENTS
Rubra (red)	1–4 days postpartum	Blood, placental and decidual debris
Serosa (pink)	4–10 days postpartum	Serous exudate, leukocytes, cervical mucus, shreds of degenerating decidua
Alba (creamy white)	10 days, persisting 1–2 weeks	Leukocytes, cellular debris

[a]Adapted from Buckley K, Kulb N: *Handbook of Maternal Child Nursing*. New York, John Wiley & Sons, 1983, p 450.

UTERINE INFECTIONS

Endometritis

In this condition the infection has not only affected the mucous membrane (endometrium) that lines the uterus but also may have spread into the smooth muscle (myometrium) (2). Signs and symptoms include tachycardia, abdominal pain, jagged temperature elevation between 101.4° F and 104.0° F, chills, and white blood cell count elevated beyond the physiological postpartum elevation. Lochia may be scant and foul smelling. (Normal lochia characteristics are listed in Table 43.3.)

Identification of the infecting microorganism is confirmed by lochial culture. At the same time, because signs and symptoms are similar, a urine culture should be obtained to rule out urinary tract infection. Prompt treatment usually resolves the infection. Treatment consists of bed rest, hydration, and appropriate antibiotics.

Pelvic Cellulitis/Parametritis

Pelvic cellulitis occurs when the infection that began as endometritis spreads to the parametrium (the extension of the subserous coat of the supracervical portion of the uterus laterally between the layers of the broad ligament) (4). Pelvic cellulitis is characterized by prolonged, sustained temperature elevations of 102–103° F, usually beginning around the 9th postpartum day. Abdominal pain may be either unilateral or bilateral. Vaginal examination reveals uterine tenderness (3, p 384).

Exudate from the infectious process may pool downward into the cul-de-sac of Douglas or upward above the inguinal ligament. The patient's reproductive system then becomes severely infected. Treatment consists of bed rest, hydration, and antibiotics. If abscess is present, it must be incised and drained. In some severe cases that do not respond to treatment, the uterus, tubes, and ovaries must be removed.

Initially, a broad spectrum antibiotic is prescribed. When lochia culture and sensitivity are available, the type of antibiotic can be adjusted. The route of administration is usually intravenous and progresses to oral once the patient is afebrile.

Generalized Peritonitis

Peritonitis occurs when the infection has spread into the peritoneal cavity and the peritoneum is inflamed. The infection may progress gradually or rapidly if a pelvic abscess ruptures.

Signs and symptoms include severe abdominal pain; high fever (105° F); weak, rapid pulse; and shallow breathing. Paralytic ileus may ensue, causing projectile vomiting and abdominal distension. Peritonitis may spread upward, causing inflammation of the pelvic veins. This, in turn, may lead to thromboembolic disease and pulmonary embolism. Peritonitis is a life-threatening condition, ending in renal failure, circulatory collapse, and death if untreated.

Treatment consists of bed rest, intravenous hydration, and appropriate antibiotic therapy. If paralytic ileus is present, a nasogastric tube should be inserted to relieve distension. If ileus is not resolved, abdominal surgery may be necessary to correct the obstruction and to drain the infectious exudate from the peritoneal cavity. Anticoagulants should be given if thromboembolic disease is present.

OTHER CAUSES OF PUERPERAL MORBIDITY

Other common nonreproductive tract causes of fever in the postpartum period are respiratory complications and urinary tract infection, including pyelonephritis (1, p 726). Diagnosis and treatment are the same as for the pregnant patient and are discussed in Chapters 15 and 16.

NURSING MANAGEMENT

Nursing care specific for patients with *perineal or uterine infection*:

☐ Apply ice packs to the perineum for the first 24 hours postpartum to reduce perineal edema and to promote healing.

☐ Provide moist heat to the perineum after the first 24 hours to increase circulation and to promote healing.

☐ Observe for perineal or rectal pain, bruising, and swelling that may indicate hematoma.

☐ Observe for redness, discharge, bruising, swelling, or poor approximation which may indicate infection.

☐ Teach the patient perineal care including:
— Importance of hand washing;
— applying perineal pad from front to back; and
— wiping from front to back.

☐ Assess lochia for color, amount, consistency, and odor; be aware that foul-smelling lochia is indicative of infection.

☐ Assess the uterine involutional process; be aware that delayed involution may indicate infection.

☐ Be aware that continuous seepage of blood in presence of a firm uterus may indicate cervical or vaginal lacerations.

☐ Teach the patient the normal amount of lochia to expect in different stages of the postpartum period and where to report abnormal findings.

☐ Assess vital signs frequently including temperature and pulse.

☐ If infection is suspected, assist with diagnostic procedures including blood and wound cultures.

☐ Administer antibiotics, as ordered.

☐ Explain all treatments and procedures to the patient and her significant others.

☐ Reassure the breastfeeding mother that she may continue nursing.

☐ Administer analgesics, as ordered.

☐ If surgery is required, explain the procedure and what treatments the patient can expect postsurgery.

Nursing diagnoses most frequently associated with *perineal or uterine infection* (see Section V):

☐ Knowledge deficit regarding etiology, disease process, treatment, and outcome.

☐ Pain.

☐ Potential altered parenting.

☐ Knowledge deficit regarding medication regimen.

THROMBOEMBOLIC DISEASE

Definition

A thrombus is a solid collection of blood components—primarily platelets and fibrin—that collects on the wall of a blood vessel (4, p 111). Because venous blood flow is slower than arterial blood flow, a thrombus is more likely to form in a vein. If the thrombus detaches from the vein, it is called an embolism. Venous thrombosis develops most often in the legs or pelvis.

The types of venous thrombosis are (1, p 731):

1. Thrombophlebitis—formation of a thrombus associated with inflammation.
2. Phlebothrombosis—formation of a thrombus without inflammatory response.

Clinically, the term *thrombophlebitis* is used to describe both entities and is used as such in this text. Today, overall incidence of thromboembolic disease in the postpartum patient is less than 1%, but this rises to 1–2% after cesarean section (2, p 874).

Etiology

Pregnancy and birth predispose a woman to development of thrombophlebitis. Specifically, the following factors are contributory (2, p 874):

1. Decreased venous return from the lower extremities and the pelvis because of both the pressure of the enlarging uterus and the relaxation of vessel smooth muscle from the effects of progesterone.
2. Increase in certain clotting factors that normally occur in pregnancy.
3. Trauma to pelvic blood vessels owing to pressure of the presenting part at birth.
4. Trauma to the mother's legs at birth due to improper positioning in the delivery table stirrups.
5. Venous stasis in the postpartum period from prolonged bed rest/failure to ambulate. Stasis is the most important predisposing factor to thrombus formation.

6. Postpartum peritonitis, which causes inflammation of pelvic blood vessels.

Thrombophlebitis may occur in superficial veins or deep veins of the legs and pelvis. Usually, it is associated with prolonged bed rest, trauma, or infection.

Superficial Thrombophlebitis

Superficial thromboembolic disease almost always involves the saphenous vein. It is characterized by a normal or slightly elevated temperature and pulse; leg pain; and warmth, tenderness, and redness at the site of the inflammation. The vein may be palpated as a hard, cord-like mass. The primary danger to the mother is development of a pulmonary embolism. Superficial thrombophlebitis rarely causes embolism. However, under no circumstances should the affected leg be massaged because it may dislodge a thrombus.

Management consists of bed rest, application of heat to the affected site, elastic stockings, and mild analgesia (3, p 387).

Deep Venous Thrombophlebitis

Deep thrombophlebitis may involve the venous system at any point from the foot to the iliofemoral region. Signs and symptoms can be abrupt in onset and dramatic in their intensity, including high fever with elevated pulse, severe leg pain, edema of the affected extremity, and decreased pedal or popliteal pulse (1, p 731). The patient may complain of calf pain when the Achilles tendon is stretched (Homans' sign). Not all cases present with the classic signs and symptoms, and symptomology is not necessarily correlated with extent of the disease. The patient runs a very real risk of pulmonary embolism. Diagnosis is confirmed by ultrasound or phlebography. Treatment consists of anticoagulation therapy and bed rest. The aim of therapy is to increase the clotting time two- to threefold. Intravenous or subcutaneous heparin is the drug of choice (2, p 875). Although any anticoagulation therapy requires special evaluation of bleeding tendencies, the postpartum patient is especially vulnerable to iatrogenic hemorrhage because of trauma during birth to the genitourinary tract. Protamine sulfate, the heparin antagonist, should be available at the bedside at all times. An-

tibiotics may be prescribed if infection is thought to be a causative factor and fever is present. In severe cases, when embolism is likely, surgical thrombectomy may be indicated. The acute phase usually subsides in 7–14 days with treatment. Low dose subcutaneous heparin or oral coumarin is continued. The patient is allowed to ambulate gradually. She should be fitted for elastic stockings, and these should be worn at all times when she is out of bed.

Because of its high molecular weight, heparin does not cross over into breast milk, and breastfeeding may be continued (5). Coumarin *does* cross over, and breastfeeding is contraindicated.

Anticoagulation therapy at low doses should continue for 6 weeks. Patients who have recurrent episodes of deep vein thrombophlebitis may be placed on permanent low dose maintenance levels of heparin or coumarin as a preventive measure.

Pulmonary Embolism

Pulmonary embolism causes partial or complete obstruction of arterial flow to the distal lung. Gas exchange is inadequate, and hypoxia occurs. If uncorrected, pulmonary hypertension and acute right heart failure may ensue (6). Symptoms vary with massive embolism; the patient obviously is in a life-threatening condition, presenting with shock, cyanosis, cerebral ischemia, and crushing substernal pain. However, symptoms may be less severe with some degree of sharp chest pain, tachycardia, tachypnea, dyspnea, air hunger, and hemoptysis (3, p 387).

Pulmonary embolism may be misdiagnosed or missed altogether. Air hunger and cerebral ischemia may cause the patient to be apprehensive and anxious. Thus, symptoms of pulmonary embolism have been attributed to psychiatric disturbances ("anxiety attack") rather than to hypoxia. Because embolism is potentially fatal, *any* symptoms need to be seriously evaluated (1, p 737). Pulmonary angiogram or lung scan will usually reveal clots or obstruction. However, they are not always conclusive. Even if diagnosis cannot be confirmed, anticoagulation therapy should be instituted. Relief of symptoms will often be rapid and complete. If anticoagulation therapy is unsuccessful, surgical removal of embolus may be necessary. Oxygen should be given. Analgesics must be used carefully to reduce pain but not to depress respiration.

NURSING MANAGEMENT

Nursing care specific for patients with
thromboembolism:

☐ During the postpartum period, ENCOURAGE EARLY AND FREQUENT AMBULATION TO PREVENT VENOUS STASIS.

☐ Assess frequently for signs of thrombophlebitis including redness, pain, heat, positive Homan's sign, increased calf circumference, elevated pulse, spiking fever, or chills. Report any signs immediately.

If thromboembolic disease is diagnosed:

☐ DO NOT WASH OR MASSAGE AFFECTED EXTREMITY.

☐ Keep the patient on complete bed rest, if ordered, and apply Ace bandages or elastic stockings, whenever she is out of bed.

☐ Administer anticoagulation therapy, as ordered, and observe for signs of heparin overdose including increased uterine bleeding, bleeding from intravenous line, etc.

☐ Check breath sounds every 4 hours, being alert for rales signaling pulmonary embolism.

☐ Assist the patient to turn, cough, and deep breathe every 4 hours.

☐ Check vital signs every 4 hours (avoid rectal temperature as this may precipitate rectal/hemorrhoidal bleeding).

☐ Check circulation of affected extremity every 4 hours.

☐ Measure calf circumference daily.

☐ Explain diagnostic procedures including risks and benefits and findings.

☐ Provide emotional support and encourage the patient to verbalize fears.

☐ Position the patient comfortably taking care to avoid venous constriction. Utilize a bed cradle to keep bedclothes off the affected extremity.

☐ If appropriate, encourage the mother to continue breastfeeding and reassure her that heparin is not excreted in the breast milk.

☐ Administer analgesics, as ordered.

☐ Facilitate maternal-infant bonding.

☐ Teach the patient measures that can prevent recurrence including:
  — Aerobic exercise;
  — Smoking cessation; and

  — Avoidance of constrictive clothing, including garters, girdles, knee-highs, or ankle stockings with elastic bands.

☐ Ensure that the patient understands her medications, the dosage, time of administration, purpose, and side effects.

☐ Teach the patient the anticoagulation precautions, if appropriate, including:
  — Avoiding vigorous nose blowing or tooth brushing;
  — Avoiding razors or other sharp instruments;
  — Refraining from contact sports;
  — Wearing shoes and slippers at all times; and
  — WEARING A MEDICAL ALERT BAND WITH NAME OF MEDICATION.

☐ Teach the patient to avoid over-the-counter drugs as these may potentiate the effects of anticoagulation therapy (e.g., those with salicylates).

☐ Teach her the symptoms to report to the physician including hematuria, vomiting, fever, pain/swelling in joints, epistaxis, bleeding gums, easy bruising, increased menstrual flow, abdominal pain, chest pain, or shortness of breath.

☐ Refer to visiting nurse service to ensure compliance with treatment regimen and to assess mother's physical ability to assume care of the child as well as the emotional adjustment to motherhood after a serious illness.

Nursing diagnoses most frequently associated
with *thromboembolic disease* (see Section V):

☐ Anticipatory grieving related to actual/perceived threat to self.

☐ Knowledge deficit regarding etiology, disease process, treatment, and outcome.

☐ Altered maternal tissue perfusion.

☐ Pain.

☐ Impaired gas exchange.

☐ Potential altered parenting.

☐ Knowledge deficit regarding medication regimen.

☐ Anxiety/fear.

DELAYED POSTPARTUM HEMORRHAGE

Definition

Delayed postpartum hemorrhage is the loss of 500 ml of blood from the uterus, cervix, vagina, or vulva occurring 24 hours after delivery until 6 weeks postpartum. Most delayed hemorrhages occur within the fourth to the ninth day postpartum. Overall incidence is 1% (2, p 495).

Etiology

Causes of delayed uterine postpartum hemorrhage are related to conditions that impede the involutional process and include (2, p 495):

1. Retained placental fragments
2. Intrauterine infection
3. Uterine submucosal myomas
4. Undiagnosed incomplete uterine inversion
5. Use of exogenous estrogens to suppress lactation (which may result in significant blood loss during the first postpartum menstrual period)

The most common causes of delayed hemorrhage are detachment of thrombi at the placental site leading to reopening of the vascular sinuses and subinvolution (7). Undiagnosed lacerations of the cervix, vagina, or vulva may result occasionally in delayed blood loss. Injury to blood vessels of the vagina or vulva without laceration of the superficial tissue causes bleeding into the connective tissue following the fascial planes, resulting in a hematoma. Infection may cause dehiscence and bleeding of the episiotomy site (7).

Signs and Symptoms

Profuse bleeding of the genital tract may lead to shock. Hematoma formation causes intense localized pain in the perineal or rectal area, and the area, if visible, is bluish and swollen.

Diagnosis

A careful, thorough pelvic examination will aid in determining the causative factors. Lacerations can be visualized. Palpation will reveal subinvolution, hematoma, fibroids, or incomplete uterine inversion. Ultrasound may be used to confirm presence of placental fragments or fibroids (7).

Maternal Outcome

Although hemorrhage may be severe, it is rarely fatal. Blood loss may result in anemia. If transfusion is required, the mother may incur the risk of infection with hepatitis B and AIDS, as well as transfusion reaction. Severe hemorrhage or shock occurring in close proximity to birth may leave the mother emotionally drained and physically exhausted. She may be unable to provide physical care for the infant, and bonding may be delayed.

Medical Management

Hospitalization is mandatory. Volume expanders and/or blood are used to replace blood loss, as needed. The specific causative factor is identified. If bleeding is uterine in origin, as is most likely, oxytoxics or prostaglandins may be used to facilitate uterine contractions. Lochial cultures should be taken and appropriate antibiotics given to control infection. If bleeding persists or if placental fragments are seen on ultrasound, curettage is performed carefully. Risks of perforation of a soft, "boggy" uterus and the potential for future development of adhesions must be weighed against the risk of continued blood loss. Curettage often does not reveal any histologic evidence of placental fragments, possibly because the fragments were evacuated during the hemorrhage. If bleeding continues after curettage and administration of oxytoxics or prostaglandins, hysterectomy may be necessary.

Degenerating submucosal uterine fibroids usually require hysterectomy to control hemorrhage. If incomplete uterine inversion is diagnosed, the uterus can be replaced manually. The uterus should be replaced under sterile conditions in an operating room with anesthesia. If manual replacement is not possible, the cervix may be incised to facilitate replacement (7, p 196).

If lacerations are seen, they should be repaired. Hematomas are evacuated, the injured blood vessels ligated, and the site of the hematoma sutured to eliminate dead space. To exert pressure on the blood vessels, the vagina may be packed with sterile gauze dressing. Vaginal packing is removed after 12 hours (7, p 202).

If the episiotomy is infected and has dehisced, appropriate antibiotics are given and the wound is allowed to heal naturally. Reconstruction of the perineum may be attempted after healing is complete and infection is eliminated.

NURSING MANAGEMENT

Nursing care specific for patients with
delayed postpartum hemorrhage:
- [ ] Monitor uterine size, consistency, placement, amount of lochia, in order to assess potential of delayed uterine bleeding.
- [ ] During the postpartum in-hospital stay, teach the mother to self-massage uterus and to report heavy bleeding.
- [ ] At discharge, give an emergency telephone number where she can call at any hour.

If the patient is actively bleeding:
- [ ] Stay with the patient.
- [ ] Massage the relaxed, boggy uterus—taking care to guard it with the other hand in order to prevent uterine inversion.
- [ ] Administer oxygen at 10–12 liters/minute, if ordered.
- [ ] Check vital signs every 15 minutes until stable; then as ordered.
- [ ] Measure intake and output.
- [ ] Save and weigh pads and linens to estimate blood loss.
- [ ] Keep the patient warm.
- [ ] Maintain patent IV; administer blood as ordered.

- [ ] Assist with diagnostic procedures and treatments.
- [ ] Briefly and simply explain procedures and plans of care.

At hospital discharge:
- [ ] Ensure that the patient is given a prescription for iron therapy and counseling regarding high dietary iron intake, if hematocrit/hemoglobin is decreased.
- [ ] Teach the patient medication regimen for oxytoxics or antibiotics, if appropriate.
- [ ] Encourage the patient to seek medical care if heavy bleeding, abdominal pain, or fever recurs.

Nursing diagnoses most frequently associated with *delayed postpartum hemorrhage* (see Section V):
- [ ] Knowledge deficit regarding etiology, disease process, treatment, and outcome.
- [ ] Fluid volume deficit.
- [ ] Altered maternal tissue perfusion.
- [ ] Pain.
- [ ] Potential altered parenting.
- [ ] Anxiety/fear.
- [ ] Impaired tissue integrity.

SUBINVOLUTION

Subinvolution is the condition in which the normal process of retrograde postpartum uterine changes are arrested or delayed. Causes of subinvolution include retained placental fragments, submucosal fibroids, and/or infection (1, p 737). Early postpartum subinvolution is characterized by a soft, "boggy" uterus that remains at the same height rather than gradually decreasing. Lochia is profuse, reddish brown. Signs and symptoms later in the puerperium include prolonged lochial flow, followed by leukorrhea and heavy, irregular bleeding. Diagnosis is by bimanual vaginal examination

that reveals a uterus that is larger and softer than normal.

Infection is diagnosed by a positive lochial culture and the presence of adnexal tenderness and pain along with pain associated with cervical movement during the postpartum pelvic examination.

Subinvolution usually is treated easily and maternal outcome is not in jeopardy. Treatment consists of methylergonovine (Methergine) or ergonovine (Ergotrate) 0.2 mg every 3–4 hours for 48–96 hours and reevaluation in 2 weeks. (Both of these are contraindicated if the patient is hypertensive.) If infection is diagnosed, appropriate antibiotic therapy is instituted. In rare cases, placental fragments may need to be evacuated surgically by D&C.

NURSING MANAGEMENT

Nursing care specific for patients with
subinvolution:
- [ ] During the postpartum in hospital stay, teach the mother signs and symptoms of uterine infection and hemorrhage, including:
  - Fever/chills;

  - Abdominal pain;
  - Foul-smelling lochia;
  - Malaise; and
  - Passage of clots.
- [ ] Encourage her to return for treatment if they occur.

NURSING MANAGEMENT

☐ If subinvolution is diagnosed, inform the patient of the diagnosis, suspected etiology, and plan for treatment.

☐ Inform the mother of regime of Ergotrate therapy including side effects such as nausea and uncomfortable uterine contractions.

☐ If antibiotic therapy is initiated, teach the patient the regime for use and potential side effects.

☐ Ensure that the patient has a follow-up gynecological appointment in 2 weeks after treatment is begun.

☐ Encourage her to return immediately if symptoms worsen.

If hospitalization is necessary:

☐ Explain the probable treatment and procedures.

☐ Ensure that child care is provided for the infant and older siblings.

☐ If appropriate, teach the patient how to use the breast pump in order to maintain lactation.

Nursing diagnoses most frequently associated with *subinvolution* (see Section V):

☐ Knowledge deficit regarding etiology, disease process, treatment, and outcome.

☐ Pain.

☐ Potential altered parenting.

☐ Knowledge deficit regarding medication regimen.

MASTITIS

Inflammation of the breast can be either sporadic or epidemic. Epidemic mastitis occurs within 2 weeks after delivery, involves glandular tissue, and is caused by nosocomial and virulent staphylococcus infection of the breastfeeding infant in the hospital nursery. It is becoming rare owing to rooming-in policy as well as early discharge, which removes the infant from sources of iatrogenic infection. The reader is referred to medical texts for further discussion of this cause of mastitis (8).

Sporadic inflammation is not an uncommon occurrence among breastfeeding mothers. It involves interlobular tissue (not the lactiferous apparatus) and usually occurs between 2–4 weeks postpartum. It may be associated with milk stasis or a cracked nipple. If staphylococci are present, they tend to be nonvirulent (2, p 878).

Signs and symptoms of sporadic mastitis include malaise, anorexia, headache, chills, and fever. The affected area of the breast is red, swollen, warm to the touch, and painful.

Before treatment milk should be expressed and cultured. However, since the sporadic inflammation is in the interlobular tissue, the culture probably will be negative. Management consists of appropriate antibiotic therapy. Most cases of mastitis resolve with use of penicillin or erythromycin. Strains of staphylococcus resistant to these drugs require alternate therapy such as cloxacillin, dicloxacillin, or cephalosporins. Mild analgesics may be prescribed. The mother should be encouraged to wear a well-fitting nursing brassiere and to nurse frequently to prevent stasis (9).

If the infection is caught early, signs and symptoms may resolve in 48 hours. However, the infection may progress to abscess in 5–10% of cases. The abscess should be incised and drained (1, p 740).

Breastfeeding may be continued during the course of treatment. In fact, breastfeeding has been shown to enhance healing. However, once an abscess is formed, breastfeeding from the affected side should be discontinued. The infant may continue to nurse on the unaffected breast. In order to prevent stasis, milk should be expressed or pumped from the affected breast. When the abscess is drained, healing is rapid, and breastfeeding may be resumed.

NURSING MANAGEMENT

Nursing care specific for patients with *mastitis*:

☐ Teach all breastfeeding mothers to avoid cracked nipples by:
  — Avoiding drying agents like soap or alcohol on the nipples;

  — Using anhydrous lanolin or vitamin E on the nipples after each nursing;
  — Proper nursing position;
  — Exposing the nipples to air and sunlight;
  — Washing nipples with clear water after nursing to prevent milk build up;

NURSING MANAGEMENT

- — Ensuring that the infant grasps the entire areola for nursing, not just the nipple;
- — Alternating nursing positions in order to change the points of maximum sucking pressure; and
- — Removing baby from the breast by inserting the finger at the side of the infant's mouth to release suction.
- ☐ Teach all breastfeeding mothers techniques to avoid milk stasis including:
  - — FREQUENT NURSING, avoiding arbitrary time limits;
  - — Wearing a well-fitting brassiere;
  - — Using warm cloths or taking a shower to relieve discomfort;
  - — Expressing milk to soften areola before nursing;
  - — Massaging firm areas of the breast while nursing; and
  - — Expressing any unused milk after nursing.
- ☐ Teach the mother to report any signs of mastitis including fever or breast redness or soreness.
- ☐ If the mother develops mastitis, reassure her about her ability to continue nursing.
- ☐ Stress the importance of good nutrition with a diet high in protein and vitamin C.

- ☐ Stress the importance of rest and adequate fluid intake.
- ☐ Encourage her to nurse frequently to prevent milk stasis.
- ☐ Observe her nursing interaction and reinforce proper techniques and correct any deficits.
- ☐ If antibiotics are prescribed, teach the mother the regimen for use, and possible side effects.
- ☐ If surgery is necessary, explain the procedure, risks, and benefits of the procedure.
- ☐ Teach the patient how to express milk manually from the affected breast or use a breast pump.
- ☐ If appropriate, encourage the patient to continue nursing on the unaffected breast.
- ☐ If the mother wishes, teach her how to wean the infant *gradually* (e.g., give up one feeding every week, beginning with the one when the breasts are the least full).

Nursing diagnoses most frequently associated with *mastitis*:
- ☐ Potential altered parenting.
- ☐ Pain.
- ☐ Anxiety/fear.
- ☐ Knowledge deficit regarding medication regimen.

SHEEHAN'S SYNDROME

Massive postpartum hemorrhage is postulated to disrupt circulation to the pituitary gland, causing varying degrees of ischemia and necrosis. This is known as Sheehan's syndrome. With as little as 10% of the gland, some degree of pituitary function can be maintained (2, p 494). Signs and symptoms of insufficient functioning include the following:

1. Lethargy
2. Polydipsia, polyphagia
3. Increased incidence of infection
4. Breast involution
5. Failure to lactate
6. Hypersensitivity to cold
7. Involution of the uterus
8. Atrophy of the external genitalia
9. Amenorrhea
10. Loss of body hair
11. Other signs of adrenal insufficiency, hypothyroidism, and diabetes insipidus

With severe pituitary necrosis, death will result. Those who survive have specific increased risk of infection from decreased or fluctuating levels of glucocorticoids (6, p 744). Medical management consists of replacement of the hormones secreted by the organs regulated by the pituitary. Depending on existing deficiencies, treatment may include vasopressin, thyroid hormones, adrenocorticotropin (ACTH), and estrogen. These hormones will need to be replaced for the rest of the patient's life (6, p 744).

TOXIC SHOCK SYNDROME

Toxic shock syndrome is an acute septic illness that affects major organs and is life-threatening. Although the exact etiology is unknown, a staphylococcus endotoxin is postulated to be the causative factor. Signs and symptoms include fever, headache, mental confusion, scarlatiniform rash, nausea, vomiting, diarrhea, oliguria, renal failure, hepatic failure, and disseminated intravascular coagulation. Circulatory collapse and death may ensue. While primarily a disease associated with menstruating women using tampons, it recently has been documented to occur in the postpartum period (1, p 719). Maternal outcome is in jeopardy. Because of the recent appearance of the syndrome, the ideal treatment has yet to be found. Currently, therapy consists of parenteral administration of β-lactamase-resistant antibiotics, fluid replacement, and other life-support measures.

A patient who has toxic shock syndrome and survives is statistically likely to develop the syndrome again.

REFERENCES

1. Pritchard J, et al.: *Williams Obstetrics*, ed 17. Norwalk, CT, Appleton-Century-Crofts, 1983, p 719.

2. Oxorn H: *Human Labor and Birth*, ed 5. Norwalk, CT, Appleton-Century-Crofts, 1986, p 872.

3. Varney H: *Nurse-Midwifery*. London, Blackwell Scientific Publications, 1980, p 267.

4. Miller B, Keane C: *Encyclopedia and Dictionary of Medical Nursing and Allied Health*, ed 3. Philadelphia, WB Saunders, 1983, p 836.

5. Briggs G, et al: *Drugs in Pregnancy and Lactation*. London, Williams & Wilkins, 1983, p 166.

6. Mahoney EA, Flynn JP (eds): *Handbook of Medical-Surgical Nursing*. New York, John Wiley and Sons, 1983, p 345.

7. Friedman E: *Obstetrical Decision Making*. St. Louis, Mosby, 1982, p 202.

8. Gibbard G: Sporadic and epidemic puerperal breast infection. *Am J Obstet Gynecol*. 65:1038, 1953.

9. Marshall B, et al.: Sporadic puerperal mastitis: an infection that need not interrupt lactation. *Am J Obstet Gynecol* 233:1377–1379, 1975.

Chapter 44
Nursing Management of the Sick Mother and/or Newborn during Transfer to Tertiary Care Center

Barbara J. Greitzer, R.N.C., P.N.P., M.S.

INTRODUCTION

Maternal and neonatal transport are vital components of a health care delivery system that offers alternative facilities for labor and delivery. It maintains the benefits of high technology maternity care and services in this age of cost containment. A carefully developed plan including trained personnel and appropriate equipment is essential for safe transport of mother or baby. It is the responsibility of each practitioner who cares for women and their newborn children to understand the principles of transport and their role in the process.

DEFINITION

Transport is the movement of a patient or patients from one health care facility to another, accompanied by health care personnel. The patient may be a pregnant woman, a newborn infant, or a mother and child. The types of health care facilities can vary widely. Primary institutions are community hospitals that are not prepared to care for a critically ill mother or infant. Physicians' offices, free-standing emergency centers, clinics, and maternity centers may be considered primary health care deliverers. Secondary health facilities are community hospitals and medical centers that have the necessary facilities and personnel to care for the majority of maternal and neonatal patients. The most highly specialized services are reserved for tertiary facilities.

TRANSPORT TEAM

The personnel required for a maternal or infant transport varies with each situation and in different regions of the country. Types of personnel that may be incorporated into the team include physicians, nurse-practitioners, midwives, nurses, respiratory therapists, nursing assistants, emergency medical technicians, ambulance drivers, and pilots. The individuals participating in the transport should be selected in advance and educated specifically for the transport process (1). It is essential that the team have experience working together, and it is imperative that the collective knowledge of the team include the expertise to provide supportive care for the wide variety of emergency conditions that may occur in transit and the ability to utilize and/or make minor repairs on equipment. One or more members of the patient's family may accompany the patient to provide emotional support during transport.

EQUIPMENT

All life support equipment utilized in transports must be battery operated. The battery life must exceed the length of the transport if the vehicle is not equipped with electrical outlets. If electrical power is available, it is necessary to assure that the equipment is compatible with the electric source. The power supplied may be 110 volt AC if the ambulance is equipped with a generator, or a 12–24 volt DC supply may be available from the batteries. However, battery power still is essential for transport from hospital unit to ambulance or aircraft and vice versa (phases II and IV—see Fig. 44.1).

Oxygen supply and suction capabilities also are important factors to consider in transit. Small "E" size oxygen or air cylinders at average flow rates last for approximately 20 minutes. Two small "E" tanks most likely will be sufficient for maternal transports. In neonatal transports two small tanks may not be sufficient. If the ambulance is equipped with its own oxygen source, the portable supply can be reserved for elevators and hallways (phases II and IV, see Fig. 44.1). Equipment for mixing air and oxygen needs to be of small size, easily secured, and operational at low flow rates. Venturi suction units or conventional suction units may be available; however, it is always prudent to have DeLee suction available, with a variety of catheter sizes, as well as a bulb syringe.

Mechanical ventilators are available as part of the transport isolette or as free-standing battery-operated units that can be anchored to the isolette (employing Velcro straps).

VEHICLES

The selection of a transport vehicle requires careful consideration of many factors. These include availability, distance to be traveled, condition of patient, weather, and geography. The least expensive and usually safest choice is an ambulance. Helicopters offer additional speed; however, they are expensive, noisy, and vibrate a great deal. This can make cardiorespiratory monitoring extremely difficult and jar respiratory or intravenous tubing loose. Fixed winged aircraft are quieter and vibrate less than helicopters. They also allow for more flexibility and ease in handling emergency situations. However, ground transportation is necessary between hospitals and airports (2).

In any vehicle chosen the essential features are a method to lift the incubator or stretcher onto the vehicle (incubators can weight 500 pounds when fully equipped), a method for securing the incubator or stretcher on board, seats with seatbelts for transport personnel (close enough to be able to observe the patient), and a communication system between the driver or pilot and the transport team. For long distance transports large "H" tanks of compressed air and oxygen and electrical outlets are necessary to sustain life support equipment.

COMMUNICATIONS

Communication is a vital component at each stage of the transport process. The phone number at which the transport team can be accessed needs to be posted clearly at all referring agencies. The dispatcher needs experience in eliciting the appropriate information in order to direct appropriate personnel and equipment to the referring center. The referring practitioner needs to be prepared with accurate historical and assessment data in order to expedite care at the perinatal institution. The perinatal institution needs to be informed of the estimated time of arrival.

Upon arrival of the transport team at the referral center, a complete report, including historical, physical, and laboratory information, is obtained from the primary caretakers. The team will need an introduction to the patient's family and the patient. Written informed consent will be obtained at this point. If the patient or family has been counseled already, unnecessary delays can be avoided.

In-transit communications between team members and between the team and the receiving institution enhance the quality of care delivered to the patient. The ambulance driver needs information on when to stop and start the vehicle and on the condition of the patient.

At the receiving institution the historical, physical, and laboratory data and current status information must be conveyed. All specimens and documentation must also be exchanged. A sample form for documenting infant status during transport is given in Figure 44.2.

Follow-up communications between referral practitioners and receiving physicians improve the interpersonal relationships while providing feedback on the quality of initial interventions. If the transport personnel are a separate group of people, they, too, need to have access to follow-up information.

MATERNAL TRANSPORT

Ideally, when it becomes evident that a mother or her fetus is in jeopardy, all efforts should be made to transport the mother prior to delivery.

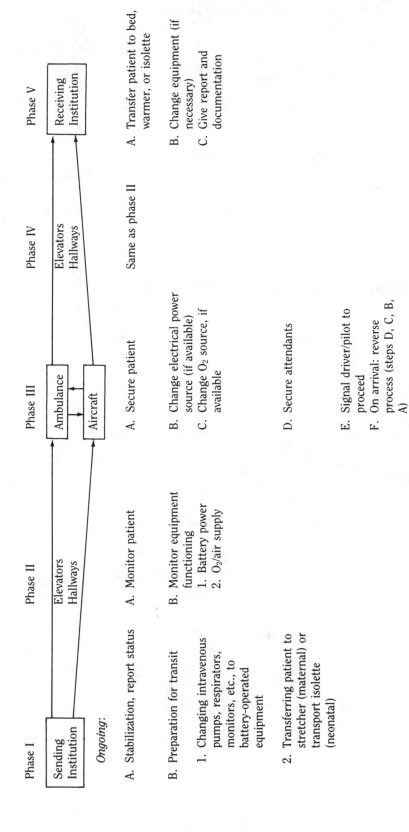

Figure 44.1. Phases of transport.

RECORD OF INFANT'S TRANSPORT

INFANT'S NAME		BIRTH WEIGHT	DATE OF BIRTH

TRANSPORTED	FROM	TO	DATE	TIME ☐ AM ☐ PM

OBSERVATIONS AT HOSPITAL/HOME PRIOR TO TRANSFER

FORM FOR INFANT TRANSPORT SERVICE. OBSTETRIC RECORD AND NEWBORN RECORD COMPLETED. IF NO. GIVE REASON:

☐ YES ☐ NO

FOOT PRINTS RECEIVED ☐ YES ☐ NO	OXYGEN CONCENTRATION %

TEMPERATURE INFANT	° ☐ RECTAL ° ☐ AXILLA	INCUBATOR

5CC MOTHER'S CLOTTED BLOOD RECEIVED ☐ YES ☐ NO	IDENTIFICATION CHECKED WITH (NAME)

BABY SHOWN TO MOTHER ☐ YES ☐ NO IF NO WHY?	FORM MNB 7 GIVEN TO (NAME)

CONDITION OF INFANT

OBSERVATIONS AND CARE OF INFANT DURING TRANSIT

OXYGEN ADMINISTERED AT_____ %

INCUBATOR TEMPERATURE _____ °

OBSERVATIONS AT RECEIVING HOSPITAL

CONDITION OF INFANT ON ARRIVAL	TIME OF ARRIVAL ☐ AM ☐ PM

INFANT IDENTIFIED AND RECEIVED BY (NAME)

5CC MOTHER'S CLOTTED BLOOD LEFT WITH (NAME)

INFANT TRANSPORT SERVICE FORMS AND FOOTPRINTS LEFT WITH: (NAME)

TEMPERATURE INFANT	° ☐ RECTAL ° ☐ AXILLA	INCUBATOR	°	OXYGEN CONCENTRATION %

DURATION OF TRANSPORT

HOSP. OF BIRTH: DEPARTURE TIME:___ AM PM TEMP. OF INCUBATOR: _____ °	OXYGEN ADMINISTERED DURING TRANSPORT ☐ YES ☐ NO
PREMATURE CENTER: ARIVAL TIME:___ AM PM TEMP. OF INCUBATOR: _____ °	IF YES, CONCENTRATION _____ DURATION _____

SIGNATURE OF TRANSPORT NURSE (IF OTHER, SIGN NAME AND SPECIFY TITLE)

21KB 10 68-10M-512088 (71)

BUREAU OF MATERNITY SERVICES AND FAMILY PLANNING
DEPARTMENT OF HEALTH—THE CITY OF NEW YORK

Figure 44.2. Sample form for documenting infant status.

Table 44.1.

INDICATIONS FOR MATERNAL TRANSPORT[a]

Premature labor
Premature rupture of membranes
Pregnancy-induced hypertension
Third trimester hemorrhage
Complicated multiple births
Poorly controlled or insulin-dependent diabetes mellitus
Severe intrauterine growth retardation
Rh isoimmunization
Infection
Severe organic heart disease
Renal disease
Drug overdose
Trauma
Acute abdomen requiring surgical intervention
Pulmonary embolus
Other significant maternal disease

[a]Adapted from American Academy of Pediatrics, American College of Obstetrics and Gynecology: *Guidelines for Perinatal Care*, 2nd ed. Washington, DC: ACOG, 1988:210-212.

Table 44.2.

CONDITIONS THAT MAY WARRANT NEONATAL TRANSPORT[a]

Gestation less than 34 weeks
Weight less that 2000 g
Neonatal infection or meningitis
Respiratory distress and metabolic acidosis (persisting after 2 hours of age)
Neonatal blood loss
Hypoglycemia
Hemolytic disease of the newborn
Neonates of mothers taking hazardous drugs
Infants of diabetic mothers
Neonatal seizures
Congenital malformation (requiring surgical intervention or observation)
Shock or asphyxia (persisting beyond 2 hours)
Neonatal cardiac disorders (with persisting cyanosis)
Any neonatal condition requiring ventilatory support for more than 1 hour
Neonates needing more than routine observation or care

[a]Adapted from American Academy of Pediatrics, American College of Obstetrics and Gynecology: *Guidelines for Perinatal Care*, 2nd ed. Washington, DC: ACOG, 1988:210-212.

In the preparation phase the transport team should be alerted to be on standby status and should be given an estimated time of departure. This will avoid any unnecessary delays. Prior to the onset of labor, maternal transport can be accomplished with traditional ambulance equipment with the attendance of a practitioner skilled in obstetrics. Once labor has been initiated, it becomes necessary to have available equipment for fetal surveillance and neonatal resuscitation as well as attendants skilled in delivery and resuscitation. If cervical dilation has exceeded 4 cm, delivery and stabilization of both the mother and infant should precede transport to prevent delivery on route (1). Table 44.1 lists indications for maternal transport to a tertiary care facility.

Should an emergency situation develop in transit, it is optimal for the vehicle to stop. Once the patient is stabilized, traveling can resume. In aircraft transports where this is not possible, every effort should be made to avoid this situation.

Brown reported that 88% of all maternal-fetal transports were carried out because of premature labor or premature rupture of membranes (3). In the management of premature labor in transport, intramuscular ritodrine hydrochloride might be prescribed. Although the FDA has not approved this route of administration of ritodrine, there is sufficient medical literature to support its use in emergency situations (3). Intramuscular therapy will obviate the necessity of intravenous administration, which is often difficult to maintain at a constant rate in transit. Ritodrine may be administered 10

mg intramuscularly and repeated every 2 hours as needed. Upon arrival at the tertiary center, intravenous ritodrine may be instituted (4).

Ensuring the safety in transit of a patient who has had premature rupture of membranes requires excellent communication between the practitioner and transport team. Assessment information such as cervical dilation, presence or absence of labor, presentation, and station will assist the transport team or dispatcher in deciding the appropriate personnel needed in this instance. Vaginal fluid obtained from the vaginal pool should be sent along with the mother for future L:S ratio and α-phosphatidylglycerol determination. If the patient is contracting, tocolytic agents may be employed to arrest labor during transit (4, p 7).

The mother will need intense support during the transport. Not only will she be anxious or fearful regarding the need for transfer and the outcome for herself and her infant, but also the transfer itself in a fast-moving vehicle or helicopter can be frightening and uncomfortable. She should be appraised of tests performed and equipment used. If the mother is in labor, breathing/relaxation techniques should be reinforced. The mother should be positioned with a roll under her right hip in order to displace the uterus off the vena cava.

NEONATAL TRANSPORT

If facilities do not exist in an institution for the care of a compromised newborn, the transport team should be activated.

Prior to transport, attention should be given to the following major needs of the neonate:

1. Temperature maintenance
2. Prevention of hypoglycemia
3. Oxygenation

It is advisable to empty the stomach to prevent aspiration during transport. Leads for fetal heart rate monitoring should be in place before putting the infant into the transport isolette. It is ideal if the infant can be photographed and a picture given to the parents prior to transport (5).

As in maternal transport, it is necessary to stabilize the infant prior to placing him or her into a transport incubator. Table 44.2 lists possible indications for neonatal transport.

The most frequent causes for neonatal transport are diseases of the respiratory tract. There are many conditions in the neonate that present with respiratory distress. Differentiating between them is not always feasible prior to transport, and often it is not necessary. Managing a baby requiring respiratory support in transport is one of the most difficult tasks the transport team is asked to do (6).

Maintaining oxygenation is of critical importance. Blood gas levels should be monitored and oxygen therapy altered accordingly. If this is not possible, oxygen should be administered at a rate just sufficient to prevent cyanosis. Assisted ventilation should be used as necessary. It is possible to maintain adequate oxygenation of the newborn via bag and mask for several hours, if necessary (5). All tubings need to be secured firmly to avoid extubation or loss of oxygen in transit. Intravenous and umbilical lines and chest tubes (if present) need to be maintained and the patient secured. These tasks must be accomplished with minimal stress on the neonate in order to maintain oxygenation.

Return transports—returning the patient to the original or local hospital after the initial problems requiring transport have been resolved—should be encouraged (6, p 27, 7). Return transports can enable the parents to visit more frequently during the convalescent stage of the infant's hospitalization. An important task for the parents at this time is to become involved increasingly in the care of their infant. This prepares them for the eventual discharge of their infant as well as promoting parent-infant bonding. The health care system also benefits from return transports by increasing the resources at the tertiary facility available to care for acute patients and by promoting the liaison between level I and II centers and the level III tertiary facility.

NURSING MANAGEMENT

Nursing care specific for a sick patient experiencing *transfer to a tertiary care center***:**

☐ Identify conditions requiring transport and facilitate the process.

☐ Determine the equipment/personnel required for transport.

☐ Ensure fully charged battery pack.

☐ Obtain written informed consent for transport.

☐ Recognize the potential need for medications (e.g., ritodrine) before/during transport.

☐ Ensure that appropriate information (e.g., diagnostic results/samples, chart, report, placenta if possible) is transported with patient.

☐ Secure patient/neonate for high speed transport (e.g., secure tubes, lines, stretcher,

isolette inside vehicle; secure patient/neonate to stretcher/isolette).

☐ Ensure that all equipment is returned to the proper institution/office/service.

☐ Educate patient/partner/family regarding the following:
  — Condition (e.g., treatment, prognosis); and
  — Rationale for transport.

☐ Assist patient/partner to inform family members of transport (e.g., why, where, when).

Nursing diagnoses most frequently associated with *transfer of sick mother/ newborn to tertiary care center* **(see Section V):**

☐ Anxiety/fear.

☐ Potential altered parenting.

REFERENCES

1. American Academy of Pediatrics/American College of Obstetrics and Gynecology: *Guidelines for Perinatal Care*. Washington, DC, AAP/ACOG, 1983, p 185.
2. Vestal K, McKenzie C: *High Risk Perinatal Nursing*. Philadelphia, WB Saunders, 1983, p 31.
3. Brown F: The management of high-risk obstetrics transfer patients. *Obstet Gynecol* 51:674–676, 1978.
4. Barden T, Peter J, Merkatz L: Ritodrine hydrochloride: a betamimetic agent for use in preterm labor. *Obstet Gynecol* 56:1, 1980.
5. Cloherty J, Stark A: *Manual of Neonatal Care*. Boston: Little, Brown & Co., 1980.
6. Bose C, Kochenour N, Brimhall D: *Current Concepts in Transport . . . Neonatal Maternal Administration*, Columbus, OH, Ross Laboratories, 1982, p 152.
7. Donn S, Faix R, Gates M: *Neonatal Transport, Current Problems in Pediatrics*. Yearbook Medical Publishers, 15:8, 1985.

Section V:
Nursing Diagnoses

INTRODUCTION

Section V details nursing diagnoses and care plans for high risk maternity patients. Nursing care of a healthy woman and her family during pregnancy, labor, birth, and the postpartum period provides, perhaps, the most rewarding professional experience. Nursing care of a woman at risk for poor maternal and/or fetal outcome is, by far, the most challenging nursing role. We are called upon to provide expert technical obstetric/medical/surgical care, while, at the same time, facilitating the family's emotional response to both the normal changes of pregnancy and the progression of serious illness. Professionals and families may be called upon to make decisions where life itself is in the balance and society gives no certain guidance for decisionmaking. The death of a mother or child during pregnancy/birth is antithetical and a grievous loss to the nurse as well as the family.

Yet, nurses who provide care for high risk women should take heart from knowing that their role, as advocate, teacher, sister, and healer, is at the very center of human experience in every culture and is profoundly needed and appreciated.

Anticipatory Grieving Related To Actual/Perceived Threat To Self

Goals:
The patient and family will verbalize feelings, utilize support systems appropriately, exhibit normal grieving behaviors, and make realistic plans.

Interventions:
- [ ] Acknowledge feelings, whether the threat of loss is real or fantasized; be aware that many women experience fear of death during pregnancy and childbirth.
- [ ] Encourage patients to discuss frightening dreams and feelings.
- [ ] Allow and encourage patient/family to express fears/concerns regarding prognosis of patient.
- [ ] Explore patient's understanding of disease process, prognosis for self/fetus; clarify misconceptions; support patient/family in decisionmaking when a choice must be made between well-being of mother or baby.
- [ ] Explain the normal stages of grief and symptoms of normal grieving; expect patient/family to proceed through them unevenly, and with digressions.
- [ ] Ensure access to clergy, if desired.
- [ ] Assist family in making plans for care of the family in the event of long-term disability or death of the patient; make necessary referrals for health care, social, or financial services.
- [ ] Refer patient/family for psychiatric evaluation or grief support group, as needed.
- [ ] Assist patient/family in preparing to share information about the anticipated loss with children, family, significant others; prepare for expected responses.
- [ ] Identify abnormal grief reactions of patient/family; make appropriate referrals.
- [ ] Be aware of own feelings related to potential loss of a patient; seek necessary support for yourself; do not abandon patient in her time of great need, but stay with her as much as possible. Allow yourself time to grieve the loss.

Desired Outcomes:
- [ ] The patient/family progresses adaptively through stages of grief;
- [ ] The patient/family utilizes appropriate support systems.
- [ ] The patient/family makes realistic plans for care of family.

Grief Loss/Related To Potential/Actual Loss Of An Infant Or Birth Of An Imperfect Child

Goals:
The patient and significant others will utilize support systems appropriately and grieve their loss adaptively.

Interventions:
- [ ] Provide a short educational booklet related to maternal concerns in pregnancy (including pregnancy loss) to all patients at the first prenatal visit.
- [ ] Encourage childbirth educators to include information on the normal crises of the childbearing period and on the fear of loss.
- [ ] Include a reference to pregnancy loss in reading lists for childbirth education groups.

☐ Assess the bereavement history of any new prenatal patient who has experienced pregnancy loss.

☐ Explore facts and feelings related to the cause of the grief reaction (e.g., previous or threatened fetal loss).

☐ Clarify misconceptions and acknowledge feelings, regardless of whether the threat of loss is real or fantasized.

☐ Be aware that grieving is the normal reaction to an actual, potential, or preceived loss.

☐ Allow and encourage patient/family to express fears/concerns regarding prognosis for self/fetus/neonate.

☐ Explore facts and feelings and clarify misconceptions related to grief reaction.

☐ If baby is born prematurely, has congenital anomalies, or is suffering effects of hypoxia, provide opportunity for maternal-neonatal contact; assess bonding if appropriate.

☐ Be aware that the birth of an imperfect child is a loss and that parents need to grieve.

☐ Acquaint the patient/family with the phenomenon of the grief-crisis reaction, including the following specifics:
  — Physical symptoms (e.g., headaches, nausea, fatigue, anorexia, abdominal flutters, pain of unknown origin);
  — Emotional symptoms (e.g., anger, depression, temporary withdrawal or denial, tearfulness, sadness, vivid dreams of labor and babies); and
  — Length of time of acute grieving (6 weeks to 6 months, with occasional regressions related to due date, holidays, anniversary of death)

☐ Explain that these reactions are expected and normal.

☐ Encourage the patient/family to express feelings; provide ample time for the family to review all pregnancy events and related feelings with the health professional.

☐ Identify positive coping behaviors that the patient presents and reinforce them.

☐ Provide assistance with the practical details of the loss, including the following specifics:
  — Encourage the parents/family to view, touch, and hold the infant after death to provide a focus for grief;

  — Help arrange for religious visitors and services as desired;
  — Review the city and private burial options;
  — Explain the application process for a death certificate;
  — Encourage the parents to name the dead infant;
  — Provide the means for a photograph of the infant to be given to the parents;
  — Give the parents a copy of the infant's footprint sheet;
  — Arrange for the parents to send burial clothes to the hospital morgue if a city/county burial is chosen; and
  — Expedite the autopsy process as indicated:
    * Explain the reason for the physician's request for autopsy;
    * Explain that it is possible the autopsy will not reveal the reason for death;
    * Support the decision of the parents regarding an autopsy; and
    * Ensure the parents will be informed of the results if an autopsy is done.

☐ Review the process of sharing the fact of the loss with siblings, family, and friends; prepare for expected responses.

☐ Acquaint the patient with follow-up resources available (e.g., support books written by bereaved parents, community self-help groups, professional crisis intervention, parent support groups for impaired infants); contact patient several times after discharge (e.g., 1 week, 4 weeks) to provide support.

☐ Ascertain that the patient has received necessary medical/genetic follow-up appointments before discharge.

☐ Identify the patient with an abnormal grief reaction (intensity of symptoms or abnormal time frame, including complete denial); refer the patient for professional psychotherapy.

Desired Outcomes:

☐ The patient and family progress adaptively through stages of grief.

☐ The patient and family utilize support systems/counseling resources to cope as needed.

Spiritual Distress Related To Values Conflict Associated With The Decision To Continue Or To Terminate A Defective Pregnancy

Goals:

The patient will make an informed decision and will experience resolution of conflicts.

Interventions:

- ☐ Ensure that all pregnant women initially are evaluated for presence of genetic or teratogenic fetal risk factors by including in the nursing history an assessment of the family tree, past reproductive performance, home and work environment, medical and/or illicit drug use including alcohol, and appropriate laboratory tests such as sickle preparation, hemoglobin electrophoresis.
- ☐ Ensure that pregnant women are screened appropriately for presence of viral infections that increase risk, such as toxoplasmosis, rubella, cytomegalovirus, herpes, hepatitis, and HIV.
- ☐ Ensure that patients with specific medical diagnoses (e.g., diabetes, chronic hypertension) understand fetal risks related to the disease process.
- ☐ Provide preventive health care teaching regarding optimizing fetal environment, including cessation of drug and alcohol use and avoidance of x-ray procedures and teratogenic substances.
- ☐ Assess your own value systems and ability to provide unbiased, complete information to a patient regarding the decision to continue or to terminate a defective pregnancy.
- ☐ Recognize that the patient has the right to receive unbiased, complete information in order to make a decision.
- ☐ Recognize that it is the *patient's* responsibility to make the decision—not the health care team's.
- ☐ If the patient is identified as having a potentially defective fetus, discuss the specifics of the deficit, percent of fetal risk, incidence of fetal mortality, extent of newborn morbidity and mortality, and care of the affected child.
- ☐ Help the patient to identify and involve at least one significant other as a support.
- ☐ Provide complete, unbiased information to the patient and significant others.
- ☐ Explain the grief reaction and help the patient begin to grieve the loss of the perfect child.
- ☐ Explore feelings of guilt and blame related to the etiology of the defect. Realize that some feelings of guilt can be reasonable if related to unhealthy life-style habits that caused the pregnancy defect (e.g., alcohol abuse, drug abuse, HIV infection due to drug abuse of spouse/partner).
- ☐ Provide an opportunity for the pregnant patient to talk to a mother whose child has the defect, if appropriate.
- ☐ Refer the patient for genetic counseling, if appropriate; advise the genetic counselor of the patient's initial response to the potential diagnosis *before* the counseling session. Follow up after the session to evaluate the patient's response to information and her decision regarding amniocentesis or chorionic villi sampling (CVS).
- ☐ Prior to amniocentesis or CVS, provide essential information, including:
  - — Risk to mother and fetus;
  - — Possibility of need to repeat procedure;
  - — Possibility of another deficit even with normal results; and
  - — Explanation of procedure.
- ☐ Assist with the procedure by:
  - — Remaining with the patient;
  - — Evaluating maternal/fetal vital signs;
  - — Maintaining sterile field; and
  - — Collecting and labeling specimen.
- ☐ After the procedure, instruct the patient where to call if there are any signs/symptoms of abnormality or emergency (e.g., vaginal bleeding or drainage, uterine contractions, fetal hyperactivity or hypoactivity, fever, chills, abdominal pain, dysuria, frequent urination).
- ☐ Inform the patient when the test results will be available (usually 1–4 weeks).
- ☐ During this waiting time, contact the patient and significant others by telephone or home visit to provide support and to allow the patient to express fear/anxiety regarding test results.
- ☐ Be aware that cultural norms regarding grieving and coping vary. Allow for ventilation of anger, frustration, and fear.
- ☐ If test results are normal, support the patient and significant others in the resolution of crisis by returning attention and educational priorities to normal changes and feelings during pregnancy.
- ☐ If test results are abnormal, help the patient through the decision-making process, discussing the consequences of the potential decision, including:

— Gains and losses to the patient;
— Gains and losses to the patient's partner/ significant other;
— Self-approval or disapproval; and
— Approval or disapproval by significant others.

☐ Be aware that religious, cultural, and personal ethical values regarding pregnancy termination vary. Explore individual values and help the patient and those most important in the decision-making process.

☐ Refer to a professional counselor if the patient requests it or if the stress of the crisis necessitates it.

☐ Support the woman and the significant others in their decision.

☐ If the patient chooses to continue the pregnancy:

— Provide ongoing counseling regarding the loss of the perfect child and guilt/blame related to a handicapped child and pertaining to the skills necessary to care for a special child;

— Alert obstetric and pediatric staff to the upcoming birth;

— Ensure public health nursing home assessment of the child's health and the family's ability to care for the special child. (Be alert to the fact that special children are at risk for child abuse/neglect.)

☐ If the patient chooses to terminate the pregnancy, provide information regarding the type of procedure, risks, the potential for viability of the fetus at termination (if appropriate), signs and symptoms of problems, and where to call for help.

☐ If appropriate, stay with the patient during the procedure.

☐ Ensure that the patient has a 2-week follow-up appointment.

☐ Contact the patient at home during these 2 weeks to help her through the grieving process.

☐ If appropriate, ensure that the products of conception are sent for genetic evaluation and that the patient knows the results of the tests.

☐ Regardless of the patient's decision, ensure that she and her partner understand the importance of preconceptual counseling and evaluation prior to attempting another pregnancy.

Desired Outcomes:

☐ The patient and partner/spouse (if appropriate) decide whether to continue or terminate the pregnancy.

☐ The patient and partner/spouse realistically grieve the loss.

☐ The patient and partner/spouse realistically assign responsibility for the defect.

Ineffective Individual Coping Related To Stress (E.g., Stress Of Pregnancy, Preexisting Medical Conditions, Life-Style Changes, Stress Related To Diagnosis Of Medical Condition During Pregnancy, Inadequate Coping Styles/Lack Of Support Systems)

Goals:

The patient will verbalize feelings and concerns; will develop at least one effective coping mechanism to deal with stress; will work with staff to implement necessary life-style changes.

Interventions:

☐ Introduce yourself and explain your role as helper/facilitator in order to establish yourself as a potential source of support for the patient.

☐ Be aware and respect cultural variations in coping styles.

☐ Make eye contact, use active listening techniques, and reflect information back for clarification/validation in order to acknowledge the patient as a person worthy of respect and support.

☐ Identify significant others on whom the patient relies for support. Involve them in a plan of care appropriate to their needs as well as patient's needs.

☐ Provide all counseling in a quiet, unhurried environment.

☐ Focus discussions by:

— Asking the patient to tell you what is the most difficult aspect of her situation— work on one stressor at a time and be concrete in developing plans to deal with the stressor.

— Acknowledging fears and feelings.

— Assisting to identify stressors/situations that elicit ineffective coping patterns.

— Discussing previously successful coping strategies, emphasizing their use.

☐ Explore the implications (maternal, fetal) of maladaptive behavior.

☐ Teach other adaptive/healthy approaches to dealing with stress (e.g., relaxation techniques, yoga, participation in consciousness-raising groups, assertiveness training, job counseling/training, body awareness).

☐ Role play new/alternative coping strategies.

☐ Involve patient with peer groups who have faced similar stressors.

☐ If ineffective coping is related to decision making, help the patient:

— Identify every possible course of action, avoiding an "either/or" process if at all possible;

— Weigh pros and cons of each decision *in writing*;

— Make concrete provisions for implementing any choices; and

— Involve all support persons in process and implementation of decisions.

☐ If ineffective coping is related to life-style changes, make sure patient is referred to and receives every resource available to help her cope (e.g., WIC, food stamps, Medicaid, home-maker services, VNS assessment/teaching, public housing, day care, job training, GED).

☐ Provide consistent support; refer patient to appropriate professional(s) (e.g., mental health clinician/clinic) as necessary.

☐ If ineffective coping is related to a diagnosis of a medical condition during pregnancy:

— Focus on the normal aspects of pregnancy and avoid making pregnancy seem a disease;

— Differentiate the normal changes of pregnancy from a disease condition;

— Concretize and compartmentalize changes necessary to deal with a disease process, making directions for the patient as simple as possible; and

— Encourage the patient to express her fear/anger regarding the diagnosis.

Desired Outcomes:

☐ The patient verbalizes the most difficult aspects of her current condition.

☐ The patient states she will integrate at least one new positive coping mechanism into her daily activities.

☐ The patient discusses fears related to potential life-style changes.

Ineffective Family Coping: Compromised

Goals:

Family members provide emotional support needed by the patient and support each other.

Interventions:

☐ Be aware that major maternal illness produces major family crises. Assess levels of stress/anxiety/ability to cope of significant others, including the children.

☐ Provide the opportunity for members of the family to express their feelings, including anger or frustration regarding their role in the patient's care.

☐ Involve significant others in all information-giving/problem-solving strategies in order to increase support persons' feelings of control and involvement.

☐ Provide referrals for visiting nurse home assessment and care/homemaker–home health aids or child care in order to relieve burden of patient care from family, if appropriate.

☐ Assess psychological status and be prepared to refer family members for professional counseling in order to prevent patient's support network from deteriorating.

☐ Teach family members nursing methods to reduce pain and to increase the patient's comfort in order to create a positive role for family support persons.

☐ If the patient is hospitalized, provide an opportunity and quiet, nonthreatening environment for family togetherness.

☐ During labor and delivery, encourage family members to become involved in the patient's care as appropriate to their needs and the patient's. Relive the birth experience with the family, and offer positive feedback for supportive behaviors.

☐ During the postpartum period, be aware of the family's need to bond. Provide a quiet, secluded atmosphere for the family to meet the newborn; provide a role model of appropriate reactions and behaviors.

Desired Outcomes:

☐ The family expresses anxiety/stresses.

☐ The family participates in patient's plan of care.

☐ The family seeks professional or peer support as needed.

Potential Altered Parenting Related To Physical Illness, Physical Or Mental Impairment, Unrealistic Expectations, Substance Abuse, Separation/Interrupted Bonding, Guilt, Possibility Of Imperfect Child, Or Birth Of More Than One Child

Goals:

The patient will describe normal infant behavior; will demonstrate caretaking skills correctly; will exhibit mothering behaviors; will identify behaviors that indicate infant attachment; will identify community support systems/groups.

Prenatal Interventions:

☐ Identify women at risk for alteration in parenting (e.g., socially isolated, battered, history of mental illness or debilitating medical illness, substance abuse, prior birth of an ill or imperfect child, diagnosed fetal abnormality in current pregnancy).

☐ Encourage the mother/family to verbalize ways the infant will impact on her/their lifestyle and career goals.

☐ Assist the woman to prepare physically and psychologically for the demands of child care, including identifying and involving support systems.

☐ Provide referrals for financial, nutritional, and psychosocial needs (e.g., social workers, nutritionists, WIC, psychologists, appropriate agencies).

☐ Refer as needed to visiting nurse service for evaluation of home, readiness for infant(s), and for monitoring of patient's status.

Postpartum Interventions:

☐ Arrange for mother-neonate and father-neonate contact in delivery room if possible. Encourage skin-to-skin contact.

☐ Point out physical features and unique behaviors of newborn.

☐ Provide a role model of caretaking skills and bonding behaviors for both parents.

☐ Encourage the mother to make eye contact with the baby and to call the baby by name.

☐ Provide an uninterrupted opportunity for parent-infant bonding; observe interaction and intervene appropriately.

☐ Encourage and support patient's mothering efforts; include father or significant others in care activities; reinforce all efforts and correct as necessary.

☐ Provide an opportunity for early breastfeeding when the mother so desires. If the infant is too ill to breastfeed and the mother desires, help her establish lactation (by using a breast pump or manual expression) and store the milk for the infant.

☐ If the newborn must be transferred to the intensive care unit, arrange for the mother/family to make frequent visits and to establish communication with pediatric caregivers.

☐ Provide a supportive environment; encourage the parents to verbalize feelings, concerns, and questions regarding caring for themselves and the infant after discharge.

☐ Ensure that the mother has the phone number of a 24-hour "parenting" hotline.

☐ Refer the parents to parenting support groups to encourage peer sharing of activities and supports.

☐ If prior or potential child abuse is suspected or if the patient is a proven substance abuser, refer her to the Bureau of Child Welfare to ensure a safe home environment for the child.

☐ For all women at risk of deviations in parenting, refer them to a visiting nurse service for assessment of maternal/newborn interaction and adequacy of infant care.

Desired Outcomes:

☐ The patient/partner begins to bond with the infant(s) as evidenced by appropriate bonding behaviors.

☐ The patient/partner discusses the parenting role in relation to new infant(s).

☐ The patient/partner demonstrates infant caretaking behaviors and skills correctly.

☐ The patient/partner has a referral to at least one community support group.

The Anxiety/Fear Related To Pregnancy, Uncertain Maternal/Fetal Outcomes, Hospitalization, Or Potential Change In Method Of Delivery

Goals:

The patient will verbalize feelings, concerns, and fears about pregnancy and prognosis for self and fetus; will experience a decrease in level of anxiety/fear.

Interventions Related to Pregnancy:

☐ Explore common causes of anxiety related to pregnancy with every pregnant patient and her support person, such as:
— Fantasies about the baby and concerns regarding the baby's health and normalcy;
— Myths related to improving outcome or having a baby;
— Body image, changes in sexuality;
— Fear of the unknown, fear of death;
— Role changes for the mother; and
— Role changes in relation to significant others.

☐ Assess level of anxiety, being aware of nonverbal cues, such as:
— Posture (e.g., hunched shoulders, arms folded across chest);
— Inability to make eye contact; and
— Movements (e.g., trembling, shaking hands, tapping fingers, wringing hands, rocking, inability to sit still.

☐ Assess level of anxiety, being aware of verbal cues, such as rapid speech, word repetition, and inappropriate laughter.

☐ Assist the patient in identifying her usual methods of coping with anxiety. Be aware of cultural variations in coping styles.

☐ Make referrals for financial and psychologic assistance (e.g., to members of clergy or specific peers).

☐ Focus on strengthening positive coping mechanisms and eliminating nonproductive or harmful strategies.

☐ Help the patient identify significant others who provide support. Involve them in the patient's care appropriate to the needs of both.

☐ Encourage the patient to express concerns/fears regarding the outcome for self and fetus.

☐ Explain the risks and benefits/rationale for all procedures to patient/family.

☐ Explain the importance of fetal testing, risks/benefits, and the expected findings of each test.

☐ Give accurate information regarding maternal/fetal status; be honest, but avoid implying hopelessness.

☐ Use therapeutic touch, if appropriate.

☐ Be aware that anxiety will decrease the patient's ability to learn/remember; provide written materials and repeat significant information to enhance the teaching and learning process. Clarify any misinformation/misunderstandings regarding treatment/procedures/outcomes.

Interventions Related to Hospitalization:

☐ Orient patient and family to the unit where the patient will be staying.

☐ Explain the necessity of strict compliance with the medical regimen.

☐ Provide the opportunity for the patient to have her personal belongings in her room to make it as home-like as possible (for a long-term stay).

☐ Provide diversionary activities that do not violate the medical need for rest.

☐ Discuss with the patient visitors who appear to upset or annoy her; restrict their visitation, if appropriate.

☐ Provide a quiet, nonstressful environment.

☐ Answer the patient's call bell promptly—anticipate her requests, if possible.

☐ Encourage support persons to visit the patient frequently.

☐ Provide for occupational therapy, if appropriate.

☐ Encourage physical activity, as appropriate, in order to provide an outlet for tension/anxiety.

☐ Use massage/techniques of therapeutic touch each day. Teach significant others these techniques.

☐ Teach the patient relaxation strategies or biofeedback.

Interventions Related to Potential Change in Method of Delivery:

☐ Discuss anticipated vaginal delivery and ensure that the patient and partner/spouse are fully aware of the possibility of cesarean section.

☐ Discuss the potential for vaginal birth after cesarean section, if appropriate.

☐ Provide privacy and a quiet environment immediately postpartum.

☐ Encourage skin-to-skin contact with the neonate at delivery and assess bonding.

☐ Encourage the patient to express disappointment regarding the method of delivery.

☐ Reassure that a cesarean delivery does not make her any less of a woman/mother.

Desired Outcomes:

☐ The patient states anxiety/fear is diminished.

☐ The patient verbalizes understanding of treatment.

☐ The patient responds positively to significant others and the care giver's efforts to support her.

☐ The patient expresses her feelings and concerns about the outcome of the pregnancy for self and fetus.

Self-Care Deficit—Feeding, Bathing/Hygiene, Dressing/Grooming, Toileting (Specify)—Related To Impaired Sensation/Mobility, Pain, Muscle Weakness, Or Mental/Emotional Impairment

Goals:

The patient will participate in activities to meet her self-care needs, and plans to correct her self-care deficits will be jointly developed.

Interventions:

☐ Involve the patient in the development of her own care plan in order to enhance sense of control.

☐ Evaluate patient's ability to perform activities of daily living (ADL); encourage patient to maintain these activities as much as possible or as close to normal as possible in order to maintain self-image/self-esteem.

☐ Provide assistance with ADL as necessary; do not develop goals beyond the patient's capacity.

☐ Provide verbal and nonverbal reinforcement for self-care activities.

☐ Provide the opportunity for the patient to express frustration or anger regarding potential or actual loss of self-control.

☐ Help to identify resources/equipment available to assist with ADL.

☐ Assist patient to schedule daily routines to provide for rest periods.

☐ Arrange necessities (e.g., bedpan, telephone, bed controls, TV remote control) for the patient confined to bed.

☐ Encourage the patient to comb her own hair and put on make-up. Praise efforts to improve attractiveness.

☐ Provide referral as needed (e.g., home health services, disability/financial assistance) to ensure patient can comply with management.

☐ Involve all team members including the patient and her family (occupational therapy, physical therapy, nutrition, social work) in evaluating problems.

☐ Refer to visiting nurse service for home assessment in order to evaluate mother's ability to perform ADL, psychologic status, compliance with iron/vitamin supplementation regimen, and follow-up of newborn status.

☐ Develop a plan of care for the infant with the patient and her family.

☐ Be prepared to refer the patient for professional counseling before discouragement or depression becomes severe.

Desired Outcomes:

☐ The patient's basic needs are met.

☐ The patient identifies self-care deficits.

☐ The patient participates in strategies to overcome deficits.

☐ The patient assesses her ability to cope with self-care deficit.

Impaired Physical Mobility Related To Pain, Deformity, Paralysis, Muscle Weakness

Goals:

The patient will perform activities of daily living (ADL); will determine schedule changes necessary to perform ADL; will be free from complications associated with restricted mobility.

Interventions:

☐ Obtain baseline data regarding daily functioning (e.g., exercise tolerance, daily routine).

☐ Develop with patient a realistic plan for maintaining optimal physical activity.

☐ Encourage assistance from family and friends.

☐ Emphasize importance of maintaining a regimen of both active and passive exercise as well as maintaining proper body alignment.

☐ Maintain bed rest as ordered; ensure use of a firm surface; assist in frequent position changes.

☐ Carry out measures to preserve function and to prevent contractures when moving and positioning the patient:

— Extend joints as tolerated; protect affected joints;

— Avoid flexing the neck;

— Protect feet from pressure of bedclothes;

— Immobilize and/or support joints and extremities; and

— Avoid quick, jarring movements.

☐ Ensure patient safety (e.g., handrails in shower/bathroom, instruction on the use of assistive devices).

☐ Inform patient that modifications in ADL may be required as energy levels and condition change.

☐ Encourage patient to make appropriate plans for care of the baby, provide referrals as needed.

Desired Outcomes:

☐ The patient performs ADL.

☐ The patient is free from skin breakdown and contractures.

Altered Sexuality Patterns Related To Pregnancy, Preexisting Condition, Or Treatment

Goals:

The patient/partner will discuss issues related to sexuality and identify mutually satisfying methods for sexual intimacy.

Interventions Related to Pregnancy:

☐ Be aware of your own feelings, beliefs, and cultural patterning regarding sexuality.

☐ Provide an opportunity for every pregnant woman to verbalize her feelings and concerns and to ask questions regarding sexuality.

☐ Be aware that assessment and evaluation of sexuality are integral parts of nursing care.

☐ Provide a private, unhurried climate for discussion.

☐ Use a vocabulary that the patient understands regarding reproductive/sexual terminology.

☐ Use open-ended questions (e.g., "Most women experience changes in sexual needs during pregnancy; what changes have you noticed?").

☐ Teach the patient the anatomy and physiology of the male and female reproductive system. Do *not* assume that it is understood already.

☐ Involve the patient's partner in discussions/teaching sessions as appropriate to the needs of both.

☐ Explore pregnancy-related changes that may alter patterns of intimacy, such as:

— Fear of harming the baby;

— Breast tenderness;

— Other physical discomforts (e.g., tiredness, heartburn, nausea, constipation);

— Inability to find a mutually comfortable position for coitus; and

— Vulvar edema.

☐ Clarify misconceptions or myths related to sexuality and pregnancy.

☐ Teach the patient/partner the potential for the patient's needing more touching behaviors, such as hugging, hand holding, and cuddling.

☐ Stress the naturalness of pregnancy and the beauty of the body during pregnancy.

☐ Teach alternative positions for coitus (e.g., woman on top, side lying).

☐ Teach alternative strategies for achieving satisfaction (e.g., mutual masturbation, increased touching behavior).

☐ Encourage discussion between the patient and her partner as to what is sexually pleasurable and how pregnancy-related changes alter both their needs for intimacy.

☐ Give the patient permission to discuss changes in sexuality during pregnancy (e.g., "Many women feel the need for more—or less—sexual activity during pregnancy. It's normal and it's perfectly okay.").

☐ During labor, allow the patient and her partner time to be alone and cuddle.

☐ Postpartum, discuss the following:

— Resumption of intercourse when vaginal bleeding has ceased and when the woman feels ready (2–6 weeks);

— Alternatives to vaginal intercourse;

— Natural fatigue in the postpartum period and relation to decreased desire for sexual intercourse; and

— Changes related to breastfeeding (e.g., vaginal dryness is related to normal decreased estrogen level and is not a reflection of decreased desire; breast milk leaking/spurting during coitus or orgasm is normal; orgasm during nursing is common/natural/normal).

Interventions Related to Preexisting Condition or Treatment:

- [ ] Explore ways the patient and her partner have restricted their sexuality based on a preexisting condition.
- [ ] Discuss with the patient/partner any expected changes in sexuality related to treatment *before* it occurs.
- [ ] Teach alternatives to vaginal intercourse if prohibited for obstetrics reasons.
- [ ] Set up counseling sessions with patient/partner to discuss fear, concerns, and alternative means of mutual gratification.
- [ ] Refer patient to mental health clinic or professional sexuality therapist as appropriate.

- [ ] Be aware that surgery involving the reproductive system (e.g., mastectomy, vulvectomy, hysterectomy) will precipitate a major self-reevaluation of a patient's feminity, sexuality, and role as a wife. Validate her need to rework these role changes and refer, if necessary.

Desired Outcomes:

- [ ] The patient and partner verbalize their sexual needs to each other.
- [ ] The patient and partner develop strategies for mutual sexual satisfaction.
- [ ] The patient and partner seek professional sexuality counseling, if appropriate.

Disturbance In Body Image, Self-Esteem

Goals:

The patient will be able to state some positive physical and psychological assets that she has.

Interventions:

- [ ] Help the patient identify and utilize support persons in her care.
- [ ] Explore the patient's feelings about her appearance, medical condition, disposition, mood swings, and self-esteem.
- [ ] Use therapeutic touch and make eye contact when talking to the patient in order to affirm individuality and worth.
- [ ] Emphasize the patient's value as an individual throughout, respecting her need for privacy and confidentiality.
- [ ] Help the patient to verbalize feelings about specific physical deficits, explore myths and misconceptions and clarify them.
- [ ] Assess the patient's ability to deal with a permanent disability. Refer her for psychological counseling as appropriate.
- [ ] Discuss how the patient perceives her significant support persons view her, and alter any misconceptions.
- [ ] Help the patient to identify her capabilities rather than her limitations.
- [ ] Encourage and praise the patient's efforts to improve her appearance.
- [ ] Encourage her to plan her activities as her strength allows, including socialization with others.
- [ ] Refer the patient to appropriate peer support groups.
- [ ] Refer the patient to a visiting nurse service for home assessment and support.

- [ ] Reinforce the fact that pregnancy is a normal process—focus on the beauty of the natural process and the body during pregnancy.
- [ ] Discuss common feelings/concerns/complaints regarding pregnancy rather than pathology.
- [ ] Involve the patient in determining her own treatment plan; provide opportunities to make realistic choices.
- [ ] Provide positive verbal and nonverbal reinforcement for realistic self-appraisal.
- [ ] Teach the patient relaxation techniques (e.g., visualization, deep breathing).
- [ ] Be prepared to provide emotional support for the patient exhibiting depression, and make referrals as necessary.
- [ ] Evaluate the effectiveness of the patient's support network on an ongoing basis. Be prepared to refer the patient and her significant others for professional counseling.
- [ ] Postpartum, relive the labor and delivery experience with the patient and significant others, pointing out every way that she was able to contribute to the process.
- [ ] Refer the patient for continuing visiting nurse service/referral and use of homemaker/home health aid as needed.

Desired Outcomes:

- [ ] The patient uses her own supports and those of family, friends, and community.
- [ ] The patient makes a realistic appraisal of her physical and emotional strengths and weaknesses.

Knowledge Deficit Regarding Pregnancy, Process Of Labor And Delivery, Concerns Of The Postpartum Period, Parenting

Goals:

The patient/significant other will understand the normal processes of pregnancy, labor, delivery, and the postpartum period, and will make appropriate plans for care of both mother and baby.

Interventions:

☐ Encourage patient/significant other to attend preparation for childbirth classes.

☐ Teach all patients the normal physiological and psychological changes of pregnancy, labor, and delivery, and postpartum; differentiate normal from abnormal signs and symptoms; inform patient where to call if abnormal symptoms are present.

☐ Review signs of impending labor (e.g., lightening, Braxton Hick's contractions, loss of mucous plug).

☐ Instruct to go to hospital if vaginal bleeding occurs, if membranes rupture, or when contractions are regular and predictable.

☐ Describe the admission procedure.

☐ Describe equipment, procedures, and medications that are likely to be used during her hospital stay.

☐ Discuss purpose/indications for analgesics and anesthetic methods available for vaginal delivery and cesarean section.

☐ Explain patient participation during actual delivery (e.g., breathing, pushing).

☐ Encourage patient/significant other to tour labor and delivery area prenatally.

☐ Describe third and fourth stages of labor.

☐ Review methods of infant feeding, including information on advantages and disadvantages of each; support patient's decision, and assist her in preparation for the method she chooses.

☐ Assist patient in making plans for medical care of the infant (i.e., to select pediatrician or clinic to care for the baby).

☐ Review available methods of contraception; assist patient in making appropriate plan for the immediate postpartum period as well as her choice for later.

☐ Evaluate knowledge of child care and normal growth and development; provide clarification and correct misconceptions.

☐ Help prepare for care of infant; consider use of public health nursing referral and/or home-makers/home health aide services, as appropriate.

☐ Review resources/support systems available (e.g., family, home health, parenting classes, peer support groups).

Desired Outcomes:

☐ The patient/significant other will be able to discuss the normal changes of childbearing.

☐ The patient/significant other will make appropriate decisions and plans for care of mother and baby.

Knowledge Deficit Regarding Etiology, Disease Process, Treatment And Expected Outcome

Goals:

The patient will describe the etiology, disease process, treatment, and expected outcome.

Interventions:

☐ Refer the patient for childbirth classes and appropriate peer support groups.

☐ Involve significant others in any explanation teaching sessions.

☐ Differentiate the normal physiologic changes of pregnancy from signs and symptoms of a disease process.

☐ Explain the etiology, the expected course of the disease during pregnancy, and the expected outcome for the patient and the fetus.

☐ Allow the patient to express concerns/fears regarding the outcome for herself and her fetus.

☐ Give the patient the opportunity to grieve the loss of a "perfect" pregnancy.

☐ Teach the patient which signs and symptoms of the disease process should be reported immediately and where to report them.

☐ Help the patient identify factors that may make the disease worsen; teach her to avoid them.

☐ Explain the risks and benefits of all maternal treatments, procedures, and tests of fetal status for both mother and baby.

□ Discuss the importance of compliance with the treatment regimen in order to effect the best outcome for mother/fetus.

□ Praise efforts to comply with the treatment regimen.

□ Be aware that the patient does have the right to refuse suggested treatments/procedures.

□ Provide written literature about the disease process and treatment to enhance the teaching/learning process. Be aware that the information may need to be repeated several times because the patient's anxiety regarding disease may impede learning.

□ Arrange for a hospital tour with significant others and demonstrate monitoring devices that may be used.

□ Refer the patient to a visiting nurse service to reinforce the learning process and compliance with the treatment regimen.

Desired Outcomes:

The patient describes the etiology, the disease process, and the expected outcomes and makes an informed decision about compliance with the treatment regimen.

Knowledge Deficit Regarding Medication Regimen

Goals:

The patient can list any/all medications prescribed with correct dose and timing and can discuss risks/benefits for her and the fetus.

Interventions:

□ Before beginning patient instruction, check for history of allergies and ascertain that the drug, dose, and route are prescribed properly for use during pregnancy.

□ Teach the patient the rationale for each drug prescribed during pregnancy, including risks, benefits, and alternatives (for both mother/fetus).

□ Explore use of over-the-counter drugs and counsel the patient not to use them at all during pregnancy unless medically ordered.

□ Teach the patient signs and symptoms of side effects or overdose and where to report them.

□ Teach the patient the generic and trade name for the drug prescribed and instruct her in proper dose.

□ Explain the need to time medication carefully in order to obtain a consistent therapeutic blood level.

□ Involve significant others in any explanation/teaching session.

□ Review the drug regimen with the patient at each prenatal visit.

□ Review specific concurrent dietary interventions related to medication with the patient and make sure that the patient can list any foods that are contraindicated.

□ Encourage the patient to wear a medical alert band, if appropriate.

□ Allow the patient to express her concerns/fears regarding drug use in pregnancy for herself and the fetus.

□ Allow the patient to express feelings of anger or powerlessness regarding a lifetime need for medication, if appropriate.

□ Refer the patient to a visiting nurse service to follow up on the teaching/learning process and compliance with medication regimen.

□ In the prenatal period, review pain relief drugs likely to be used during labor and delivery, including uses and benefits to herself and her fetus, and alternatives to medications; prepare her to make an informed choice in labor.

□ Review the medication regimen carefully before delivery to ascertain whether or not breastfeeding may be initiated or is contraindicated and inform the patient.

□ If the patient in labor will need medication usually not kept in stock on the labor floor, inform the care coordinator in advance so that the medication can be made available to the patient.

Desired Outcomes:

□ The patient takes the prescribed medication correctly and side effects/overdose are minimized or reported promptly.

Altered Nutrition: More Than Body Requirements Related To Decreased Metabolic Rate, Excessive Dietary Intake, Lack Of Knowledge

Goals:

The patient will consume a diet adequate to meet the demands of pregnancy without gaining excessive weight.

Interventions:

☐ Plot weight gain at each prenatal visit on a standard graph to check appropriateness of weight gain.

☐ Evaluate cause of excessive weight gain (e.g., excessive dietary intake, edema, maternal illness); report to physician/counsel as appropriate.

☐ Conduct diet history; counsel patient regarding nutritional requirements for pregnancy and expected weight gain based on pre-pregnancy weight.

☐ Refer to dietician, as needed, for counseling regarding specific diets (e.g., diabetic exchange).

☐ Emphasize the importance of normal weight gain during pregnancy and the need to delay weight loss until after delivery.

☐ Monitor progress at each prenatal visit by interim diet history and weight gain evaluation; praise positive efforts.

☐ Screen for associated complications (e.g., thyroid disorders, diabetes mellitus, hypertension).

☐ Be alert to labor and delivery complications in the obese woman (e.g., dysfunctional labor, shoulder dystocia, macrosomic infant resulting in birth injury, birth asphyxia); be prepared to assist in management of any complications that occur; alert pediatrician to attend delivery if necessary.

☐ Postpartually, discuss health risks of overweight and encourage plan for weight loss.

☐ Refer to a peer support group, such as Weight Watchers.

☐ Refer for professional counseling or other appropriate assistance when psychosocial stress is identified.

Desired Outcomes:

☐ The patient maintains appropriate weight gain for pregnancy.

☐ The patient maintains diet adequate to meet nutritional demands of pregnancy.

☐ The patient establishes sound plan for weight loss after delivery.

Altered Nutrition: Less Than Body Requirements Related To Decreased Intake, Increased Nutritional Demand, Lack Of Knowledge Of Normal Pregnancy Requirements

Goals:

The patient will increase nutrition intake to meet her requirements.

Interventions:

☐ Conduct a diet history (including questions regarding pica, smoking, use of alcohol, bulemia) and assess economic resources available to purchase food.

☐ Counsel patient based on diagnosis, dietary history, maternal prepregnancy weight, weight gain pattern and age (teens vs. elderly gravida).

☐ Refer to dietician, as needed, for additional counseling regarding specific diets (e.g., diabetic exchange, high iron).

☐ Refer to food/financial assistance programs as needed.

☐ Refer to professional counseling or other appropriate assistance when psychosocial stress is identified.

☐ Screen for associated complications (e.g., thyroid disorders, hypertension, anemia).

☐ For patients experiencing difficulty consuming an adequate volume to meet nutritional requirements:

— Encourage small, frequent meals and snacks;

— Advise that soft or liquid high protein foods may be easier to manage;

— Discourage consumption of high calorie, low nutritive value foods; and

— Discourage foods that may make the patient feel nauseated or bloated.

☐ Monitor progress at each prenatal visit by interim diet history and weight gain evaluation; praise progress.

- [ ] Obtain maternal weight under the same conditions at each prenatal visit (e.g., same scale, same time of day, same clothing).
- [ ] Monitor fetal growth at each visit by measuring fundal growth/estimating fetal weight.
- [ ] Monitor lab studies to rule out folic acid deficiency and anemias.

Desired Outcomes:
- [ ] The patient exhibits normal weight gain and normal fetal growth.
- [ ] The patient reports diet history adequate to meet her nutritional requirements.

Pain

Goals:

The patient will be as free from pain as possible; will verbalize pain relief.

Interventions:
- [ ] Take a pain history: location, frequency, type (e.g., throbbing, knife-like), duration, self-help relief measures, activity that worsens pain, and relief achieved with medication.
- [ ] Teach self-help pain relief measures (e.g., relaxation techniques, therapeutic touch/massage, accupressure, imaging, music, whirlpool/water therapy). Encourage family members to participate in implementation of those the patient finds effective.
- [ ] Work with the patient and the physician to develop a plan for pain medication management that maximizes both relief and ability to perform activities of daily living but that minimizes adverse effects on fetus.
- [ ] Teach the patient to ask for and to take medication before pain becomes severe.
- [ ] Ensure that the patient's environment is free from noxious, painful stimuli:
  - Quiet: removed from hospital/home traffic;
  - Temperature: appropriate to patient's condition and neither too hot nor too cold;

  - Bed linen: dry, clean, unwrinkled—use lamb's wool underpads; and
  - Bedside area: clean, neat and uncluttered—used tissues or bedpans removed.
- [ ] Before painful procedures or surgery, explain that pain relief medications will be available and encourage the patient to report pain and ask for medication at once.
- [ ] After surgery:
  - Position mother to decrease stress on the incision;
  - Provide comfort measures (e.g., warm blankets, cold compresses of ice packs, mouth care);
  - Splint the incision before the patient is asked to turn, cough, or deep breathe;
  - Keep the patient and significant others informed of her condition and fetal wellbeing; and
  - Encourage significant others to visit and provide support as soon as possible.

Desired Outcomes:
- [ ] The patient notifies staff when pain begins.
- [ ] The patient states that she has some relief from pain.
- [ ] The patient identifies and utilizes at least one self-help measure to relieve pain.

Potential For Infection

Goals:

The patient will be free from infection and will receive appropriate treatment for any early signs and symptoms of an infection.

Interventions:

Assess every pregnant patient at every prenatal visit for signs and symptoms of common prenatal infections:
  - Upper respiratory: cough, shortness of breath, dyspnea, fever;
  - Urinary tract: fever, chills, dysuria, hematuria, frequency; and

  - Reproductive tract: leaking of fluid, vulvar burning, itching, increased vaginal fluid, malodorous discharge.
- [ ] Teach the patient measures to prevent common prenatal infection:
  - Respiratory: discontinue smoking, wash hands frequently, avoid exposure to people with colds;
  - Urinary tract: drink eight glasses of water daily, never ignore the urge to void, maintain perineal hygiene; void and then drink at least two glasses of water after

sexual intercourse, drink 4 ounces of cranberry juice at bedtime daily.

— Reproductive tract: wear cotton underwear, cleanse the perineal area from front to back, avoid rubbing or scratching the perineum, limit sexual partners, and use condoms if partner's reproductive health status is unknown; and

— Encourage every prenatal patient to take prenatal vitamins and to consume a daily food source of vitamin C in her diet.

☐ Stress the importance of both daily exercise and rest/sleep in prevention of infection.

☐ Encourage every pregnant patient to obtain an oral thermometer, and teach every patient to read the temperature scale and where to report fever.

☐ Identify patients with a history of infection or at risk for a specific infection. Ensure that appropriate screening is conducted (e.g., monthly urine cultures for patients at risk of urinary tract infections). Teach the patient all signs and symptoms and where to report them.

☐ Be aware that chronic anemia (unexplained by other causes) may be a sign of a chronic subclinical infection.

☐ Be aware that stress related to physical activity, a disease process, the ability to cope, and lack of support systems predisposes the patient to infection by depleting the immune system.

☐ Act as an advocate on the patient's behalf during any treatment/procedure/vaginal examination to maintain sterile technique. Do *not* permit the procedure to proceed if sterile technique is violated; ensure proper preparation, regowning, regloving, and redraping as necessary.

☐ If the patient is diagnosed as having an infection, teach the patient the name of the prescribed medication and the importance of taking medication on time to maintain a therapeutic blood level.

☐ Review the medication prescribed, its appropriateness during pregnancy, and check for allergies before administering.

☐ Reinforce the need for rest and a diet high in protein and vitamin C and the need for at least eight glasses of water daily.

☐ Ensure that a test of cure is performed after the course of medication.

Desired Outcomes:

☐ The patient has a normal temperature.

☐ The patient is free from signs of infection or reports fever or other signs of infection promptly.

☐ The patient is free from sequelae of infection.

Impaired Skin Integrity Related To Pregnancy, Preexisting Conditions, Immobility

Goals:

The patient will be free from skin lesions; will be free from discomfort associated with broken skin surfaces.

Interventions:

☐ Be alert for systemic disease that may have dermatologic manifestations (e.g., lupus erythematosus, syphilis, hepatic disease).

☐ Teach all pregnant patients basic preventive skin care:

— Avoid drying agents (e.g., alcohol, alcohol-containing lotions/astringents);

— Use lanolin-based lotion/oil daily after shower or bath and apply when skin is wet to increase absorption;

— Wear loose-fitting clothes appropriate to climate and avoid irritating fabrics like wool;

— Restrict use of soap;

— Increase intake of fluids to at least eight glasses of water daily; and

— Maintain humidified environment (in winter use humidifier or place pans of water near radiator to increase moisture in air).

☐ For pruritus associated with normal pregnancy, suggest a warm bath with one half cup of baking soda, or cornstarch, or a cup of Aveeno Oilated Oatmeal Powder.

☐ Teach the patient to report skin lesions promptly.

☐ Teach the patient to apply topical treatments, if ordered. Stress good handwashing techniques.

☐ Teach the patient to maintain a sterile technique for broken skin surfaces.

☐ Teach the patient signs and symptoms of secondary infection (e.g., redness, edema, pain, discharge).

☐ Avoid exposing lesions to harmful ultraviolet rays—i.e., sun; teach the patient to use a sunscreen and to cover lesions.

☐ Provide skin care for the bedridden patient:
- Turn patient every 2 hours, massage pressure areas when turned, use a rotation schedule and post it above the patient's bed with a written sign-off for each position;
- Provide passive range-of-motion exercises when the patient is turned in order to enhance circulation;
- Use sheep skins, alternating pressure mattress, waterbed, or bedside cradle to maintain even pressure on skin surfaces.

- Keep bed clean, dry, and free from crumbs or other debris that may irritate skin, and
- Observe patient carefully for decubitus and treat promptly.

Desired Outcomes:
☐ The patient utilizes preventive measures to maintain skin integrity.
☐ The patient reports skin lesions promptly.
☐ The patient complies with treatment regimens if appropriate.

Altered Maternal Tissue Perfusion

Goals:
The patient will maintain adequate tissue perfusion and will be free from preventable complications.

Interventions:
☐ Assess all perinatal patients for and report signs/symptoms of impaired tissue perfusion:
- Cerebral (e.g., changes in behavior, mentation, level of consciousness; restlessness; anxious, fearful behavior; complaints of headaches, visual disturbances, altered proprioception; seizures);
- Cardiopulmonary (e.g., irregular or slow pulses; change in pattern of cardiac monitor, blood pressure; edema; shortness of breath; cyanosis);
- Renal (e.g., decreased output, excess fluid intake, hematuria);
- Gastrointestinal (e.g., abdominal pain, blood in vomitus, melena, bleeding gums); and
- Peripheral (e.g., color of skin, mucous membranes, nail beds; capillary refill; temperature of skin; bruising, petechiae; change in ability to move, sensations; tremors; decreased healing).
☐ Refer the patient for a visit from a religious representative if the patient so desires.
☐ Assist with monitoring maternal status based on maternal status; set-up/participate in diagnostic/monitoring procedures (e.g., blood test for kidney and liver function, cardiac monitor, pulmonary artery catheter [Swan-Ganz], central venous pressure) and treatment as needed.
☐ Administer medications as ordered/necessary; monitor their effectiveness (administer blood if necessary, observe carefully for reaction).
☐ Provide oxygen as ordered/necessary; monitor effectiveness.

☐ Maintain intravenous therapy and intake and output to maintain hydration status.
☐ Encourage patient to remain in left lateral position to enhance uteroplacental blood flow.
☐ Keep patient warm and comfortable; keep skin clean and dry.
☐ Discourage sudden movements (e.g., stooping over, rising suddenly from bed) to avoid orthostatic changes.
☐ Prepare for emergencies; have emergency equipment (e.g., cardiac arrest cart, intravenous lines and fluids) and aids for delivery (e.g., forceps) available; notify operating and pediatric staff of delivery complications as necessary.
☐ Communicate and collaborate with staff/colleagues in intensive or cardiac care units as needed.
☐ If altered tissue perfusion is diagnosed and the patient is hospitalized:
- Discuss physical activity and stress levels; prioritize nursing care with the patient in order to provide rest periods as necessary and minimize stress if possible;
- Keep the environment as quiet and relaxed as possible;
- Involve significant others in the plan of care, but limit the number of visitors;
- Explain all treatments and procedures; and
- Encourage verbalization of fears and concerns for self and fetus.

Desired Outcomes:
☐ The patient maintains stable vital signs, level of consciousness, and cardiac perfusion.
☐ The patient maintains a controlled state of underlying disease status.
☐ The patient participates in the treatment regimen.

Altered Fetal Tissue Perfusion

Goals:

The fetus will be delivered in the best possible condition and will be free from preventable complications.

Interventions:

☐ Encourage patients in their third trimester or during labor and delivery to maintain left-lateral position whenever possible.

☐ Ensure that the high risk patient has a patent intravenous line prior to delivery.

☐ Be alert to indications for using electronic fetal monitoring (e.g., prematurity, postmaturity, meconium-stained amniotic fluid, fetal heart rate abnormalities heard on auscultation, high risk pregnancy).

☐ Explain electronic fetal monitoring to patient/spouse/partner (e.g., specific indications, equipment, and procedure), nursing support, and patient needs throughout labor (e.g., comfort measures, continuing presence).

☐ Apply the external fetal monitor as indicated:
   — Position the patient in a semi-Fowler's position;
   — Place the tocodynamometer over the uterine fundus;
   — Locate the fetal heart tones with a fetoscope;
   — Place the ultrasound transducer, with coupling gel, over the spot where fetal heart tones were heard;
   — Adjust the belts so they are secure but not uncomfortable for the patient;
   — Inform the patient what activities she may perform with the monitor in place;
   — Tell the patient to get assistance in moving about (from nurse); and
   — Readjust the placement of the tocodynamometer and ultrasound transducer if they become dislodged, the patient changes position, or as necessary with fetal rotation and descent during labor.

☐ Apply the fetal scalp electrode as indicated; insert the intrauterine catheter as indicated if properly trained/supervised; or assist the physician with the application of internal fetal monitoring equipment:
   — Turn on the monitor or let it warm up;
   — Apply the fetal scalp electrode over a bony area, not over a fontanelle or suture;
   — Fill the pressure catheter with sterile water before insertion to prevent the introduction of air into the uterus;
   — Insert the pressure catheter between the cervix and the fetal presenting part until the tip is approximately level with the umbilicus (i.e., when the black line on the catheter is at the introitus);
   — Flush the catheter with sterile water once it is in place;
   — Flush the strain gauge on the monitor and place it at about the same level as the tip of the catheter in the uterus;
   — Attach the catheter and stopcock to the strain gauge;
   — Open the stopcock to air to adjust the pressure line on the monitor readout to 0 and turn the stopcock so the catheter is "on" to the strain gauge; and
   — Place the leg plate securely on the patient's thigh (with conductive paste);
   — Attach the wires of the fetal scalp electrode, matching the colors of the wires with the colors of the terminals on the leg plate;
   — Secure the catheter and leg plate if necessary to the mother's thigh with tape; and
   — Take the mother's temperature hourly to observe for infection.

☐ Verify the accuracy of the fetal monitor tracing by auscultating fetal heart tones and palpating uterine contractions initially to establish the baseline and at least every hour.

☐ Evaluate the fetal monitor tracing at least every 15 minutes; notify the physician of any abnormalities in the contraction pattern or fetal heart rate.

☐ When early decelerations are present, observe for signs/symptoms of cephalopelvic disproportion (CPD) (see Chapter 35) as early decelerations early in labor may indicate CPD.

☐ When late decelerations or bradycardia is present:
   — Notify the physician;
   — Turn the patient to her left side to enhance uteroplacental blood flow;
   — Start IV infusion or increase the rate of flow to ensure adequate uterine perfusion;
   — Discontinue oxytocin;
   — Give oxygen by mask at 6–8 liters/minute to enhance fetal oxygenation (the effectiveness of this step is questionable, but since it carries no risk and may be beneficial, it is often tried);

— Take maternal temperature to rule out hypothermia (for bradycardia);

— Assess for imminent delivery; and

— Alert neonatal resuscitation team to attend delivery; assist with resuscitation.

☐ When variable decelerations are noted:

— Notify the physician;

— Turn the patient to whatever position relieves cord compression (e.g., left side, right side, hands and knees, Trendelenburg);

— Perform vaginal examination to rule out cord prolapse (or, if decelerations are severe, to lift presenting part and relieve pressure on cord);

— Observe for imminent delivery; and

— Employ nursing actions for late decelerations if the decelerations are severe and cannot be relieved by position changes.

☐ When fetal tachycardia is present:

— Notify the physician;

— Take maternal temperature to rule out fever;

— Assess maternal hydration status and start intravenous infusion if necessary, or increase the rate to ensure adequate hydration;

— Evaluate whether medication that might increase the baseline fetal heart rate (e.g., ritodrine hydrochloride, atropine) has been used; and

— Position the patient on her left side to maximize uteroplacental blood flow.

☐ When decreased baseline variability is present:

— Evaluate whether medications (especially analgesics) may be suppressing variability; if so, continue to observe; allow time for medication to be metabolized;

— Evaluate in early labor whether the fetus is sleeping; attempt to waken by abdominal palpation, gently moving fetal buttocks back and forth; and

— Utilize nursing actions for late decelerations or bradycardia if variability does not improve.

☐ Document indications for fetal monitoring, the type instituted, and the time begun.

☐ Document any abnormalities noted on the fetal heart rate tracing.

☐ Document all nursing actions instituted in response to fetal heart rate or uterine contraction abnormalities (e.g., notification of physician).

☐ Document fetal response to treatment measures instituted.

☐ Document all events/procedures that might affect the fetal heart rate or uterine contraction tracing (e.g., vaginal examinations, rupture of membranes, medications, maternal vital signs).

☐ Document directly on the fetal monitor strip:

— Identifying information (e.g., number of strip, patient's name, age, parity, gestational age, date, time, indication for monitoring and type, estimated fetal weight, presentation and position of fetus);

— Maternal position;

— Maternal vital signs as they are taken (at least hourly);

— Time of last vaginal examination and findings;

— Status of membranes, time of rupture, whether spontaneous or artificial, characteristics of fluid;

— Medications (e.g., time, dose, route);

— Other events (e.g., vomiting, coughing);

— Evaluation of tracing by physician (e.g., time, physician's name);

— Time of fetal blood gas sampling and results; and

— Measures to correct abnormalities in the fetal heart rate or uterine contractions.

☐ After the delivery of a baby who had a fetal scalp electrode, cleanse the puncture site with providone iodine or another acceptable solution. Notify nursery personnel to observe the baby for abscess at the site.

☐ Alert the postpartum staff to monitor the patient for postpartum infection.

Desired Outcomes:

☐ The fetus is delivered in the best possible condition.

Fluid Volume Deficit Related To Trauma, Blood Loss

Goals:

The patient will take in sufficient fluids to regain fluid balance; will have good skin turgor, moist mucous membranes; will be free from signs/symptoms of dehydration/shock.

Interventions:

☐ *Never* perform a vaginal or rectal examination on a maternity patient with vaginal bleeding until cause of bleeding is diagnosed.

☐ Postpartum assess uterine tone and the amount of lochia carefully; checks sites of incision/laceration carefully for bleeding or hematoma formation; massage uterine fundus if not firm, guarding the uterus.

☐ If patient is bleeding or has had significant blood loss:

— Maintain calm, quiet bedside atmosphere;

— Continuously inform the patient of her status, prognosis, and treatment plan;

— Keep the patient warm;

— Maintain bed rest; advise the patient that she will receive nothing by mouth until stable; when able to tolerate oral fluids, encourage increased intake;

— Monitor fluid balance by keeping strict intake and output records; insert a Foley catheter if necessary.

— Ensure that a patent intravenous line is in place with a 16- or 18-gauge catheter; two lines may be required if bleeding is profuse; check site at least every 4 hours for tenderness, swelling;

— Assess blood loss at least every 15 minutes until stable; weigh pads, sheets, etc. for a more accurate assessment of blood loss.

— Send blood specimen for type- and cross-match for at least 2 units of blood and administer as ordered, observing for transfusion reaction.

— Check vital signs at least every 15 minutes until the patient is stable; observe for signs and symptoms of shock (e.g., cool, clammy skin, thirst, anxiety);

— Check hematocrit every 4 hours, or as needed; and

— Monitor blood clotting status:

   * Observe for signs and symptoms of bleeding disorders (e.g., petechiae, bleeding gums); and

   * Evaluate serial clotting studies.

☐ If patient exhibits shock, place in Trendelenberg position, administer oxygen, and intravenous fluids.

Desired Outcomes:

☐ The patient maintains a normal pulse rate and blood pressure.

☐ The patient has moist mucous membranes and good skin turgor.

Potential For Trauma Related To Seizures

Goals:

The patient will not injure self or fetus during seizure.

Interventions:

☐ Explain the risks/benefits and alternatives for patient/fetus to seizure medication during pregnancy and encourage the patient to comply with treatment regimen.

☐ For hospitalized patient with potential for seizure:

— Pad siderails of bed;

— Provide airway at bedside;

— Ensure anticonvulsant appropriate for diagnosis (e.g., Valium, magnesium sulfate) is drawn up and ready for administration;

— Ensure oxygen and suction apparatus are at bedside and functional; and

— Start and maintain patent intravenous line.

☐ When patient experiences a seizure:

— Stay with patient; send someone else to notify physician and other staff;

— Protect patient from injury (e.g., move objects away, place pad or pillow under head if on floor);

— Loosen tight clothing (e.g., belt or collar);

— Insert oral airway;

— Turn patient's head to side to prevent aspiration of muclus or saliva; and

— Administer oxygen; suction mouth and airway after the seizure, as required.

☐ Monitor maternal and fetal heart rate frequently during and after seizure.

☐ Document type of seizure, activity, treatment and time.

☐ After seizure, explain to patient what has happened, implications for patient and baby, and anticipated treatment to prevent further seizure activity.

Desired Outcomes:

☐ The patient is free from injury due to seizures.

Ineffective Airway Clearance Due To Preexisting Condition, Ineffective Breathing Patterns, Or Impaired Gas Exchange

Goals:

The patient will maintain a patent airway, will maintain adequate pulmonary function, and will be free from respiratory distress.

Interventions:

☐ Evaluate complaints of breathlessness carefully to differentiate between pathology and the normal complaints of pregnancy.

☐ Evaluate for signs and symptoms of respiratory distress (e.g., nasal flaring, tachypnea or bradypnea, retractions, use of accessory muscles of respiration, diminished chest wall movement, labored breathing, air hunger, altered levels of consciousness).

☐ Assess breath sounds for presence of rales, rhonchi, and wheezes.

☐ Check blood pressure, pulse, respiration, color of mucus membranes and nail beds, and level of consciousness as appropriate to patient's state. Take rectal temperature in order to avoid air hunger that would occur with oral thermometer.

☐ Monitor fetal status.

☐ Remain with the patient; provide explanations for all treatments and procedures.

☐ Maintain a quiet, nonthreatening environment.

☐ Limit the amount of speaking for the patient; ask questions that can be answered by a nod of the head.

☐ Review underlying predisposing pulmonary conditions for patient's diagnosis and develop care plan for them.

☐ Maintain a patent airway (e.g., turn, cough, and deep breathe every 2 hours; suction prn; provide oxygen therapy via cannula to decrease feeling of suffocation associated with mask).

☐ Assist in proper collection and transport of arterial blood gas samples. Ensure up-to-date charting of values.

☐ Be prepared for respiratory arrest and assist with intubation, if necessary. Alert anesthesiologist if there is a possibility of arrest.

Desired Outcomes:

☐ The patient maintains a patent airway.

☐ The patient has normal color, respiratory rate, breath sounds, and arterial blood gases.

☐ The patient is free from signs of respiratory distress or recovers with no sequelae from respiratory distress.

Impaired Tissue Integrity Related To Trauma, Surgery, Delivery

Goals:

The patient will remain free of hemorrhage, infection; and will engage in self-help measures to promote healing.

Interventions:

☐ Observe site of incision/trauma for hemorrhage and signs/symptoms of infection (e.g., swelling, redness, warmth, drainage).

☐ Monitor vital signs for evidence of infection, unobserved bleeding.

☐ Keep suture line clean and dry; change dressing as necessary, maintaining sterile technique.

☐ Maintain position of comfort; administer analgesic medications, as ordered.

☐ Splint abdominal incisions when coughing or moving.

☐ Teach self-care of site (e.g., to keep dry, covered).

☐ For the patient with episiotomy/perineal laceration:

— Apply ice packs for first 24 hours;

— After the first day, use warm sitz bath or heat lamp three times daily to promote healing;

— Use peri-bottle for perineal cleansing;

— Apply and remove sanitary napkins from front to back;

— Use topical anesthetic sprays, as needed;

— Do not ignore urge to defecate because the fear of tearing stitches is unfounded; and

— Delay resumption of sexual intercourse until vaginal bleeding has stopped and there is no perineal discomfort.

☐ Teach the patient after cesarean section positions to hold or nurse infant comfortably.

Desired Outcomes:

☐ The patient utilizes self-help measures to promote comfort and healing.

☐ The patient remains free of infection and hemorrhage.

Excess Fluid Volume Related To Salt Retention, Protein Loss

Goals:

The patient/fetus will retain a sufficient circulating fluid volume; will be free from the complications of fluid excess.

Interventions:

- ☐ Monitor blood pressure, heart rate, respirations, weight. Evaluate urine for protein and I+O.
- ☐ Assess for pitting edema, deep tendon reflexes and clonus, fetal heart tones, and patient's subjective symptoms of complications of preeclampsia/eclampsia (e.g., severe headaches, visual disturbances epigastric pain) frequently.
- ☐ Encourage patient to assume a position at least three times daily for at least 30 min. to enhance return of extracellular fluid to circulation and renal perfusion (e.g., left lateral position with legs elevated on pillows so they are higher than the heart).

- ☐ Teach the patient to:
  - — Maintain adequate fluid intake, at least 8 glasses daily;
  - — Salt foods to taste; avoid excessively salty foods. Teach patient how to read food labels to evaluate sodium content of foods; and
  - — Maintain moderate exercise, e.g., walking.
- ☐ Encourage patients to consume at least 80 grams of protein per day.
- ☐ For the rare patient who is on a salt-restricted diet (e.g., cardiac or renal disease), teach to use other herbs and spices to flavor foods.

Desired Outcomes:

- ☐ The patient is free from independent edema.
- ☐ The patient has normal hematocrit, adequate urinary output/blood pressure.

Altered Patterns Of Urinary Elimination Related To Pregnancy, Infection, Calculi, Lacerations, Lack Of Bladder Tone, And Sensations

Goals:

The patient will regain normal pattern of urinary elimination; will be free from infection.

Interventions:

- ☐ Teach all pregnant women measures to prevent urinary tract infection (UTI):
  - — Drink at least 8 glasses of fluid per day to assist mechanical movement of bacteria out of the bladder;
  - — Void frequently; never ignore the urge to void;
  - — After urinating or defecating and while bathing, always wipe the perineal area from front to back; and
  - — Void before and after sexual intercourse.
- ☐ Screen pregnant women for UTI according to protocol, ensuring that the patient understands how to collect a clean catch urine specimen.
- ☐ Teach all patients to report signs/symptoms of urinary infection (e.g., urgency, burning or pain on urination, malodorous urine, fever).
- ☐ For patients with UTI:
  - — Teach patient to avoid bladder irritants (e.g., alcohol, coffee, tea, spices);

  - — Administer antibiotics as ordered; teach patient the importance of completing the full course of treatment.
  - — Encourage the patient to drink a large glass of cranberry juice daily at bedtime to acidify urine, and
  - — Ensure that a test of cure is performed after treatment for UTI.
- ☐ During labor, encourage patient to void at least every 2 hours to prevent infection, bladder trauma, or interference with uterine contractions.
- ☐ After delivery, assess bladder status when checking fundal height and consistency. Encourage patient to void as often as necessary to prevent infection and excessive uterine bleeding.
- ☐ For the patient who is unable to empty bladder:
  - — Assist patient to the bathroom, if possible; if not, assist her to an upright position on the bedpan, and ensure privacy;
  - — Provide measures to assist her to void (e.g., the sound of running water, placing hands in warm water, pouring warm water over the perineum); and
  - — If unable to void, catheterize her.

☐ Maintain strict sterile technique when catheterizing the patient.

☐ Strain urine per protocol if stones are suspected.

Desired Outcomes:

☐ The patient remains free of infection.

☐ The patient is able to void as needed to keep bladder empty.

Index

Page numbers in *italics* denote figures; those followed by "t" denote tables.

Maternal death rate, 5–6
  causes of, 5–6, 7t
  decline in, 5
  definition of, 3
  by race, 5, 7t
Maternal role, 480t–481t
  factors affecting adjustment to, 480t
  postpartum blues and, 481t
  stages in adjustment to, 480t–481t
Maternity nurse, 9–14
  developing individualized actions of, 18–19
  high risk perinatal responsibilities of, 13–14
  patient/family assessment by, 18
  role of, 9–10
Maximal midexpiratory flow, definition of, 182t
Maximal voluntary ventilation, definition of, 182t
Mean arterial pressure, 142, 147
Mean corpuscular hemoglobin, 75, 76t
Mean corpuscular hemoglobin concentration, 75, 76t
Mean corpuscular volume, 75, 76t
Meconium, amniotic fluid level of, 56
Meconium staining, 445–448, 446
  breech presentation and, 412
  conditions associated with, 446
  definition of, 445
  diagnosis of, 447
  incidence of, 446
  maternal and fetal outcome of, 447
  medical management of, 447
  nursing diagnoses for, 448
  nursing management of, 447–448
  pathophysiology of, 446
  in postdates pregnancy, 366–368
  signs and symptoms of, 446–447
Meiosis, definition of, 283
Melphalen, side effects of, 236t
Mental retardation, 178
Meperidine, for hypertonic labor, 390–391
Mepivacaine, effects on fetus and neonate, 428
Mercury, teratogenicity of, 278
Mesoderm, tumors of, 228, 229t
Metabolic acidosis, fetal, 438
Metaethics, definition of, 28
Methadone addiction. See Narcotic addiction
Methergine. See Methylergonovine
Methotrexate
  for chorioadenoma destruens, 238
  for choriocarcinoma, 237t
Methyldopa, 154
Methylergonovine, 420
Methysergide, for migraine prophylaxis, 161
Metropolitan height-weight tables, 294t
Migraine, 159–161
  definition of, 159
  diagnosis of, 160
  etiology of, 160
  incidence of, 159
  maternal and fetal outcome of, 161
  medical management of, 161
  nursing diagnoses for, 161
  nursing management of, 161
  types of, 159
Minerals, daily requirements for, 286t
Minute volume, definition of, 182t
Miscarriage, 20. See also Abortion, spontaneous;
    Pregnancy loss
  emotional impact of, 24
Mitosis, definition of, 283

Mitral stenosis, 98–99
  cardiac output in, 98
  during labor and delivery, 98–99
  management of, 98
  valvotomy for, 98
Mitral valve prolapse, 100
Mitral valve replacement surgery, 99
Morals. See also Ethics
  definition of, 28
  development of, 29
  reasoning process related to, 29
Morning sickness, 119, 120t–121t. See also Hyperemesis
    gravidarum
Mortality rates, definition of, 3
Mosaicism, 275
  definition of, 283
Motor vehicle accidents, 223
Mucolytics, for asthma, 184t
Mucomyst. See Acetylcysteine
Mullerian duct cyst, 230
Multifactorial, definition of, 283
Multiple gestation, 377–381
  cesarean delivery for, 380
  death of one fetus in, 25
  definition of, 377
  diagnosis of, 377
  etiology of, 377
  fertility drugs and, 377, 384
  incidence of, 377
  loss of, 377
  maternal and fetal outcome of, 377–378, 378t
  medical management of, 378–380
  nursing diagnoses for, 381
  nursing management of, 380
  nutritional requirements of, 378, 379
  polyhydramnios and, 336, 336t
  signs and symptoms of, 377
Muscle relaxants, placental transport of, 428
Mutation, definition of, 283
Myasthenia gravis, 165–168
  crises of, 165–166, 166t
  definition of, 165
  diagnosis of, 166
  etiology of, 165
  maternal and fetal outcome of, 166–167
  medical management of, 167t, 167–168
  nursing diagnoses for, 168
  nursing management of, 168
  signs and symptoms of, 165–166, 166t
Myocardial infarction, 100
Myoma
  cervical, 230
  uterine, 233–234
Myopathy, peripartal, 100

Narcotic addiction, 205–208
  detoxification regimen for, 207t, 207–208
  heroin, 205
  medical complications of, 206, 206t
  medical management of, 207t, 207–208
  methadone, 205
  neonatal withdrawal syndrome, 206t, 206–207
  signs and symptoms of, 205–206
  tolerance and withdrawal from, 205
Narcotics, for hypertonic labor, 390–391
Nausea/vomiting, 119
  causes of, 121t